D0086258

Essentials of Dental Radiography

for Dental Assistants and Hygienists

SEVENTH EDITION

3, 4, 11, 20, 21

8, 9, 10, 17, 18, 19

Orlen N. Johnson, BS, DDS, MS
Associate Professor of Dental Radiology
College of Dentistry
University of Nebraska Medical Center
Lincoln, Nebraska

Michael A. McNally, DDS
Aurora, Colorado

Christine E. Essay, BS, RDH
Lincoln, Nebraska

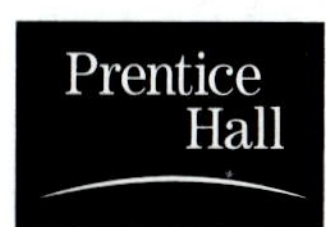

Upper Saddle River, New Jersey 07458

Library of Congress Cataloging-in-Publication Data
Johnson, Orlen N.
Essentials of dental radiography for dental assistants and hygienists / Orlen N. Johnson, Michael A. McNally, Christine E. Essay.— 7th ed.
p. ; cm.
Includes bibliographical references and index.
ISBN 0-13-093231-0
1. Teeth—Radiography. 2. Dental assistants.
[DNLM: 1. Radiography, Dental. 2. Dental Assistants. 3. Dental Hygienists. WN 230 J68e 2003] I. McNally, Michael A. II. Essay, Christine E. III. Title.
RK309 .D44 2003
617.6'307572—dc21

2002008646

Notice: Care has been taken to confirm the accuracy of the information presented in this book. The authors, editors, and the publisher, however, cannot accept any responsibility for errors or omissions or for the consequences for application of the information in this book and make no warranty, express or implied, with respect to its contents.

The authors and the publisher have exerted every effort to ensure that drug selections and dosages set forth in this text are in accord with current recommendations and practice at time of publication. However, in view of ongoing research, changes in government regulations, and the constant flow of information relating to drug therapy and drug reactions, the reader is urged to check the package inserts of all drugs for any change in indications of dosage and for added warnings and precautions. This is particularly important when the recommended agent is a new and/or infrequently employed drug.

The authors and publisher disclaim all responsibility for any liability, loss, injury, or damage incurred as a consequence, directly or indirectly, of the use and application of any of the contents of this volume.

Publisher: Julie Levin Alexander
Assistant to Publisher: Regina Bruno
Acquisitions Editor: Mark Cohen
Assistant Editor: Melissa Kerian
Editorial Assistant: Mary Ellen Ruitenberg
Marketing Manager: Nicole Benson
Product Information Manager: Rachele Strober
Director of Production and Manufacturing: Bruce Johnson
Managing Production Editor: Patrick Walsh
Production Liaison: Cathy O'Connell
Production Editor: Jessica Balch, Pine Tree Composition
Manufacturing Manager: Ilene Sanford
Manufacturing Buyer: Pat Brown
Design Director: Cheryl Asherman
Design Coordinator: Maria Guglielmo-Walsh
Interior Designer: Pine Tree Composition
Cover Designer: Keven Kall
Composition: Pine Tree Composition
Printer/Binder: Von Hoffman
Cover Printer: Coral Graphics

Pearson Education Ltd., London
Pearson Education Australia Pty. Limited, Sydney
Pearson Education Singapore, Pte. Ltd.
Pearson Education North Asia Ltd., Hong Kong
Pearson Education Canada, Ltd., Toronto
Pearson Educación de Mexico, S.A. de C.V.
Pearson Education—Japan, Tokyo
Pearson Education Malaysia, Pte. Ltd.
Pearson Education, Upper Saddle River, New Jersey

Copyright © 2003 by Pearson Education, Inc., Upper Saddle River, New Jersey 07458. All rights reserved. Printed in the United States of America. This publication is protected by Copyright and permission should be obtained from the publisher prior to any prohibited reproduction, storage in a retrieval system, or transmission in any form or by any means, electronic, mechanical, photocopying, recording, or likewise. For information regarding permission(s), write to: Rights and Permissions Department.

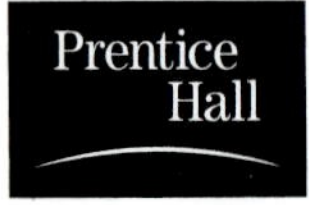

10 9 8 7 6 5 4 3 2 1
ISBN 0-13-093231-0

CONTENTS

PREFACE

Since the sixth edition was published in 1999, there have been numerous technique and equipment changes that make another revision of this book essential. The text has been updated to include the latest trends in research and clinical methods.

Essentials of Dental Radiography has been written in a clear, easy-to-understand manner for the dental assistant and dental hygiene student. The book is a balanced, flexible approach that presents a clearly written treatment of one of the most important techniques used in dental diagnosis. This basic text provides an excellent balance of both the essential fundamental theories and the day-to-day clinical procedures practiced in the modern dental office. The inclusion of learning objectives and review questions in each chapter makes it easier for both teachers and students to use.

This book is an in-depth introduction to dental radiography—the art and science of producing radiographs the dental practitioner requires to make a diagnosis and complete the patient's treatment plan. Whereas the book is written primarily for college students of dental assisting and dental hygiene, the important topics with which it deals concern everyone who works in the vicinity of equipment that produces x-radiation. It is appropriate for one- and two-semester lecture-laboratory classes in introductory and advanced dental radiographic techniques.

Essentials of Dental Radiography is also adaptable for courses of various lengths offered by commercial dental assisting training schools and may serve as a handy review for dentists, dental hygienists, dental assistants, and dental radiography technicians who must prepare for radiation safety or licensing examinations. It is also useful to the on-the-job trainee who is unable to enroll in a formal training program and must rely on self-study. This book will be a valuable addition to the library of any dental practitioner, dental assistant, or dental hygienist.

The twenty-eight chapters of the seventh edition have been organized into eight easily manageable sections.

- History and Radiation Basics
- Biological Effects of Radiation and Radiation Protection
- Dental X-ray Film and Processing Techniques
- Radiographic Anatomy and Mounting Radiographs
- Intraoral Techniques
- Extraoral Techniques
- Dental Radiographer Fundamentals
- Radiographic Interpretation

Teachers who have used former editions of this text in their classes will recognize immediately that a thorough revision has taken place. Each change, whether brief or complex, has been made to eliminate data that are no longer pertinent, to improve the presentation, or to add information that is required to qualify the student in the latest acceptable radiographic techniques.

Outstanding features and specific improvements in this edition include the following:

- More than 100 new radiographs, diagrams, photographs, or tables have been added or improved to replace outdated illustrations and to clarify new techniques.
- Four completely new chapters (Chapter 12, Mounting and Viewing Dental Radiographs; Chapter 19, Digital Radiography; Chapter 27, Periodontal Disease; and Chapter 28, Dental Caries) were written to present the material in depth.
- The book has been written in a manner to make it "reader friendly." Simple explanations are used to assist the reader in retaining the concept presented.
- Color has been used to improve readability.
- Contents of each chapter are listed at the beginning of the chapter.
- Key words are located in the front of each chapter. Each key word is highlighted in boldface color as it is introduced in the text.
- Helpful reminders have been added to appropriate chapters.
- Objectives have been written for each chapter to assist the reader in focusing on the most important topics of the material presented.
- Changes were made to the glossary. Several obsolete terms were removed and more than ninety new terms were added.
- Review questions have been revised, added, or deleted where deemed necessary. Answers to the review questions are located at the end of the text.

Flexibility should be the keynote for using this book. Some may wish to study the chapters in a different sequence or omit chapters that do not conform to their course outline. Some teachers prefer to begin with the chapters on radiation safety; others begin with the clinical phases and cover the theory last. The decision on where to start may hinge on the number of hours available for radiography, whether there is a separate lecture and laboratory class, and the type of students enrolled.

No claim is made to presenting original knowledge or techniques in this text. In many instances the material presented has been known for many years and is common knowledge in dental radiography. In some instances new subject matter has been derived from a condensation of lecture presentations and syllabuses made available at the workshops and symposiums conducted at the annual professional meetings.

Many authors have permitted the use of materials and illustrations from their writings. These are all gratefully acknowledged. Though it is virtually impossible to thank all that have so generously helped with this edition, we give special thanks to Nancy O. Johnson, Phoenix, Arizona, for her legal expertise and help with Chapter 25, Regulations and Legal Aspects. We thank Karen Knap, University of Nebraska Medical Center (UNMC), for her clerical assistance.

Credit is also due to Eastman Kodak Company, Gendex Corporation, Planmeca Incorporated, Dentsply/Rinn Corporation, Dexis, and Siemens Medical Systems, as well as other manufacturers, for technical assistance and permission to use their illustrations and diagrams.

We thank the editorial and proofreading staff of Prentice Hall for their assistance and unending help.

We give thanks to Joelene I. Johnson for spending many hours on the computer, skillfully typing, correcting grammar and misspelled words, and suggesting constructive changes.

And finally, we wish to express our appreciation to our spouses, Joelene, Annette, and John, for their patience, encouragement, and support.

Orlen N. Johnson, BS, DDS, MS
Michael A. McNally, DDS
Christine E. Essay, BS, RDH

PART I: History and Radiation Basics

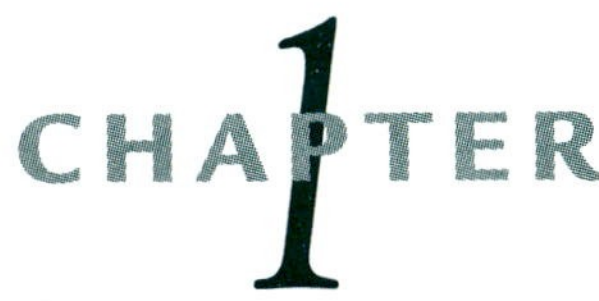

History of Dental Radiography

OBJECTIVES

By the end of this chapter the student should be able to:

- Define the key words.
- State who discovered x-rays and the date.
- Name the pioneers of radiography and identify their contributions.
- Discuss the history of dental x-ray equipment.
- Discuss the history of dental x-ray film.
- Identify the two techniques used in making dental radiographs.
- List the uses of dental radiographs.

KEY WORDS

Computed tomography (CT)	Radiograph
Cone	Radiography
Digital imaging	Roentgen ray
Magnetic resonance imaging (MRI)	Roentgenograph
Panoramic radiography	Tomography
Position indicating device (PID)	X-ray

Introduction

Modern dentistry is progressing so rapidly that changes in equipment and methods of practice are constantly taking place. One of these methods is radiography, the art and science of making x-ray pictures called **radiographs.**

For over a century, the dental profession has recognized that radiographs are valuable tools for diagnosing clinical findings. Although many new diagnostic aids have been developed during the past decades, x-ray continues to be the basis for most diagnostic procedures and has become an essential procedure in the practice of dentistry. As public demand for dental care increased, the duties of dental assistants and hygienists have expanded to include the exposure, processing, and mounting of x-ray films.

Radiography is the making of radiographs by exposing and processing x-ray film. The purpose of dental radiography is to provide the dental team with a radiograph of the best possible diagnostic quality.

Good radiographs seldom happen by chance: They are the result of comprehensive education and practice of skills. All individuals working with radiographic equipment should be thoroughly trained and versed in the theory of x-ray production. They should understand the operation of the x-ray unit and the various techniques commonly used to expose and process the films, as well as patient management, quality control, infection control, and radiation safety procures.

The purpose of this chapter is to introduce and present the history of dental radiography.

History of Dental Radiography

The **history of dental radiography** begins with the discovery of the x-ray. The x-ray revolutionized the methods of practicing medicine and dentistry by making it possible to visualize internal body structures.

Discovery of the X-ray

Professor **Wilhelm Conrad Roentgen's** (pronounced "rent´gun") experiment in Bavaria (Germany) on a Friday afternoon, **November 8, 1895,** produced a tremendous advance in science. Professor Roentgen's curiosity was aroused during an experiment with a vacuum tube called a Crookes tube (named after William Crookes, an English chemist). He observed that a fluorescent screen near the tube began to glow when the tube was activated by passing an electric current through it. Examining this strange phenomenon further, he noticed that shadows could be cast on the screen by interposing objects between it and the tube. Further experimentation showed that such shadow images could be permanently recorded on photographic film (Figure 1–1). For his work, Dr. Roentgen was awarded the first Nobel Prize for physics in 1901.

In the beginning, Roentgen was uncertain of the nature of this invisible ray that he had accidentally discovered. When he later reported his findings at a scientific meeting he spoke of it as an **x-ray** because the symbol ***x*** represented the unknown. After his findings were reported and published, fellow scientists honored him by calling the invisible ray the **roentgen ray** and the image produced on photosensitive film a **roentgenograph.** Whether the image is called an x-ray picture, a roentgenograph, or a radiograph makes no difference—the terms are interchangeable. The patient is best acquainted with the word x-ray; scientists and professionals generally prefer radiograph.

Because a photographic negative and an x-ray film have basic similarity and the x-ray closely resembles the radio wave, the prefix *radio-* and the suffix *-graph* have been combined into **radiograph.** The latter term is used in professional offices because it is more descriptive than x-ray and easier to pronounce than roentgenograph.

Early Pioneers

A few weeks after Professor Roentgen announced his discovery, **Dr. Otto Walkhoff,** a German physicist, was the first to expose a prototype of a **dental radiograph.** This was accomplished by covering a small, glass photographic plate with black paper to protect it from light and then wrapping it in a sheath of thin rubber to prevent moisture damage during the 25 minutes that he held the film in his mouth. A similar exposure can now be made in 1/10 second. The resulting radiograph was experimental and had little diagnostic value because it was impossible to prevent film movement, but it did prove that the x-ray would have a role in dentistry. The length of the exposure made the experiment a dangerous one for Dr. Walkhoff, but the dangers of overexposure were not known at that time.

We will probably never know who made the first dental radiograph in the United States. It was either **Dr. William Herbert Rollins,** a dentist and physician of Boston, **Dr. William James Morton,** a physician of New York, or **Dr. C. Edmund Kells,** a dentist of New Orleans.

Dr. Rollins was one of the first to alert the profession to the need for radiation hygiene and protection and is considered by many to be the **father of the science of radiation protection.** Unfortunately, his advice was not taken seriously by many of his fellow practitioners for a long time.

Dr. Morton is known to have taken radiographs very early on skulls. He gave a lecture on April 24, 1896, be-

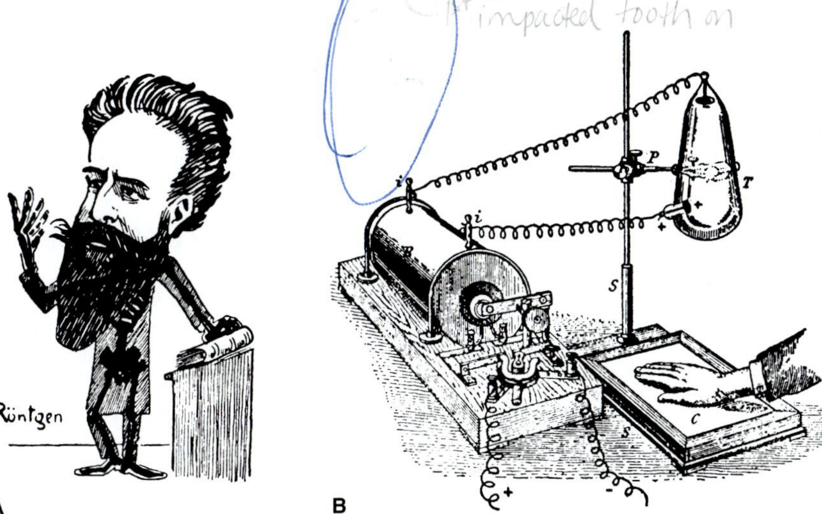

FIGURE 1–1. **Early sketches. (A)** Caricature of Professor Roentgen. **(B)** Initial equipment by Professor Roentgen. (Courtesy of Heinz Moos Verlag, Munich, and Siemens Corporation, Dental Division, West Germany)

fore the New York Odontological Society calling attention to the possible usefulness of roentgen rays in dental practice. One of Dr. Morton's radiographs revealed an impacted tooth, which was otherwise invisible. Dr. Morton took the first whole body radiograph in 1897 on a 30-year-old female using a 3 × 6 ft (0.91 × 1.83 m) sheet of film.

Most people claim **Dr. Kells** took the first dental radiograph on a living subject in the United States. He was the first to put the radiograph to practical use in dentistry. Dr. Kells made numerous presentations to organized dental groups and was instrumental in convincing many dentists that they should use dental radiography as a diagnostic tool. At that time, it was still customary to send the patient to a hospital or physician's office on those rare occasions when dental radiographs were prescribed. Unfortunately, Dr. Kells lost his life—as did some other pioneers in radiography—from excess radiation.

Two other dental x-ray pioneers should be mentioned, **William David Coolidge** and **Howard Riley Raper.** The most significant advancement in radiology came in 1913 when **Dr. Coolidge,** working for the General Electric Company, introduced the hot cathode tube. The x-ray output of the Coolidge tube could be predetermined and accurately controlled. **Professor Raper,** Indiana Dental College, wrote the first dental textbook, *Elementary and Dental Radiology*, and introduced bitewing radiographs in 1925.

Because x-rays are invisible, the pioneers in the field of radiography were not aware that continued exposure to them produced accumulations of radiation effects in the body and, therefore, could be dangerous to both patient and radiographer. When radiography was in its infancy, it was common practice for the dentist to help the patient hold the film in place while making the exposure. The dentist was needlessly exposed to unnecessary radiation. Frequent repetition of this practice endangered the dentist's health and occasionally led to permanent injury or death. Fortunately, although the hazards of prolonged exposure to radiation are not completely understood, scientists have learned how to reduce them drastically by proper use of fast film and safer x-ray machines.

Today, when almost half of the radiation-producing equipment used in the United States is in dental offices, it is worth noting that initially few hospitals and only the most progressive physicians and dentists possessed x-ray equipment. This limited use of dental radiography can be attributed to the fact that the early equipment was primitive and sometimes dangerous. Also x-rays were used for entertainment purposes by charlatans at fairgrounds so people often associated it with quackery. Resistance to change, ignorance, apathy, and fear delayed the widespread acceptance of radiography in dentistry for years.

Table 1–1 lists the early dental radiology pioneers.

Dental X-ray Machines

Dental x-ray machines manufactured before 1920 were an electrical hazard to the dentist and patient because of the open, uninsulated high-voltage supply wires. In 1919, William David Coolidge and General Electric intro-

TABLE 1–1. **Early Dental Radiology Pioneers**

Name	Event	Year
W. C. Roentgen	Discovered x-rays.	1895
C. E. Kells	May have taken first dental radiograph in U.S.	1896
W. J. Morton	May have taken first dental radiograph in U.S.	1896
W. H. Rollins	May have taken first dental radiograph in U.S. Published "X Light Kills," warning of x-ray dangers.	1896 1901
O. Walkhoff	First to make a dental radiograph.	1896
W. A. Price	Suggested basics for both bisecting and paralleling techniques.	1904
A. Cieszynski	Applied "rule of isometry" to bisecting technique.	1907
W. D. Coolidge	Introduced the hot cathode tube.	1913
H. R. Raper	Wrote first dental x-ray textbook. Introduced bitewing radiographs.	1913 1924
F. W. McCormack	Developed paralleling technique.	1920
G. M. Fitzgerald	Designed a "long-cone" to use with the paralleling technique.	1947

duced the Victor CDX shockproof dental x-ray machine. The x-ray tube and high-voltage transformer were placed in an oil-filled compartment that acted as a radiation shield and electrical insulator. Modern x-ray machines use this same basic construction. Variable, high-kilovoltage machines were introduced in the middle 1950s allowing increased target-film distances to be used, which in turn spread the use of the paralleling technique.

Within the last 30 years, major progress has been made in restricting the size of the x-ray beam. One such development is the replacing of the pointed **cone** through which x-rays pass from the tube head toward the patient with open cylinders. When the pointed cones were first used, it was not realized that the x-rays were scattered through contact with the material of the cones. Because cones were used for so many years, many still refer to the open cylinders or rectangular tubes as cones. The term **position indicating device (PID)** is more descriptive of its function of directing the x-rays, rather than of its shape. A further improvement has been the introduction of rectangular lead-lined PIDs. They limit the size of the x-ray beam that strikes the patient to the actual size of the dental film. Such a PID is shown in Figure 1–2.

Panoramic radiology became popular in the 1960s with the introduction of the panoramic x-ray machine. Panoramic units are capable of exposing the entire denti-

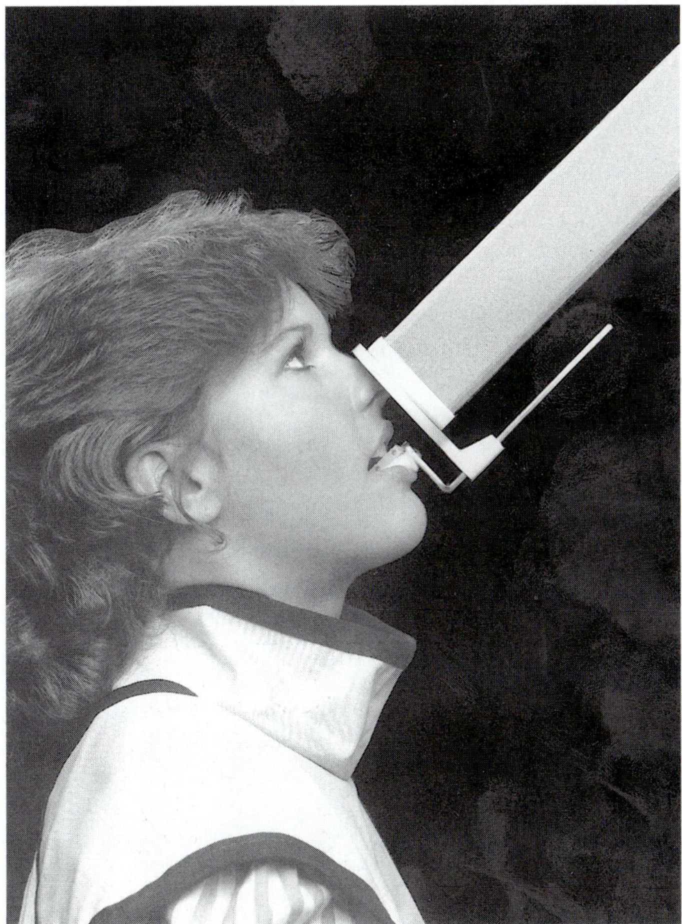

FIGURE 1–2. **Rectangular instrumentation** for reduced tissue exposure. The radiographer first places the x-ray film on a holder and positions it in the oral cavity, and then brings the position indicating device (PID) into alignment with the aiming device. The lead-lined PID limits the size of the x-ray beam to an area just large enough to expose the film. Note the patient is draped with a lead apron and thyroid collar. (Courtesy of Dentsply/Rinn Corporation)

tion and surrounding structures on a single film. Today, many dental offices have a panoramic x-ray machine.

Dental X-ray Film

Early dental x-ray film packets consisted of glass photographic plates wrapped in black paper and rubber. In 1913, the Eastman Kodak Company marketed the first hand-wrapped, moisture-proof dental x-ray film packet. It wasn't until 1919 that the first machine-wrapped dental x-ray film packet became commercially available (Kodak).

Early film had emulsion on only one side and required long exposure times. Today, both sides of the dental x-ray film is coated with emulsion and require only about 1/16th the amount of exposure required 40 years ago.

The film base has also greatly improved. Early base material was cellulose nitrate, which was highly flammable. In the 1920s, cellulose acetate replaced the nitrate base and was used until the early 1960s when polyester (Dacron) was introduced. With the introduction of automatic film processors, it was necessary to have a thinner base that did not warp.

Dental X-ray Techniques

Two basic techniques are employed in intraoral radiography. The first and earliest technique is called the **bisecting technique.** The second and newer technique is referred to as the **paralleling technique.** The paralleling method is the technique of choice and is taught in all dental assisting, dental hygiene, and dental schools.

In 1904, **Dr. Weston A. Price** suggested the basics of both the bisecting and paralleling methods. As others were working on the same problems and were unaware of Price's contributions, the credit for developing the techniques went to others.

In 1907, **A. Cieszynski,** a Polish engineer, applied the *Rule of Isometry* to dental radiology and is given credit for suggesting the **bisecting technique.** The bisecting technique was the only method used for many years.

The search for a less complicated technique that would produce better radiographs more consistently resulted in the development of the **paralleling technique** by **Dr. Franklin McCormack** in 1920. **Dr. G. M. Fitzgerald,** Dr. McCormack's son-in-law, designed a "long-cone" and made the paralleling technique more practical in 1947.

Modern Use of Dental Radiography

Few dental offices today are without x-ray units; many even have a unit in each operatory. In fact, most dentists have supplemented their conventional-type x-ray unit with a panoramic-type x-ray machine (Figure 1–3) that

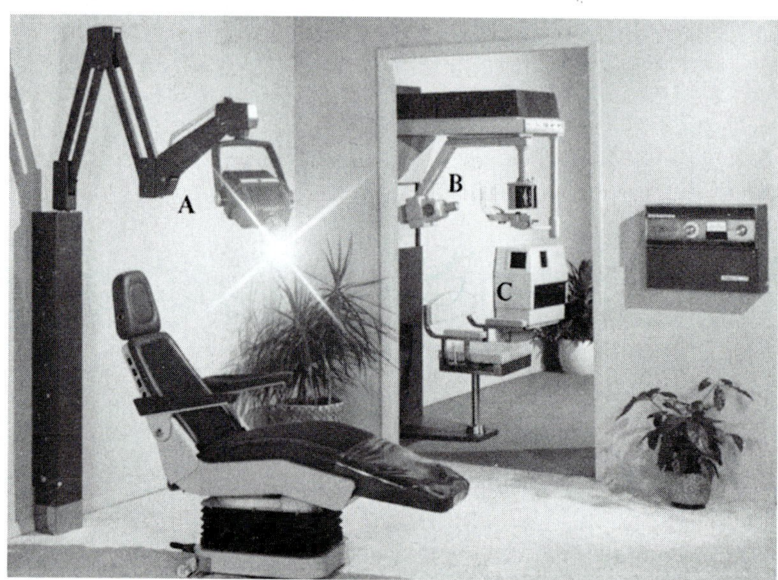

FIGURE 1–3. **X-ray room in modern dental office** showing dental chair with (**A**) conventional x-ray unit in foreground, and (**B**) panoramic-type x-ray unit and (**C**) automatic processor suitable for daylight use in background. (Courtesy of General Electric Company, Medical Systems Division)

can produce a radiograph of the entire dentition and surrounding structures on a single film. The use of radiography enables the dentist to practice better dentistry (Table 1–2). It is difficult to imagine how any modern dental practice could be carried on without radiography. At the same time, no diagnosis can be based only on radiographic evidence. A visual and digital examination must always be made as well.

Radiography, aided by the introduction of transistors and computers, is benefited by the incorporation of minicomputer technology that permits significant radiation reduction in modern x-ray units.

The use of tomography in medicine and dentistry is increasing. **Tomography** is a method of radiography by which a single selected plane is radiographed, with the outlines of structures in other planes eliminated. This principle is used in most panoramic-type x-ray machines.

New imaging techniques which include magnetic resonance imaging (MRI), computed tomography (CT), and digital imaging (see Chapter 19) have expanded the field of dental radiology.

Magnetic resonance imaging (MRI) is a new technique for obtaining cross-sectional pictures of the human body without exposing the patient to x-rays. The patient is placed within a large MRI machine that generates a static magnetic field. The nuclei of certain atoms within the body react to the magnetic field, and a picture is obtained. Non-ionizing radiofrequency energy is used to produce the images instead of x-rays. In dentistry, MRIs are used to visualize soft tissue components of the temporomandibular joint and to view pathologic conditions.

Computed tomography (CT) scanning has been used in radiology since the early 1970s. CT images are computer-generated and need no film or film-screen combinations. However, x-radiation is used as the energy source. Originally called CAT scans, CTs are used in dentistry for diagnosing lesions and planning implant cases.

TABLE 1–2. **Uses of Dental Radiographs**

- To detect, confirm, and classify dental diseases and lesions
- To detect and evaluate trauma
- To evaluate growth and development
- To detect missing and extra teeth
- To document the dental condition of a patient
- To educate the patient about their dental health

MRI units and CT scanners are not found in dental offices, but dental radiographers should be familiar with them. Dental patients may be referred for such images, and copies may be sent to the office for interpretation.

The introduction of a computed approach with instant images (both radiographic and photographic) has the potential to greatly improve the quality of dental care. This recent and exciting advance in dental radiography is called **digital imaging** (see Chapter 19). Digital imaging systems used in dentistry replace film with an alternative sensor. Image sensors now are comparable to film in dimensions of the exposed field of view and approach film in overall radiographic quality. Their advantages include a reduction in radiation dosage averaging around 80%, and there is no need for the purchase of film and processing chemistry, or the disposal of spent chemicals hazardous to the environment.

The discovery of x-radiation has already revolutionized the practice of dentistry. Future technological advances undoubtedly will increase the use of radiography in the years ahead and make it safer.

CHAPTER SUMMARY

Professor Wilhelm Conrad Roentgen's discovery of the x-ray on November 8, 1895 revolutionized the methods of practicing medicine and dentistry by making it possible to visualize internal body structures. The usefulness of x-ray as a diagnostic tool was recognized almost immediately and many dental radiology pioneers contributed to the advancement of the profession. The use of radiographs in medical and dental diagnostic procedures is now essential.

Trained technicians, dental assistants, and dental hygienists now make most dental radiographs. It is of vital importance that the person making the x-ray exposure understands how x-rays are produced, controlled, and used to achieve the best diagnostic results.

Improved equipment, advanced techniques, and better-trained personnel make it possible to obtain radiographs with high diagnostic value and minimal risk of unnecessary radiation to patient or operator.

REVIEW QUESTIONS

For questions 1–5, match each term with its definition.

- **a.** Digital imaging
- **b.** Position indicating device (PID)
- **c.** Radiograph
- **d.** Radiography
- **e.** X-ray

_____ 1. An image produced on photosensitive film by exposing the film to x-rays and then developing the film so that a negative is produced.

_____ 2. A method of making a radiographic image using a computer.

_____ 3. The radiant energy of short wavelength discovered by Wilhelm Conrad Roentgen and designated as x-ray by him. This form of radiant energy has the power to penetrate substances that are ordinarily opaque and to record shadow images on photographic film.

_____ 4. Any device attached to the tube head at the aperture to direct the useful beam of radiation.

_____ 5. The making of radiographs by exposing and processing x-ray film.

6. Who discovered the x-ray?

   (a) C. Edmund Kells
   (b) Franklin McCormack
   (c) Wilhelm Conrad Roentgen
   (d) William Rollins

7. When were x-rays discovered? _____

8. Who is believed to have exposed the prototype of the first dental x-ray film?

   (a) William Rollins
   (b) Otto Walkhoff
   (c) Wilhelm Conrad Roentgen
   (d) C. Edmund Kells

9. Who is considered by many to be the father of the science of radiation protection?

   (a) William Rollins
   (b) William Morton
   (c) C. Edmund Kells
   (d) Franklin McCormack

10. What proportion of all x-ray equipment in the United States is believed to be owned by dentists?

    (a) 15%
    (b) 35%
    (c) 50%
    (d) 85%

11. Who is given credit for suggesting the bisecting technique?
    (a) William Rollins
    (b) A. Cieszynski
    (c) William Morton
    (d) Otto Walkhoff

12. Who is given credit for developing the paralleling technique?
    (a) W. D. Coolidge
    (b) H. R. Raper
    (c) Franklin McCormack
    (d) William Morton

13. What is the most important use of radiography in dental practice?
    (a) For therapy
    (b) For diagnosis
    (c) For patient education
    (d) For control of pain

14. In which method of radiography is a single plane selected to be radiographed?
    (a) Digital imaging
    (b) Tomography
    (c) Radioisotope scanners
    (d) Magnetic resonance imaging

BIBLIOGRAPHY

Eastman Kodak. *Radiation Safety in Dental Radiography*. Rochester, NY: Eastman Kodak, 1998.

Langland, O. E. & Langlais, R. P. *Principles of Dental Imaging*. Philadelphia: Williams & Wilkins, 1997.

White, S. C. & Pharoah, M. J. *Oral Radiology Principles and Interpretation*, 4th ed. St. Louis: Mosby, 2000.

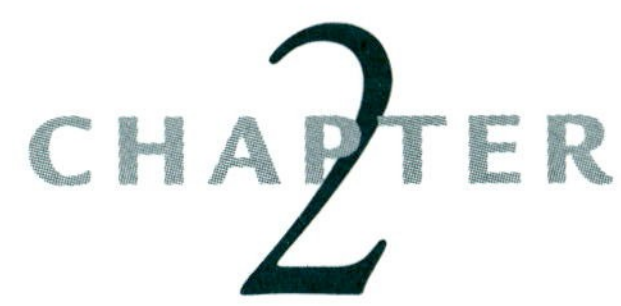

Characteristics of Radiation

OBJECTIVES

By the end of this chapter the student should be able to:

- Define the key words.
- Draw and label a typical atom.
- Describe the process of ionization.
- Explain radioactivity.
- Discuss the difference between particulate radiation and electromagnetic radiation and give two examples of each.
- State examples of electromagnetic radiation
- List the properties of electromagnetic radiation.
- Compare x-ray wavelength to its penetrating power.
- List the properties of x-rays.
- Explain how x-rays are produced.
- List and describe the possible interactions of dental x-rays with matter.
- Define the terms used to measure x-radiation.
- Explain background radiation.

KEY WORDS

Absorbed dose
Absorption
Alpha particle
Angstrom (Å)
Atom
Background radiation
Beta particle
Bremsstrahlung radiation
Characteristic radiation
Coherent scattering
Compton effect (scattering)
Coulombs per kilogram (C/kg)
Decay
Dose equivalent
Electromagnetic radiation
Electromagnetic spectrum
Electron
Element
Energy levels
Exposure
Frequency
Gamma rays
Gray (Gy)
Hard radiation
Ion
Ion pair
Ionizing radiation
Ionization
Isotope
Kinetic energy
Modifying factor (Quality factor)
Molecule
Neutron
Particulate radiation
Photoelectric effect
Photon
Proton
Rad
Radiation
Radiolucent
Radiopaque
Rem
Roentgen (R)
Sievert (Sv)
Soft radiation
Velocity
Wavelength

Introduction

The scientist conceives the world to consist of matter and energy. Matter is defined as anything that occupies space and has mass. Thus all things that we see and recognize are forms of matter. Energy is defined as the ability to do work and overcome resistance. Heat, light, electricity, and x-radiation are forms of energy. Matter and energy are closely related. Energy is produced whenever the state of matter is altered by either natural or artificial means. The difference between water, steam, or ice is the amount of energy associated with the molecules. Such an energy exchange is produced within the x-ray machine and will be discussed later.

Atomic Structure

To understand radiation, we must understand atomic structure. Currently we know of 105 basic **elements** occurring either singly or in combination in natural forms. Typical elements of interest in radiography are aluminum, beryllium, copper, lead, oxygen, samarium, radium, and tungsten. Each of these elements is made up of atoms. An **atom** is the smallest particle of an element that still retains the properties of the element. If any given atom is split, the resulting components no longer retain the properties of the element. Atoms are generally combined with other atoms to form molecules. A **molecule** is the smallest particle of a substance that retains the properties of that substance. A simple molecule such as sodium chloride (table salt) contains only two atoms, whereas a complex molecule like DNA (desoxyribonucleic acid) may contain hundreds of atoms.

Atoms are extremely minute and are composed of three basic building blocks: **electrons, protons,** and **neutrons.**

- **Electrons** have little mass or weight, a charge of −1, and are constantly in motion orbiting the nucleus.
- **Protons** weigh about 1,840 times as much as electrons, and have a charge of +1. The number of protons in the nucleus of an element determines its atomic number and is designated by the symbol Z.
- **Neutrons** can be thought of as a combination of one proton and one electron, having a mass approximately equal to the proton and have no charge. The total number of protons and neutrons in the nucleus of an atom is the mass number and is designated by the letter A.

The atom's arrangement in some ways resembles the solar system (Figure 2–1). The atom has a nucleus as its center or sun, and the electrons revolve around it like planets. The protons and neutrons form the central core or nucleus of the atom. The electrons orbit around the nucleus in paths called shells or energy levels. Normally, the atom is electrically neutral, having equal numbers of protons in its nucleus and electrons in orbit.

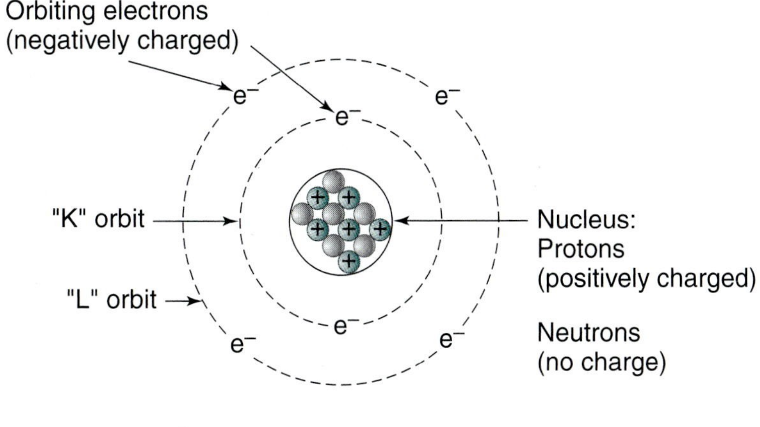

FIGURE 2–1. **Diagram of carbon atom.** In the neutral atom, the number of positively charged protons in the nucleus is equal to the number of negatively charged orbiting electrons. The innermost orbit or energy level is the K shell, the next is the L shell, and so on.

Atoms of the same element all have the same number of protons. For example, every atom of carbon has 6 protons. The number of protons determines the chemical element. The number of neutrons, however, in combination with the fixed number of protons may differ from one atom of an element to another. Atoms of the same element, having different numbers of neutrons in combination with the fixed number of protons, are called **isotopes.**

Isotopes of an element have the same atomic number (number of protons) but vary by the number of neutrons in the nucleus (Figure 2–2). For example, carbon 10 has 6 protons and 4 neutrons in its nucleus, carbon 12 has 6 protons and 6 neutrons in its nucleus, and carbon 14 has 6 protons and 8 neutrons in its nucleus. Some isotopes, like carbon 14, are radioactive.

Most elements are now believed to have one or more isotopes. Over 1,500 of these have already been identified. Of these, more than half are unstable and radioactive. Instability in an atom can be natural or man-made; either type is important to medicine and dentistry.

The nucleus of all atoms except hydrogen contains at least one proton and one neutron (hydrogen in its simplest form has only a proton). Some atoms contain a very high number of each. The electrons and the nucleus normally remain in the same relative position to one another. To accommodate the electrons revolving about the nucleus, the larger atoms have several concentric orbits at various distances from the nucleus. These are referred to as "electron shells," which some chemists now call **energy levels.** (The number of electrons in each of these spherical layers of energy varies but is generally 2 in the first shell, a maximum of 8 in the second, 18 in the third, 32 in the fourth, 50 in the fifth, 72 in the sixth, and 98 in the seventh.) The innermost level is referred to as the K shell, the next as the L shell, and so on (Figure 2–1). No known atom contains more than 7 shells.

Electrons are maintained in their orbits by the positive attraction of the protons known as binding energy. The binding energy of an electron is strongest in the intermost K shell and becomes weaker in the outer shells.

Ionization

Atoms that have gained or lost electrons are electrically unstable and are called **ions.** An ion is defined as a charged particle. The formation of ions is easier to understand if we review the normal structural arrangement of the atom. The atom normally has the same number of protons (positive charges) in the nucleus as it has electrons (negative charges) in the orbital levels. When one of these electrons is removed from its orbital level in a neutral atom, the remainder of the atom loses its electrical neutrality.

An atom from which an electron has been removed has more protons than electrons, is positively charged, and is called a positive ion. The negatively charged electron that has been separated from the atom is a negative ion. The positively charged atom ion and the negatively charged electron ion are called an **ion pair. Ionization** is the formation of ion pairs. When an atom is struck by an x-ray photon, an electron may be dislodged and an ion pair created (Figure 2–3). As high-energy electrons travel on, they push out (like charges repel) electrons from the orbits of other atoms, creating additional ion pairs. These unstable

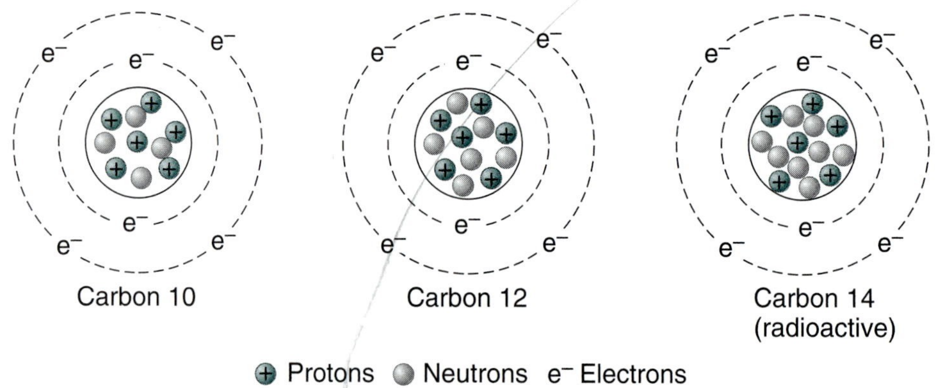

FIGURE 2–2. **Isotopes of carbon element.** Isotopes of an element have the same number of protons but vary by the number of neutrons in the nucleus. Carbon 10 has six protons and four neutrons in its nucleus. Carbon 12 has six protons and six neutrons in its nucleus and carbon 14 has six protons and eight neutrons in its nucleus.

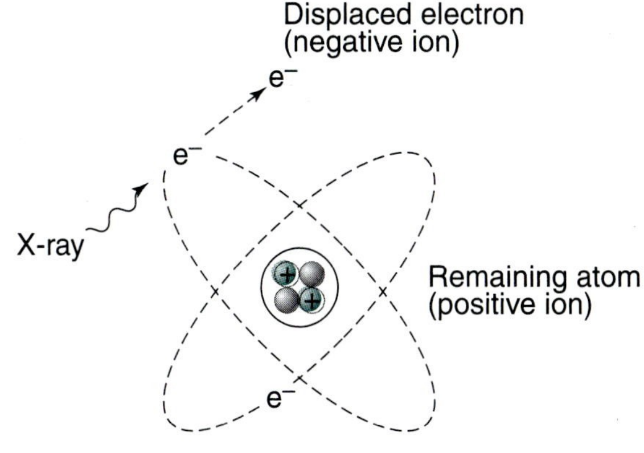

Protons Neutrons e^- Electrons

FIGURE 2–3. **Ionization** is the formation of ion pairs. When an atom is struck by an x-ray, an electron may be dislodged and an **ion pair** results.

ions attempt to regain electrical stability by combining with another oppositely charged ion.

Ionizing Radiation

Radiation is defined as the emission and movement of energy through space in the form of electromagnetic radiation (x and gamma rays) or particulate radiation (alpha and beta particles). Any radiation that produces ions is called **ionizing radiation.** Only a portion of the radiation portrayed on the electromagnetic spectrum, the x-rays and the gamma and cosmic rays, are of the ionizing type. In dental radiography, our concern is limited to the possible changes that may occur in the cellular structures of the tissues as the ions are produced by the passage of x-rays through the cells. The mechanics of biologic tissue damage is explained in Chapter 5.

Radioactivity

Radioactivity is defined as the process whereby certain unstable elements undergo spontaneous disintegration (decay) in an effort to attain a stable nuclear state. Unstable isotopes are radioactive and attempt to regain stability through the release of energy, by a process known as **decay.** This decay process involves the giving off of two distinct forms of radiation: **particulate radiation,** consisting of bits of matter traveling at high speeds (also called corpuscular radiation), and **electromagnetic radiation,** which is a combination of electric and magnetic energy and is emitted in the form of rays or waves.

Particulate radiation originates from radioactive isotopes and is given off in the form of alpha particles, beta particles, and neutrons.

- **Alpha particles** contain two protons and two neutrons and are positively charged.
- **Beta particles** are high-speed, negatively charged electrons.
- **Neutrons** have no charge.

The electromagnetic radiation emitted from a radioactive isotope is called **gamma radiation. Gamma rays** have properties similar to x-rays but occur naturally, whereas x-rays are man-made.

To understand radioactivity, we must realize that while most elements are stable, a few undergo constant spontaneous changes. As we have already seen, each atom of an element has an equal number of protons and electrons. However, variations occur in some elements. For example, the majority of hydrogen atoms contain no neutrons, but two rarer isotopes exist. The first of these, deuterium, contains a neutron in its nucleus and is stable. The second and much rarer form, tritium, contains two neutrons and is unstable and radioactive. Each isotope of a specific atom has the same chemical properties. They differ only in mass and weight (Figure 2–4).

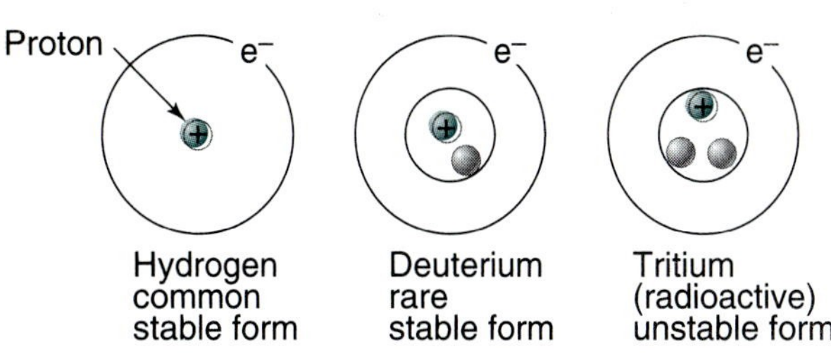

Protons Neutrons e^- Electrons

FIGURE 2–4. **Isotopes of hydrogen.** Approximately 1 in 14,000 hydrogen atoms contain one neutron in the nucleus (deuterium). Another rare hydrogen atom is tritium, which contains two neutrons in the nucleus. All of these isotopes have the same chemical properties, but they differ in physical mass and weight. Unstable isotopes seek to become stable by a release of energy through a process known as decay. This process involves giving off two kinds of radiation: (1) corpuscular, or particular radiation and (2) electromagnetic radiation.

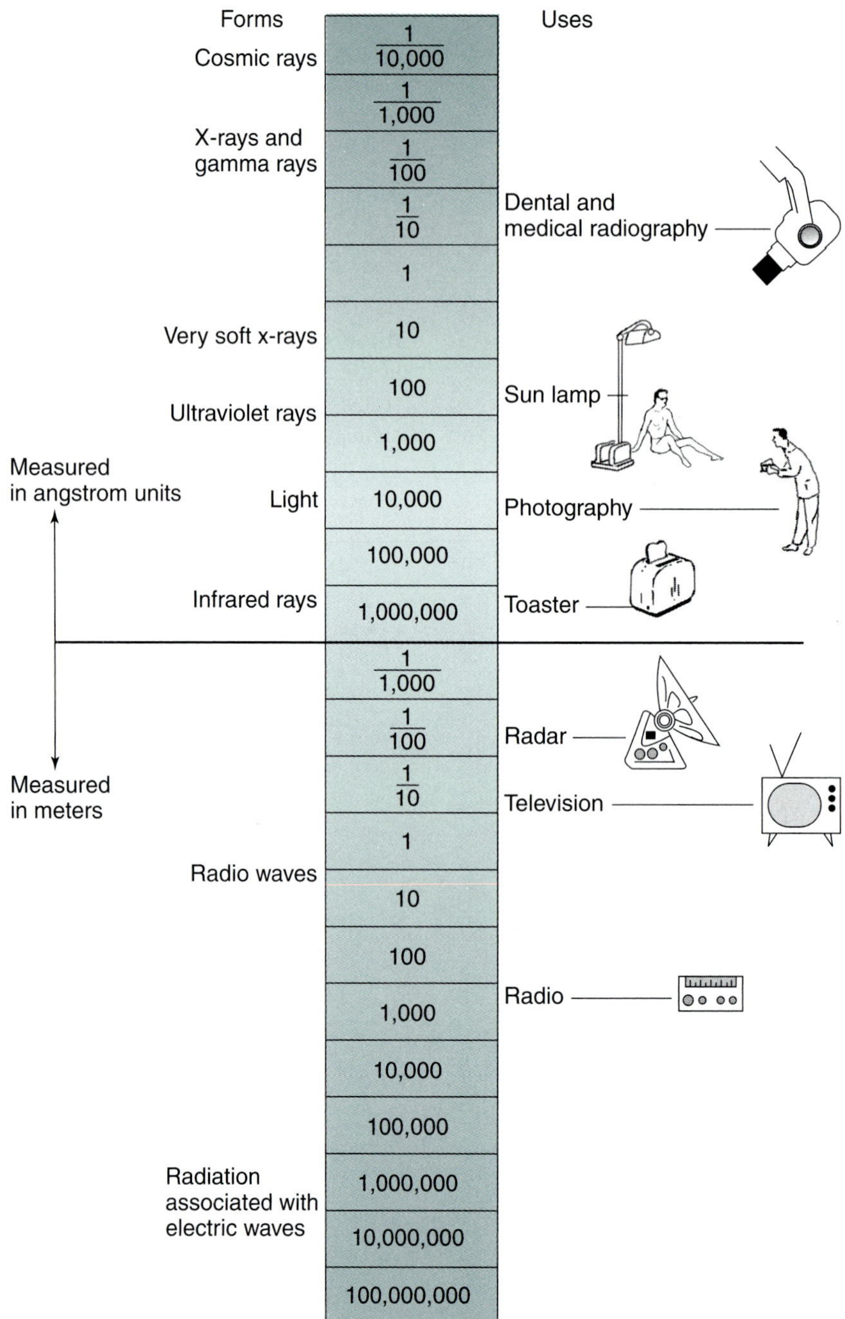

FIGURE 2–5. **The Electromagnetic Spectrum.** Electromagnetic radiations are arranged in an orderly fashion according to their energies in what is called the **electromagnetic spectrum.**

Radioactive isotopes are frequently used in hospitals and are also being used by dentists in some research and teaching centers.

Scientists have learned to produce several types of radiations that are identical to natural radiations. Ultraviolet waves are produced artificially for sun lamps or fluorescent lights and for numerous other uses. One of the most recent manmade radiations is the laser beam, whose potential is not fully known at this time.

Electromagnetic Radiation

Electromagnetic radiation is the movement of wave-like energy through space as a combination of electric and magnetic fields. Electromagnetic radiations are arranged in an orderly fashion according to their energies in what is called the **electromagnetic spectrum** (Figure 2–5). All energies of the electromagnetic spectrum share the following properties:

- Travel at the speed of light
- Have no electrical charge
- Have no mass or weight
- Pass through space as particles and in a wave-like motion
- Give off an electrical field at right angles to their path of travel and a magnetic field at right angles to the electric field
- Have energies that are measurable and different

Electromagnetic radiations display two seemingly contradictory properties. They are believed to move through space as both a particle and a wave. The particle or quantum theory assumes the electromagnetic radiations are particles or quanta. These particles are called photons. **Photons** are bundles of energy that travel through space at the speed of light. The wave theory assumes that electromagnetic radiation is propagated in the form of waves similar to waves resulting from the disturbance in water. Electromagnetic waves exhibit the properties of wavelength, frequency, and velocity.

- **Wavelength** is the distance between two similar points on two successive waves, as illustrated in Figure 2–6. The symbol for wavelength is the Greek letter lambda (λ). Wavelength may be measured in the metric system or in **angstrom (Å)** units (1 Å is about 1/250,000,000 in. or 1/100,000,000 cm). The shorter the wavelength, the more penetrating the radiation.

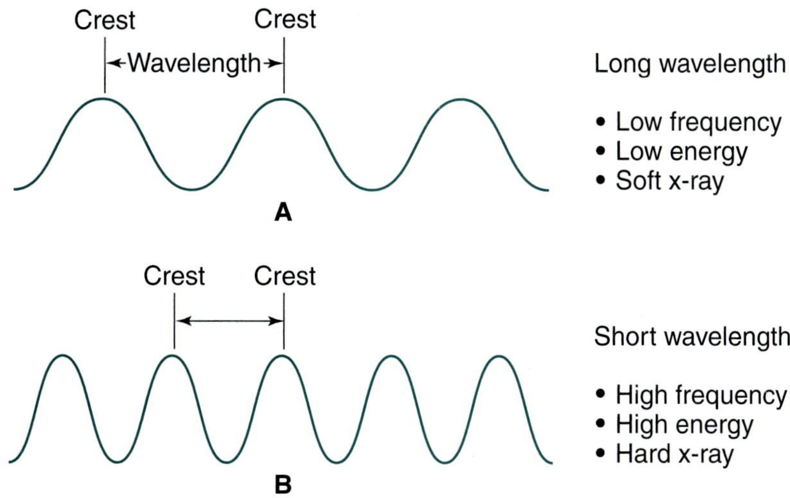

FIGURE 2–6. **Differences in wavelengths and frequencies.** Only the shortest wavelengths with extremely high frequency and energy are used to expose film in dental radiography. **Wavelength** is determined by the distances between the crests. Observe that this distance is much shorter in (**B**) than in (**A**). The photons that comprise the dental x-ray beam are estimated to have over 250 million such crests per inch. **Frequency** is the number of crests of a wavelength passing a given point per second.

- **Frequency** is a measure of the number of waves that pass a given point per unit of time. The symbol for frequency is the Greek letter nu (ν). The special unit of frequency is the hertz (Hz). One hertz equals 1 cycle per second. The higher the frequency, the more penetrating the radiation.
- Wavelength and frequency are inversely related. When the wavelength is long, the frequency is low, resulting in low-energy, **soft x-rays** (Figure 2–6). And when the wavelength is short, the frequency is high, resulting in high-energy, **hard x-rays.**
- **Velocity** refers to the speed of the wave. In a vacuum, all electromagnetic radiations travel at the speed of light (186,000 miles/sec or 3×10^8 m/sec).

The **electromagnetic spectrum** consists of an orderly arrangement of all known radiant energies (see Figure 2–5). X-radiation is a part of the electromagnetic spectrum, which also includes cosmic rays, gamma rays, ultraviolet rays, visible light, infrared, television, radar, microwave, and radio waves. The longest wavelengths, which are those used for low-frequency communications, are so long that they are best measured in kilometers (each kilometer is 1,000 m or about 5/8 mile). The shortest cosmic rays are measured in **angstrom (Å)** units.

No clear-cut separation exists between the various radiations represented on the electromagnetic spectrum; consequently, overlapping of the wavelengths is common. Each form of radiation has a range of wavelengths. This accounts for some of the longer infrared waves being measured in meters while the shorter infrared waves are measured in angstrom units. It therefore follows that all x-radiations are not the same wavelength. The longest of these are the Grenz rays, also called **soft radiation,** that have only limited penetrating power and are unsuitable for exposing dental radiographs. The wavelengths used in diagnostic dental radiography range from about 0.1 to 0.5 Å and are classified as **hard radiation,** a term meaning radiation with great penetrating power. Even still shorter wavelengths are produced by super-voltage machines when still greater penetration is required, as in some forms of medical therapy and industrial radiography.

Properties of X-rays

X-rays are believed to consist of minute bundles (or quanta) of pure electromagnetic energy called **photons**. These have no mass or weight, are invisible, and cannot be sensed. Because they travel at the speed of light (186,000 miles/sec or 3×10^8 meters/sec), these x-ray photons are often referred to as "bullets of energy." X-rays have the following properties. They

- Are invisible
- Travel in straight lines
- Travel at speed of light
- Have no mass or weight
- Have no charge
- Interact with matter causing ionization
- Can penetrate opaque tissues and structures
- Can affect photographic film emulsion (causing a latent image)
- Can affect living tissue

X-ray photons have the ability to pass through gases, liquids, and solids. The ability to penetrate materials or tissues depends on the wavelength of the x-ray and the thickness and density of the object. The composition of the object or the tissues determines whether the x-rays will penetrate and pass through it or whether they will be absorbed in it. Materials that are extremely dense and have a high atomic number will absorb more x-rays than thin materials with low atomic numbers. This partially explains why dense structures such as bone and enamel appear **radiopaque** (white or light gray) on the radiograph, whereas the less dense pulp chamber, muscles, and skin appear **radiolucent** (dark gray or black).

Production of X-rays

X-rays are generated in an x-ray tube located in the tube head (see Chapter 3). X-rays are produced whenever high-speed electrons are abruptly stopped or slowed down. Bodies in motion are believed to have **kinetic energy** (from the Greek word *kineticos*, "pertaining to motion"). In a dental x-ray tube, the kinetic energy of electrons is converted to electromagnetic energy by the formation of bremsstrahlung (German for "braking radiation") and characteristic radiation.

Bremsstrahlung radiation is produced when high-speed electrons are stopped or slowed down by the tungsten atoms of the dental x-ray tube. Referring to Figure 2–7, observe that the impact from both (A) and (B) electrons produce bremsstrahlung. When a high-speed electron collides with the nucleus of an atom in the target metal, as in (A), all of its kinetic

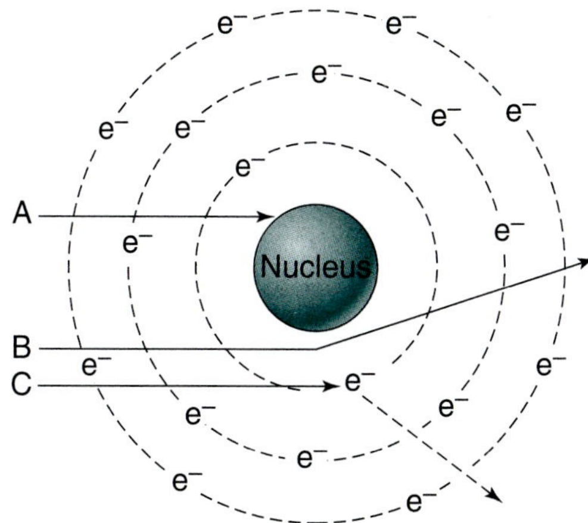

FIGURE 2-7. **Bremsstrahlung and characteristic radiation.** High-speed electron (**A**) collides with the nucleus and all of its kinetic energy is converted into a single x-ray. High-speed electron (**B**) is slowed down and bent off its course by the positive pull of the nucleus. The kinetic energy lost is converted into an x-ray. The impact from both A and B electrons produce **bremsstrahlung** radiation. **Characteristic** radiation is produced when high-speed electron (**C**) hits and dislodges a K shell (orbiting) electron. Another electron in an outer shell quickly fills the void and an x-ray is emitted. Characteristic radiation only occurs above 70 kVp with a tungsten target.

energy is transferred into a single x-ray photon. In (B) a high-speed electron is slowed down and bent off its course by the positive pull of the nucleus. The kinetic energy lost is converted into an x-ray. The majority of x-rays produced by dental x-ray machines are formed by Bremsstrahlung.

Characteristic radiation is produced when a bombarding electron from the tube filament collides with an orbiting K electron of the tungsten target as shown in Figure 2–7 (C). The K-shell electron is dislodged from the atom. Another electron in an outer shell quickly fills the void, and an x-ray is emitted. The x-rays produced in this manner are called characteristic x-rays. Characteristic radiation can only be produced when the x-ray machine is operated at or above 70 kilovolts (kVp) because a minimum force of 69 kVp is required to dislodge a K electron from a tungsten atom. Characteristic radiation is of minor importance because they account for only a very small part of the x-rays produced in an x-ray machine.

Interaction of X-rays with Matter

A beam of x-rays passing through matter is weakened and gradually disappears. Such a disappearance is referred to as **absorption** of x-rays. When so defined, absorption does not imply an occurrence such as a sponge soaking up water, but rather refers to the process of transferring the energy of the x-rays to the atoms of the material through which the x-ray beam passes. The basic method of absorption is ionization.

When a beam of x-rays pass through matter, four possibilities exist:

1. **No interaction.** The x-ray can pass through an atom unchanged and no interaction occurs (Figure 2–8). In dental radiology about 9% of the x-rays pass through the head without interaction.
2. **Coherent scattering** (unmodified scattering, also known as Thompson scattering). When a low-energy x-ray passes near an atom's outer electron, it may be scattered without loss of energy (Figure 2–8). The incoming x-ray interacts with the electron by causing the electron to vibrate at the same frequency as the incoming x-ray. The incoming x-ray ceases to exist. The vibrating electron radiates another x-ray of the same frequency and energy as the original incoming x-ray. The new x-ray is scattered in a different direction than the original x-ray. Essentially, the x-ray is scattered unchanged. **Coherent scattering** accounts for about 8% of the interactions of matter with the dental x-ray beam. Coherent scattering does not create film fog because it is totally absorbed within the patient.
3. **Photoelectric effect.** The **photoelectric effect** is an all-or-nothing energy loss. The x-ray imparts all of its energy to an orbital electron of some atom. This dental x-ray, since it consisted only of energy in the first place, simply vanishes. The electromagnetic energy of the x-ray is imparted to the electron in the form of kinetic energy of motion and causes the electron to fly from its orbit with considerable speed. Thus, an ion pair is created (Figure 2–9). Remember, the basic method of the interaction of x-rays with matter is the formation of ion pairs. The high-speed electron (called a photoelectron) knocks other electrons from the orbits of other atoms (forming secondary ion pairs) until all of its energy is used up. The positive ion atom combines with a free electron and the absorbing material is restored to its original condition. The photoelectric effect interaction takes place about 30% of the time.

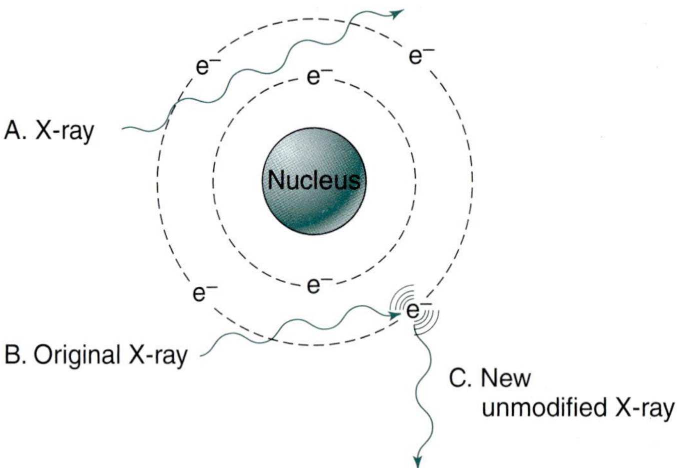

FIGURE 2–8. **X-rays interacting with atom.** X-ray (**A**) can pass through an atom unchanged and no interaction occurs. Incoming x-ray (**B**) interacts with the electron by causing the electron to vibrate at the same frequency as the incoming x-ray. The incoming x-ray ceases to exist. The vibrating electron radiates new x-ray (**C**) with the same frequency and energy as the original incoming x-ray. The new x-ray is scattered in a different direction than the original x-ray.

4. **Compton effect.** The **Compton effect** (often called Compton scattering) is similar to the photoelectric effect in that the dental x-ray interacts with an orbital electron and ejects it. But in the case of Compton interaction, only a part of the dental x-ray energy is transferred to the electron and a new, weaker x-ray is formed and scattered in some new direction (Figure 2–10). The new x-ray may even travel in a direction opposite to that of the original x-ray. The new x-ray may undergo another Compton scattering or it may be absorbed by a photoelectric effect interaction. The positive ion atom combines with a free electron and the absorbing material is restored to its original condition. Thus, it is important to remember that the Compton effect causes x-rays to be scattered in all directions and areas of the dental office. So we must protect ourselves from these scattered x-rays by standing at least 6 ft (1.8 m) from the head of our patient.

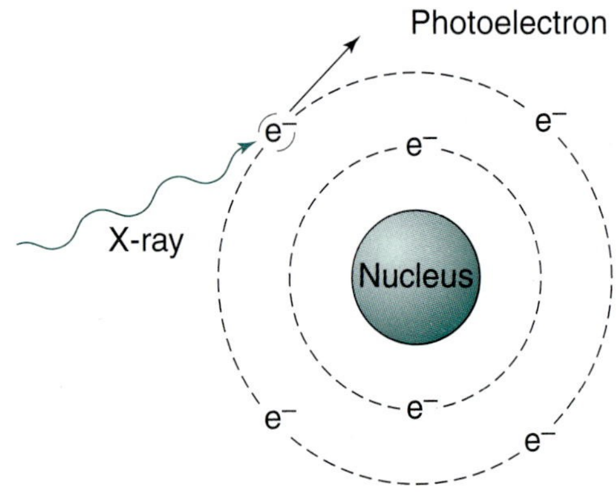

FIGURE 2–9. **Photoelectric effect.** The incoming x-ray gives up all of its energy to an orbital electron of the atom. The x-ray is absorbed and simply vanishes. The electromagnetic energy of the x-ray is imparted to the electron in the form of kinetic energy of motion and causes the electron to fly from its orbit. Thus, an ion pair is created. The high-speed electron (called a photoelectron) knocks other electrons from the orbits of other atoms forming secondary ion pairs.

A question often asked is, "Do x-rays make the material they pass through radioactive?" The answer is no. Dental x-rays have no effect on the nucleus of the atoms they interact with. Therefore, equipment, walls, and patients do not become radioactive after exposure to x-rays.

Units of Radiation

The terms used to measure x-radiation are based on the ability of the x-ray to deposit its energy in air, soft tissues, bone, or other substances. These terms can be quite confusing to anyone lacking a strong background of mathematics and physics. The requirements for in-depth stud-

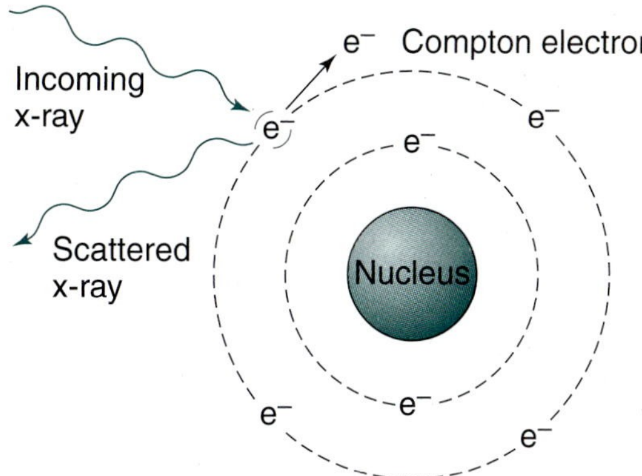

FIGURE 2–10. **Compton scattering.** Compton scattering is similar to the photoelectric effect in that the incoming x-ray interacts with an orbital electron and ejects it. But in the case of Compton interaction, only a part of the x-ray energy is transferred to the electron and a new, weaker x-ray is formed and scattered in some new direction. The new x-ray may undergo another Compton scattering or it may be absorbed by a photoelectric effect interaction.

ies of these terms will vary depending on the educational level of the student. The authors have made every attempt to simplify the definitions and explanations that follow. Those desiring additional information are urged to refer to the glossary for more complete explanations.

The International Commission on Radiation Units and Measurements (ICRU) has established standards that clearly define radiation units and radiation quantities. At the present time, two sets of terms are used for units of radiation (Table 2–1). The older system, referred to as the traditional units, is being phased out. Gaining greater acceptance is the metric equivalent known as the Systeme Internationale (SI). The **traditional** units are:

1. **Roentgen (R)**
2. **Rad** (radiation absorbed dose)
3. **Rem** (radiation equivalent in man)

The **Systeme Internationale (SI)** units are:

1. **Coulombs per kilogram (C/kg)**
2. **Gray (Gy)**
3. **Sievert (Sv)**

The American Dental Association requires the use of SI terminology on national board examinations. In this book, we will use the new SI units first, followed by the traditional units.

A "quantity" may be thought of as a description of a physical concept such as time, distance, or weight. The measure of the quantity is a "unit" such as minutes, miles (kilometers), or pounds (kilograms).

For practical x-ray protection measurement three quantities are used. They are:

1. **Exposure**
2. **Absorbed dose**
3. **Dose equivalent**

Exposure

Exposure can be defined as the measurement of ionization in air produced by x- or gamma rays. The units for measuring exposure are coulombs per kilogram (C/kg) and the roentgen (R).

Coulomb per kilogram (C/kg): A coulomb is a unit of electrical charge. Therefore, the unit C/kg measures electrical charges (ion pairs) in a kilogram of air.

Roentgen (R): One roentgen is the amount of x- or gamma rays that will produce 2.08×10^9 (about 2 billion) ion pairs in 1 cc of air at standard conditions of pressure and temperature (Figure 2–11).

The roentgen only applies to x- or gamma radiation and only measures ion pairs in air. It does not measure the radiation absorbed by tissues or other materials. Therefore, it is not a measurement of dose. An exposure does not become a dose until the radiation is absorbed in the tissues.

TABLE 2–1. **Radiation Measurement Terminology**

Quantity	Systeme International (SI) Unit	Traditional Unit
Exposure	coulombs per kilogram (C/kg)	roentgen (R)
Absorbed dose	gray (Gy)	rad
Dose equivalent	sievert (Sv)	rem

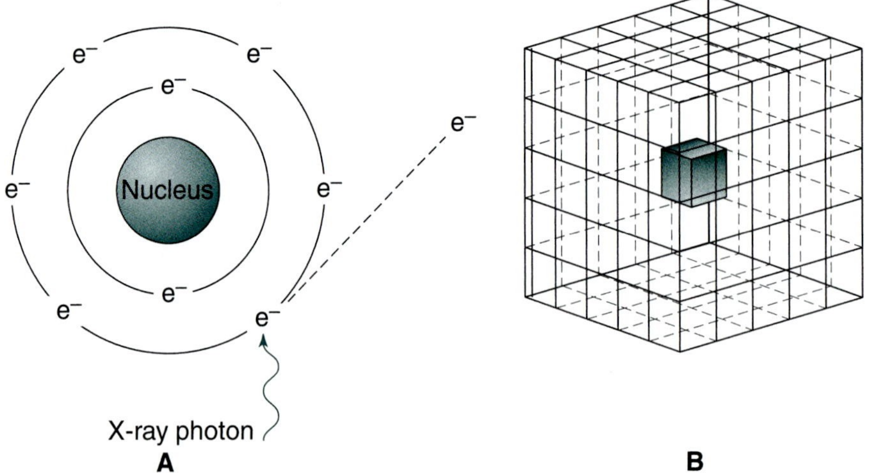

FIGURE 2–11. **Schematic representation.** (**A**) Ionization of an oxygen atom. (**B**) One roentgen is the amount of radiation that will produce about 2 billion oxygen ion pairs in 1 cubic cm of air surrounded by an infinite amount of air.

Absorbed Dose

Absorbed dose is defined as the amount of energy deposited in any form of matter (such as wood, bracket table, air, teeth, muscles, and so on), by any type of radiation (alpha or beta particles, gamma or x-rays). The units for measuring the absorbed dose are the **gray (Gy)** and the **rad** (radiation absorbed dose).

Gray (Gy): A unit for measuring absorbed dose that is replacing the rad. One gray equals 1 joule (J) (a unit of energy) per kilogram of tissue. One gray equals 100 rads.

Rad (radiation absorbed dose): A special unit of absorbed dose equal to 0.01 J/kg of tissue. For x-rays absorbed in the soft tissues, the rad is approximately numerically equivalent to the roentgen.

Dose Equivalent

Dose equivalent is a term used for radiation protection purposes to compare the biological effects of the various types of radiation. Dose equivalent is defined as the product of the absorbed dose times a biological-effect modifying factor. Because the *modifying factor* (see glossary) for x-rays is 1, the absorbed dose and the dose equivalent are equal. The units for measuring the dose equivalent are the **sievert (Sv)** and the **rem** (roentgen equivalent man).

Sievert (Sv): A unit used to measure the dose equivalent. One sievert equals 1 Gy times a biological-effect modifying factor. Because the modifying factor for x- and gamma radiation equals 1, the number of sieverts is identical to the absorbed dose in grays for these radiations. One sievert equals 100 rems.

Rem (roentgen equivalent [in] man): A unit used to measure the dose equivalent. One rem equals one rad times a biological-effect modifying factor. Because the modifying factor for x- and gamma radiation equals 1, the number of rems is identical to the absorbed dose in rads for these radiations. One rem equals 0.01 sievert.

Fortunately, in dental radiology, grays and sieverts are equal, while roentgens, rads, and rems are considered to be numerically equal; however, it should be pointed out that only x-rays and gamma rays are measured in coulombs per kilogram or roentgens. Grays or rads and sieverts or rems are used to measure all radiations: gamma and x-rays, alpha and beta particles, neutrons, and high-energy protons.

A simplified comparison of the terms explains the coulomb per kilogram or roentgen as a measurement of x-ray exposure in air; the gray or rad represents the amount of energy the tissues absorb; and the sievert or rem represents the relative biological effect of radiation absorbed in the body tissues.

Because units of measurement in dental radiology are fairly large, smaller multiples of these units are commonly used. For example, the word *milli* means "one-thousandth of" and we express a smaller dose of a gray as a milligray (mGy).

An internationally accepted system of writing and abbreviating units has been accepted. To avoid confusion with the name of the person for whom a unit may be named, the word is capitalized when referring to the person (Roentgen) but when referring to the unit, the word is written in lowercase (roentgen). The abbreviation for the unit is, however, capitalized (R).

Background Radiation

Radiation is briefly defined as the process by which energy in the form of electromagnetic waves or particulate emissions is sent out of atoms as they undergo internal change. This energy is emitted and propelled outwardly from its source in all directions (unless the direction is controlled as in the x-ray machine). This may occur spontaneously as with unstable elements such as radium or uranium or under man-made conditions.

Background radiation is defined as ionizing radiation that is always present in our environment. The human race has always been subjected to exposure from natural background radiations originating from the following sources:

- Cosmic radiations from outer space
- Terrestrial radiations from the earth and its environments
- Background radiations from naturally occurring radionuclides (unstable atoms that emit radiations) that are deposited in our bodies by inhalation and ingestion

Natural background radiation levels for the United States range from about 0.9 mSv (millisievert) or 90 mrem (millirem) to 2 mSv or 200 mrem per year. The exact amount varies according to locality, the amount of radioactive material present, and the intensity of the cosmic rays—this intensity varies according to altitude and latitude. For example, persons living near sea level in Philadelphia receive less background radiation than persons living in the mile-high city of Denver.

The whole body is exposed to background radiation, whereas in dental radiography only a small area of the head is directly exposed. For purposes of comparison, it is of interest that a typical single x-ray film subjects the average patient's body (reproductive organs) to no more than 0.002 mSv (0.2 mrem).

CHAPTER SUMMARY

The three basic building blocks of an atom are protons, neutrons, and electrons. Protons and neutrons make up the central nucleus, which is orbited by the electrons. The number of protons determines the chemical element. Isotopes are atoms of the same element that varies by the number of neutrons in the nucleus. Some isotopes are radioactive.

Ionization is the formation of charged particles called ions. A positive ion and a negative ion are called an ion pair.

Radioactivity is defined as the process whereby unstable atoms undergo decay (emit radiation) to attain a stable nuclear state. The decay process involves two forms of radiation: particulate (alpha and beta particles) and electromagnetic (gamma rays).

Electromagnetic radiation is the movement of wave-like energy through space. Electromagnetic waves exhibit the properties of wavelength, frequency, and velocity. Short-wavelength x-rays, called hard radiation, are very penetrating. Long-wavelength x-rays, called soft radiation, have limited penetrating power. The electromagnetic spectrum consists of an orderly arrangement of all known radiant energies.

X-rays are invisible, travel in straight lines at the speed of light, interact with matter causing ionization, affect photographic film, and affect living tissue. X-rays are produced whenever high-speed electrons are abruptly stopped or slowed down. They may pass through a patient with no interaction, or they may be absorbed by the photoelectric effect or scattered by either Compton scattering or coherent scattering.

For practical x-ray measurement three quantities are used. They are exposure, absorbed dose and dose equivalent. The units for measuring exposure are coulombs per kilogram (C/kg) and the roentgen (R). The units for measuring the absorbed dose are the gray (Gy) and the rad (radiation absorbed dose). The units for measuring the dose equivalent are the sievert (Sv) and the rem (roentgen equivalent man).

The ever-present background radiation consists of cosmic radiation, terrestrial radiations, and naturally occurring radionuclides that are deposited in our bodies by inhalation and ingestion.

REVIEW QUESTIONS

1. What term describes the smallest particle of a substance that retains the properties of that substance?
   (a) Element
   (b) Molecule
   (c) Photon
   (d) Isotope
2. Draw and label a typical atom.
3. Which of these subatomic particles carries a negative electric charge?
   (a) Electron
   (b) Neutron
   (c) Nucleus
   (d) Proton
4. What term describes an alternate form of an atom that does not contain the same number of neutrons?
   (a) Ion
   (b) Neutron
   (c) Photon
   (d) Isotope
5. Which term describes the process by which unstable atoms undergo decay in an effort to obtain nuclear stability?
   (a) Radioactivity
   (b) Radiolucent
   (c) Ionization
   (d) Absorption
6. Which of these electromagnetic radiations has the shortest wavelength?
   (a) Radar
   (b) Ultraviolet
   (c) Infrared
   (d) X-rays
7. Which of these forms of radiation has the greatest penetrating power?
   (a) X-ray
   (b) Infrared
   (c) Ultraviolet
   (d) Radio wave

8. Which of these forms of radiation is least capable of causing ionization of body tissue cells?
   (a) Cosmic rays
   (b) X-rays
   (c) Gamma rays
   (d) Infrared

9. Which x-ray wavelength has the most penetrating power?
   (a) 0.1 Å
   (b) 0.5 Å
   (c) 0.8 Å
   (d) 1.0 Å

10. Which form of radiation causes ionization of body tissue cells?
    (a) Radar
    (b) Radio
    (c) X-ray
    (d) Microwaves

11. What term best describes the process of transferring the energy of the x-rays to the atoms of the material through which the x-ray beam passes?
    (a) Compton scattering
    (b) Photoelectric effect
    (c) Absorption
    (d) Bremsstrahlung

12. Which of these terms is the unit used to measure radiation exposure?
    (a) Curie
    (b) Gray (rad)
    (c) Sievert (rem)
    (d) Coulombs per kilogram (roentgen)

13. The Systeme Internationale (SI) unit that is replacing the rem is:
    (a) Coulomb/kilogram
    (b) Gray
    (c) Sievert
    (d) Rad

14. Define background radiation.

15. What is the average background radiation to an individual in the United States?
    (a) 0–1.0 mSv (0–100 millirem) per year
    (b) 1–2 mSv (100–200 millirem) per year
    (c) 3–4 mSv (300–400 millirem) per year
    (d) 4–5 mSv (400–500 millirem) per year

BIBLIOGRAPHY

Bushberg, J. T., Seibert, J. A., Leidholdt, E. M. Jr., & Boone, J. M. *The Essential Physics of Medical Imaging*, Baltimore, MD: Williams & Wilkins, 1994.

Langland, O. E., Sippy, F. H., & Langlais, R. P. *Textbook of Dental Radiology*, 2nd ed. Springfield, IL: Charles C. Thomas, 1984.

White S. C. & Pharoah, M. J. *Oral Radiology Principles and Interpretation*, 4th ed. St Louis: Mosby, 2000.

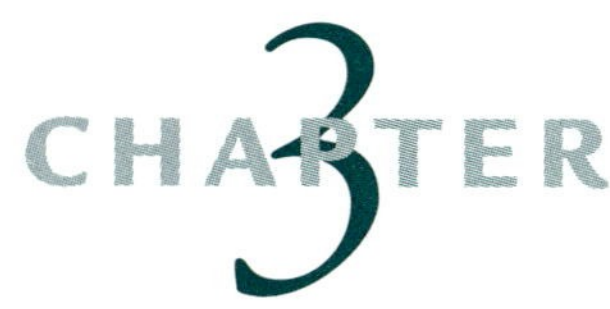

The Dental X-ray Machine: Components and Functions

OBJECTIVES

By the end of this chapter the student should be able to:

- Define the key words.
- Identify the major components of an x-ray machine.
- List the four controls on most dental x-ray machines.
- List the components of the tube head.
- Draw and label a typical dental x-ray tube.
- Discuss the principles of x-ray tube operation.
- Explain the function of the mA, kVp, and timer control devices.
- Name the three transformers, describe their functions, and state their locations.
- Identify, in sequence, the steps that must be followed in operating the dental x-ray machine.

KEY WORDS

Alternating current (AC)
Ammeter
Amperage
Ampere (A)
Anode
Autotransformer
Cathode
Collimator
Control panel
Dead-man switch
Direct current (DC)
Duty cycle
Electrical circuits
Electricity
Electrode
Extension arm
Filament
Filter
Focal spot
Focusing cup
Half-value layer (HVL)
Incandescence
Impulse
Intensity
Kilovolt
Kilovolt peak (kVp)
Line-focus principle
Line switch
Milliampere (mA)
Port
Primary beam
Radiator
Rectification
Self-rectifying
Step-down transformer
Step-up transformer
Target
Thermionic emission
Timer
Transformer
Tube head
Tungsten
Voltage
Volt
Voltmeter
X-ray tube
Yoke

Introduction

The x-ray machine has undergone a long period of development. The unreliable gas tubes used in the early machines gave way to the vastly improved Coolidge hot cathode vacuum tube, a thermionic emission (the creation of ions by heat) tube invented by Dr. W. D. Coolidge in 1913. The first shock-proof machines were introduced in 1923. Few changes were made until the mid-1950s when the variable kilovoltage machines were introduced. At the suggestion of A. G. Richards, the recessed tube design was introduced in 1966. New technology employing miniaturized solid-state transformers and rare-earth materials for filtration of the x-ray beam has resulted in a modern dental x-ray machine that is safe, compact, easy to position, and simple to operate.

Many manufacturers, domestic and foreign, offer a variety of x-ray machine models and accessories. All x-ray machines—whether mobile or stationary; whether mounted on the wall, the floor, or the ceiling—operate on similar principles. The greatest differences among them are their size, voltage range, controls, and whether the voltage varies or is constant.

The purpose of this chapter is to discuss the conventional dental x-ray machine, its components and functions.

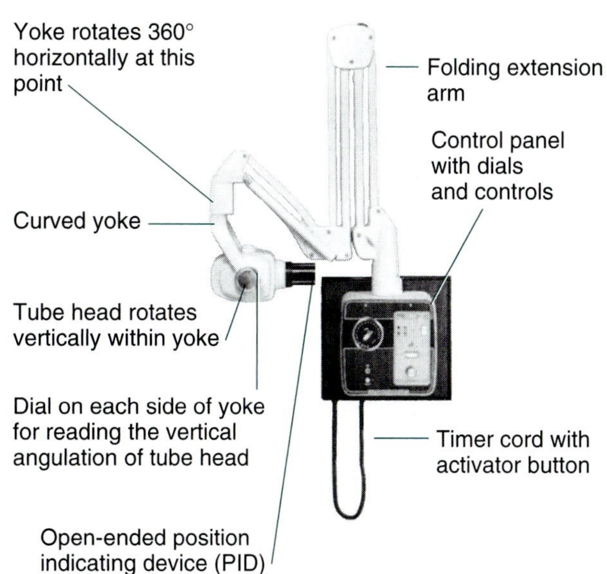

FIGURE 3–1. **Typical wall-mounted dental x-ray machine.** (Courtesy of Ritter-Midwest Division of Sybron Corporation)

X-ray Machine Components

Dental x-ray machines vary in size and appearance but have similar structural components (Figure 3–1). The typical dental x-ray machine consists of three parts:

1. The **control panel,** which contains the regulating devices.
2. The **extension arm** or bracket, which enables the tube head to be positioned quickly.
3. The **tube head** contains the x-ray tube from which x-rays are generated.

Dental x-ray machines may be mounted on the wall, on the floor, on the dental unit, or on a mobile base.

Control Panel

The **control panel** (see Figure 3–2) may be a part of the x-ray machine or it may be remote from the unit, mounted on a shelf or wall. One control panel may serve two or more tube heads. Control panels vary greatly according to the manufacturer.

The electric current enters the control panel either through a cord plugged into a grounded outlet in the wall or through a direct connection to a power line in the wall. It continues to and through the hollow extension arm and the **yoke,** entering the tube head from one or both sides at a point where the tube head attaches to the yoke. All areas are heavily insulated to protect the patient and the operator from electrical shock.

Four major controls must be operated on most variable-type dental x-ray machines: the line switch to the electrical outlet, the milliampere selector, the kilovoltage selector, and the timer.

Line Switch

The **line switch** may be a toggle switch that can be flicked on or off with light finger pressure, or it may be an ON/OFF push button. It is generally located on the side or face of the cabinet or control panel. An indicator light turns on indicating the machine is operational. Additionally, all new x-ray machines are now required by federal law to give off an audible signal when x-rays are produced. In the ON position, this switch energizes the circuits in the control panel but not the low- or high-voltage circuits. In the OFF position, the transformers are totally disconnected from the supply of electric current.

Milliammeter (mA) Selector

The **milliammeter (mA)** (or **milliamperage selector,** as it is often called) measures the amount of current passing

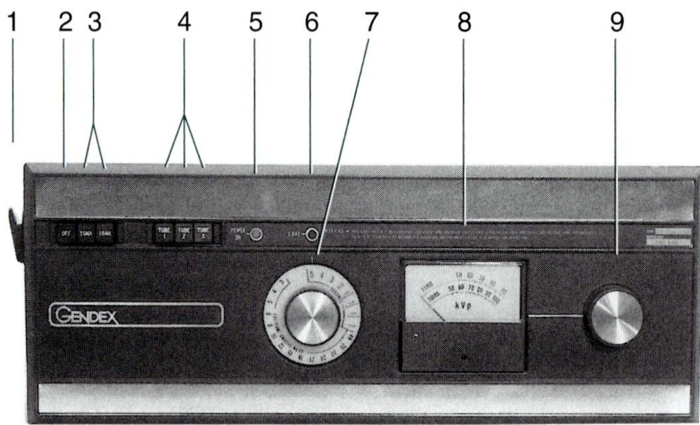

FIGURE 3–2. **Control panel** of Gendex dental x-ray machine. (**1**) Exposure button holder, (**2**) main on/off switch, (**3**) mA control, (**4**) x-ray tube selector, (**5**) power on light, (**6**) x-ray emission light, (**7**) timer control, (**8**) kVp meter, (**9**) kVp control (autotransformer). This basic master **control unit** accommodates three remote tube heads. Positive interlocks assure operation of only one tube head at a time. This unit permits variable kVp and mA selection for settings of 50 kVp to 90 kVp at 15 mA and 50 kVp to 100 kVp at 10 mA.

through the wires of the circuit. Mathematically, amperage is a linear factor expressed in the first power. That means that if amperage is doubled, the radiation produced is also doubled. The milliampere selector may be a knob or push button (Figure 3–2). On a preset x-ray machine, it is connected directly to the ON/OFF switch. On some machines a needle on the control panel dial indicates that current is available for operation.

Kilovolt Peak (kVp) Selector

The **voltmeter** measures the electromotive force (the difference in potential or voltage across the x-ray tube) (Figure 3–2). A **kilovolt peak selector,** in the form of push buttons, knobs, or dials, controls the tabs that slide over the turns of the wire in the autotransformer and enables the operator to change the peak kilovoltage. Mathematically, voltage is an exponential factor. For example, doubling the kilovoltage would result in far more than twice as much penetrating power. For practical purposes, an increase from 65 kVp to 80 kVp is sufficient to double the penetrating power of the x-rays that are produced.

Timer

The **timer** serves to regulate the duration of the interval that the current will pass through the x-ray tube (Figure 3–2). Some of the older x-ray machines that are still in use have mechanical or electric timers that are not sufficiently accurate for modern high-speed film and techniques. Units equipped with a vacuum-type electronic timer are accurate up to 1/60-sec intervals. Time settings of less than a second may be indicated in fractions and in **impulses** (there are 60 impulses in a second). For example, the frequently used 1/10-sec exposure lasts 6 impulses, 1/5 sec for 12 impulses, and so forth. Newer x-ray machines with electronic digital timers are accurate to 1/100-sec intervals and work well with digital radiography systems.

The timer is set by turning the selector knob or depressing the marked push button. An activator button is located on the handle of the timer cord or the control panel. All dental x-ray machines are required to be equipped with an exposure switch of the **"dead-man"** type, which automatically terminates the exposure when the finger ceases to press on the timer button. This makes it necessary to maintain firm pressure on the button during the entire exposure. Failure to do so results in the formation of an insufficient number of x-rays to properly expose the film. Ideally, the timer cord should be sufficiently long to enable the operator to step into an area of radiation safety, normally at least 6 ft (1.83 m) from the source of the x-ray beam. Timer switches may also be installed outside the room where the x-ray machine is housed. By observing the dial on the milliammeter and listening to the audible sound, it is possible to determine whether x-rays are being generated.

The present trend is toward simpler and automated controls. An example of this is the electrical timer that automatically resets itself and does not have to be altered unless a change in the exposure time is desired.

The operation of each x-ray machine is explained fully in the operating manual provided by the manufacturer. All persons operating an x-ray machine should study the manual until they are thoroughly familiar with the operational capability and maintenance requirements of the machine.

Extension Arm

A folding **extension arm** is a support from which the tube housing is suspended (Figure 3–1). The extension arm is hollow to permit the passage of electrical wires to the tube. It folds up like a bracket and can be swiveled from side to side. The extension arm allows for moving and positioning the tube head.

After use, fold the extension arm bracket up as far as it will go. The tube head is finely counterbalanced in its suspension from the extension arm. This balance can be disturbed if the tube is left suspended for prolonged time periods with the extension arm stretched out.

Tube Head (Tube Housing)

The **tube head** (sometimes called tube housing)(Figure 3–3) is a tightly sealed heavy metal housing that contains the dental x-ray tube, insulating oil, and step-up and step-down transformers. The metal housing performs several important functions:

1. It protects the x-ray tube from accidental damage.
2. It increases the safety of the x-ray machine by grounding its high-voltage components (the x-ray tube and the transformers) to prevent shock.
3. It prevents overheating of the x-ray tube by providing a space filled with oil, gas, or air to absorb the heat created during the production of x-rays.
4. It absorbs any x-rays produced except the primary beam that exits through the port.

The tube head is attached to the extension arm by means of a yoke that can revolve 360 degrees horizontally where it is connected. In addition, the tube head can be rotated vertically within the yoke. The tube head

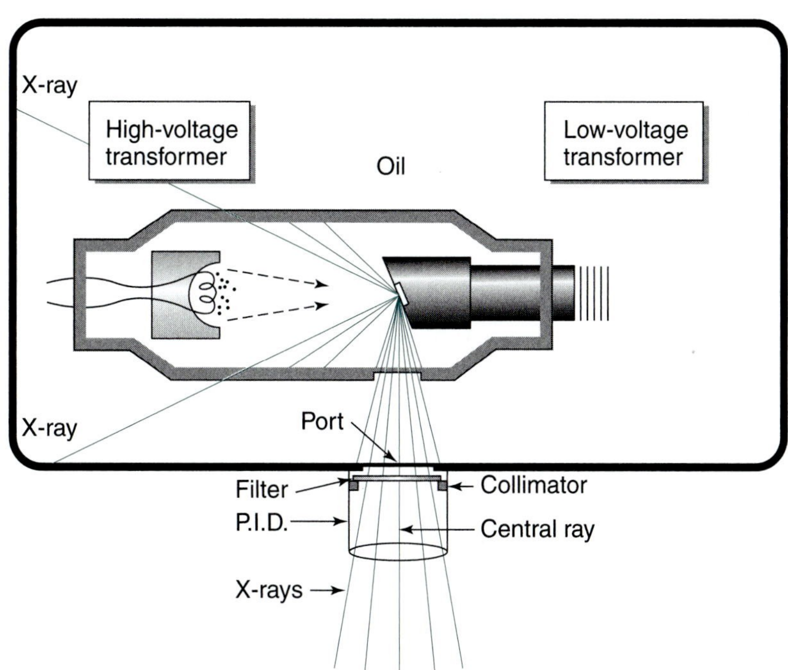

FIGURE 3–3. **Dental x-ray tube head,** containing dental x-ray tube, transformers, and oil. When an electric current is applied to the high-voltage circuit (between the cathode and the anode), each electron is propelled from the cathode to the target on the anode, producing heat and x-rays. X-rays are emitted in all directions. Most of the x-rays travel towards the port because of the 20-degree angle of the anode target. These x-rays make up the primary x-ray beam and exit the tube head via the port. The central ray is the x-ray in the center of the primary beam. **PID** (position indicating device)

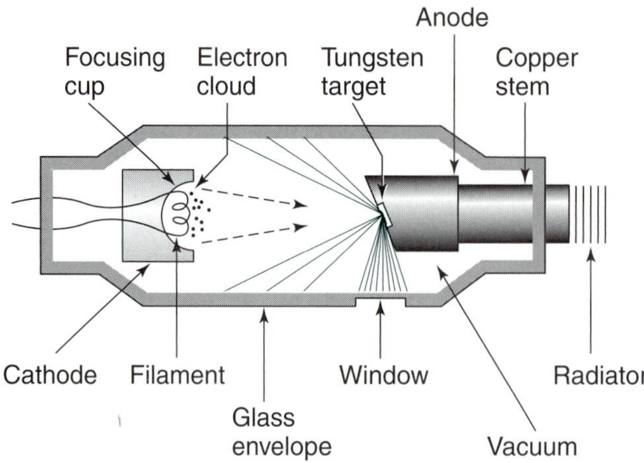

FIGURE 3–4. **Drawing of a typical dental x-ray tube.**

is made of cast metal (often aluminum) and protectively lined with lead to prevent the escape of radiation in any direction except toward the position indicating device (PID). The PID attaches to the tube head at the port.

The X-ray Tube

X-rays are produced when a stream of high-speed electrons are stopped or slowed down. Therefore, three conditions must exist for x-rays to be produced:

1. A source of free electrons
2. High voltage to impart speed to the electrons
3. A target that is capable of stopping the electrons

The **x-ray tube** (Figure 3–4) and the circuits within the machine are designed to create these conditions.

The earliest tubes used in radiography were glass bulbs from which the air had been only partially evacuated and replaced with hydrogen or some other gas. An **anode** (the positive electrode) and a **cathode** (the negative electrode) were sealed within the tube, and the two protruding arms of the electrodes permitted the passage of the current through the tube. The electron supply depended on the ionization of gases within the tube when it was in operation. The current flowing between these electrodes from cathode to anode was called the cathode stream. Because the air evacuation was only partial, these early tubes operated quite erratically, working well one day and not at all the next. A major breakthrough was the invention in 1913 of the Coolidge vacuum tube, an improved model that is still used in today's x-ray machines.

The design of the Coolidge vacuum tube eliminated the need for gas to create electrons, replacing gas with an incandescent filament in the cathode. Now, electrons are created at the filament wire of the cathode. This process, known as **thermionic emission,** occurs whenever a wire is heated to **incandescence** (glowing red with heat). A familiar example of this phenomenon is the tungsten electric light bulb we all use. The radiographer, by adjusting the milliamperage, can accurately control the thermionic emission.

The **x-ray tube,** located inside the tube head, is a glass bulb from which the air has been pumped out to create a vacuum (Figure 3–5). The vacuum offers a minimum resistance to the stream of electrons flowing across the space between the cathode and anode. In most dental x-ray tubes, the space between the electrodes is less than 1 in. (25.4 mm). The cathode and the anode are con-

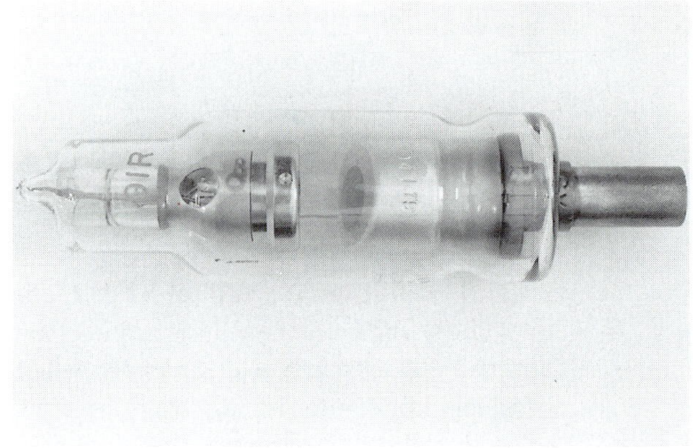

FIGURE 3–5. **Photograph of a dental x-ray tube.**

nected to the outside of the tube by massive copper wires, which permit a high-voltage current to flow across the tube when the x-ray machine is in operation. On x-ray machines of conventional design, the tube is located in front of the transformers (Figure 3–3); on those employing the Richards design, the tube is recessed behind the transformers (see Figure 3–6).

Cathode

The purpose of the **cathode** is to supply electrons necessary to produce x-rays. The cathode, or negative electrode, consists of a thin, spiral filament of tungsten wire about 1/2 in. (12.7 mm) long. This **filament** wire, when heated to incandescence (red hot and glows), produces the electrons (Figure 3–7). Tungsten's high atomic number makes it possible to liberate electrons easily from their orbital shells when the metal is heated. The wire filament is recessed into a molybdenum **focusing cup,** which directs the electrons toward the target on the anode (Figure 3–8).

Anode

The purpose of the **anode** is to stop the high-velocity electrons, converting their kinetic energy into x-rays (electromagnetic energy). The anode, or positive **electrode,** consists of a copper bar with a **tungsten** button imbedded in the end that faces the focusing cup of the cathode. On dental x-ray machines, this tungsten button, called the **target,** is set into the copper at an angle of 20 degrees to the cathode. The angle assures that most of the x-rays (the primary beam) are produced in one direction.

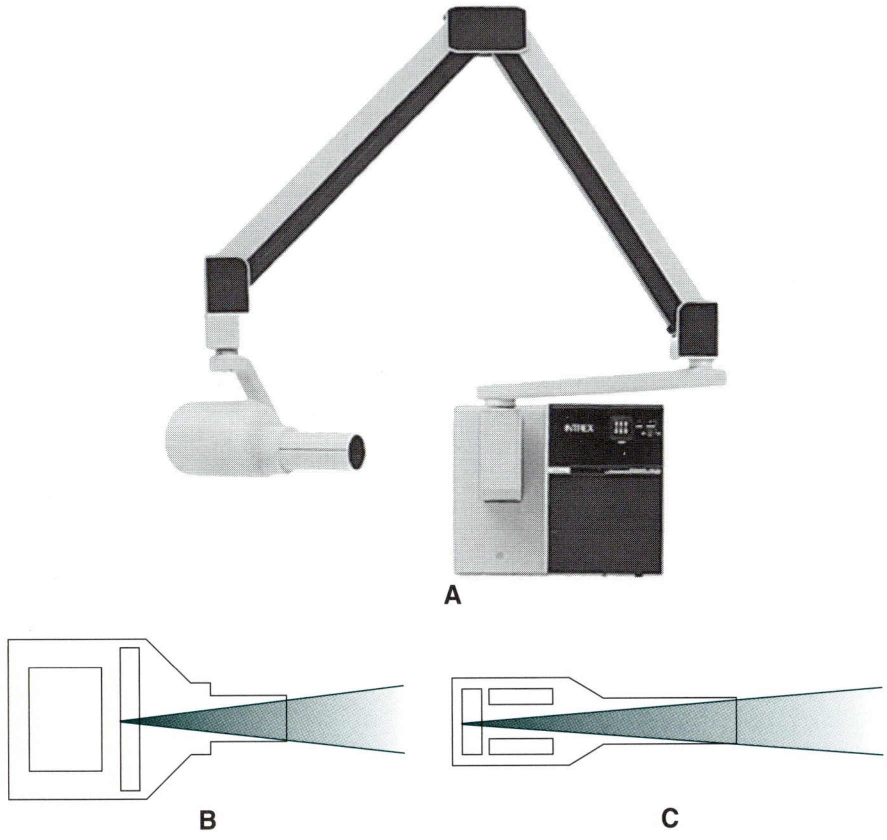

FIGURE 3–6. **Comparison of conventional and recessed tube position within tube head.** (**A**) Intrex recessed tube x-ray machine. (**B**) Conventional position with tube in front of transformer. Because x-ray source is in front, the beam pattern quickly flares out. (**C**) Recessed tube of Intrex machine with miniaturized transformers. Because x-ray source is at the rear, a relatively more parallel x-ray beam is produced. (Courtesy of S.S. White Dental Products International)

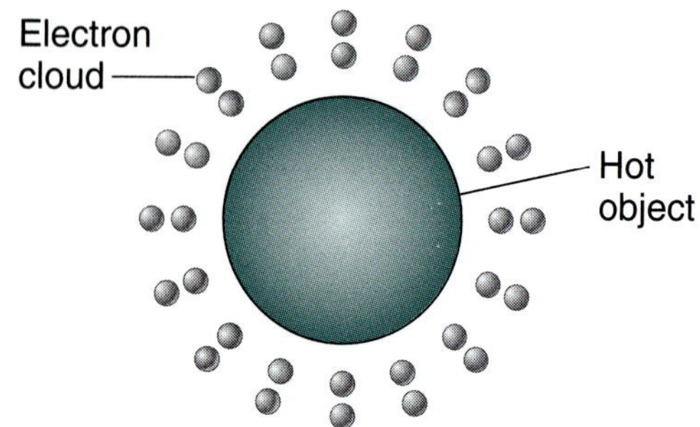

FIGURE 3–7. **Cross section of a filament wire.** The filament wire in the cathode is heated to incandescence (**thermionic emission**). The attached electrons are literally boiled out of the wire and become available as a source of free electrons, thus fulfilling the first requirement for x-ray production. The milliamperage selected by the operator will determine the size of the electron cloud and therefore the number of electrons available to be accelerated across to the target of the anode.

When the tube is in operation, a cloud of electrons first forms around the filament wire of the cathode as the tube warms. Later, when the high-voltage current is applied, these electrons are attracted and propelled toward a rectangular area on the surface of the target is known as the focal spot.

Focal Spot

The **focal spot** is a small rectangular area on the target of the anode to which the focusing cup directs the electron beam. X-rays originate at the focal spot. Its size (about 1 × 3 mm) is controlled by the manufacturer. The smaller the focal spot, the sharper the radiographic image. A small focal spot not only improves the sharpness on the radiograph but also concentrates the electrons and creates enormous heat. To prevent damage to the tube, the size of the focal spot is effectively reduced by the application of the line-focus principle.

Line-focus Principle

The purpose of the **line-focus principle** (Figure 3–9) is to generate x-rays over a large area for better heat dissipation and still have a small source of x-rays to increase sharpness of the image. To create a small focal spot and yet distribute the electrons over the surface of a larger target, the target is placed at an angle with respect to the electron beam. The electron stream is focused and directed onto a narrow rectangle on the face of the target on the anode. If one were to stand directly beneath the x-ray tube and look up at it, the rectangular focal spot (**actual focal spot**) would appear square (**effective focal spot**).

- **Actual focal spot** is a rectangle (about 1 × 3 mm or smaller).
- **Effective focal spot** is a square (about 1 × 1 mm or smaller).

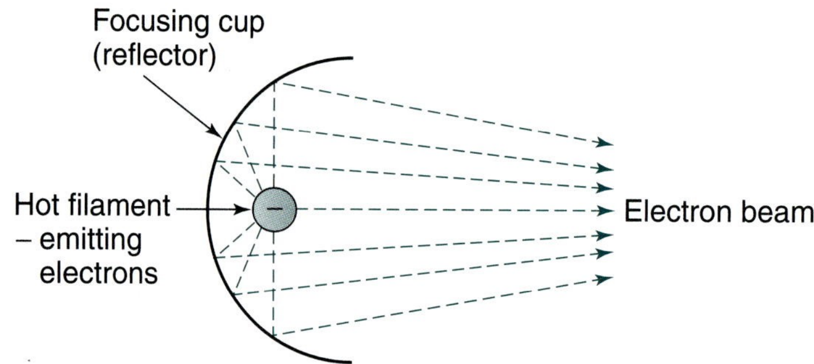

FIGURE 3–8. **Formation of electron beam by focusing cup.** A reflector, or focusing cup, within the cathode structure into which the filament is placed, focuses the electron beam in a similar manner as light is focused by a flashlight reflector. When the high-voltage circuit is activated, the free electrons are accelerated toward the focal spot on the anode target at approximately half the speed of light.

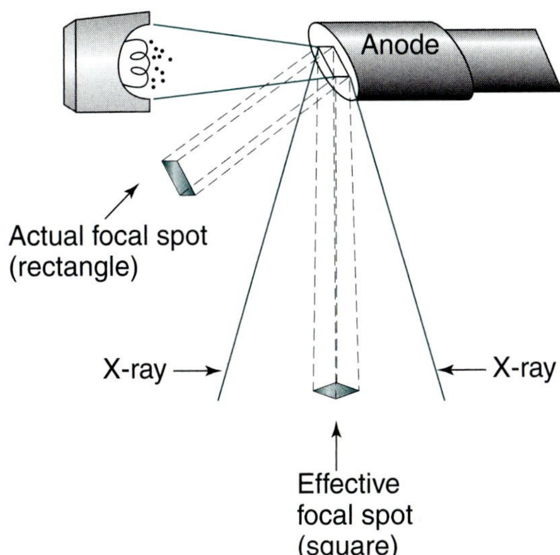

FIGURE 3–9. **Line-focus principle.** Representation of the anode, focal spot, and x-ray beam. As seen from points within the x-ray beam, **the focal spot appears as a square** of approximately 0.8 mm × 0.8 mm. This square is the source of radiation or **effective focal spot** for the beam of radiation. **The actual focal spot is rectangular** and has a considerably greater area (approximately 0.8 mm × 1.8 mm).

Principles of X-ray Tube Operation

Before x-ray production can begin, the machine must be turned on and the necessary settings made on the control panel. The **amperage** selected determines the available number of free electrons at the cathode filament. The **kilovoltage** selected determines their speed of travel toward the target on the anode. The **time** selected determines the duration of the exposure.

The process of x-ray production is initiated by firmly pressing the exposure button. This permits the current to enter the filament circuit to form the electron cloud. After a time delay of less than 1/2 sec the filament is fully heated, and the electron cloud is formed. The high voltage now automatically enters the cathode-anode circuit, speeding the free electrons across the tube to the focal spot on the target. These high-velocity electrons are stopped by the tungsten atoms in the target. This energy is converted into 99% heat and 1% x-rays.

The metal tungsten (symbol W and atomic number 74—also known as wolfram) is ideally suited for use in the filament and target because it can withstand extremely high temperatures (melting point 3370°C). Because it is subjected to such extreme heat and has low thermal conductivity, the tungsten button is always imbedded in a core of copper.

Copper is highly conductive and carries the heat off to the **radiator,** which is just outside the tube (refer to the tube diagram in Figure 3–4). In an oil-cooled tube, the large mass of copper conducts the heat out of the tube into a radiator that transfers the heat to the oil surrounding the tube. In an air-cooled tube the heat is transferred through the copper and the radiator into the air inside the tube head.

The x-rays produced by the energy exchange within the tube are emitted in all directions within the tube housing. Many of these rays are absorbed by the glass tube, oil, air, wires, transformers, and the tube head lining. A window (a thin area in the glass envelope) is located at a point where the emission of x-rays is most intense. In turn, this window is aligned with an opening in the tube housing called the **port** that is covered by a permanent seal of glass, beryllium, or aluminum.

If the tube head is properly sealed, the port is the only place through which the x-rays can escape the tube head (Figure 3–3). These x-rays make up the primary beam. The PID fits over the port and can be moved to aim the primary beam of x-rays in the desired direction. Upon completion of the predetermined exposure, the high-voltage current is automatically shut off, and x-ray production stops.

The X-ray Beam

X-rays are produced in 360-degree direction at the focal spot of the target. However, because of the 20-degree angle of the anode, a high concentration of x-rays travel towards the port of the tube head. Only a beam of radiation the size of the port seal is allowed to exit the tube head. The other x-rays are stopped (absorbed) by the contents and walls of the tube head. After the beam exits through the port, the lead **collimator** (explained in Chapter 6) further restricts the x-ray beam to the desired size.

The x-ray beam is **cone-shaped** because x-rays travel in diverging straight lines as they radiate from the focal spot. This beam of x-rays is called the **primary beam** or the useful beam. The primary beam is the original useful beam of x-rays that originates at the focal spot and emerges through the port of the tube head. The **central ray** is the x-ray in the center of the primary beam.

The primary beam consists of x-rays of many different energies. Only x-rays with sufficient energy to penetrate oral structures are useful for diagnostic radiology. X-rays of low penetrating power (long wavelength) add to the patient dose but not to the information on the film. To remove the soft x-rays, a thin sheet of aluminum, called a **filter,** is placed in the path of the x-ray beam. Filtration is explained in detail in Chapter 6.

The **intensity** of the x-ray beam refers to the quantity and quality of the x-rays. **Quantity** refers to the number of x-rays in the beam. **Quality** refers to the energy or penetrating ability of the x-ray beam. **Intensity** is defined as the product of the number of x-rays (quantity) and the energy of the x-rays (quality) per unit of area per unit of time. Intensity of the x-ray beam is affected by milliamperage (mA), kilovoltage (kVp), exposure time, and distance.

Half-value Layer

The **half-value layer (HVL)** of an x-ray beam is the thickness (measured in millimeters) of some material, usually aluminum, that will reduce the intensity of the beam by one half. Measuring the HVL determines the penetrating quality of the x-ray beam. The HVL is more accurate than kilovoltage to describe the x-ray beam quality and penetration. Two similar x-ray machines operating at the same kilovoltage may not produce x-rays of the same quality and penetration. The half-value layer is used by radiological health personnel when determining filtration requirements.

Electricity

Since electricity is necessary to produce x-rays, we need to understand some basic electrical concepts. **Electricity** has been defined as electrons in motion. An electric current is a movement of electrons through a conducting medium (such as copper wire). Amperage is the measurement of the number of electrons moving through a wire conductor. Voltage is the measurement of electrical force that causes electrons to flow through a conductor. Both amperage and voltage can be adjusted by the radiographer.

Amperage

Amperage measures the number of electrons that move through a conductor. The **ampere** (abbreviated **A**) is the unit of quantity of electric current. An increase in amperage results in an increase in the number of electrons that are available to travel from the cathode to anode when the tube is activated. This results in a production of more x-rays. Only a small current is required to operate the x-ray machine; therefore, the term **milliampere** (abbreviated **mA**), denoting 1/1,000 of an ampere, is used. The majority of dental x-ray machines operate in ranges from 7 to 15 mA. On some x-ray units, the milliamperage can be selected by the operator; on others, it is preset by the manufacturer.

Voltage

Voltage is the electrical pressure (sometimes called potential difference) between two electrical charges. In radiography the voltage determines the speed of the electrons when traveling from cathode to anode. This speed of the electrons, in turn, determines the energy (penetrating power) of the x-rays produced. When the voltage is increased, the electrons travel faster and produce the hardest type of radiation.

The **volt** (abbreviated **V**) is the unit of electromotive force used to measure the electric potential. It is defined as the electromotive force sufficient to cause 1 A of current to flow against a resistance of 1 ohm (the ampere is a measure of amount of current, the ohm is a measure of resistance). Because dental x-ray equipment operates at very high voltages, it is customary to express voltage in terms of **kilovolts.** The kilovolt equals 1,000 V and is abbreviated **kV.** The voltage varies during an exposure, producing a polychromatic beam (x-rays of many different energies) containing high-energy rays and also containing soft rays that have barely enough energy to escape from the tube. The highest voltage to which the current in the tube rises during an exposure is called the **kilovolt peak** (abbreviated **kVp**). Thus if the x-ray machine controls are set at 75 kVp (75,000 V), the maximum x-ray energy that can be produced during this exposure is 75 kVp. Dental x-ray machines currently manufactured operate within a range from 60 kVp to 90 kVp.

Electric Current

Electric current can flow in either direction along a wire or conductor. It can flow steadily in one direction (**direct current**) or flow in pulses and change directions (**alternating current**).

Direct Current

Direct current (abbreviated **DC**), flows continuously in one direction. Such a unidirectional current is used in flashlight batteries, for example, but cannot be used in

the dental x-ray machine unless modifications are made to the machine.

Alternating Current

The ordinary household current used in the United States is a 110-V and 60-cycle **alternating current** (abbreviated **AC**), which changes its direction of flow 60 times per second (Figure 3–10). Thus the alternating current has two phases—one positive and the other negative—and alternates between these phases. Most dental x-ray machines operate on 110- or 220-V alternating current.

Although it is customary to describe the cathode as the negative electrode and the anode as the positive electrode, this is not quite the case. During the time that the x-ray tube is producing x-rays, the cathode and the anode each change from negative to positive 60 times per second. Since free electrons are available only at the cathode filament, x-rays can be produced only when the electrons flow across the gap from cathode to anode during the phase when the anode is positive. Theoretically, when the cycle reverses, any available electrons flow back to the cathode. However, x-rays cannot be produced when the anode is in the negative phase because no free electrons are available at the target on the anode to be carried back across the gap to the cathode, and the current is thus blocked from traveling in that direction.

This alternation in current direction occurs every 1/120 sec (twice during each full cycle) on x-ray machines

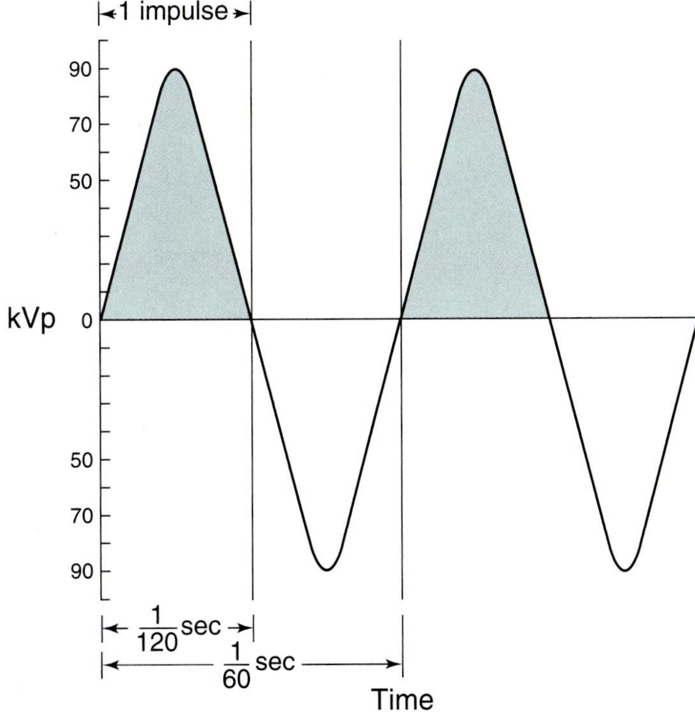

FIGURE 3–10. **Sine wave of 60-cycle alternating current operating at 90,000 V (90 kVp).** Ordinary household electric current is called 60-cycle alternating current because the current changes its direction of flow 60 times a second. During the time that the x-ray tube is producing x-rays, the cathode and the anode each change from negative to positive 60 times per second. The crest of the wave represents the maximum voltage when the current is moving in one direction, while the trough of the wave represents the maximum voltage when the current is moving in the other direction. The total cycle takes place in 1/60 sec. This alternation in current direction occurs every 1/120 sec (twice during each full cycle) on x-ray machines of conventional design. It produces the x-rays in a series of bursts, or **impulses,** rather than in a continuous flow.

of conventional design. It produces the x-rays in a series of bursts or **impulses** rather than in a continuous flow.

The term **rectification** is used to describe the process in which the current is unidirectional. Because no special rectifying tubes or devices are used, x-ray equipment that operates only to produce x-rays during half of each cycle is known as **self-rectifying.**

Electrical Circuits

An **electrical circuit** is a path of electrical current. There are two electrical circuits used in producing dental x-rays (Figure 3–11).

1. A **filament circuit** provides low voltage (3–8 V) to the filament of the x-ray tube.
2. A **high-voltage circuit** that provides the high voltage (60–90 kilovolts) necessary to accelerate the electrons from the cathode filament to the anode target.

Transformers

A **transformer** is an electromagnetic device for changing the alternating current and consists of two coils of electric wire wound on an iron core (Figure 3–12). Transformers are required to decrease (step down) or increase (step up) the ordinary 110-V current that enters the x-ray machine. The primary coil (input) is connected to the alternating current supply, and the secondary coil (output) is connected to the tube circuit. The wires in these coils are insulated from one another.

When the current is flowing, a magnetic field around the primary coil induces an electric current in the secondary coil. The secondary voltage created can be accurately predicted. The number of wire turns in each coil determines whether the voltage is decreased or increased. For example, if there are ten times more turns on the primary than on the secondary coil, the voltage is decreased tenfold; if the ratio is reversed, the voltage increases tenfold.

Step-down Transformer

A **step-down** (low-voltage) **transformer** (Figure 3–12) decreases the voltage to approximately 5 V, just enough to heat the filament and form the electron cloud.

Step-up Transformer

A **step-up** (high-voltage) **transformer** (Figure 3–12) increases the voltage as required by the technique the radiographer is using. The high-voltage current, 60–90 kVp,

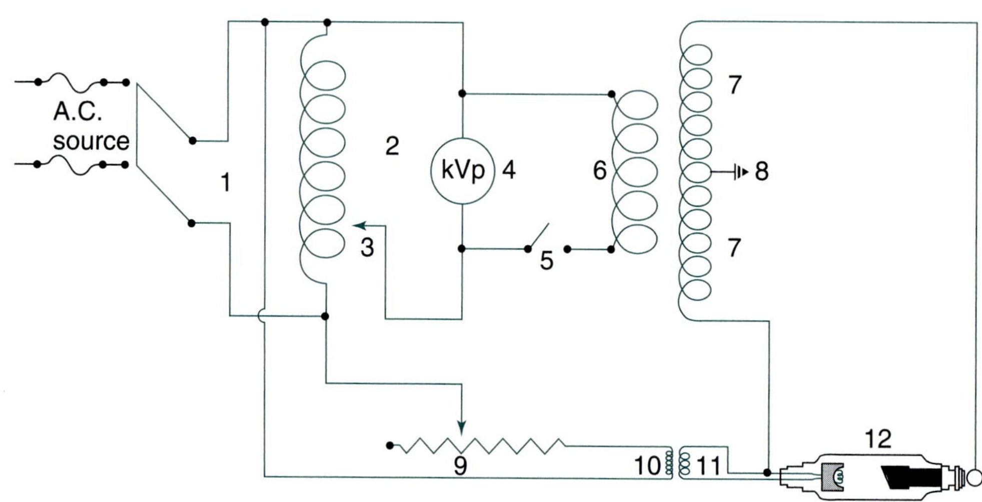

FIGURE 3–11. **Simplified diagram of the basic electrical circuits and parts of a dental x-ray machine.**

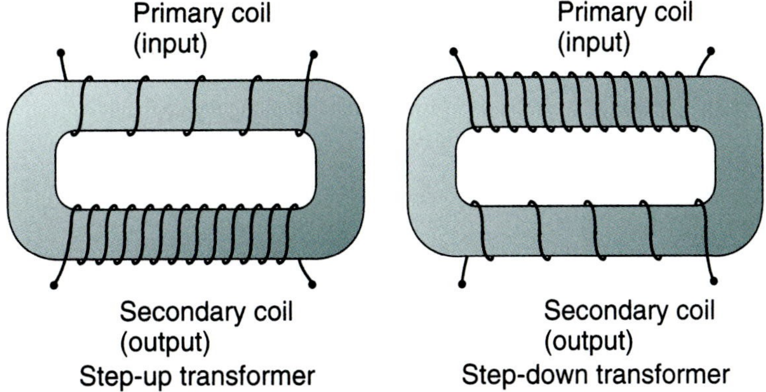

FIGURE 3–12. **Step-up and step-down transformers** are located in the tube head.

current begins to flow through the cathode-anode circuit when the activator button on the line switch is depressed. X-rays are produced during the half of the cycle when the cathode is negative and the anode is positive.

The step-up and step-down transformers are located in the tube head (Figure 3–3).

Autotransformer

An **autotransformer** (Figure 3–13) is a voltage compensator that corrects minor fluctuations in the current flowing through the wires. The output of the autotransformer is regulated by the kVp selector dial on the control panel. The kVp dial selects the desired voltage and applies it across the primary of the high voltage transformer.

Like the other transformers, the autotransformer has an iron core but is wound with only a single coil that does the work of two. The action of the autotransformer is based on self-induction in a single coil rather than on mutual induction produced between two coils with different numbers of turns.

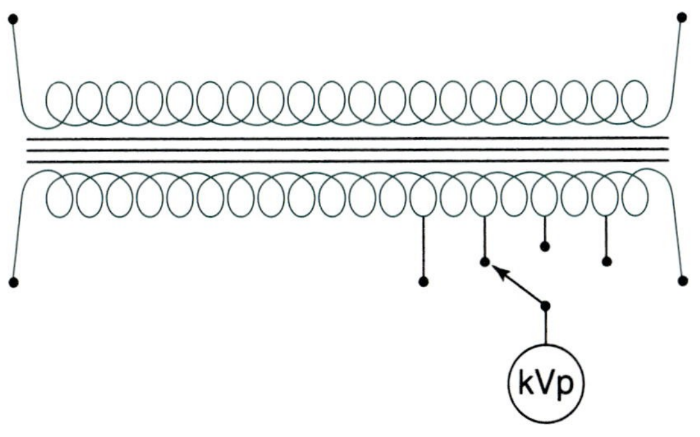

FIGURE 3–13. **Autotransformer** is located in the control panel.

The autotransformer is located in the control panel. By turning a knob on the control panel the operator causes a selector switch to slide over a series of tabs that regulate the voltage by either decreasing or increasing it. This action is comparable to fine tuning on a radio.

Many transformers used in conventional x-ray machines are heavy and bulky. The trend is toward using lighter weight and miniaturized solid-state components. This has the added advantage of reducing the size and the weight of the tube head, thus making it easier for the operator to position it.

Operation of the Dental X-ray Machine

A summation of the fundamentals of x-ray generation is in order before considering the procedures for operating the x-ray machine.

In review, the line switch of the x-ray machine is turned on and the exposure button at the end of the timer cord is held down until the exposure is completed. The line current enters the filament circuit of the x-ray machine. A step-down transformer reduces the voltage before it enters the filament circuit and heats the filament of the cathode to incandescence, separating electrons from their atoms.

The degree to which the filament is heated depends on the milliamperage that is selected, the higher the mA, the more electrons in the electron cloud. These electrons are now in a state of excitation as they hover around the filament wire. After a time delay of less than 1/2 sec, the line current enters the cathode-anode high-voltage circuit. A step-up transformer then increases the voltage to impart sufficient force to propel the free electrons to the focal spot on the anode where the energy conversion takes place, resulting in the production of x-rays.

The x-ray beam formed at the focal spot is polychromatic, consisting of x-rays of various wavelengths. The higher the voltage, the greater the penetration power of the x-rays that are formed.

Procedures for Operating the X-ray Machine

Whenever x-ray exposures are made on patients, it is assumed here and in all subsequent instructions that:

- The patient is properly positioned.
- The patient has received verbal instructions.
- The patient has been draped with a protective lead apron.
- All equipment is sanitized.
- The operator's hands have been washed and gloved.
- Infection control procedures are followed (see Chapter 22).

To achieve consistent results, the x-ray machine operator should always follow an orderly procedure:

1. Turn on the line switch or depress the ON button. A red light will indicate that the machine is ready to operate.
2. Unless the machine is preset by the manufacturer, select the milliamperage and kilovoltage best suited for the exposure to be made. If the machine has a dial (or dials), a needle will point to the mA and kVp that are available.
3. Set the timer for the desired exposure time.
4. Place the x-ray film packet in the patient's mouth. The film is usually held in place by a film-holding device.
5. Adjust the position indicating device (PID) so that the central beam of radiation is directed toward the center of the film at the proper horizontal and vertical angulations.
6. Pick up the timer cord and move to an area of safety at least 6 ft (1.83 m) away or behind the cover of structural shielding such as a lead-lined wall or partition. While watching the patient to see that they do not move, press the timer button and hold it down firmly until the exposure is completed. On new x-ray machines, an audible signal is heard and a light is visible for the duration of the exposure.
7. Watch the needle on the milliammeter while the exposure is being made. If it fails to move or go to the proper position, it indicates a malfunction caused either by a temporarily overloaded circuit or by failure to keep a firm pressure on the timer button.
8. On most machines, the timer resets itself automatically and is ready for the next exposure unless a changed setting is desired. Although unlikely, it is possible to damage the x-ray tube through excessive repetition of prolonged exposures at short intervals, thus overheating the tube. To avoid abusing the equipment, consult the manufacturer's instructions regarding the tube ratings and **duty cycle**—the length of time that the tube may be energized in a given period.
9. Remove the film from the patient's mouth after each exposure. After the final exposure, turn off the line switch and fold the extension arm bracket up as far as it will go. The tube head is finely counterbalanced in its suspension from the extension arm. This balance can be disturbed if the tube is left suspended for prolonged time periods with the extension arm stretched out.
10. Turn off the x-ray machine at the end of each working day.

CHAPTER SUMMARY

All x-ray machines, regardless of size and voltage range, operate similarly and have the same components (control panel, extension arm, and tube head) and electrical parts (x-ray tube, low- and high-voltage circuits, and a timing device).

The control panel may be a part of the x-ray machine or it may be remote from the unit, mounted on a shelf or wall. There are four major controls that must be operated on most variable-type dental x-ray machines, the line switch to the electrical outlet, the milliampere selector, the kilovoltage selector, and the timer.

A folding extension arm is a support from which the tube housing is suspended The tube head is a tightly sealed heavy metal housing that contains the dental x-ray tube, insulating oil, and step-up and step-down transformers.

Three conditions must exist to produce x-rays: (1) a source of free electrons; (2) high voltage to accelerate them; and (3) a target to stop them. The dental x-ray tube creates these conditions.

X-rays are produced only when the unit is turned on and a firm pressure is maintained on the activator button.

Electric current is a movement of electrons through a conducting medium. This flow may be in either direction along a wire but is always from negative to positive. The standard 110- or 220-V alternating current is modified by step-up and step-down transformers within the tube housing. The current reverses direction from negative to positive 60 times per second as the voltage flows across the tube from cathode to anode. With most machines, x-rays are formed only during that phase of the cycle when the cathode is negatively charged; however, with some machines the potential is constant.

Most dental x-ray units operate in ranges of 7 to 15 mA and between 60 and 90 kVp. The milliamperage determines the quantity of x-rays that can be produced in a predetermined time interval, and the kilovoltage determines the quantity and quality (penetrating power) of the rays. The operator can vary the mA and kVp settings on many machines, but some are preset by the manufacturer and only the time interval can be changed.

For maximum effectiveness in exposing radiographs, the patient is first positioned and draped with a protective lead apron, and all controls on the x-ray unit are set as desired before the film is positioned. Following an orderly sequence in positioning the film packets reduces the likelihood of errors and retakes.

REVIEW QUESTIONS

1. Draw and label a typical dental x-ray tube.

2. The tube head contains the:

   (a) Rectifier tube, x-ray tube, and oil.
   (b) Voltmeter, ampmeter, and insulation.
   (c) Transformers, x-ray tube, and oil.
   (d) Diode, timer, and x-ray tube.

3. The hot cathode tube was invented by:

   (a) Roentgen.
   (b) Rollins.
   (c) Coolidge.
   (d) Ciesynski.

4. List the three conditions that must exist for x-rays to be produced.

   (1) source of free electrons
   (2) high voltage to accelerate them
   (3) a target to stop them

5. Which of these must be charged negatively during the time that the x-ray tube is operating in order to produce x-rays?
   (a) The anode
   (b) The radiator
   (c) The cathode
   (d) The aperture

6. Which part of the x-ray tube is heated when the electric current is allowed to flow through the low-voltage circuit?
   (a) The focal spot
   (b) The tube housing
   (c) The anode target
   (d) The cathode filament

7. The process of heating the cathode wire filament until red hot and electrons boil off is called thermionic emission.

8. What metal is used for the filament in the x-ray tube?
   (a) Lead
   (b) Copper
   (c) Molybdenum
   (d) Tungsten

9. What percent of the kinetic energy inside the x-ray tube is converted into x-rays?
   (a) 1%
   (b) 50%
   (c) 75%
   (d) 99%

10. What metal is used for the target in the x-ray tube?
    (a) Copper
    (b) Tungsten
    (c) Aluminum
    (d) Molybdenum

11. The shape of the "effective" focal spot is square.

12. Which term describes the opening in the tube housing that allows the primary beam to escape?
    (a) Focal spot
    (b) Port
    (c) Filament
    (d) Focusing cup

13. Which term describes the electrical pressure (difference in potential) between two electrical charges?
    (a) Voltage
    (b) Amperage
    (c) Ionization
    (d) Rectification

14. Why are x-rays not formed during the alternating phase when the anode is negative?
    (a) Because there are no free electrons at the anode
    (b) Because the tube is evacuated
    (c) Because the voltage is too low
    (d) Because the radiator absorbs the electrons

15. What should be done to increase the quantity of free electrons inside the tube so more x-rays can be generated?
    (a) Decrease the kilovoltage
    (b) Increase the milliamperage
    (c) Increase the kilovoltage
    (d) Decrease the milliamperage

16. Which term best describes an x-ray beam that is composed of a variety of wavelengths?
    (a) Collimated
    (b) Short-scale
    (c) Filtered
    (d) Polychromatic

17. Which of these terms describes an electromagnetic device within the x-ray tube head for changing the voltage of alternating current?
    (a) Rectifier
    (b) Transformer
    (c) Voltage regulator
    (d) Alternator

18. If the x-ray machine timer is calibrated in impulses instead of fractions of a second, how many impulses are equivalent to 2/5 sec?
    (a) 6
    (b) 15
    (c) 24
    (d) 40

19. Fill in the blanks.
    (a) 30 impulses equals ________ second.
    (b) 42 impulses equals ________ second.
    (c) 1/4 second equals ________ impulses.
    (d) 3/10 second equals ________ impulses.

20. Which of the following is used to decrease the voltage in the filament circuit?
    (a) Voltage regulator
    (b) Autotransformer
    (c) Step-up transformer
    (d) Step-down transformer

BIBLIOGRAPHY

Bushberg, J. T., Seibert, J. A., Leidholdt, E. M. Jr., & Boone, J.M. *The Essential Physics of Medical Imaging*. Baltimore, MD: Williams & Wilkins, 1994.

Eastman Kodak. *Successful Intraoral Radiography*. Rochester, NY: Eastman Kodak, 1998.

White S. C. & Pharoah, M. J. *Oral Radiology Principles and Interpretation*, 4th ed. St. Louis: Mosby, 2000.

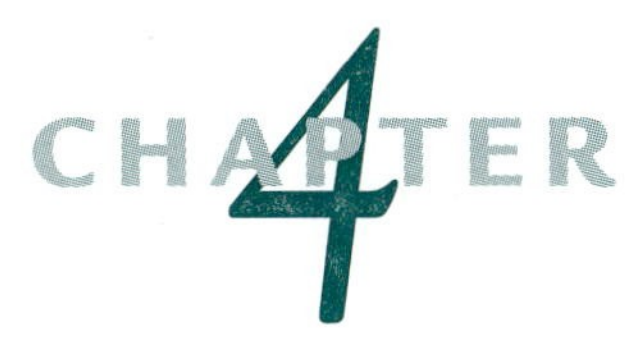

Producing Quality Radiographs

OBJECTIVES

By the end of this chapter the student should be able to:

- Define the key words.
- Identify the basic requirements of an acceptable diagnostic radiograph.
- Differentiate between radiolucent and radiopaque areas on a dental radiograph and give an example of each.
- Describe radiographic density and contrast.
- Summarize the factors affecting the radiographic image.
- Differentiate between subject contrast and film contrast.
- List the geometric factors that affect image sharpness.
- List the rules for casting a shadow image.
- List the factors that influence magnification and distortion.
- Describe how mA, kVp, and exposure time affect film density.
- Discuss how kVp affects contrast.
- Differentiate between short-scale contrast and long-scale contrast.
- Explain target-surface, object-film, and target-film distances.
- Explain the Inverse Square Law and give two examples where it is used.

KEY WORDS

Central ray (CR)
Contrast
Control factors
Definition
Density
Distortion
Exposure chart
Exposure time
Extraoral radiography
Film contrast
Focal spot
Grid
Intensifying screen
Intensity
Intraoral radiography
Inverse square law
Intensifying screen
Kilovoltage peak (kVp)
Long-scale contrast
Magnification
Milliampere (mA)
Milliampere/second (mAs)
Movement
Object-film distance
Penumbra
Position indicating device (PID)
Radiographic contrast
Radiolucent
Radiopaque
Sharpness
Short-scale contrast
Subject contrast
Target-film distance
Target-object distance
Target-surface distance

Introduction

There are three basic requirements for an acceptable diagnostic radiograph (Figure 4–1).

1. All parts of the structures radiographed must be shown on the film as close to their natural shapes and sizes as the patient's oral anatomy will permit. Distortion and superimposition of structures should be at a minimum.
2. The area examined must be shown completely, with enough surrounding tissue for the dentist to distinguish between the structures shown.
3. The film itself must be high in quality with proper density, contrast, and definition.

The quality of a radiograph depends upon both the physical factors and the subjective opinion of the individual who reads it. The purpose of this chapter is to describe the physical factors involved in producing quality radiographs. This includes the factors that affect the radiographic image, the rules for casting a shadow image, and the effect of varying the **control factors.**

Terminology

The following terms need to be explained when discussing quality radiographs: **radiolucent, radiopaque, density, contrast,** and **sharpness.**

When a dental radiograph is viewed on a light source images appear that are black, white, and various shades of gray in between. The terms used to describe the black and white areas are **radiolucent** and **radiopaque.**

Radiolucent

Radiolucent refers to the portion of a processed radiograph that is dark or black (see Figure 4–1). Structures that appear radiolucent permit the passage of x-rays with little or no resistance. Soft tissues and air spaces are examples that appear radiolucent on a radiograph.

Radiopaque

Radiopaque refers to that portion of a radiograph that appears light or white (see Figure 4–1). Structures that appear radiopaque are dense and absorb or resist the passage of x-rays. Enamel, dentin, and bone are examples of radiopaque structures.

Radiolucent and radiopaque are relative terms. For instance, even though both enamel and dentin are radiopaque, dentin is more radiolucent (appears darker) than enamel.

Three visual image characteristics that directly influence the quality of the radiograph are **density, contrast,** and **sharpness.**

Density

Density, also known as film blackening, is the amount of light transmitted through the film (see Figure 4–2). If a great deal of light is transmitted through the film, the radiograph is said to have little density. If the radiograph is very dense (black), little light will be transmitted through the film. The blackness in a dental radiograph is caused when x-rays strike sensitive crystals in the film emulsion and subsequent processing causes the crystals to

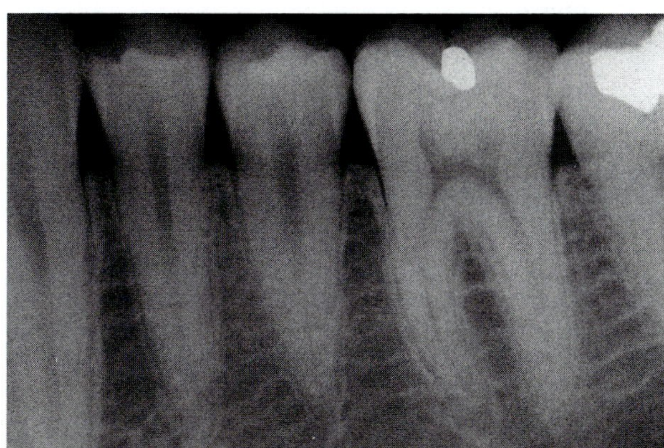

FIGURE 4–1. **An acceptable diagnostic radiograph.**

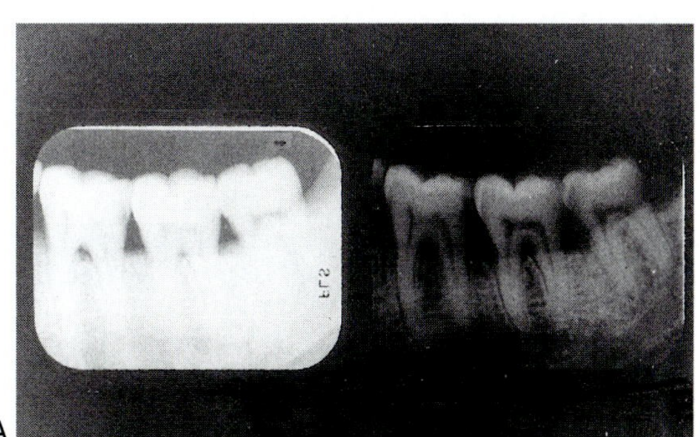

FIGURE 4–2. **Radiographic density.** Radiograph (**A**) is underexposed and appears too light (white). Radiograph (**B**) is overexposed and appears too **dense** (**dark**).

turn black. Thus the degree of darkening of the radiograph is increased when the milliamperage or the exposure time is increased and more x-rays are produced to reach the film emulsion.

Radiographs need just the right amount of density to be viewed properly. If the density is too light or too dark, the images of the teeth and supporting tissues cannot be visually separated from each other. The ideal radiograph has the proper amount of density for the interpreter to view black areas (radiolucent), white areas (radiopaque), and the gray areas.

Contrast

Contrast refers to how sharply dark and light areas are differentiated (see Figure 4–3). A film with good contrast will contain black, white, and many shades of gray. A radiograph that shows just a few shades is said to have short-scale contrast, while one that shows many variations in shade is said to possess long-scale contrast.

The term **short-scale contrast** (see Figure 4–4) describes a radiograph in which the density differences between adjacent areas are large. The contrast is high because there are fewer shades of gray and more black against white. The gray tones indicate the differences in absorption of the x-ray photons by the various tissues of the oral cavity or the head. The radiograph is **radiolucent** (dark) where the tissues are soft or thin and **radiopaque** (white) where the tissues are hard or thick. Such radiographs result when low (60–70) kVp is applied. Some dentists prefer radiographs, with short-scale contrast, thinking that dental caries are easier to recognize; however, fine detail may be difficult to distinguish.

The term **long-scale contrast** (Figure 4–4) describes a radiograph in which the density differences between adjacent areas are small. The contrast is low and very gradual because there are many shades of gray. Such radiographs result when high (80–90) kVp is applied. More detailed information can be obtained from such radiographs, provided that a view box with variable light control is used. The proper kVp to use is strictly a matter of individual preference.

In the past it was thought that high-kVp techniques resulted in a lower dose to the patient. That is not necessarily so. High-kVp techniques do result in lower *expo-*

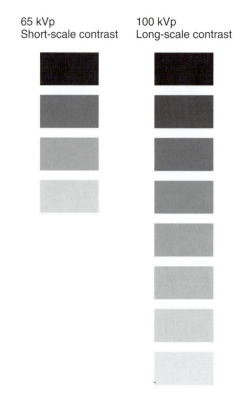

FIGURE 4–3. **Penetrometer** tests demonstrate radiographically that a much **longer contrast scale** results from the use of 100 kilovolt techniques. Dental radiographs made using 100 kVp have **long-scale contrast.** Radiographs made using 65 kVp have **short-scale contrast.** (Courtesy of General Electric Company, Medical Systems Division)

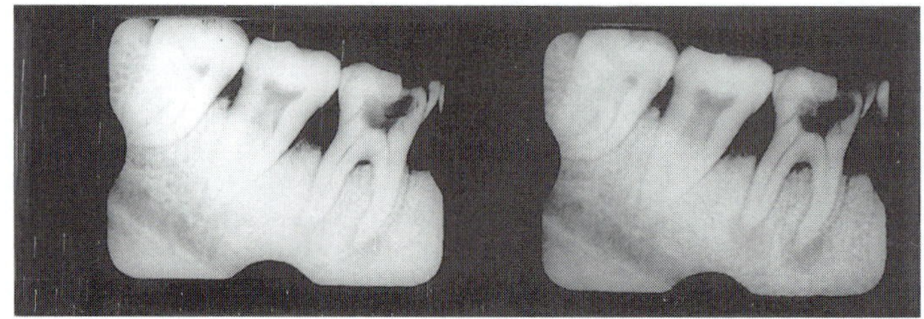

FIGURE 4–4. **Radiographic contrast.** Radiograph (**A**) made using 60 kVp, has high contrast. Radiograph (**B**) made using 90 kVp, has low contrast.

sures to the patient, but not lower *doses* (see Chapter 2 to understand the difference between exposure and dose). Compared to high-kVp techniques, low-kVp techniques result in a higher entrance dose but a lower exit dose to the patient's head. This is because the x-rays are less penetrating. High-kVp techniques result in a lower entrance dose but a higher exit dose because the x-rays are more penetrating. The total dose to the patient is essentially the same with either kVp technique, only the dose is distributed through the patient's head differently. From the radiological health aspect, it doesn't matter which technique the dentist uses.

Sharpness

Sharpness (definition) is a geometric factor that refers to the detail and clarity of the outline of the structures shown on the radiograph. Unsharpness is generally caused by movement of the patient, film, or the tube head during exposure.

Factors Affecting the Radiographic Image

The dental radiographer must have a working knowledge of the factors that effect the radiographic image. The detail and visibility of a radiograph depends upon two independent factors—**radiographic contrast** and **sharpness** (definition) (see Table 4–1).

Radiographic Contrast

Radiographic contrast can be defined as the visible difference between densities on a radiograph. It depends upon two separate factors:

1. **Subject contrast** is the result of differences in absorption of the x-ray by the tissues under examination.
2. **Film contrast** is a characteristic of the film and processing.

Subject Contrast

The three factors that affect the subject contrast are: the **subject** (patient), **kilovoltage,** and **scatter radiation.**

1. **Subject (patient).**
   Subject contrast is the result of differences in absorption of the x-rays by the tissues under examination. The subject to be radiographed must have contrast. A radiograph of a 1-in. sheet of plastic would show no contrast since the plastic is of uniform thickness and composition (Z number). Patients have contrast because human tissues vary in size, thickness, and density.
2. **Kilovoltage (kVp).**
   There is an inverse relationship between **kVp** and **contrast** (see Figure 4–4). In relative terms, higher kilovoltages produce lower subject contrast. The blacks are grayer, the whites are grayer, and there are more steps (or shades) of gray in between. Lower kilovoltages produce higher subject contrast. The blacks are blacker, the whites are whiter, and there are fewer steps (or shades) of gray in between.
3. **Scatter radiation.**
   Remember Chapter 2, where we learned that Compton scattering occurs whenever x-rays interact with matter such as the tissues of the patient's head. These scattered x-rays add a uniform exposure to the radiograph, thereby decreasing the contrast. For **intraoral radiography** (inside the mouth), a collimator (lead washer) is used to keep the beam size as small as possible to help reduce scatter radiation. For **extraoral radiography** (outside the mouth), grids are used to

TABLE 4–1. **Summary of Factors That Affect the Radiographic Image**

Detail—Visibility			
Radiographic Contrast		Sharpness (Definition)	
Subject Contrast	Film Contrast	Geometric Factors	Crystal Size
Subject	Film type	Focal spot size	Crystal size
kVp	Exposure	Target–film distance	
Scattered radiation	Processing	Object–film distance	
		Motion	
		Screen thickness	
		Screen–film contact	

absorb scattered x-rays. A **grid** is a mechanical device composed of thin strips of lead alternating with a radiolucent material (plastic). The grid is placed between the patient and the film in order to absorb scattered x-rays.

Film Contrast

Film contrast is the inherent contrast built into the film by the manufacturer. Film contrast is affected by **film type, exposure,** and **processing.**

1. **Film type.**
   Each film has its own built-in contrast. Film contrast is determined by the film manufacturer.
2. **Exposure.**
   An underexposed or an overexposed film will result in poor contrast and reduce viewing quality of the radiograph. The radiographer must always use the proper exposure factors to produce quality radiographs.
3. **Processing.**
   Processing is extremely important (see Chapter 8). In order that maximum film contrast be obtained, it is essential that proper processing be utilized. Film processing is under the control of the radiographer. If improper development time or temperature is used, the radiograph will not have the contrast the manufacturer built into it.

Sharpness (Definition)

Sharpness (also known as **definition**) refers to the clarity of the outline of the structures on the image of a radiograph. Sharpness is the result of two separate factors—**geometric factors** and **crystal size** (see Table 4–2).

Geometric Factors

The geometric factors that contribute to the radiographic image are: focal spot size, target-film distance, object-film distance, movement, screen thickness, and screen-film contact.

1. **Focal spot size.**
   As explained in Chapter 3, the **focal spot** is the small area on the target that converts bombarding electrons into x-rays. The smaller the focal spot area, the sharper the image appears (see Figure 4–5). Large focal spots create more **penumbra** (partial shadow) and therefore loss of image sharpness (see Figure 4–6). Ideally, the focal spot should be a point source, and then no penumbra would be present. However, a single point source would create extreme heat and burn out the tube.
2. **Target-film distance.**
   The **target-film distance** (source-film) is the distance between the source of x-ray production (the focal spot) and the film. PIDs are used to establish the target-film distance. The longer the target-film distance,

TABLE 4–2. **Factors Influencing Sharpness**

Factors	Modify	Sharpness
Focal spot size	Small focal spot Large focal spot	Increase sharpness Decrease sharpness
Target-film distance	Long target-film distance Short target-film distance	Increase sharpness Decrease sharpness
Object-film distance	Short object-film distance Long object-film distance	Increase sharpness Decrease sharpness
Movement	No movement Movement	Sharp image Fuzzy image
Screen thickness	Thin screen Thick screen	Increase sharpness Decrease sharpness
Screen-film contact	Close contact Poor contact	Increase sharpness Decrease sharpness
Film crystal size	Small crystals Large crystals	Increase sharpness Decrease sharpness

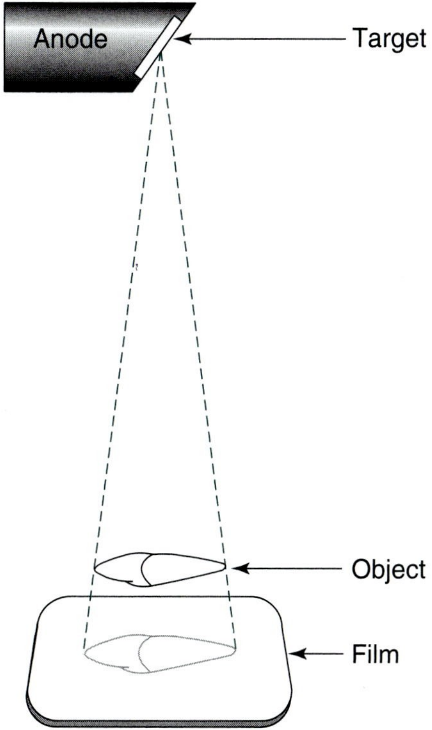

FIGURE 4–5. Using a **small focal spot** on the target, a **long target–film distance,** and a **short object–film distance** will result in a sharp image.

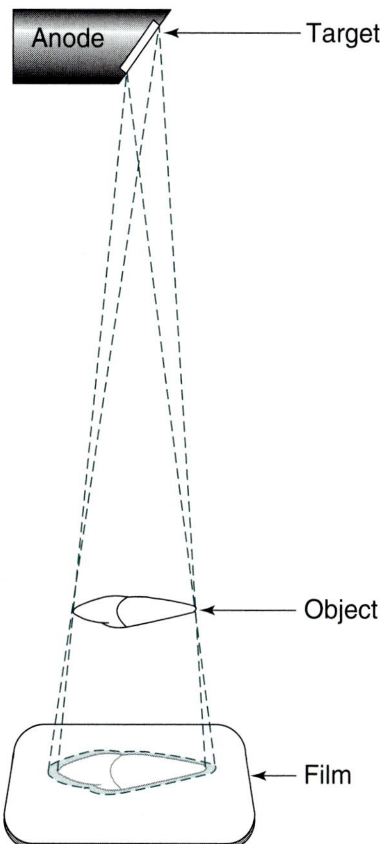

FIGURE 4–6. **Large focal spot** on the target results in more penumbra (partial shadow) and therefore loss of image sharpness.

the less divergent the x-ray beam. A long target-film distance has x-rays in the center of the beam that are nearly parallel. Therefore, the image on the radiograph will be sharper (see Figure 4–5). Also a longer target-film distance will result in less image magnification (explained later in this chapter).

3. **Object-film distance.**
   The **object-film distance** is the distance between the object being radiographed (tooth) and the dental x-ray film. The film should always be placed as close to the teeth as possible. The closer the proximity of the film to the teeth, the sharper the image and the less magnification (image enlargement). The image will become fuzzy (more penumbra) and magnified, as the object-film distance is increased (see Figure 4–7).
4. **Movement.**
   Movement may involve the patient, the film, or the tube head (source of radiation). If any, or combination, of the three occurs, there will be a loss of image sharpness (see Figure 4–8).

Helpful Hint

- Always make sure the tube head (PID) stops vibrating and the patient does not move when exposing the film.

5. **Screen thickness.**
   Intensifying screens (often referred to as simply screens), used in extraoral radiography, are made of crystals that emit light when struck by x-rays. The light, in turn, exposes the screen film. Intensifying screens require less radiation to expose a film, therefore exposing the patient to less radiation. However, screens decrease the sharpness of the radiographic image (see Figure 4–9). The thicker the screen, the less radiation required to expose the film, and the less sharp the image. The loss in sharpness is compen-

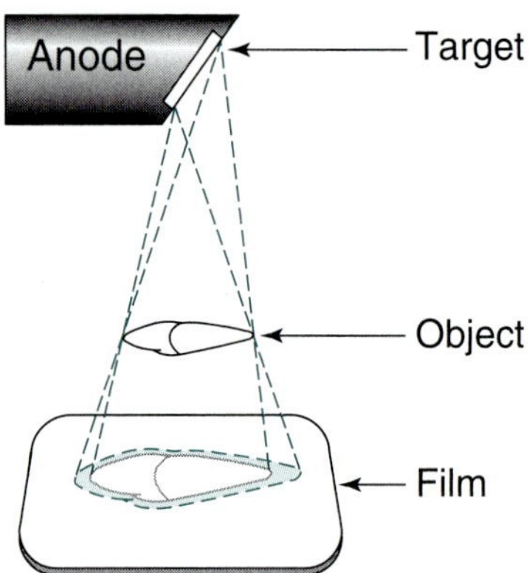

FIGURE 4–7. **Large focal spot** on the target **and large object–film distance** results in more penumbra (partial shadow) and therefore loss of image sharpness.

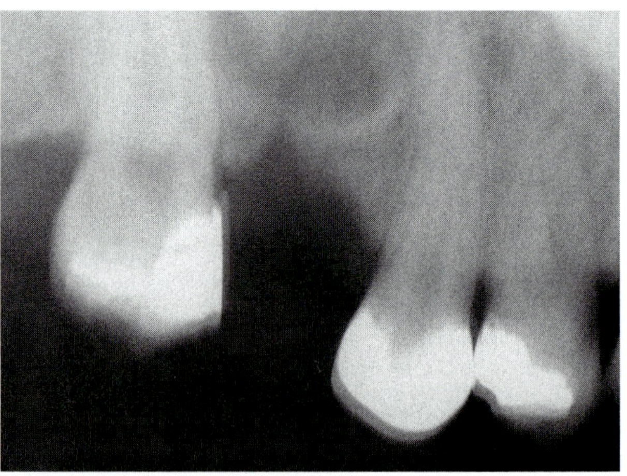

FIGURE 4–8. **Blurry, unsharp image caused by movement** of the patient, the film, or the tube head.

sated for by the reduction in patient exposure. Generally, the radiographer should use the highest speed screen and film combination that is consistent with good diagnostic results. Intensifying screens are explained in detail in Chapter 8.

6. **Screen-film contact.**
   The film should be in close physical contact with the intensifying screen. Poor screen-film contact results in the wider spread of light and fuzziness (more penumbra) of the image. Intensifying screens should be examined periodically for proper screen-film contact.

Crystal Size

Sharpness is influenced by the size of the **crystal** in the emulsion of the film. The smaller the size of the crystal, the sharper the radiographic image.

X-ray film emulsion contains crystals that are struck by x-rays when exposed. Sharpness of the radiographic image is relative to the size of the crystals. High-speed film requiring less radiation for exposure uses larger crystals that produce less image sharpness. Again, the loss of sharpness is compensated for by the reduction in patient exposure. Image definition (sharpness of details) is more distinct when crystals are small. Blurriness occurs because larger crystals do not produce object outlines as

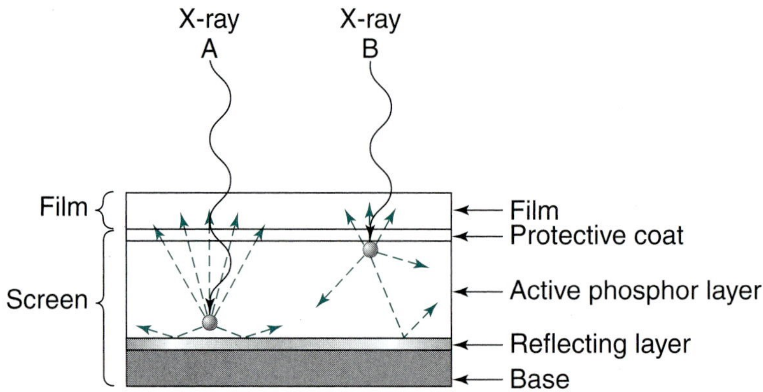

FIGURE 4–9. **Screen thickness. X-ray A** strikes a crystal far from the film and the divergent light exposes a wide area of the film resulting in unsharpness. **X-ray B** strikes a crystal close to the film resulting in less divergence of the light that exposes the film and therefore a sharper image. The thicker the screen, the less sharp the image.

well as small crystals. Dental x-ray film is explained in detail in Chapter 7.

Rules for Casting a Shadow Image

Now that you have learned the factors affecting the clarity of the image, the factors to reproduce the size and shape of the objects accurately will be discussed.

A radiograph is a two-dimensional image of three-dimensional objects. Therefore, it is necessary to apply the rules for creating a shadow image to produce a quality radiograph.

Rules for casting a shadow image

1. Small focal spot
2. Long target-object distance
3. Short object-film distance
4. Object and film must be parallel
5. Central ray of x-ray beam must be perpendicular to the object and film

- **Small focal spot** to reduce the size of the penumbra resulting in a sharper image and slightly less magnification.
- **Long target-object distance** to reduce the penumbra and magnification.
- **Short object-film distance** to reduce penumbra and magnification.
- **Object and film** must be parallel to each other to prevent distortion.
- **Central ray of x-ray beam** must be perpendicular to the object and the film to prevent distortion.

Two geometric factors—**magnification** and **distortion**—influence the quality of a dental radiograph. Both must be minimized to produce an accurate radiographic image.

Magnification (Enlargement)

Magnification is the increase in size of the image on the radiograph compared to the actual size of the object.

In Chapter 3, we learned that x-rays travel in diverging straight lines as they radiate from the focal spot of the target. Because of these diverging x-rays, there is some magnification present in every radiograph (see Figure 4–10).

Magnification is mostly influenced by the **target-object distance** and the **object-film distance.** The target-object distance is determined by the length of the **position indicating device (PID).** When a long PID is used, the x-rays in the center of the beam are more parallel, resulting in less image magnification. The object-film distance should be kept to a minimum. Always place the

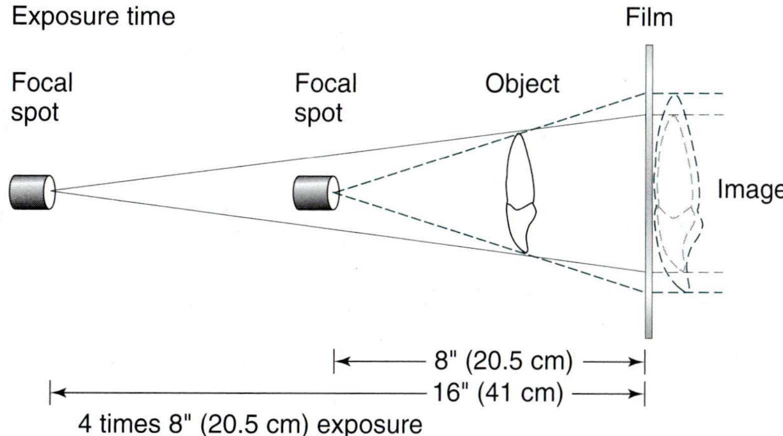

FIGURE 4–10. **Magnification.** Comparison of 8-in. (20-cm) and 16-in. (41-cm) target–film (T/F) distance. The image is magnified (enlarged) when the T/F distance is shortened and the object (tooth)-to-film distance is held constant. Ideally, the distance from the target to the object should be as long as possible and the object (tooth)-to-film distance should be as short as possible. When using the 16-in. (41-cm) T/F distance, the exposure time must be lengthened to four times that required at 8-in. (20-cm) T/F distance. (Courtesy of Dentsply/Rinn Corporation)

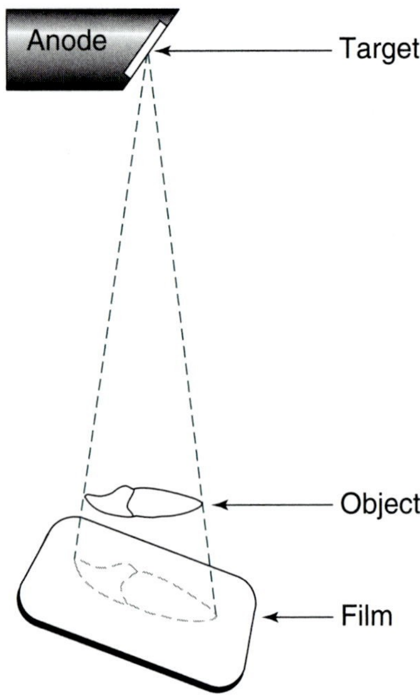

FIGURE 4–11. **Object and film are not parallel, resulting in distortion.**

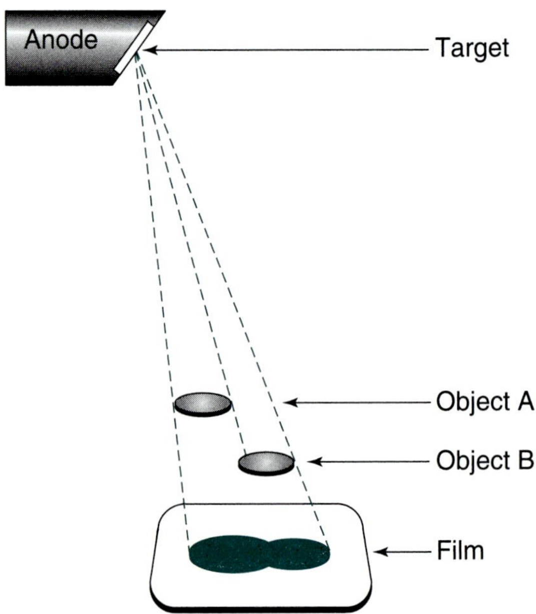

FIGURE 4–12. **Central ray of x-ray beam is not perpendicular to the objects and film resulting in distortion and overlapping** of object A and object B. Note object A is magnified larger than object B because object A is a greater distance from the film than object B.

film as close to the tooth as possible to decrease magnification.

Increasing the target-object distance and decreasing the object-film distance will minimize image magnification. Note that these two methods for reducing magnification also increase image sharpness.

Distortion

Distortion is the result of unequal magnification of different parts of the same object. Distortion (of the image) refers to the true size and shape of the object being radiographed. Distortion results when the film is not parallel to the object (see Figure 4–11) and when the central ray of the x-ray beam is not perpendicular to the object and film (see Figure 4–12).

To minimize image distortion, always position the film parallel to the tooth and align the central ray of the x-ray beam perpendicular to the tooth and film.

Effects of Varying the Control Factors

Two visual characteristics of the radiographic image, **density** and **contrast,** have a tremendous influence on the diagnostic quality of the radiograph. We need to understand how the control factors affect the density and contrast.

The three **control factors** on the x-ray machine, the **milliamperage,** the **exposure time,** and the **kilovoltage,** are known either as the control factors, the exposure factors, or the radiation beam factors.

Whenever one of the control factors is altered, one or a combination of the other factors must be proportionally altered to maintain radiographic density (see Table 4–3). For example, exposure time may be decreased when milliamperage or kilovoltage is increased.

Distance, an additional variable factor, is explained later in this chapter.

Variations in Milliamperage (mA)

The amount of electric current used in the x-ray machine is expressed in **milliamperes (mA).** The mA selected by the operator determines the quantity or number of x-rays that are generated within the tube. The density of the radiograph is affected whenever the operator changes the milliamperage. Increasing the mA increases (darkens) the density of the radiograph, whereas decreasing the mA decreases (lightens) the density of the radiograph.

TABLE 4–3. **Effect of Varying Controls on Film Density**

Control Adjustment[a]	Film Density
Increase mA	Darker
Decrease mA	Lighter
Increase time	Darker
Decrease time	Lighter
Increase kVp	Darker[b]
Decrease kVp	Lighter[b]

[a]When any control factor is increased, or decreased, one or more of the other control factors must be adjusted to maintain optimum film density.
[b]Varying kVp, varies both film density and film contrast. Increase kVp for less contrast; decrease kVp for more contrast.

Variations in Exposure Time

Exposure time is the interval that the x-ray machine is fully activated and x-rays are produced. The principal effect of changes in exposure time is on the density of the radiograph. Increasing the exposure time darkens the radiograph, while decreasing exposure time lightens it. Opinions differ on optimum density and contrast because visual perception varies from person to person. Some dentists may prefer lighter radiographs and others may prefer darker radiographs. Thus the operator should consult with the dentist concerning density preference. Of the three controls, exposure time is easiest to change. In fact, some x-ray machines have fixed milliamperage and kilovoltage, so time is the only control factor that can be changed.

Milliampere-seconds (mAs)

Since both milliamperage and exposure time are used to regulate the number of x-rays generated and have the same effect on radiographic density, it is common practice to combine them into a common factor **milliampere-seconds (mAs).** Combining the milliamperage with the exposure time is an effective way to determine the total radiation generated.

A simple formula for determining this total is: **mA** multiplied by the **exposure time** (in seconds or impulses) equals **mAs.**

$$\text{mA} \times \text{s} = \text{mAs}$$

PROBLEM. Let us consider a practical problem using this formula. The exposure factors in a dental office are: 10 mA, 0.6 sec, 90 kVp, and 16-in. (41-cm) target-film distance. The dentist decides to increase the mA to 15 and leave the kVp and target-film distance constant. What is the new exposure time?

SOLUTION. The only exposure factor changed is the mA. The dentist is going to increase the mA from 10 mA to 15 mA. We need to compensate for the increase in mA by decreasing the exposure time.

$$\text{mA} \times \text{s} = \text{mAs}$$
$$10 \text{ mA} \times 0.6 \text{ sec.} = 6 \text{ mAs}$$
$$15 \text{ mA} \times ? \text{ sec.} = 6 \text{ mAs}$$
$$? \text{ sec.} = \frac{6 \text{ mAs}}{15 \text{ mAs}}$$
$$? \text{ sec.} = 0.4 \text{ sec}$$

ANSWER. The new exposure time is 0.4 sec.

Notice the mA increased, and the exposure time decreased. Why would a dental office want to do this? Perhaps, with a shorter exposure time, there would be less time for possible patient movement.

Variations in Kilovoltage (kVp)

The quality of the radiation (wavelength or energy of the x-ray photons) generated by the x-ray machine is determined by the **kilovoltage peak (kVp).** The more the kVp is increased, the shorter the wavelength and the higher the energy and penetrating power of the x-rays produced. Increasing the kVp also increases the number (quantity) of x-rays produced. Therefore, the number of x-rays that enter the emulsion coating of the x-ray film also increases, resulting in increased density of the radiograph. As the kVp of the x-ray beam is increased, the density of the radiograph is held constant by reducing the milliampere-seconds (mA or exposure time). Exposure time is usually the easiest control factor to change.

Radiographic Contrast

Kilovoltage is the only exposure factor that directly influences the contrast of a dental radiograph. As we learned earlier in this chapter, **radiographic contrast** refers to the difference in the amount of light transmitted through two or more adjacent film areas. Two terms, **short-scale contrast** and **long-scale contrast,** are used to describe contrast when the kilovoltage is varied.

SHORT-SCALE CONTRAST. The term **short-scale contrast** (see Figure 4–3) describes a radiograph in which the differences between adjacent areas are large. The contrast is high because there are few shades of gray, more black against white. The gray tones indicate the differences in absorption of the x-ray photons by the various tissues of the oral cavity or the head. The film is **radiolucent** (dark) where the tissues are soft or thin and **radiopaque** (white) where the tissues are hard or thick. Such radiographs result when low (60 to 70) kVp is applied. Some dentists prefer radiographs with short-scale contrast, thinking that dental caries are easier to recognize; however, fine detail may be difficult to distinguish.

LONG-SCALE CONTRAST. The term **long-scale contrast** (see Figure 4–3) describes a radiograph in which the density differences between adjacent areas are small. The contrast is low and very gradual because there are many shades of gray. Such radiographs result when high (80 to 90) kVp is applied. More detailed information can be obtained from such radiographs, provided that a view box with variable light control is used.

No standard kVp technique is used in all dental offices. Most dental offices use 70 to 90 kVp. The proper kVp to use is strictly a matter of individual preference. The customary procedure required to maintain film density is either to reduce the milliampere/seconds when higher kilovoltage is applied or to increase the milliampere/seconds when lower kilovoltage is applied. Thus one factor balances the other.

Effects of Variations in Distances

The operator must take into account several distances in making x-ray exposures:

- The distance between the x-ray source (at the focal spot on the target) and the surface of the patient's skin
- The distance between the object to be x-rayed (usually the tooth) and the film
- The distance between the x-ray source and the recording plane of the film

Various terms are used in dental literature to describe these distances. The terms target-surface (skin), anode-surface, focus-surface, tube-surface, and source-surface are synonymous, as are target-film, anode-film, focus-film, and source-film. In this text, the terms **target-surface** distance, **target-film** distance, and **object-film** distance are used (see Figure 4–13).

Target-surface (Skin) Distance

Generally, whenever the film is positioned intraorally, the length of the **target-surface distance** depends on the length of the position indicating device used. PIDs are classified as being short or long. All intraoral techniques

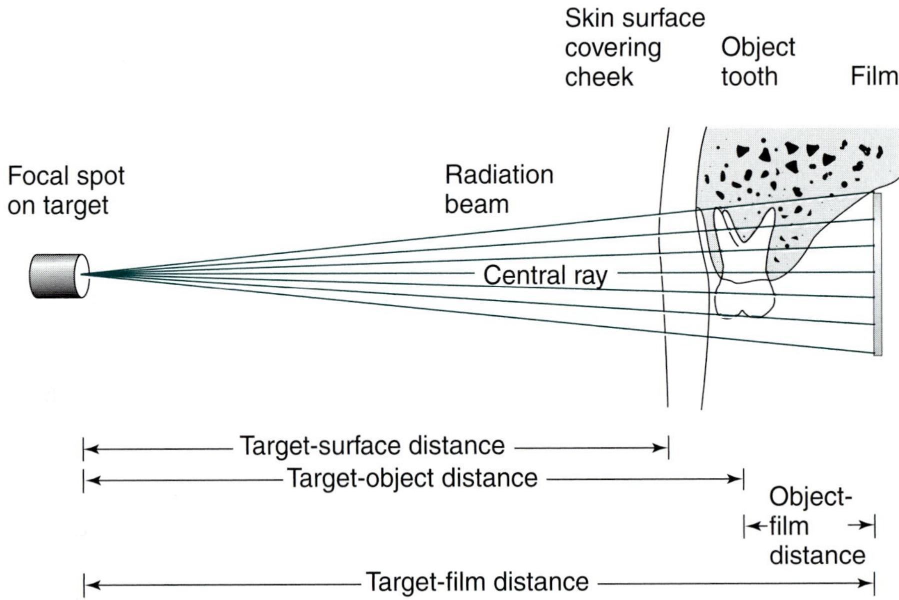

FIGURE 4–13. **Distances.** Relationship among target, skin surface, object (tooth), and x-ray film distance.

require that the end of the PID should almost touch the skin. This is necessary to standardize measurements.

The *National Bureau of Standards Handbook 76* sets the minimum target-surface distance at 7 in. (18 cm) for x-ray machines operating at above 50 kVp and at 4 in. (10 cm) for those that operate at 50 kVp or lower. No maximum distances are set. In extraoral radiography, where larger films are positioned outside the face, target-film distances of up to 72 in. (183 cm) are occasionally used.

Object-film Distance

The **object-film distance** depends largely on the method that is employed to hold the film in position behind the teeth. When the bisecting technique is used, the film is pressed against the lingual tissues as close as the oral anatomy will permit. This results in the object-film distance being shorter in the area of the crown where the tooth and film may touch than in the area opposite the root, where the thickness of the bone and gingiva may cause a divergence between the long axis of the tooth and the film. The least divergence occurs in the mandibular molar areas. The greatest divergence is in the maxillary anterior areas where the palatal structures may curve sharply.

With the paralleling technique, most film holders are designed so that the film is held parallel to the average long axes of the teeth being x-rayed. This necessitates positioning the film sufficiently to the lingual of the teeth to avoid impinging on the supporting bone and gingival structures. This technique results in object-film distances that are often more than 1 in. (25 mm).

Target-film Distance

The **target-film distance** is the sum of the target-object and the object-film distance (see Figure 4–13). The quality of the radiograph image improves whenever the target-film distance is increased. Magnification is reduced, and sharpness of detail (definition) is increased. Increasing the target-film distance reduces the fuzzy outline (penumbra) that is seen around all radiographic images.

In most intraoral procedures, either an 8-in. (20-cm) or a 16-in. (41 cm) distance is used. In the 8-in. (20-cm) technique, a short PID is used and the film may be positioned in direct contact with the lingual tissues. In the 16-in. (41-cm) technique, a longer PID is used and the film is positioned far enough from the teeth to enable it to be held parallel. These techniques are described in detail in Chapter 14.

The location of the x-ray tube within the tube housing makes a big difference in the target-film distance when the aiming device (PID) is attached. On the conventional x-ray machine, either a short or long PID can be attached. When the tube is recessed, enough space is gained within the tube head so that a long target-film distance is achieved with a short PID (see Figure 3–7).

Inverse Square Law

The x-ray photons, traveling in straight lines, spread out (diverge) as they radiate away from the source (target). It follows that the **intensity** of the beam is reduced (Figure 4–14). This is based on the **inverse square law,** which states that "the intensity of radiation varies inversely as the square of the distance from its source."

The inverse square law may be written as:

$$\frac{I_1}{I_2} = \frac{(D_2)^2}{(D_1)^2}$$

where: I_1 is the original intensity.
I_2 is the new intensity.
D_1 is the original distance.
D_2 is the new distance.

The inverse square law is used when we consider distance as a means of protection and when we change the length of the PID (change the target-film distance).

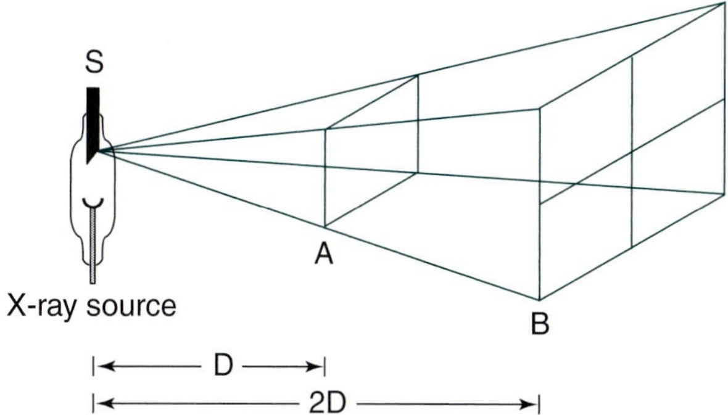

FIGURE 4–14. **Inverse square law.** Relationship of distance (D) to the area covered by x-rays emitted from the x-ray tube. X-rays emerging from the tube travel in straight lines and diverge from each other. The areas covered by the x-rays at any two points are proportional to each other as the square of the distances measured from the source of radiation. (Reproduced with permission from Wuehrmann AH, Manson-Hing LR. *Dental Radiology.* 5th ed. St. Louis: Mosby, 1981)

Let us solve a problem where we consider distance as a means of protection.

PROBLEM. A dental radiographer stands 3 ft (0.9 m) from the source of radiation where the measured intensity is 100 milliroentgens (mR) per minute. The radiographer is asked to move to a new location 6 ft (1.8 m) from the source of radiation. What is the intensity at the new location?

SOLUTION.

$$I_1 = 100 \text{ mR/min}$$
$$D_1 = 3 \text{ ft}$$
$$D_2 = 6 \text{ ft}$$

Find I_2.

$$\frac{100}{I_2} = \frac{6^2}{3^2}$$

$$I_2 \times 6^2 = 100 \times 3^2$$

$$I_2 = \frac{100 \times 9}{36} = 25 \text{ mR per minute}$$

ANSWER. The intensity at the new location is 25 mR/min

The radiographer's new location only receives one fourth the exposure of the old location and is a safer place to stand.

mAs-distance Relationship

Since the x-rays emerging from the tube travel in straight lines and diverge from one another, it follows that the intensity of the beam is reduced unless a corresponding increase is made in one or a combination of the exposure factors. Such changes in exposure factors are essential to maintaining optimum film density. Because milliamperage and time are the main factors influencing film density, the following formula can be used to determine the **mAs-distance relationship:**

$$\frac{\text{Original mAs}}{\text{New mAs}} = \frac{\text{Original distance}^2}{\text{New distance}^2}$$

For example, if a film of the same speed is used in two exposures and the mA and the kVp are left unchanged, it would only be necessary to increase the exposure time when the target-film distance is doubled. In that event, by applying the formula given, the exposure time must be increased fourfold.

Usually time is the easiest exposure factor to change. This formula is useful for obtaining a multiplying factor for changing the exposure time when only the target-film distance is altered.

Exposure Charts

Many operators readily memorize the exposure factors they need to know for the particular technique they are using. Several excellent **exposure charts** are available through the manufacturers of the films or the x-ray equipment. These show at a glance how much exposure time is required for a film of any given film speed when used with all possible combinations of exposure time, milliamperage, and peak kilovoltage. The charts should be displayed beside the control panel. Many health departments require that exposure charts be posted by the control panel.

Some recent x-ray machine models incorporate the most commonly used film speeds and other exposure factors into the dial of the control panel. In that case, the operator only has to set the pointer to the desired combination for a film of a given speed; all the rest is done automatically when the timer button is depressed.

CHAPTER SUMMARY

An acceptable diagnostic radiograph must show the areas of interest—the designated teeth and surrounding bone structures—completely and with minimum distortion and maximum sharpness. The degree of density and contrast is optional.

The dental radiographer must have a working knowledge of the factors that affect the radiographic image. The detail and visibility of a radiograph depends upon two factors—radiographic contrast and sharpness (definition). Radiographic contrast is composed of both subject contrast and film contrast. Sharpness is determined by geometric factors and crystal size of the film emulsion.

To create a sharp image, the radiographer must use a small focal spot, long target-film distance, short object-film distance, and limit patient and film movement.

Two geometric factors, magnification and distortion, influence the quality of a dental radiograph. To minimize magnification, use a long target-film distance and a short object-film distance. Distortion results when the film is not parallel to the object and when the central ray is not perpendicular to the tooth and film.

On many x-ray units it is possible to vary the exposure factors: milliamperage, exposure time, and kilovoltage. Some units are preset, and only one or two factors can be altered. The radiographer can take advantage of the exposure factors to produce radiographs that have the desired sharpness, density, and contrast.

The Inverse Square Law explains how distance affects the intensity of the x-ray beam.

REVEW QUESTIONS

1. What target-film distance would produce a radiograph with the least image magnification?
   (a) 4 in. (10 cm)
   (b) 7 in. (18 cm)
   (c) 8 in. (20 cm)
   (d) 16 in. (41 cm)
2. Which term describes the white areas on the processed radiograph?
   (a) Density
   (b) Penumbra
   (c) Radiolucent
   (d) Radiopaque
3. Subject contrast is affected by:
   (a) Processing procedures.
   (b) Type of film.
   (c) Scatter radiation.
   (d) Crystal size.
4. As crystals in the film emulsion increase in size, image sharpness:
   (a) Increases.
   (b) Decreases.
   (c) Stays the same.
   (d) None of the above.
5. What term best describes the amount of light transmitted through a film?
   (a) Definition
   (b) Contrast
   (c) Density
   (d) Penetration

6. What factor has the greatest effect on film sharpness?
   (a) Movement
   (b) Filtration
   (c) Kilovoltage
   (d) Amperage

7. What term best describes a fuzzy shadow around the outline of the radiographic image?
   (a) Magnification
   (b) Penumbra
   (c) Detail
   (d) Distortion

8. Distortion is caused when:
   (a) Object and film are parallel.
   (b) Object and film are not parallel.
   (c) Using a short object-film distance.
   (d) Using a long target-film distance.

9. Which is most likely to produce a radiograph with long-scale contrast?
   (a) kVp is increased.
   (b) kVp is decreased.
   (c) mAs is increased.
   (d) mAs is decreased.

10. Which of these radiographs would show the most contrast between two adjacent areas?
    (a) Exposed at 60 kVp
    (b) Exposed at 70 kVp
    (c) Exposed at 80 kVp
    (d) Exposed at 90 kVp

11. The dental radiograph will appear lighter if one increases the:
    (a) mA.
    (b) kVp.
    (c) Exposure time.
    (d) Target-film distance.

12. In order to increase the contrast on a radiograph, it is necessary to:
    (a) Lengthen the target-film distance and increase the exposure time.
    (b) Increase the kVp and decrease the exposure time.
    (c) Increase the exposure time and decrease the developing time.
    (d) Decrease the kVp and increase the mA.

13. Selection of proper kVp is influenced most by which two of the following?
    (a) Size of film
    (b) Size of patient
    (c) Developing temperature
    (d) Density of the tissues
    (e) Diameter of the primary beam
    (f) Amount of decay of teeth

14. The ray in the middle of the x-ray beam is called the ________ ________.

15. The differences in density appearing on a radiograph is called ________.

16. The exposure factors in a dental office are: 10 mA, 0.9 sec, 70 kVp, and 16-in. (41-cm) target-film distance. The dentist decides to increase the mA to 15 and leave the kVp and target-film distance constant. What is the new exposure time?

17. Based on the inverse square law, what happens to the intensity of the x-ray beam when the target-film distance is doubled?
    (a) Intensity is doubled.
    (b) Intensity is not affected.
    (c) Intensity is half as great.
    (d) Intensity is one-quarter as great.

18. A radiographer stands 3 ft (0.9 m) from the head of the patient while exposing dental film. A radiological health inspector measures the exposure at that position and finds it to be 40 mR/min. The inspector requires the radiographer to move to a new location 6 ft (1.83 m) from the head of the patient. What is the exposure at the new location?

BIBLIOGRAPHY

Eastman Kodak. *Successful Intraoral Radiography*. Rochester, NY: Eastman Kodak, 1998.

Langland, O. E., Sippy, F. H., & Langlais, R. P. *Textbook of Dental Radiology*, 2nd ed. Springfield, IL: Thomas, 1984.

White, S. C. & Pharoah, M. J. *Oral Radiology Principles and Interpretation*, 4th ed. St Louis: Mosby, 2000.

PART II: Biological Effects of Radiation and Radiation Protection

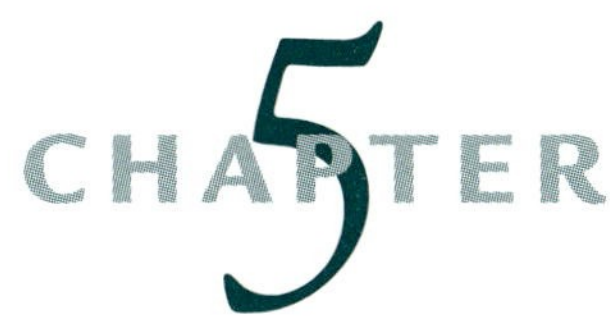

Effects of Radiation Exposure

OBJECTIVES

By the end of this chapter the student should be able to:

- Define the key words.
- Compare the theories of biological damage and the possible effect of radiation on somatic and genetic cells.
- Identify the body cells in the order of their radiosensitivity.
- Identify the factors that determine radiation injuries.
- List the sequence of events that may follow exposure to radiation.
- Identify the three areas in the head and neck that are most affected by radiation.
- List the possible short- and long-term effects of irradiation.
- Discuss the risk versus benefit of dental radiographs.
- Identify the effects of oral radiation therapy.

KEY WORDS

Acute radiation syndrome (ARS)	Law of B and T
As low as reasonably achievable (ALARA)	Lethal dose (LD)
Direct-hit theory	Period of injury
Dysphagia	Radioresistant
Genetic mutations	Radiosensitive
Indirect-action theory	Recovery period
Ionization	Risk
Latent period	Somatic cell
	Xerostomia

Introduction

The fact that ionizing radiation produces biological damage has been known for many years. The first x-ray burn was reported just a few months following Roentgen's discovery of x-rays in 1895. As early as 1902, the first case of x-ray-induced skin cancer was reported in the literature.

As we have seen in Chapter 2, x-rays belong to the ionizing portion of the electromagnetic spectrum. X-rays have the ability to detach and remove electric charges from the complex atoms that make up the molecules of body tissues. This process, known as **ionization,** creates an electrical imbalance within the normally stable cells. Because disturbed cellular atoms or molecules generally attempt to regain electrical stability, they often accept the first available opposite electrical charge. In such cases, the undesirable chemical changes become incompatible with the surrounding body tissues. During ionization, the delicate balance of the cell structure is altered, and the cell may be damaged or destroyed.

The purpose of this chapter is to explain the theories of radiation injury, to discuss the factors that determine radiation injury, to explain the short and long term effects of radiation, to discuss the risks of radiation exposure, and to detail the effects of oral radiation therapy.

Concerns with Potential Radiation Effects

Many dental patients are concerned with the safety of x-ray procedures. Such concerns are shared by the dentist and radiologists. Public concern increased by the testing of atomic weapons and by the accident at the nuclear power plant at Three Mile Island. These events have generated unfavorable attitudes toward the use of x-rays in dentistry and medicine and have resulted in the passage of several laws including the Consumer-Patient Radiation Health and Safety Act of 1981. The subsequent nuclear disaster at Chernobyl, The Ukraine, in 1986 increased this concern.

Some of the public concern is warranted but much is the result of sensational and unsubstantiated newspaper or magazine articles. The trained professionals in the field of radiation are doing everything that is possible to avoid repeated exposures and to keep radiation to a minimum by following all possible safety procedures.

It should be understood that radiation may occur **naturally** or be **manmade.** Naturally caused radiation includes cosmic rays and those rays given off by radioactive elements in the earth. This is called **background radiation** and varies from place to place, generally being lowest at sea level and highest in the mountains. Background radiations are of small concern to us because apparently we can live with them and certainly can do very little about them.

What concerns us more are the manmade radiations caused by emissions from industrial atomic waste, from military testing of atomic weapons, and from certain commercial products. Of special concern are radiations used in industry, medicine, and dentistry. These account for some 90% of the manmade radiations to which the general public is exposed.

Any exposure to radiation is believed to have at least a little biological effect on the exposed person. Unfortunately, we do not yet fully understand all these effects or their future consequences. Scientists believe that some of these effects are cumulative, especially if exposure is too great and the intervals between exposures too frequent for the body cells to repair themselves. Unless the damage is too severe or the subject is in extremely poor health, many body cells (**somatic cells**) have a recovery rate of almost 75% during the first 24 hours; after that, repair continues at the same rate.

In determining whether or not an exposure is potentially harmful, the radiographer should consider the quantity and the duration of the exposure and which body area is to be irradiated. Continued exposure over prolonged periods alters the ability of the genetic cells (eggs and sperm) to reproduce normally. Present evidence indicates that chromosome damage is cumulative, increasing in effect by each successive additional radiation exposure, and genetic cells cannot repair themselves. Radiation may alter the genetic material in the reproductive cells so that **mutations** (abnormalities) may be produced in future generations. The use of lead aprons, thyroid collars, and proper safety techniques protect the patient from any conceivable damage.

There have been no reports of radiation injuries caused by normal dental procedures since safety rules have been adopted. The benefits of dental radiographs far outweigh the minor risks to the patient.

Theories of Biological Effect Mechanisms

There are two generally accepted theories on how radiation damages biological tissues: (1) the **direct-hit** (or target) **theory** and (2) the **indirect-action** (or poison-water) **theory** (see Figure 5–1).

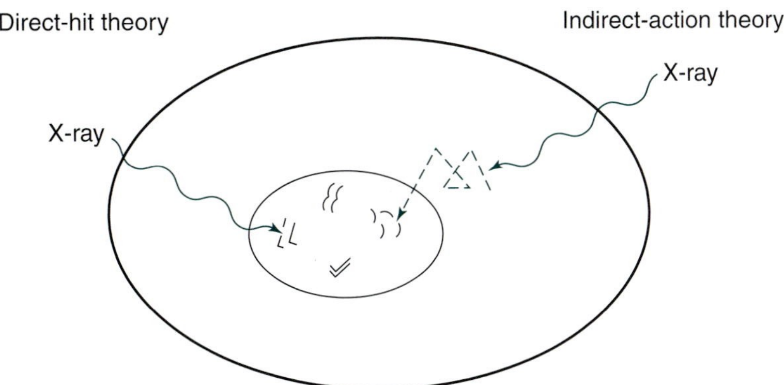

FIGURE 5–1. **Direct-hit theory and indirect-action theory.** In the direct-hit theory, x-ray photons collide with large molecules and break them apart by **ionization.** The indirect-action theory is based on the assumption that radiation can cause chemical damage to the cell by **ionizing** the water within it.

- **Direct-hit theory:** According to the **direct-hit theory,** x-ray photons collide with important cell chemicals and break them apart by **ionization** and thus critical damage to large molecules (see Figure 5–2). Most x-ray photons, however, probably pass through the cell with little or no damage. A healthy cell can repair any minor damage that might occur. Moreover, the body contains so many cells that the destruction of a single cell or a small group of cells will have no observable effect.
- **Indirect-action theory:** The **indirect-action theory** is based on the assumption that radiation can cause chemical damage to the cell by **ionizing** the water within it (see Figure 5–3). Since about 80% of body weight is water and ionization can dissociate water into hydrogen and hydroxyl radicals, the theory proposes that new chemicals such as hydrogen peroxide could be formed under certain conditions.

These chemicals act as a poison to the body, causing cellular dysfunction. Fortunately, when the water is broken down during irradiation, the ions have a strong tendency to recombine immediately to form water again instead of seeking out new combinations. This tendency holds cellular damage to a minimum. Under ordinary circumstances, even when a new chemical is formed, other cells that are not affected can take over the functions of the damaged cells until recovery takes place. Only in extreme instances, where massive irradiation has taken place, will entire body areas be destroyed or death result. However, it should be remembered that cellular destruction is not the only biological effect; the potential exists for the cell to become malignant.

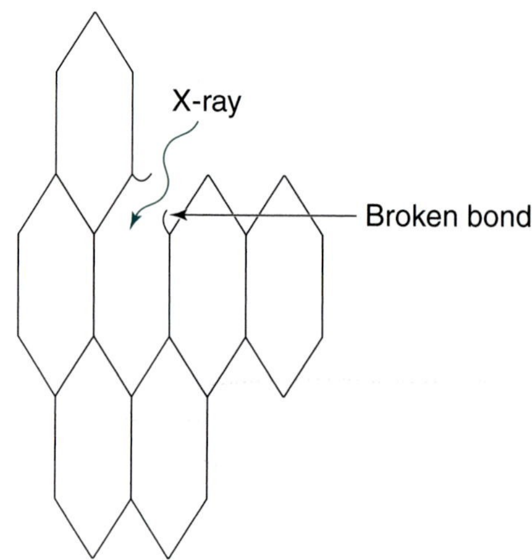

FIGURE 5–2. **Direct-hit theory. Radiation breaks the bonds** connecting atoms in molecules **causing ionization,** thus producing harmful effects.

Much about radiation effects remains to be discovered. Moreover, most of our radiation research is conducted with experimental animals. Not all species have the same radiosensitivity. Much of what we know about human's sensitivity to radiation is derived from studies of survivors that received large doses of whole-body radiation from atomic bombs at the end of World War II or from certain nuclear accidents. Conceivably, future research may demonstrate that human beings are not as sensitive to radiation damage as we now believe. But until we have such evidence, commonsense dictates improving radiographic safety techniques in every way possible.

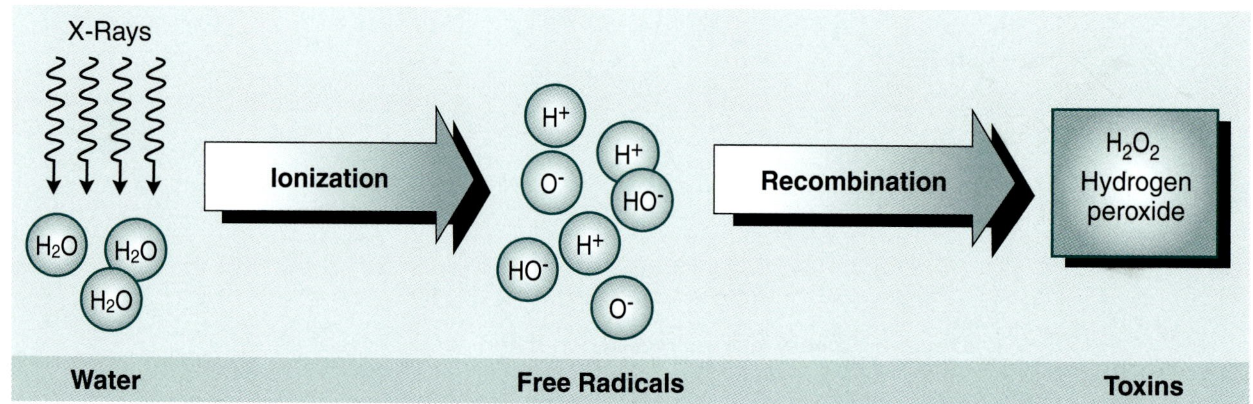

FIGURE 5–3. **Indirect-action theory. X-rays ionize water,** resulting in the formation of **free radicals,** which recombine to form **toxins.**

Cell Sensitivity to Radiation Exposure

The terms**radiosensitive** and**radioresistant** are used to describe the degree of susceptibility of various cells and body tissues to radiation. The cell is most susceptible to radiation injury during mitosis (cell division). All cells are not equally sensitive to radiation. The relative sensitivity of cells to radiation was first described in 1906 by two French scientists, Bergonie and Tribondeau, and is known as the**Law of B and T.** The law states that "the radiosensitivity of cells and tissues is directly proportional to their reproductive capacity and inversely proportional to their degree of differentiation."

The first half of the Law of B and T means that actively dividing cells, such as white blood cells, are more sensitive than slowly dividing cells. Embryonic and immature cells are more sensitive than mature cells of the same tissue. The second half of the Law of B and T means the more specialized a cell is, the more radioresistant the cell.

Based on these factors, it is possible to **rank** various kinds of **cells** in **descending order of radiosensitivity:**

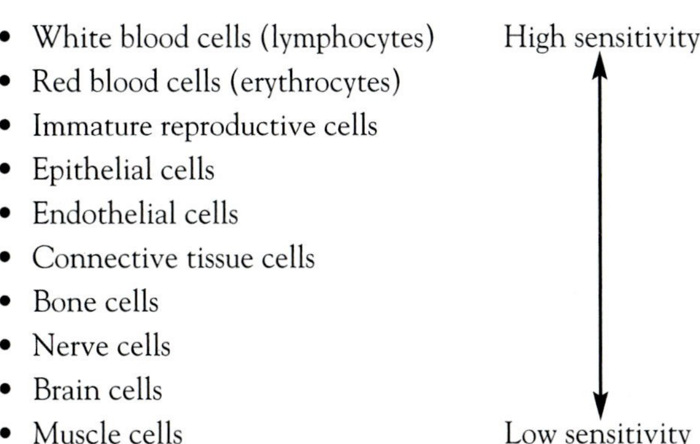

• White blood cells (lymphocytes)
• Red blood cells (erythrocytes)
• Immature reproductive cells
• Epithelial cells
• Endothelial cells
• Connective tissue cells
• Bone cells
• Nerve cells
• Brain cells
• Muscle cells
High sensitivity
Low sensitivity

The facial and oral structures, composed largely of bone, nerve, and muscle tissue, are fairly radioresistant. In dental radiography, exposure is limited to a very small area, and the amount of radiation is minimal. Specific measures for making radiation safe for both patient and operator are described in Chapter 6.

The Dose-response Curve

For drugs, radiation, or any other biologically harmful agent, it is useful to plot the dosage administered with the response or damage produced, in order to establish acceptable levels of exposure. In plotting these two variables, a **dose-response curve** is produced. With radiation, it is important to consider the nature and shape of this curve. Two possibilities are illustrated in Figure 5–4.

Unfortunately, radiobiologists have been unable to determine radiation effects at very low levels of exposure (for instance, below 10 roentgens) and cannot be certain whether or not a threshold effect exists. It is felt that somatic effects (changes in the irradiated individual) could be threshold, whereas genetic effects (changes in hereditary material affecting future generations) could be considered nonthreshold effects. This is as yet highly controversial and may need to be revised later.

To be on the safe side, radiation protection groups take the conservative approach and consider all radiation effects as being nonthreshold. This assumption has been made in the establishment of radiation protection guides and in radiation control activities. The concept that every dose of radiation produces damage and should be kept to the minimum necessary to meet diagnostic requirements is known as the**ALARA** concept, where ALARA stands for **"as low as reasonably achievable."**

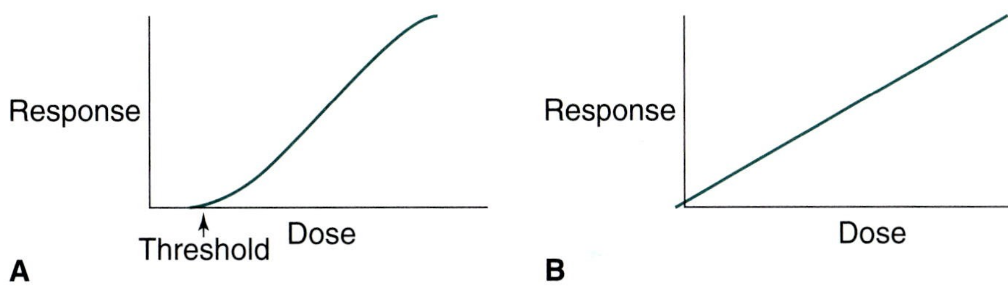

FIGURE 5–4. **Diagram of dose-response curve.** (**A**) A typical **"threshold"** curve. The point at which the curve intersects the base line (horizontal line) is the threshold dose that is the dose below which there is no response. If an easily observable radiation effect, such as erythema (reddening of the skin) is taken as "response," then this type of curve is applicable. (**B**) A linear **"non-threshold"** curve, in which the curve intersects the base line at its origin. Here it is assumed that any dose, no matter how small, causes some response.

Factors that Determine Radiation Injury

The factors that determine the amount of radiation injury are total dose, dose rate, area exposed, variation in species, individual sensitivity, variation in cell sensitivity, variation in tissue sensitivity, and age.

- **Total dose:** The total dose of radiation depends on the type, energy, and duration of the radiation. The greater the dose, the more severe the probable biological effect.
- **Dose rate:** The rate at which the radiation is administered or absorbed is very important in the determination of what effects will occur. Since a considerable degree of recovery occurs from the radiation damage, a given dose will produce less effect if it is divided (thus allowing time for recovery between dose increments) than if it is given in a single exposure. For instance, an exposure of 1 R/week for 100 weeks would result in far less injury than a single exposure of 100 R. This principle is utilized in determining doses for radiation therapy.
- **Area exposed:** The amount of injury to the individual depends on the area or volume irradiated. The larger the area exposed, other factors being equal, the greater the injury to the organism. This is why it is recommended to expose as small an area as practical. In dentistry we use a very small (2.75 in. or 7 cm) beam diameter to limit the beam of radiation to the area of diagnostic concern, and this area can be further limited by the use of rectangular collimation (see Figure 1–2).
- **Variation in species:** Various species have a wide variation of radiosensitivity. Lethal doses for plants and microorganisms are usually hundreds of times higher than those for mammals.
- **Individual sensitivity:** Individuals vary in sensitivity within the same species. For this reason the **lethal dose (LD)** for each species is expressed in statistical terms, usually as the LD 50/30 for that species, or the dose required to kill 50% of the individuals in a large population in a 30-day period. For humans, the LD 50/30 is estimated to be 4.5 grays (Gy) or 450 rads (grays and rads are units of absorbed dose, more completely described in Chapter 6) of whole-body radiation.
- **Variation in cell sensitivity:** Within the same individual, a wide variation in susceptibility to radiation damage exists among different types of cells and tissues. As the Law of B and T pointed out, the cells that rapidly divide or have a potential for rapid division are more sensitive to radiation than those that do not divide. Furthermore, primitive or nonspecialized cells are more sensitive than those that are highly specialized. Within the same cell families, then, the immature forms, which are generally primitive and rapidly dividing, are more radiosensitive than the older, mature cells, which have specialized in function and have ceased to divide.
- **Variation in tissue sensitivity:** Some tissues (organs) of the body are more radiosensitive than others. For instance, blood-forming organs such as the spleen and red bone marrow are more sensitive than the highly specialized heart muscle.

  In dental radiology, the most critical areas in the head and neck are the **mandible (red bone marrow),** the **lens of the eye,** and the **thyroid gland.** The mandible contains an estimated 15 g of red bone marrow. This is only about 1% of the total amount of red bone marrow in the adult body. The lens of the eye is of interest because it is occasionally in the primary beam during some maxillary exposures. The thyroid gland is relatively radiosensitive. However, during dental radiographic procedures it is generally out of the range of the primary beam and is only exposed by scatter radiation. The risk can be further reduced by the use of a thyroid collar or shield (see Figure 6–8).
- **Age:** Younger, more rapidly dividing cells are more radiosensitive than older, mature cells so it follows that children may be more susceptible to injury than adults from an equal dose of radiation. Also, in children the distance from the oral cavity to the reproductive and other sensitive organs is less than for adults. Therefore the dental doses to the critical organs may be higher than they would be for an adult. This is why it is wise to use leaded aprons and thyroid collars to protect all patients.

Sequence of Events Following Radiation Exposure

The **sequence of events** following radiation exposure are **latent period, period of injury,** and **recovery period,** assuming, of course, that the dose received was nonlethal.

- **Latent period:** Following the initial radiation exposure, and before the first detectable effect occurs, a time lag called the **latent period** occurs. The latent period may be very short or extremely long, depending on the initial dose. Effects that appear within a

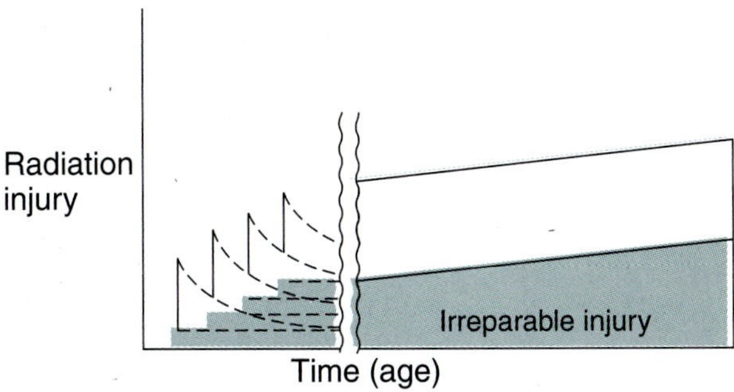

FIGURE 5–5. **Concept of accumulated irreparable injury.** After exposure to radiation cell recovery can take place. However, there may be a certain amount of damage from which no recovery occurs, and it is this **irreparable injury** that can give rise to later long-term effects.

matter of minutes, days, or weeks are called short-term effects and those that appear years, decades, and even generations later are called long-terrn effects. Again, this relates to the types of cells involved and their corresponding rates of mitosis (cell division).

- **Period of injury:** Following the latent period, certain effects can be observed. One of the effects seen most frequently in growing tissues exposed to radiation is the stoppage of mitosis, or cell divisions. This may be temporary or permanent, depending upon the radiation dosage. Other effects include breaking or clumping of chromosomes, abnormal mitosis, and formation of giant cells.
- **Recovery period:** Following exposure to radiation, some **recovery** can take place. This is particularly apparent in the case of the short-term effects. Nevertheless, there may be a certain amount of damage from which no recovery occurs, and it is this **irreparable injury** that can give rise to later long-term effects (Figure 5–5).

Short- and Long-term Effects of Radiation

The **effects of radiation** are classified as either **short-term** or **long-term** effects.

Short-term Effects

Short-term effects of radiation are those seen minutes, days, or months after exposure. When a very large dose of radiation is delivered in a very short period of time, the latent period is short. If the dose of radiation is large enough (generally over 1.0 Gy or 100 rads, whole-body), the resultant signs and symptoms that comprise these short-term effects are collectively known as the **acute radiation syndrome (ARS).** The ARS symptoms include erythema (redness of the skin), nausea, vomiting, diarrhea, hemorrhage, and hair loss. The acute radiation syndrome is not a concern in dentistry, because our x-ray machines could not produce the very large exposures necessary to cause it.

Long-term Effects

Long-term effects of radiation are those that are seen years after the original exposure. The latent period is much longer (years) than that associated with the acute radiation syndrome (hours or days). Delayed radiation effects may result from a previous acute, high exposure that the individual has survived or from chronic low-level exposures delivered over many years. In dentistry, we are potentially exposed to these chronic low levels of radiation. From the public health point of view, the possibility of long-term effects on the large number of people receiving low, chronic exposures is cause for greater concern than the short-term radiation effects from acute exposures that involve only a few individuals.

There is no unique disease associated with the long-term effects of radiation. However, there is a statistical increase in the incidence of certain already existing conditions. Because of the low normal incidence of these conditions, one must observe large numbers of exposed persons in order to evaluate this kind of an increase.

The long-term effects observed have been somatic damage, which may result in an increased incidence of cancer, embryological defects, cataracts, life span shortening, and genetic mutations. The first four conditions are somatic effects and only involve the individual exposed. Genetic mutations involve hereditary material and may have an adverse effect for many generations after the original exposure.

- **Cancer:** Anything that is capable of causing cancer is called a *carcinogen*. X-rays, like certain drugs, chemicals, and viruses, have been shown to have carcinogenic effects. Carcinogenic mechanisms are not clearly understood. Moreover, cancer is probably "caused" by the simultaneous interaction of several factors, and the presence of some of these factors without the others may not be sufficient to cause the disease.

  Some explanations for the carcinogenic action of x-rays include the following: x-rays activate viruses already present in cells; x-rays damage chromosomes, and certain diseases (such as leukemia) are associated with chromosomal injury; x-rays cause mutations in somatic cells, which may result in uncontrolled growth of cells; and x-rays ionize water, which results in chemical "free radicals" that may cause cancer.

Any one or a combination of these theories may explain how cancer is caused. X-radiation is only one of a number of possible carcinogens involved, and the precise mechanism is not yet understood. Much of the evidence that x-radiation is carcinogenic comes from studies of early radiation workers, including dentists, who were exposed to large amounts of radiation (see Figures 5–6 and 5–7).

- **Embryological defects:** The immature, undifferentiated, rapidly growing cells of the embryo are highly sensitive to radiation. The first trimester of a pregnancy when the fetus undergoes the period of major organogenesis (formation of organs) is especially critical. High doses of radiation may cause birth abnormalities, stunting of growth, and mental retardation. It is fortunate for dentistry that the dose from a dental x-ray examination is no more than 0.0003 to 0.003 milligrays (0.03 to 0.3 millirads). Of course, the use of a leaded apron reduces this potential dose to zero.
- **Cataracts:** When the lens of the eye becomes opaque, it is called a **cataract.** Various agents, including x-rays, have been known to cause cataracts. It takes at least 2 Gy (200 rads) of x-radiation to cause cataract formation. The dose to the eye from dental radiographic procedures is in the order of milligrays (millirads). Dental x-rays have never been reported to cause cataracts.

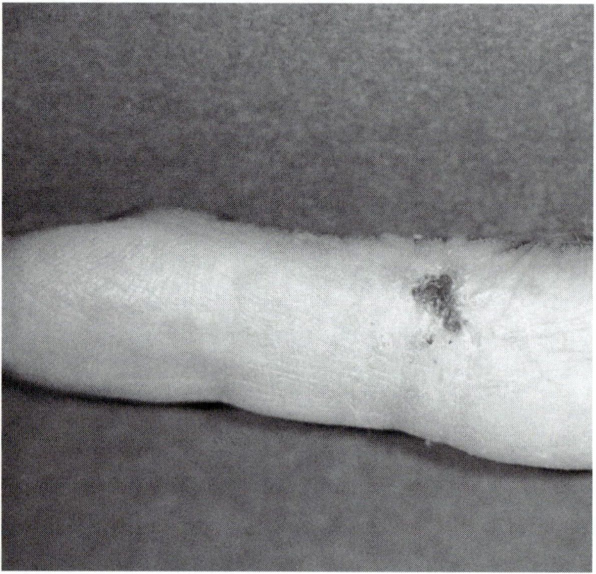

FIGURE 5-6. **Ulcerated lesion** (early carcinoma) on finger of dentist who admitted holding films for his patients.

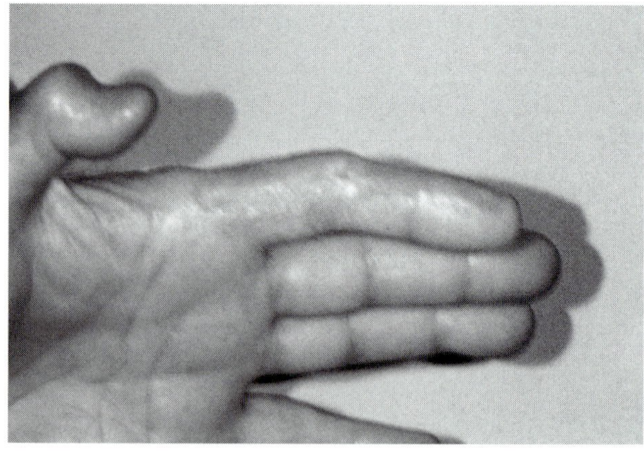

FIGURE 5-7. **Radiation injury** on finger of dentist caused by holding films in the mouth of patients. Many of these lesions become squamous cell carcinoma (cancer).

- **Life-span shortening:** Life-span shortening effects caused by x-radiation have been demonstrated in animal experiments. The effect seems to be caused by premature aging. However, life span shortening has never been demonstrated in humans.
- **Genetic mutations:** X-radiation is known to sometimes cause changes in the genetic material of cells. These changes are referred to as **genetic mutations.** The genetic material is the means by which hereditary traits are passed from one generation to another. Drugs, chemicals, and even elevated body temperatures are also capable of causing mutations. Genetic effects are especially important, because there may be no level of radiation that will not produce at least some effect.

While humans may not have evolved if it were not for genetic mutations parity induced by naturally occurring radiations, most geneticists agree that the majority of genetic mutations are harmful. Because of their damaging effects, they are gradually eliminated from the population by natural means, since individuals with this damage are less likely to reproduce themselves successfully than are normal individuals. The more severe the condition produced by the mutation, the more rapidly it will be eliminated. As a balance to this natural elimination of harmful mutations, new ones are constantly occurring. Natural background radiation probably accounts for a small proportion of naturally occurring mutations.

Since the scattered radiation reaching the gonads from dental radiography is less than .0001 that of the exposure to the surface of the face, the dental contribution to genetic mutations is extremely small ranging from 0.0 to about 0.002 milligrays (0.2 millirad) per radiograph. By using a lead apron and thyroid collar, the dose is essentially reduced to zero.

Risk Estimates

A **risk** may be defined as the likelihood of injury or death from some hazard. The primary risk from dental radiography is radiation-induced cancer.

Risk estimates vary, depending upon several factors, such as speed of film, collimation, and the technique used. The potential risk of a full mouth dental x-ray examination inducing cancer in a patient has been estimated to be 2.5 per 1,000,000 examinations.

Every day we assume hundreds of risks such as climbing stairs, crossing the street, riding a bicycle, and driving a car. Activities with a fatality risk of 1 in 1,000,000 include riding 300 miles in an automobile, traveling 1,000 miles in an airplane, or smoking 1.4 cigarettes a day (Table 5–1). Obviously we accept these risks every day without the benefit of diagnostic radiographs.

- **Risk versus benefit:** Dental radiographs should be taken only when the benefit outweighs the risk of biologic injury to the patient. When dental radiographs are properly prescribed (see Chapter 6), exposed, and processed, the health benefits to the patient far outweigh any risk of injury.

Effects of Oral Radiation Therapy

So much has been said and written about radiation hazards that, for the peace of mind of both patient and operator, it must be emphasized that the exposures used in dental radiation are so minimal that, unless repeated hundreds of times in rapid succession, it would be virtually impossible to create the conditions described in the previous section.

TABLE 5-1. **One in One Million Fatality Risk**

Risk	Nature
Smoking 1.4 cigarettes/day	Cancer
Riding 10 miles on a bicycle	Accident
Travel 300 miles by auto	Accident
Travel 1,000 miles by airplane	Accident

This, however, is not the case when radiation is applied therapeutically to treat cancer lesions. After 6 or more weeks of treatment, during which the patient may receive doses of 2 Gy (200 rads) daily for five days a week at the site of the malignancy, the total localized dose is in the range of 60 Gy (6,000 rads). Remember that this is a local and not a whole-body dose. A person could not survive such a dose to the entire body.

Such tremendous doses over a short time period cause many adverse responses in the normal tissues surrounding the lesion being treated. Since oral radiation therapy has assumed an ever increasingly prominent role in cancer treatment, all members of the dental team—particularly the dental assistant or hygienist who frequently is the first one to see the patient in a professional capacity—should be aware of the complications and discomforts that are common with the irradiated patient.

Complications can appear soon after initiation of radiation therapy and continue at unspecified intervals over a period of years. During the 5 years following the initiation of treatment, the patient goes through **three clinical stages:**

1. An **acute clinical period** during the first 6 months.
2. A **subacute clinical period** during the second 6 months.
3. A **chronic clinical period** that lasts from the second through the 5th year.

Hopefully, recovery is complete by this time, but there may be a recurrence of the malignancy or a radiation-induced growth at a later time.

Obviously, the patient undergoes the greater degree of discomfort and emotional stress during the acute stage. Not only is the cancer irradiated but also the highly radiosensitive tissues of the mucosa that line the oral vestibule, pharynx, larynx, salivary glands, and tongue. If such patients require dental treatment, they must be handled with great care. The mouth is painful and sensitive to touch, and the danger of complications arising from trauma or infection must be considered. Patients lose their appetite and sense of taste. The saliva becomes thick and ropy, and the mouth feels dry (**xerostomia**). Swallowing becomes difficult (**dysphagia**), the tongue may be swollen, and the throat feels congested. Mucositis, an inflammation and sluffing of the mucous membranes, is common.

The dryness of the mouth continues through most of the subacute stage. The oral mucosa becomes blanched and takes on a spider web appearance with red markings, and ulcers may appear. More serious, from a dental view, is that radiation caries may develop around the cervical portions of the teeth.

Salivary gland function and taste response generally return during the chronic stage. However, ulcers may continue, and a necrosis (cellular death) of the alveolar bone—a condition called osteoradionecrosis (bone death)—may occur. This is often accompanied by an inflamed appearance of the gingiva, looseness of the teeth, and extreme pain.

Obviously, there is a major concern whenever the necessity arises to expose additional radiographs on any patient who is currently receiving or has already undergone radiation therapy. The patient is extremely reluctant to receive additional radiation, no matter how minimal, and the dentist may be hesitant to order any additional radiographs. Likewise, the radiographer making the exposure may feel apprehensive about the procedure.

The dental staff must communicate with the patient that the concerns for radiation safety are shared. Although the irradiated patient may already have received large therapeutic doses of radiation, there should be no hesitation in exposing additional radiographs provided that they are deemed to be necessary to make a diagnosis. The additional radiation that the patient would receive is minimal, and its use is justified if the patient benefits.

CHAPTER SUMMARY

Ionizing radiation has the potential to produce biological damage because x-rays can detach subatomic particles from larger molecules and create an electrical imbalance within a normally stable cell. This potential for cellular damage is of great concern to everyone—the general public and those who work with radiation.

Everyone is exposed to some background and manmade radiations. Our concern is to keep dental radiation as low as possible, consistent with obtaining the desired diagnostic information. Genetic and somatic cell reaction to the ionization that occurs during radiation exposure depends on the age, size, and health of the patient, the output of the x-ray machine, the duration of the exposure, the degree of tissue radiosensitivity, and the area of exposure, local or whole-body.

There are two generally accepted theories on how radiation may cause damage to cellular tissues: (1) the direct-hit or target theory, and (2) the indirect-action or poison-water theory. Whether cell damage from radiation is physical or chemical, it has been established that minor damage is soon repaired by a healthy body. Our main concern is that damage to genetic cells may result in altering the chromosomes and creating mutations in future generations. This can be avoided by draping the patient with a protective lead apron.

The terms radiosensitive and radioresistant are used to describe the degree of susceptibility of various cells and body tissues to radiation. Most facial tissues are fairly radioresistant.

The dose-response curve is a method used to plot the dosage of radiation administered with the response produced in order to establish responsible levels of radiation exposure. The conservative view that every dose of radiation potentially produces damage and should be kept to a minimum is expressed by the ALARA concept—"as low as reasonably achievable."

The factors that determine the amount of radiation injury include total dose, dose rate, area exposed, variation in species, individual sensitivity, variation in cell sensitivity, variation in tissue sensitivity, and age. The lethal dose for each species is expressed in statistical terms—the LD 50/30 for that species.

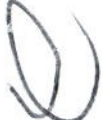

In dental radiology, the most critical areas in the head and neck are (1) the red bone marrow in the mandible, (2) the lens of the eye, and (3) the thyroid gland.

Assuming that the dose received is not lethal, the sequence of events following radiation exposure are (1) a latent period, (2) a period of injury, and (3) a recovery period.

The effects of radiation exposure may be short- or long-term. Short-term effects often include erythema and general discomfort. Long-term effects may result in an increased incidence of cancer, embryological defects, cataracts, life-span shortening, and genetic mutations. Since dental exposures are very minimal there is little danger if radiation safety techniques are followed. The potential risk of injury caused by normal dental radiographic procedures is very small. Health benefits to the patient far outweigh any risk involved.

Many patients receive large amounts of radiation during treatment for cancer. Such therapy produces many complications and discomforts, which may include dryness of the mouth, swollen tongue, difficulty in swallowing, looseness of teeth, and pain. Radiographs should be taken on irradiated patients only if deemed necessary for the patient's welfare. The auxiliary must exercise extreme care in film placement as the patient's mouth may have many unhealed lesions.

REVIEW QUESTIONS

1. Which term best describes radiation of natural origin?
   (a) Background radiation
   (b) Scatter radiation
   (c) Ionizing radiation
   (d) Leakage radiation

2. The primary cause of biological damage from radiation is:
   (a) Ionization.
   (b) Direct effect.
   (c) Indirect effect.
   (d) Genetic effect.

3. Direct injury from radiation ocurrs when:
   (a) X-rays ionize water and form toxins.
   (b) X-rays pass through the cell.
   (c) X-rays strike critical cell molecules.
   (d) All of the above.

4. Indirect injury from radiation occurs when:
   (a) X-rays ionize water and form toxins.
   (b) X-rays pass through the cell.
   (c) X-rays strike critical cell molecules.
   (d) All of the above.

5. Which of these cells is most radiosensitive?
   (a) Muscle cells
   (b) Nerve cells
   (c) Red blood cells
   (d) Mature bone cells

6. Which of these cells is most radioresistant?
   (a) Red blood cells
   (b) Muscle cells
   (c) Epithelial cells
   (d) White blood cells

7. Which of the tissues that may be in the path of the dental x-ray beam is most radioresistant?
   (a) Lens of the eye
   (b) Thyroid gland
   (c) Red bone marrow in mandible
   (d) The enamel of the teeth

8. The tissue which is most sensitive to radiation is:
   (a) Skin.
   (b) Muscle.
   (c) Bone.
   (d) Lymphoid.

9. Which of these factors has no effect on determining the extent of radiation injury?
   (a) The area exposed
   (b) The age of the patient
   (c) The type of film used
   (d) The dose rate

10. According to the Law of B and T, cells with a high reproductive rate are described as:
    (a) Radiopaque.
    (b) Radiolucent.
    (c) Radioresistant.
    (d) Radiosensitive.

11. Gamma ray therapy of tumors has its greatest effect on cells that are:
    (a) Hyperplastic.
    (b) Hypertrophied.
    (c) Highly differentiated.
    (d) Undergoing active mitosis.

12. Which of these is not an event that follows major exposure to radiation?
    (a) A dose-response period
    (b) A latent period
    (c) A period of injury
    (d) A recovery period

13. Which of these is the earliest detectable symptom of excessive radiation exposure?
    (a) Erythema
    (b) Xerostomia
    (c) Alopecia
    (d) Dysphagia

14. Which of these is not considered to be a possible long-term effect of exposure to radiation?
    (a) Cataracts
    (b) Arthritis
    (c) Embryological defects
    (d) Genetic mutations

15. Approximately how much smaller is the radiation exposure in the area of the gonads than at the surface of the face?
    (a) .10
    (b) .01
    (c) .001
    (d) .0001

16. Radiation injuries that do not appear in the person irradiated but occur in future generations are called:
    (a) Long-term effects.
    (b) Somatic effects.
    (c) Genetic effects.
    (d) Threshold effects.

17. The earliest detectable physical change caused by a large radiation exposure is:
    (a) Shortening of the life span.
    (b) Sterility.
    (c) Presence of mutations.
    (d) A drop in lymphocyte count.

18. Those effects which appear within a matter of minutes, days, or weeks are called:
    (a) Acute effects.
    (b) Latent effects.
    (c) Long-term effects.
    (d) Accumulated effects.

19. The two theories explaining how radiation damages biological tissues are __________ and __________.

20. ALARA stands for __ ___ __ ________ ________.

BIBLIOGRAPHY

Carl, W. Local and systemic chemotherapy: Preventing and managing oral complications. *J. Am. Dent. Assoc.* 1993; 124:119–123.

Eastman Kodak. *Radiation Safety in Dental Radiography*. Rochester, NY: Eastman Kodak, 1998.

Khan, F. M. *The Physics of Radiation Therapy*, 2nd ed. Baltimore: Williams & Wilkins, 1994.

Mettler, F. A. & Upton, A. C. *Medical Effects of Ionizing Radiation*, 2nd ed. Philadelphia: Saunders, 1995.

National Academy of Sciences, National Research Council. *The Effects on Populations of Exposure to Low Levels of Ionizing Radiation* (BEIR III report). Washington, DC: National Academy Press, 1980.

National Cancer Institute. *Consensus Development Conference on Oral Complications of Cancer Therapies: Diagnosis, Prevention and Treatment.* Bethesda, MD: National Institutes of Health; 1990. National Cancer Institute monograph no. 9.

National Council on Radiation Protection and Measurements. *Implementation of the Principle of as Low as Reasonably Achievable (ALARA) for Medical and Dental Personnel.* Washington, DC: 1991. NCRP report no. 107.

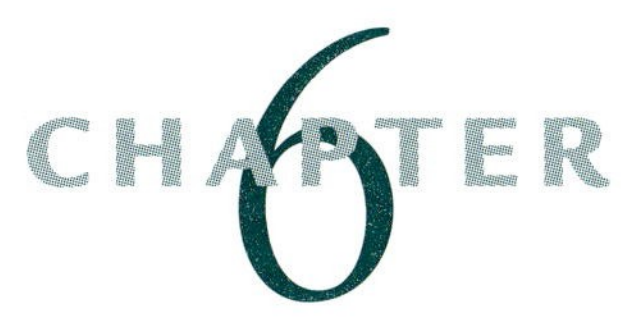

Radiation Protection

OBJECTIVES

By the end of this chapter the student should be able to:

- Define the key words.
- Explain the ALARA concept.
- Summarize the radiation protection methods for the patient.
- Summarize the radiation protection methods for the operator.
- Describe a collimator, discuss its use, and state the recommended diameter of the beam at the patient's skin.
- Describe a filter, discuss its use, and state filtration requirements above and below 70 kVp.
- Explain inherent, added, and total filtration.
- Discuss the use of the lead apron and thyroid collar.
- Discuss the importance of film handling and processing.
- Describe personnel monitoring devices used to detect radiation.
- Discuss maximum permissible dose (MPD) and state the MPD for radiation workers and for the general public.

KEY WORDS

Added filtration
Area monitoring
As low as reasonably achievable (ALARA)
Collimation
Collimator
Depth dose
DXTTR (phantom)
Entrance (skin) dose
Exit dose
Exposure factors
Fast film (high speed)
Film badge
Film holder
Filter
Filtration
Inherent filtration
Lead apron
Leakage radiation
Maximum permissible dose (MPD)
Monitoring
Monitoring badge
Personnel monitoring
Pocket dosimeter
Position indicating device (PID)
Primary beam
Primary radiation
Protective barrier
Radiation protection supervisor
Scatter radiation
Secondary radiation
Thermoluminescent dosimeter (TLD)
Thyroid collar
Timer
TLD badge
Total filtration

Introduction

As partially explained in Chapter 5, any radiation exposure, however slight, carries a potential for biological damage to the patient and operator. The dental team shares the public's concern over the effects of needless or unnecessary radiation. Since the hazard increases with the amount of radiation, everything must be done to keep radiation exposures as low as possible.

One of the cardinal principles in radiography is to use the least radiation needed to perform the task. This is called the **ALARA** concept—**As Low As Reasonably Achievable**—economic and social factors being taken into account.

In this chapter we discuss methods to minimize x-ray exposure to both the dental patient and the radiographer. Also, guidelines for prescribing dental radiographs and guides for maintaining safe radiation levels are discussed.

Protection Measures for the Patient

Using proper patient protection techniques, the radiation dose to the dental patient is very small. Patient protection techniques should be used at all times to keep radiation exposures as low as possible (see Table 6–1).

Guidelines for Prescribing Dental Radiographs

The initial step in keeping the patient's exposure to a minimum is the proper **prescribing (ordering) of the radiographs** by the dentist. The decision to use dental radiographs as diagnostic aids rests on the professional judgment of the dentist. Guidelines developed by an expert panel of dentists convened by the Public Health Service and adopted by the American Dental Association have been published to help the dentist decide when, what type, and how many radiographs should be taken (Table 6–2). The recommendations are subject to clinical judgment and may not apply to every patient. They are to be used by the dentist only after reviewing the patient's health history and completing a clinical examination. These guidelines do not need to be altered because of pregnancy.

The guidelines suggest that all new patients have a recent full-mouth radiographic examination before treatment begins. Recall patients should not have radiographs made as a "matter of routine," but only after determining their diagnostic needs. For instance, a decay-prone teenager may need radiographs more often than a middle-aged patient.

TABLE 6–1. **Summary Protections Methods for Patient**

Proper Prescribing
Safe Equipment
Collimation
Filtration
Open end, lead-lined PID
Modern timers
Preparing the Patient
Lead Aprons
Thyroid Collar
Exposing the Film
Fast Film
Film-holding devices
Proper Exposure Factors
Proper Technique
Optimum Film Processing

Safe Equipment

Using **proper equipment** is the next step in reducing exposure to the patient. Today, virtually all dental x-ray equipment in the United States is safe from a radiological health point of view. The Federal Performance Standard for Diagnostic X-ray Equipment became effective on August 1, 1974. The provisions of the Standard requires that all x-ray equipment manufactured after that date meet certain radiation safety requirements including collimation, filtration, position indicating device (PID), and timer.

Collimation

Collimation is the control of the size and shape of the useful beam. This is done by using a collimator, which is a lead diaphragm or washer (see Figure 6–1). The function of the **collimator** is to reduce the size of the x-ray beam and thus the volume of irradiated tissue.

The collimator is placed in the path of the **primary beam** as it exits the tube housing at the port (see Figure 6–2). Collimators may have either a round or a rectangular opening. Rectangular collimators restrict the beam to the approximate size of the film (see Figure 6–3). Most dental x-ray machines have round openings. Federal regulations require that round opening collimators restrict the x-ray beam to 2.75 in. (7 cm) at the patient end of the PID (see Figure 6–4). Figure 6–5 shows the circular collimator is larger than the outline of a number-2 film.

Collimation reduces **scatter radiation** (sometimes called **secondary radiation**). Scattered radiation is radiation that has been deflected from its path by impact during its passage through matter.

Collimation is the second most important factor (next to fast film) in reducing unnecessary radiation.

TABLE 6–2. **Guidelines for Prescribing Dental Radiographs**

Patient category	Child		Adolescent	Adult	
	Primary dentition (prior to eruption of first permanent tooth)	Transitional dentition (following eruption of first permanent tooth)	Permanent dentition (prior to eruption of third molars)	Dentulous	Edentulous
New patient					
All new patients to assess dental diseases and growth and development	Posterior bitewing examination if proximal surfaces of primary teeth cannot be visualized or probed posterior bitewings or panoramic	Individualized radiographic examination consisting of periapical/occlusal views and examination and posterior bitewings	Individualized radiographic examination consisting of posterior bitewings and selected periapicals. A full-mouth intraoral radiographic examination is appropriate when the patient presents with clinical evidence of generalized dental disease or a history of extensive dental treatment.		Full-mouth intraoral radiographic examination or panoramic examination
Recall patient					
Clinical caries or high-risk factors for caries	Posterior bitewing examination at 6-mo intervals or until no carious lesions are evident		Posterior bitewing examination at 6- to 12-mo intervals or until no carious lesions are evident	Posterior bitewing examination at 12- to 18-mo intervals	Not applicable
No clinical caries and no high-risk factors for caries	Posterior bitewing examination at 12- to 14-mo intervals if proximal surfaces of primary teeth cannot be visualized or probed	Posterior bitewing examination of 12- to 24-mo intervals	Posterior bitewing examination at 18- to 36-mo intervals	Posterior bitewing examination at 24- to 36-mo intervals	Not applicable
Periodontal disease or a history of periodontal treatment	Individualized radiographic examination consisting of selected periapical and or bitewing radiographs for areas where periodontal disease (other than nonspecific gingivitis) can be demonstrated clinically		Individualized radiographic examination consisting of selected periapical and bitewing radiographs for areas where periodontal disease (other than nonspecific gingivitis) can be demonstrated clinically		Not applicable
Growth and development assessment	Usually not indicated	Individualized radiographic examination consisting of a periapical occlusal or panoramic examination	Periapical or panoramic examination to assess developing third molars	Usually not indicated	Usually not indicated

Courtesy of the US Department of Health and Human Services

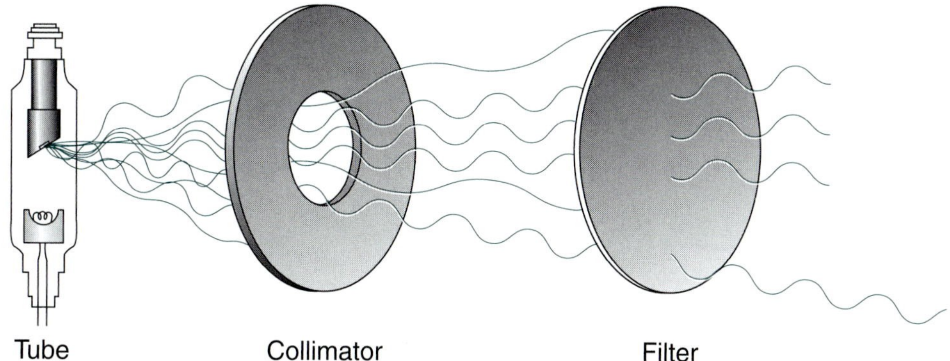

FIGURE 6–1. **Collimator and filter.** The **collimator** is a lead washer that restricts the size of the x-ray beam. The **filter** is an aluminum disc that filters (removes) the long wavelength x-rays.

Two important advantages of collimation are:

- Collimation reduces the radiation dose to the patient by reducing the volume of tissue exposed.
- Collimation reduces scatter radiation that causes poor contrast of the radiograph (see Chapter 4).

Filtration

Filtration is the absorption of the long wavelength, less penetrating, x-rays of the polychromatic x-ray beam by passage of the beam through a sheet of material called a **filter** (see Figure 6–1). A filter is an absorbing material (usually aluminum) placed in the path of the x-ray beam in order to remove a high percentage of the soft x-rays (the longer wavelengths).

In the dental x-ray machine, these filters are disks of pure aluminum that vary in thickness. Filters may be sealed into the tube head or inserted into the port where the PID attaches. Pure aluminum or its equivalent will not hinder the passage of high-energy x-rays but will absorb a

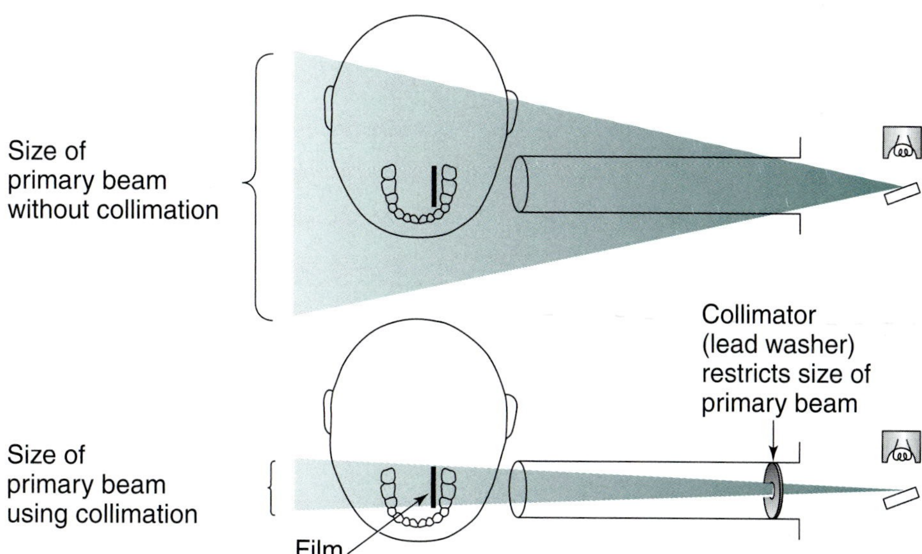

FIGURE 6–2. **Effect of collimation on primary beam.** Lead collimators control the shape and size of the primary beam. The beam is limited to the approximate size of the film.

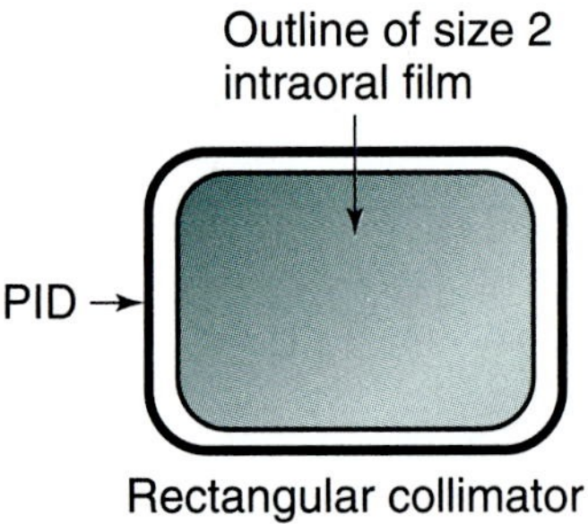

FIGURE 6-3. **The rectangular collimator** restricts the beam to the approximate size of a #2 film.

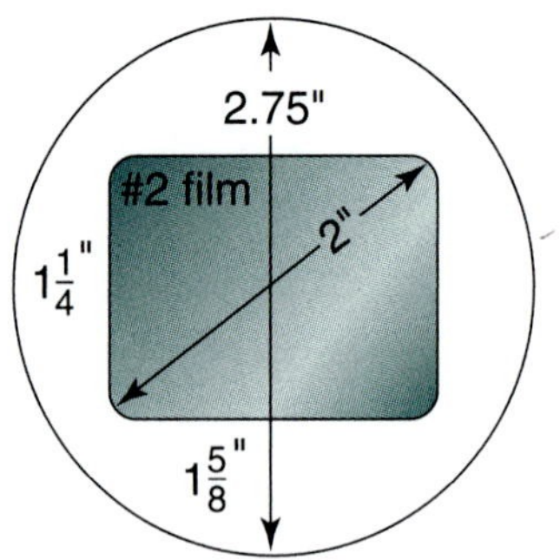

FIGURE 6-5. **Beam Size.** The 2.75 in (7 cm) **beam size** adequately exposes a #2 size intraoral film.

high percentage of the low-energy x-rays. The latter do not contribute to the radiographic image. However, they are harmful to the patient because they are absorbed by the skin and increase the patient's dose (see Figure 6–6).

Any material the x-ray beam passes through, filters the beam. Filtration may be built into the tube head (inherent) or it may be added.

Inherent filtration is the filtration built into the machine by the manufacturer. This includes the glass of the x-ray tube, the insulating oil, and the material that seals the port. All x-ray units have some built-in filtration. Usually the inherent filtration is not sufficient to meet state and federal standards, requiring filtration be added.

Added filtration is the placement of aluminum discs in the path of the x-ray beam between the port seal of the tube head and the PID. When the inherent filtration is not sufficient to meet present safety standards, a disk of aluminum of the appropriate thickness (usually 0.5 mm) can be inserted between the port of the tube head and the PID. Several manufacturers have introduced x-ray units in which the traditional aluminum filter is replaced with samarium, a rare-earth metal.

Total filtration is the sum of the inherent and added filtration expressed in millimeters of aluminum equivalent. Beam filtration must comply with state and federal laws. Present safety standards require an equivalent of 1.5 mm aluminum for x-ray machines operating in ranges below 70 kVp and a minimum of 2.5 mm aluminum for machines operating at or above 70 kVp.

Position Indicating Device (PID)

The **position indicating device (PID)** is an extension of the tube housing and is used to direct the primary x-ray beam. The length of the PID helps to establish the desired target-surface distance. PID's may be shaped as cones, cylinders, or rectangular tubes. Some dental radiographers use the term **beam indicating device (BID).** The term PID will be used in this textbook.

The pointed plastic cone was originally designed as an aiming device. The tip of the cone indicated the central ray and was aimed at the center of the film packet.

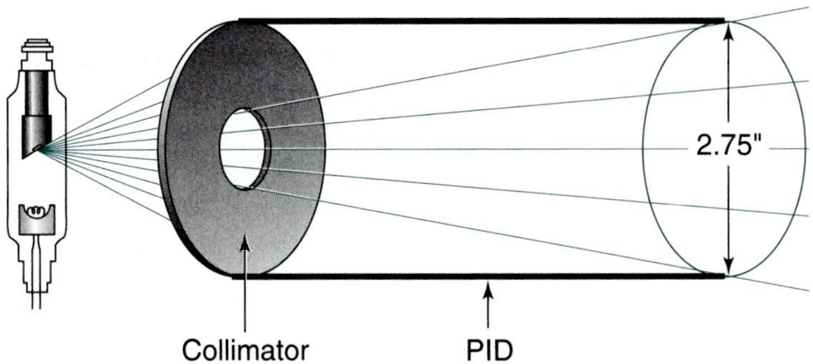

FIGURE 6-4. **The collimator** restricts the size of the primary beam to 2.75 in. (7 cm) at the end of the PID.

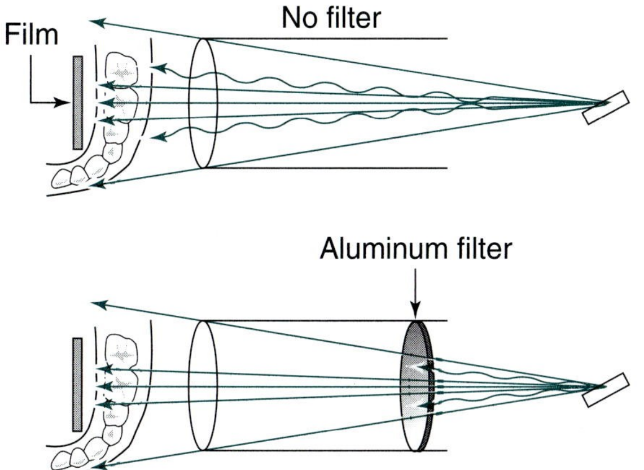

FIGURE 6–6. **Effect of filtration on skin exposure.** Aluminum filters selectively absorb the long wavelength x-rays.

When the pointed cones were first used, it was not realized that many of the x-rays were deflected through contact with the material of the cones, thus producing scatter radiation. Pointed plastic cones are no longer used in dentistry.

Today most PIDs are open-ended round cylinders. Rectangular, lead-lined PIDs are the most effective in reducing exposure to the patient. Because cones were used for so many years, many still refer to the open cylinders or rectangular tubes as cones. The term **position indicating device (PID)** is more descriptive of its function of directing the x-rays, rather than of its shape.

Modern PIDs are open-end and most commonly available in 8 in. (20 cm), 10 in. (25 cm), 12 in. (30 cm), and 16 in. (41 cm). All intraoral techniques require that the end of the PID should almost touch the skin. This is necessary to establish the desired target-surface distance. Longer distance is recommended because the rays are more parallel (see Chapter 4) and the beam is less divergent resulting in less tissue exposed (see Figure 6–7).

Timers

A **timer** is a device that can be set to predetermine the duration of time that the current flows through the x-ray machine to produce x-rays. Modern x-ray units are equipped with a vacuum-type electronic timer or timers with a transistorized circuit that are accurate up to 1/60-sec intervals. Some of the older x-ray machines that are still in use have mechanical timers that are not sufficiently accurate for modern high-speed film. Old spring wound mechanical timers are inconsistent when set for time intervals under one second. They should be replaced with modern timers.

Tube Head Drift

The **tube head** should be **stable** and not **drift,** or move, in any direction after it is positioned for an exposure (see Figure 6–8). Movement can cause a blurred image, or the x-ray beam may not be aligned with the film, resulting in a cone cut. If the tube head drifts, the extension arm should be adjusted or repaired immediately. The radiographer should never hold the PID or the tube head in place during an exposure.

Equipment Modifications for Safety

Some older x-ray machines lack adequate filtration, collimation, and PIDs. Their mechanical timers are not ac-

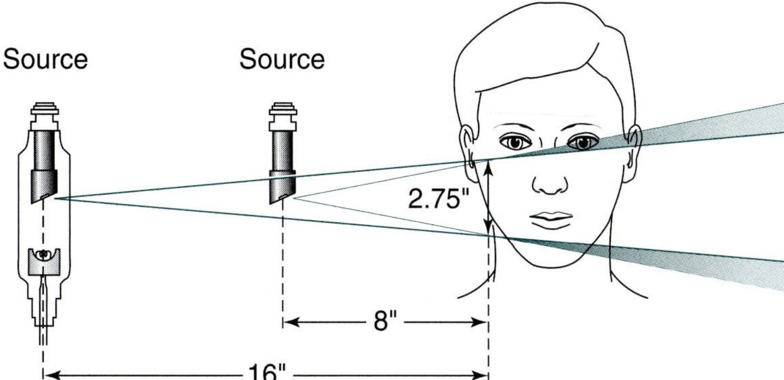

FIGURE 6–7. **Source-Film Distance.** The **longer** the **source-film distance,** the more parallel the rays and the less tissue exposed. Note the beam size at the end of the PID is 2.75 in. (7 cm).

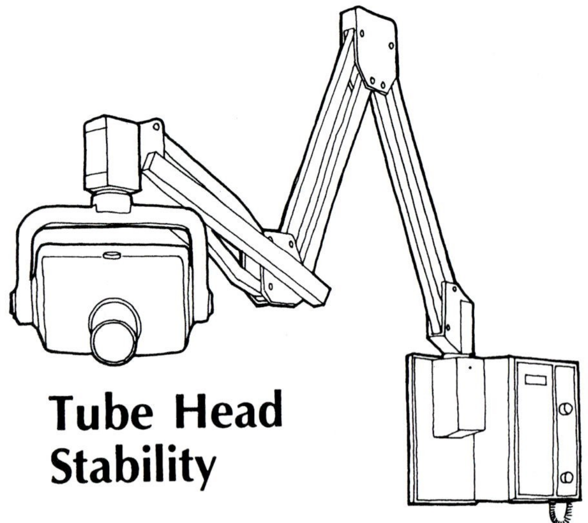

FIGURE 6–8. **Tube head should be stable and not drift after positioning for exposure.**

curate enough to measure the short exposure times used with high-speed films. Thus, they often fail to meet recommended safety standards. Some of these machines should be replaced, whereas others can be modified to make them safer.

The addition of aluminum disks of the proper thickness to meet the recommended standards will increase the filtration and reduce harmful low-energy radiation. Proper collimation will restrict the size of the primary beam. Replacing the closed plastic cone with an open-ended PID (especially one with lead lining) further reduces scatter radiation. And replacing the mechanical timer with an electronic one will permit shorter exposure times. These modifications can be made at a modest expense and improve both safety and the diagnostic quality of the radiograph.

Preparing the Patient

Discuss with the patient the radiation protection methods used to keep exposure to a minimum. Explain what radiographs will be taken and why they are necessary.

Lead Apron

A **lead apron** is an apron made of .25-mm lead or lead-equivalent materials (see Figure 6–9). It is placed over the patient's body to protect the reproductive organs and other radiosensitive tissues from scatter radiation. All patients should be draped with a lead apron in preparation for all x-ray exposures.

Lead aprons should be stored flat or hung unbent. **DO NOT FOLD OR BEND LEAD APRONS.** The material may crack and become defective.

Several states have laws requiring the use of a lead apron over the abdominal area. Even if it is not legally required, the use of a lead apron is important, especially for women in the reproductive age and for children. Keeping with the ALARA concept, lead aprons should be used on all patients.

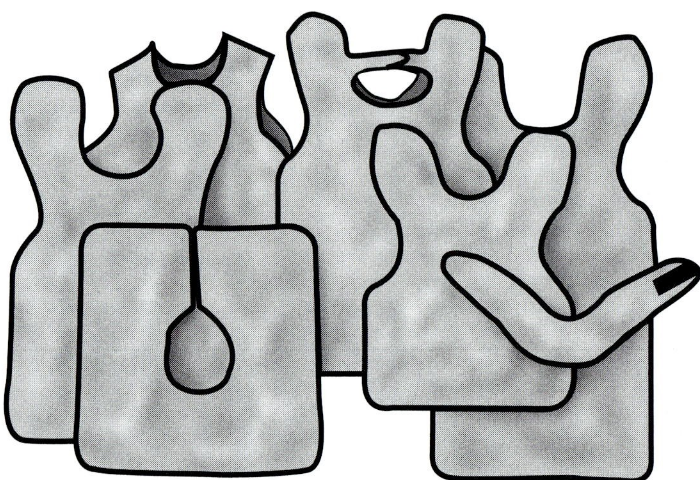

FIGURE 6–9. **Lead aprons and thyroid collars.** This assortment shows aprons and collars in child and adult sizes. The thyroid collar may be separate or be a part of the larger lead apron. (Courtesy of Dentsply/Rinn Corporation)

Thyroid Collar

Additional protection can be derived from the use of a **thyroid collar** (see Figure 6–9). The thyroid collar contains lead or lead-equivalent material and protects the radiosensitive thyroid gland in the neck region. The thyroid collar may be used separately or as part of the lead apron. Its use is not appropriate when using rotational panoramic equipment because the collar or upper part of the apron to which it is attached may obscure diagnostic information or interfere with the rotation of the panoramic unit.

Exposing the Film

Another radiation safeguard is to use the largest film that can be placed comfortably in the patient's mouth, so that fewer films and exposures are needed. However, this is not always practical. Sometimes smaller films are needed to avoid bending, which distorts the image.

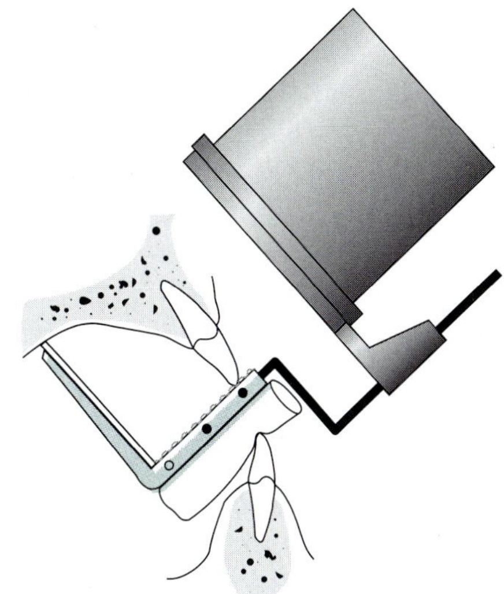

FIGURE 6–10. **Anterior film-holding device.** (Courtesy of Dentsply/Rinn Corporation)

Fast Film (High-Speed Film)

Fast film requires less radiation for exposure and is essential from the standpoint of exposure reduction. In fact, high-speed film is the single most effective method of reducing unnecessary radiation to the patient. Currently, intraoral dental x-ray film is available in three speed groups, D, E and F, and are the only film speed groups that should be used. E-speed film, when compared to D-speed film, is twice as fast and therefore requires only one-half the exposure time. The new F-speed film will reduce radiation exposure 20% compared to E-speed film. The American Dental Association recommends the use of speed group E or faster and that film slower than speed group D should not be used.

Film-Holding Devices

Film-holding devices that align the x-ray beam with the film in the patient's mouth are recommended (see Figure 6–10). These devices stabilize the film in the mouth and reduce the possibility of cone cutting. Filmholders should never be held in place by the radiographer. The use of film holders affords the patient additional protection by reducing the number of retakes and avoids having the patient hold the film with the fingers.

Proper Exposure Factors

Operating the dental x-ray machine includes selecting the **proper exposure factors**—kilovoltage (kVp), milliamperage (mA), and time. Proper exposure factors should be used for optimum density and contrast of the radiograph.

The selection of either high (90 kVp) or low (70 kVp) kilovoltage should be made depending on contrast preference. As we learned in Chapter 4, both milliamperage (mA) and time control the density of the radiograph. If either is too great, the film will be overexposed (too dark). If either is too small, the film will be underexposed (too light). Both overexposed and underexposed radiographs result in unnecessary exposure to the patient. Exposure charts should be posted near the control panel.

Proper Technique

The student should make every effort to master the technique of making radiographs. Techniques used most often are paralleling (right angle), bisecting angle, anterior and posterior bitewing, and occlusal. Poorly made radiographs that are nondiagnostic need to be retaken resulting in unnecessary radiation. Both the dental radiographer and the dentist should perfect their technique so that retakes are unnecessary.

Optimum Film Processing and Handling

Proper darkroom procedures should be followed (see Chapter 8). Always **process** film using time-temperature techniques in an adequately equipped darkroom. Some dental offices overexpose and underdevelop the film in order to save time. This results in needless exposure to the patient and films of inferior quality.

Films should be **handled properly** to prevent scratches and artifacts (see Chapter 9). Nondiagnostic radiographs must be retaken and results in unnecessary radiation to the patient.

Protection Measures for the Operator

Basic radiation protection methods for the radiographer are time, distance and shielding. One should spend the least amount of time, at the greatest distance, with the most shielding, to receive the least exposure to radiation. All the radiation protection measures we have discussed to protect the patient also benefit the operator (see Table 6–3).

Time

In dentistry, the time factor is very small because of the fast film used. Exposure times for dental radiographs are only fractions of a second.

TABLE 6-3. **Summary Methods to Protect the Operator**

Patient Protection Measures and:
Time
Use fast film.
Distance
Stand at least 6 ft (1.82 m) from the head of the patient.
Stay out of the primary beam.
Never hold film for the patient.
Never hold the tube head.
Shielding
Use protective barriers, if necessary

Distance

Distance is an important safeguard for operator protection. The operator should always stand as far away as practical—at least 6 ft (1.8 m)—from the head of the patient (the source of scatter radiation) while making the exposure. The intensity of the x-radiation diminishes the farther the x-rays travel (see Figure 6–11). A careless op-

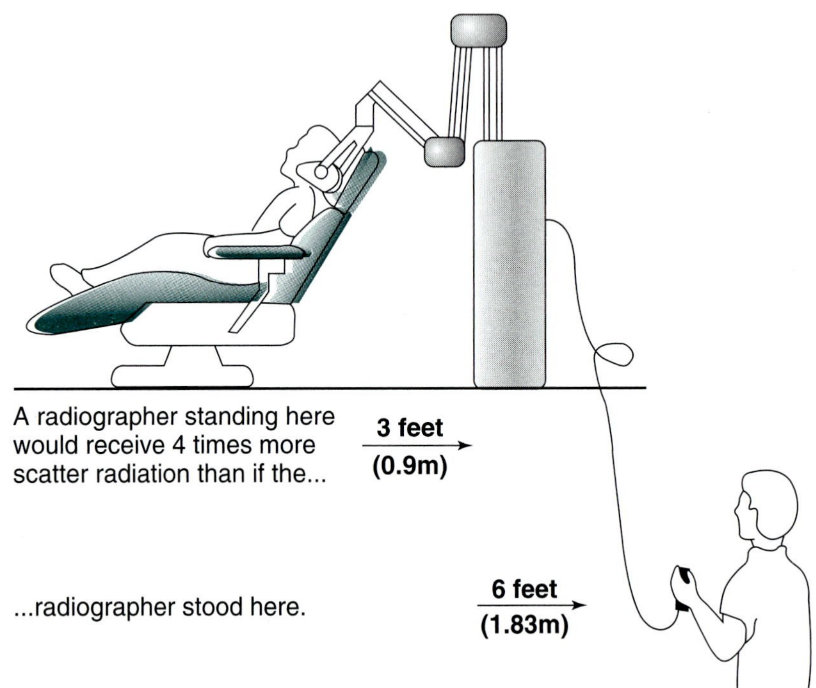
A radiographer standing here would receive 4 times more scatter radiation than if the...
3 feet
(0.9m)
...radiographer stood here.
6 feet
(1.83m)

FIGURE 6-11. **Distance** is an effective means of reducing exposure from scatter radiation.

erator who stands close to the patient while making an exposure can receive unnecessary scatter radiation. Another important rule is never to hold the film for the patient or stabilize the tube head or the PID.

The safest place for the operator to stand is from 90 to 135 degrees out of the primary beam, behind the bulkiest part of the patient's head (see Figure 6–12). The head thus absorbs most of the primary beam and much of the scatter radiation. All persons not directly concerned with the x-ray exposure should leave the room.

Shielding

Shielding is rarely necessary in a dental office because of the use of fast film and small beam diameter. When shielding is required, the National Council on Radiation Protection and Measurements (NCRP) report number 35, "Dental X-ray Protection" should be consulted. Lead-lined walls, thick or specially constructed partitions between the rooms, or specially constructed lead screens afford excellent protection for the operator.

Radiation Measuring Devices

The problem of radiation measurement is complicated because radiation-measuring instruments can measure only radiation received at the skin surface but not that within the body. One may attach a measuring device to the skin surface at one side of the face to determine the **entrance dose** (also called **skin exposure**) and attach another meter to the other side of the face to determine the **exit dose.** However, one may only estimate the **depth dose,** or amount of dose between entrance and exit, by considering such factors as the distance from the point of entrance or exit, the quality of the radiation, and the types of intervening tissues. Computers are now being used to estimate depth doses.

The same holds true when attempting to estimate radiation to genetic tissues. The size and sex of the patient make a difference, the gonads of a child being closer to the source of radiation than those of an adult and the female reproductive organs being better protected by the abdominal structures than those of the male.

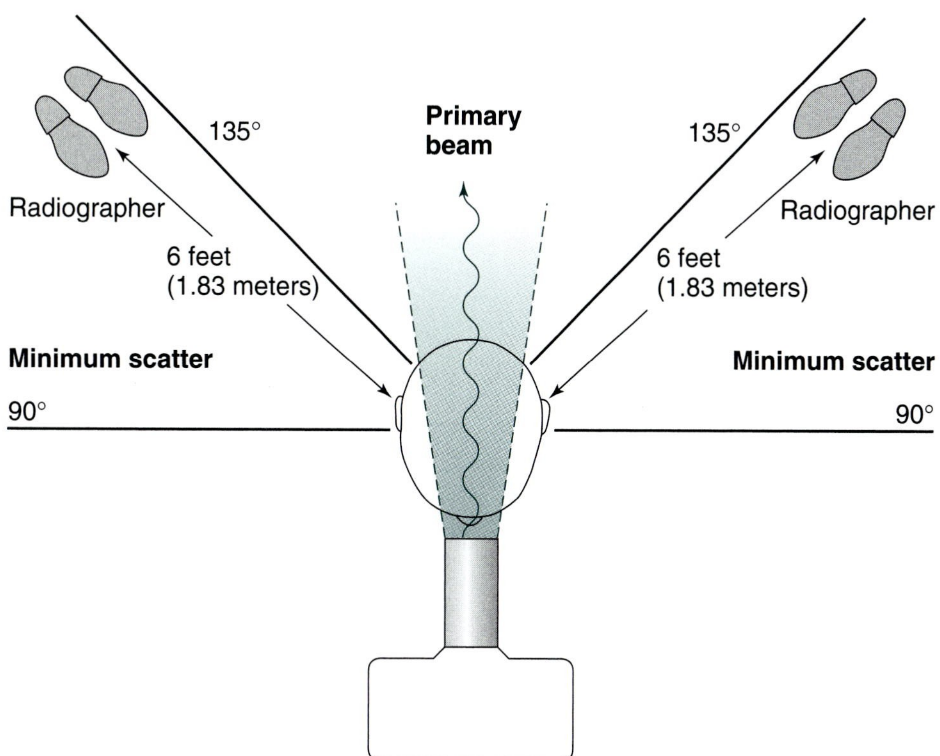

FIGURE 6–12. Always **stand** at least 6 ft (1.83 m) from the head of the patient at 135° angle, out of the primary beam.

Figures dealing with exposure and dosage can be very misleading. It makes a difference whether all of the body is exposed or only a small area of the face. Obviously the dose received in an internal organ is less than that received by the skin because the intervening tissue absorbs some of the radiation. Also, the strength of the radiation beam diminishes inversely proportionally to the square of the distance from the source. Another variable is the density of the structures through which the rays are directed.

Although effects of radiation on patients are difficult to determine and depth doses difficult to measure, it is possible to measure accurately the amount of radiation on a monitoring badge or similar device. These will be described later in this chapter.

Structural Modifications

A **protective barrier** is a radiation absorbing material used to reduce radiation exposure. Many states have the following protective barrier requirements for dental rooms containing x-ray machines.

1. All areas struck by the useful beam must be provided with protective barriers.
2. Protective barriers must be provided between the x-ray rooms and nearby operatories or hallways.
3. Each installation must be arranged so that the operator can stand at least 6 ft (1.8 m) from the patient and away from the x-ray beam or provide a protective barrier for the operator.

When these conditions cannot be met by relocating the x-ray machines or equipment in adjacent operatories, structural modifications must be made. In many cases structural materials of ordinary walls will suffice as a protective barrier without additional special shielding material. A wall made of two thicknesses of 5/8-in. (16 mm) gypsum board (1/4 in. or 32 mm total) can be assumed to provide protection from scattered radiation if the following conditions are met:

1. The occupiable areas protected by the wall are at least 6 ft (1.8 m) from the dental x-ray chair.
2. The use of the x-ray equipment does not exceed 60 sec/week of "on time" at 90 kVp or 100 sec per week of "on time" at 65 kVp.

The average dental office can usually meet these conditions by proper planning. Gypsum board or plastered walls will provide adequate protection. The primary beam can be directed toward an outside wall or into an unoccupied area. When a receptionist sits immediately adjacent to the wall receiving the primary beam, additional structural shielding in the form of lead sheathing with a thickness of 1/32 in. (0.8 mm) may be needed. When properly located, such lead shielding is almost always adequate in the dental office. The thickness and locations or those barriers should be determined by an individual qualified in x-ray shielding design.

Radiation Monitoring

The only way to make sure that x-ray equipment is not emitting too much radiation and people are not receiving more than the maximum permissible dose is to use monitoring devices. In radiography, **monitoring** is defined as periodic or continuing measurement to determine the dose rate in a given area or the dose received by a person.

Radiation has four qualities that make accurate measurements possible: It affects photographic emulsions, produces ionization in air, produces a rise in temperature, and causes certain salts to fluoresce. All measuring devices make use of one of these qualities.

Area Monitoring

Area monitoring involves making an on-site survey to measure the output of the dental x-ray unit, to check for possible high-level radiation areas in the room, and to determine if any radiation is passing through walls. Special equipment is needed to detect the exact amount of ionizing radiation at any given area. Numerous firms specialize in monitoring. In some regions, this service may be performed at the dentist's request by qualified state personnel.

Personnel Monitoring

Personnel monitoring requires office staff members to wear a device that measures how much radiation they are receiving. Monitoring devices vary in cost and effectiveness. Some merely indicate that radiation has been received; others show the amount, and still others measure the amount and type of radiation. In hospitals, industrial plants, and some dental offices, everyone working around radiation is required to wear a monitoring device at all times while on duty. The monitoring badge (discussed later in this chapter) is sufficiently accurate and economical to be worn in the dental office. More and more dentists are providing monitoring devices and services for themselves and their employees. Monitoring badges are mandatory in several states.

Personnel Monitoring Devices

A **personnel monitoring device** is a device worn by a person working around radiation used to measure and monitor radiation exposure. The personnel monitoring device does not "protect" the wearer form radiation. But it does alert the wearer to exposures higher than anticipated. If this happens, the wearer should reevaluate the radiation safety procedures in the dental office.

The forerunner of these devices used in the dental office was an unexposed film to which a paper clip was attached. One wore it in a pocket with the clip and the exposure side of the film facing toward the outside. The film was developed at intervals ranging from 1 to 3 months. Although extremely simple and economical, the shortcoming was that this homemade film badge showed only that radiation had been received and failed to record the amount of radiation.

Film Badge

The **film badge** is a descendant of the paper clip device. Firms provide a film badge service on a subscription basis. Each subscriber is supplied with a badge loaded with a radiosensitive film. The plastic or metal holder is lined with various thickness of filters of different materials that make it possible to measure the types of radiation received. Film badges are not accurate at very low exposures.

Thermoluminescent Dosimeter (TLD)

Film badges are being replaced by a radiation detection device called a **thermoluminescent dosimeter (TLD)** (from the Greek word *therme*, meaning heat, and the Latin words *lumen*, meaning light, and ascent, meaning any giving off of light caused by absorption of radiant energy). Those devices have crystals, usually lithium fluoride, that absorb energy when exposed to radiation. When the crystals are heated, after being exposed to radiation, energy in the form of visible light is given off. The total light emitted is proportional to the amount of radiation (energy) absorbed by the crystals. TLDs are extremely accurate.

TLD Badges

Several manufacturers make **TLD badges** and offer a monitoring service that includes periodic reports to the subscriber. The typical TLD badge (see Figure 6–13) is small, lightweight, has a clip for attachment to the clothes or uniform, and should be worn throughout the workday.

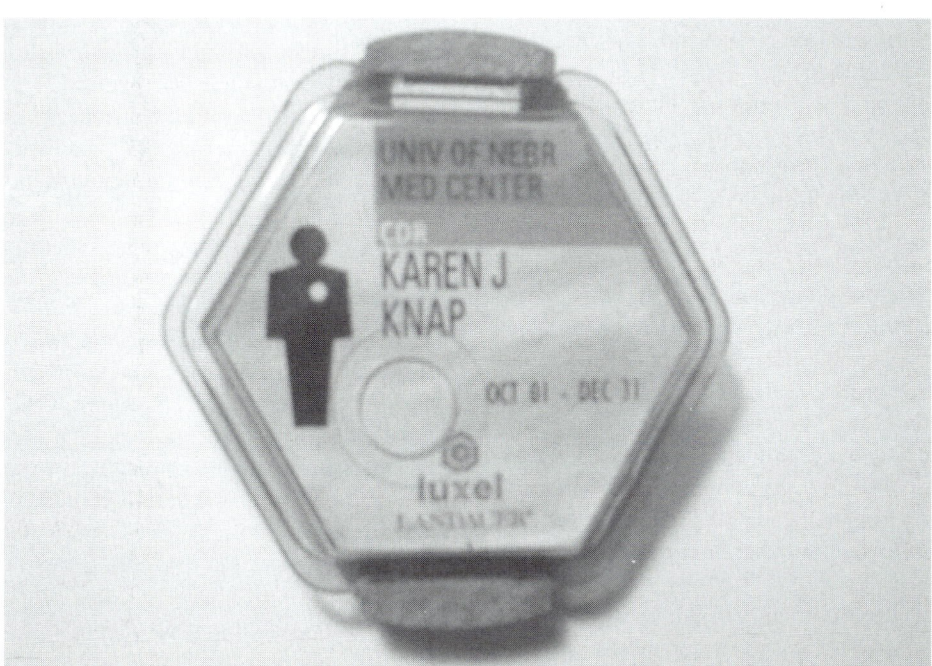

FIGURE 6-13. A **TLD badge** that is worn by the radiographer and used for radiation measurement.

These badges are easy to load and have no dials to set or read. Each badge is identified by a number, the wearer's name, and the dates on which the badge will be used. All that is necessary is to periodically replace the packet of crystals and mail it in to be read. At agreed monitoring periods, generally 1 month, the subscriber receives an easy-to-read report that compares each person's exposure reading with the maximum allowable level. The monitoring firm updates the subscriber's records to keep the wearer in full compliance with all federal and state safety regulations.

The wearing of TLD badges is not mandatory in every state; however, for maximum protection, a TLD badge is recommended for each person working directly with radiation or other personnel subject to radiation exposure.

Studies on Radiation Exposure

As early as 1902, some studies were undertaken to determine the effect of radiation exposure on the body and to consider setting limits on radiation exposure. The international Commission on Radiation Protection was formed in 1928, and in 1929 the National Council on Radiation Protection and Measurements (NCRP) was created in the United States. The American Dental Association (ADA), through its various committees and affiliated organizations, works closely with all organizations interested in radiation safety. It will send its publications to those who write for them.

The NCRP has proposed two sets of limits, one for occupationally exposed persons working in radiography or with radioactive materials (dentists, dental assistants, dental hygienists, and radiography technicians) and the other for the general population. These limits do not apply to medical or dental radiation used for diagnostic or therapeutic purposes. The maximum limits were set higher for workers than for the public, but the suggested limits of the maximum permissible accumulated dose for both groups were purposely set far lower than it was believed the body could safely accept.

Over the years, the acceptable limits have been constantly revised downward; they are now about 700 times smaller than those originally proposed in 1902. Many aspects of tissue damage from radiation are still not clearly understood.

Although the NCRP and similar organizations have no legal status, their suggestions and recommendations are highly regarded. Many regulatory bodies have used them to formulate legislation controlling the use of radiation in the dental office. Three publications are recommended for obtaining additional information concerning radiation protection: (1) NCRP Report No. 35 [*Dental X-ray Protection*, Washington, DC, 1970]; (2) NCRP Report No. 39 [*Basic Radiation Protection Criteria*, Washington, DC, 1971]; and NCRP Report No. 91 [*Recommendations on Limits for Exposure to Ionizing Radiation*, Washington, DC, 1987]. (See this chapter's Bibliography for further listings.)

Guides for Maintaining Safe Radiation Levels

Radiation Safety Legislation

The Tenth Amendment gives the states the constitutional authority to regulate health. Because many federal agencies are involved in the development and use of atomic energy, the federal government has preempted the control of radiation. Certain provisions of the Constitution and Public Law 86-373 have enabled the states to assume this preempted power and pass laws that spell out radiation safety measures to protect the patient, the operator, or anyone (the general public) near the source of radiation. In fact, even counties and cities have passed ordinances to protect their citizens from radiation hazards. Most states and a few localities require periodic inspection or monitoring of the equipment and its surroundings.

The entry of the federal government into the regulation of x-ray machines began in 1968 with the enactment of the Radiation Control for Health and Safety Act, which standardizes the performance of x-ray equipment. Subsequently the Consumer-Patient Radiation Health and Safety Act of 1981 was passed requiring the various states to develop minimum standards for operators of dental x-ray equipment.

Since the laws concerning radiation control vary greatly, individuals working with x-rays are urged to become familiar with the major provisions of their own state or local radiation code and observe its requirements. Regardless of laws, failure to observe safety procedures cannot be justified morally. Many excellent booklets and articles on radiation safety and radiation hygiene methods are available. Especially recommended are National Council on Radiation Protection and Measurements (NCRP) Report Nos. 35, 39, and 43, which are available at nominal cost. These are listed in the bibliography.

Maximum Permissible Dose (MPD)

The National Council on Radiation Protection and Measurements (NCRP) developed radiation protection guides referred to as the **maximum permissible dose (MPD)** for the protection of radiation workers and the general public. Maximum permissible dose is defined as the dose equivalent of ionizing radiation that, in the light of present knowledge, is not expected to cause detectable body damage to average persons at any time during their lifetime. The guides represent doses far below those at which any effects have ever been observed.

Radiation Workers

The maximum permissible dose (MPD) for dentists and dental personnel is the same as for other **radiation workers.** According to these guidelines, the whole-body dose may not exceed **50 mSv (5 rem) per year.** There is no established weekly limit, but state public health personnel usually use a weekly dose of 1.0 mSv (0.1 rem) when inspecting dental offices. There are some exceptions to these guidelines; the skin of the whole body, the hands and forearms, and the feet and ankles may receive larger doses.

The 50 mSv (5 rem) yearly limit for radiation workers has two very important exceptions. It does not apply to persons under 18 years or to any female members of the dental team—whether dentist, assistant, or hygienist—who are known to be pregnant. Persons under 18 years are classified as part of the general public and can accumulate only 5 mSv (0. 5 rem) per year. In the case of pregnant women, it is recommended the fetus be limited to 5 mSv (0.5 rem), not to be received at a rate greater than 0.5 mSv (0.05 rem) per month. The wearing of a monitoring device, while not mandatory, is a good procedure in these circumstances.

The reports from any monitoring service are the most reliable permanent records of accumulated doses. If a worker's monitoring device indicates that the average weekly or monthly levels are frequently exceeded, there is justifiable cause for concern. All techniques should be reviewed for errors, and the x-ray machine should be tested for leakage.

An older accumulated lifetime radiation dose, referred to as the maximum accumulated dose (MAD) is obsolete and is no longer used. Its formula for occupational workers was $(N - 18) \times 5$ rem/year, where N referred to the worker's age in years.

General Public

The general public is permitted **5 mSv (0.5 rem) per year** or one-tenth the dose permitted radiation workers. This was done because workers represent only a small fraction of the total population. Also it was believed that if they suffer greater genetic damage than the general population, the damaged hereditary material would be so diluted in the general population that it will not result in a disastrous mutation level. Radiation necessary for medical or dental diagnostic purposes is not counted in the permissible amounts of radiation.

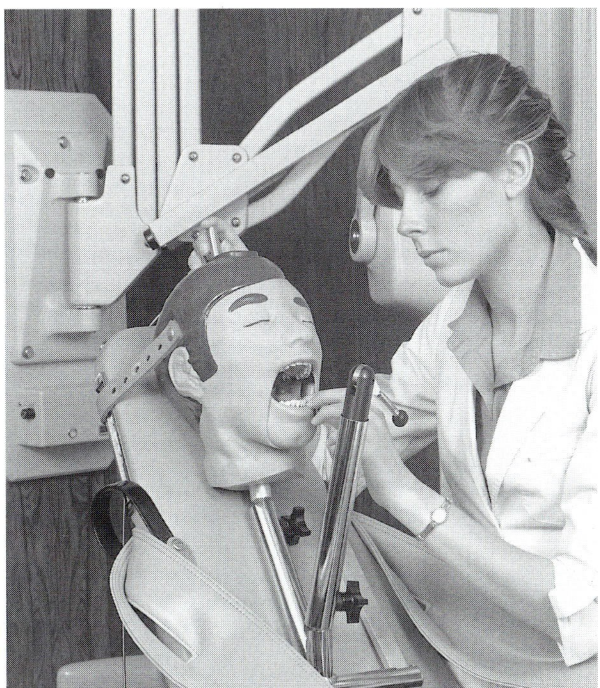

FIGURE 6–14. **Dental x-ray teaching and training replica (DXTTR).** The phantom (pronounced "dexter") is used by students to gain proficiency in making dental radiographs before exposing patients. (Courtesy of Dentsply/Rinn Corporation)

Guides for Students

Guides are also established for students. Until the student gains some degree of proficiency, all radiographic exposures must be made on a skull, dummy, or **phantom** known as **DXTTR**—dental x-ray teaching training replica—pronounced "dexter" (see Figure 6–14).

Helpful Reminders

- Avoid the primary beam.
- Never hold film in the patient's mouth.
- Stand at least 6 ft from the patient's head.
- Never overexpose or underdevelop dental x-ray film.
- Always use a lead apron.

CHAPTER SUMMARY

One of the cardinal principles in radiography is to use the least radiation needed to perform the task. This is called the **ALARA** concept—**A**s **L**ow **A**s **R**easonably **A**chievable—economic and social factors being taken into account.

The initial step in keeping the patient's exposure to a minimum is the proper prescribing (ordering) of the radiographs by the dentist.

Collimation is the control of the size and shape of the useful beam. Federal regulations require that round opening collimators restrict the x-ray beam to 2.75 in. (7 cm) at the patient end of the PID.

Filtration is the absorption of the long wavelength, less penetrating, x-rays of the x-ray beam by passage of the beam through a sheet of material called a **filter.** Present safety standards require an equivalent of 1.5 mm aluminum for x-ray machines operating in ranges below 70 kVp and a minimum of 2.5 mm aluminum for machines operating at or above 70 kVp.

The **position indicating device (PID)** is an extension of the tube housing and is used to direct the primary x-ray beam. The length of the PID helps to establish the desired target-surface distance. PID's may be shaped as cones, cylinders, or rectangular tubes.

Discuss with the patient the radiation protection methods used to keep exposure to a minimum. Explain what radiographs will be taken and why they are necessary.

All patients should be draped with a lead apron in preparation for all x-ray exposures.

Fast film requires less radiation for exposure. Use speed group D, E or F.

Operation of the dental x-ray machine includes selection of the proper **exposure factors**—kilovoltage (kVp), milliamperage (mA), and time. Proper exposure factors should be used for optimum density and contrast of the radiograph.

Always process film using time-temperature techniques in an adequately equipped darkroom. Radiographs should be handled properly to prevent scratches and artifacts.

The operator should always stand as far away as practical—at least 6 ft. (1.8 m)—from the head of the patient (the source of scatter radiation) while making the exposure.

A TLD badge is recommended for each person working directly with radiation or other personnel subject to radiation exposure.

The maximum permissible dose (MPD) is 50 mSv (5 rem) per year for radiation workers and 5 mSv (0.5 rem) for the general public, radiation workers who are pregnant, and children under 18 years of age.

REVIEW QUESTIONS

1. Who has the legal responsibility for all acts and services performed in the dental office?
   (a) The dental hygienist
   (b) The dental technician
   (c) The dental assistant
   (d) The dentist

2. Which of these terms best describes the x-rays that are coming directly from the focal spot on the target of the x-ray tube?
   (a) Filtered beam
   (b) Secondary beam
   (c) Primary beam
   (d) Scatter beam

3. Who is the only person who should be in the path of the primary beam?
   (a) The dentist
   (b) The patient
   (c) The dental assistant
   (d) The receptionist

4. In normal dental radiographic procedures, the principal hazard to the operator is produced by:
   (a) Direct radiation.
   (b) Scattered radiation.
   (c) Gamma radiation.
   (d) Alpha radiation.

5. What is a device that restricts the size of the x-ray beam called?
   (a) A dosimeter
   (b) A filter
   (c) A collimator
   (d) A primary barrier

6. What material is the collimator made of?
   (a) Copper
   (b) Tungsten
   (c) Samarium
   (d) Lead

7. The purpose of the collimator is to:
   (a) Shape the x-ray beam.
   (b) Remove many of the long wavelength x-rays.
   (c) Increase the energy of the x-ray beam.
   (d) Increase scatter radiation.

8. The purpose of the filter is to:
   (a) Shape the x-ray beam.
   (b) Remove many of the long wavelength x-rays from the primary beam.
   (c) Remove many of the short wavelength x-rays from the primary beam.
   (d) Prevent tube head leakage.

9. What is the minimum total filtration that is required by an x-ray machine that can operate in ranges above 70 kVp?
   (a) 1.5 mm of aluminum equivalent
   (b) 5/8 in. (16 mm) of gypsum
   (c) 2.5 mm of aluminum equivalent
   (d) 1/32 in. (0.8 mm) of lead

10. What is the recommended minimum distance that the operator should stand from the source of the radiation?
    (a) 16 in. (41 cm)
    (b) 3 ft (0.91 m)
    (c) 6 ft (1.83 m)
    (d) 9 ft (2.74m)

11. What is the recommended size of the diameter of the primary beam at the end of the PID (at the skin of the patient's face)?
    (a) 2.75 in. (7 cm)
    (b) 3.25 in. (8.2 cm)
    (c) 4.50 in. (11.4 cm)
    (d) 5 in. (12.7 cm)

12. Total filtration is the sum of the ______ and ______ filtration expressed in millimeters of ______

13. The collimator is used to control the ______ and ______ of the useful beam.

14. The filter is an absorbing material usually made of ______.

15. The filter is placed in the path of the beam of radiation in order to remove a high percentage of the ______ wavelength x-rays.

16. A dentist is using a personnel monitoring service to measure radiation exposure. The monitoring report indicates that the TLD badge received 4.75 mSv (475 millirems) in the preceding month. The dentist should:
    (a) Stop taking radiographs immediately.
    (b) Use a slower film to reduce the mAs.
    (c) Report to a physician for a blood count.
    (d) Reevaluate the office radiation safety procedures.

17. The maximum permissible whole-body dose for dental personnel is:
    (a) 10 mSv (1 rem) per month.
    (b) 50 mSv (5 rem) per year.
    (c) 5 mSv (0.5 rem) per year.
    (d) 0.5 mSv (.05 rem) per year.

18. The maximum permissible dose for the general public is ______.

BIBLIOGRAPHY

ADA Council on Scientific Affairs. *An Update on Radiographic Practices: Information and Recommendations*. J. Am. Dent. Assn. 2001;132:234–238.

Eastman Kodak: *Radiation Safety in Dental Radiography*. Rochester, NY: Eastman Kodak, 1998.

National Council on Radiation Protection and Measurements. *Implementation of the Principle of As Low As Reasonably Achievable (ALARA) for Medical and Dental Personnel*. Washington, DC: NCRP, 1991. NCRP report no. 107.

National Council on Radiation Protection and Measurements. *Recommendations on Limits for Exposure to Ionizing Radiation*. Washington, DC: NCRP, 1987. NCRP report no. 91.

National Council on Radiation Protection and Measurements. *Review of NCRP Dose Limit for Embryo and Fetus in Occupationally Exposed Women*. Washington, DC: NCRP; 1977. NCRP report no. 53.

National Council on Radiation Protection and Measurements. *Review of the Current State of Radiation Protection Philosophy*. Washington, DC: NCRP; 1975. NCRP, report no. 43.

National Council on Radiation Protection and Measurements: *Basic Radiation Protection Criteria*. Washington, DC: NCRP; 1971. NCRP report no. 39.

National Council on Radiation Protection and Measurements. *Dental X-ray Protection*. Washington, DC: NCRP, 1970. NCRP report no. 35.

U.S. Department of Health and Human Services: *The Selection of Patients for X-ray Examinations: Dental Radiographic Examinations*. Rockville, MD: U.S. Department of Health and Human Services; 1987. HHS Publication (FDA) 88–8273.

PART III: Dental X-ray Film and Processing Techniques

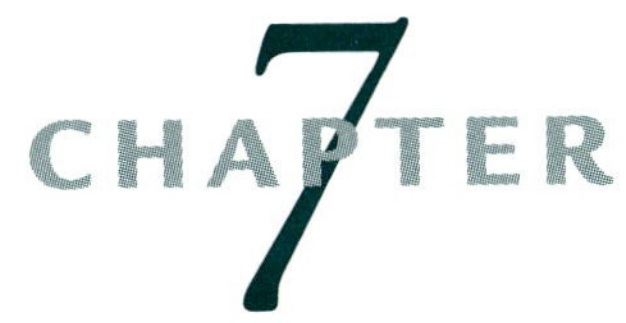

Dental X-ray Film

OBJECTIVES

By the end of this chapter the student should be able to:

- Define the key words.
- Discuss the composition of dental x-ray film.
- Describe latent image formation.
- Differentiate between screen and nonscreen films.
- Identify the contents in dental x-ray film packets.
- Identify and compare the various intraoral films according to size, customary usage, and film speed.
- Differentiate between intraoral and extraoral films.
- Identify the parts and intended use of the extraoral cassette.
- Describe duplicating film.
- Discuss correct methods of film storage and protection.

KEY WORDS

Bitewing radiograph
Cassette
Duplicating film
Emulsion
Extraoral film
Film packet
Film sensitivity
Film speed
Halide
Identification dot
Intensifying screen
Intraoral film
Latent image
Nonscreen film
Occlusal radiograph
Pedodontic film
Periapical radiograph
Phosphors
Screen film

Introduction

The films used in dental radiology are photographic films that have been adapted to dental use. A photographic image is produced on the film when it is exposed to x-rays that have passed through the teeth and oral structures. X-ray film serves as an image receptor by recording the image.

The purpose of this chapter is to explain film composition and latent image, to describe the types of intraoral and extraoral film, and to discuss film protection and storage.

Composition of Dental X-Ray Films

Dental x-ray films are very similar to those used in photography; in fact, the first dental radiograph was made on a photographic plate a few weeks after Roentgen announced the discovery of the x-ray. Dr. Otto Walkhoff, given credit for taking the first dental x-ray picture, inserted an ordinary glass photographic plate, protected against light and moisture by an inner wrapping of black paper and an outer wrapping of rubber dam, into his mouth and exposed it. Although film emulsions and film packing have undergone many changes since that time, the fundamentals have not. The films used in dental radiography are photographic films that have been especially adapted in size, emulsion, film speed, and packaging to dental uses. Figure 7–1 is a schematic cross-sectional drawing of dental x-ray film.

Film Base

The purpose of the **film base** is to provide support for the fragile emulsion and to provide strength for handling.

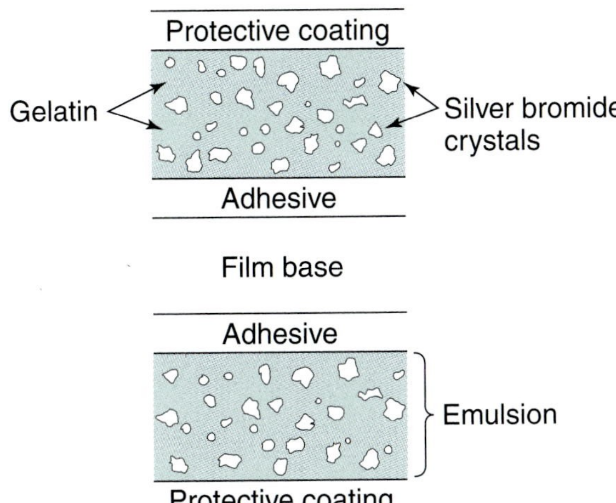

FIGURE 7–1. **Schematic cross-section drawing of dental x-ray film.** The rigid, but flexible **film base** is coated on both sides with an **emulsion** consisting of **silver bromide** (or other halide) **crystals** embedded in **gelatin.** Each emulsion layer is attached to the base by a thin layer of **adhesive.** The emulsion layers are covered by a supercoating of gelatin to protect the emulsion from scratching and rough handling.

Films used in dental radiography have a thin, flexible, clear or blue-tinted polyester base. The blue tint enhances contrast and image quality. The base is 0.008-in. (0.2-mm) thick—the thickness deemed necessary for proper handling and manipulation—and is covered with a photographic emulsion on both sides.

Emulsion

The **emulsion** is composed of **gelatin** in which **crystals** of silver halide salts are suspended. **Halides** are compounds of a halogen (fluorine, chlorine, bromine, or iodine) with another element—in photography, silver. Silver is most frequently combined with bromine in dental films. Each emulsion layer is attached to the base by a thin layer of adhesive. A supercoating of gelatin to protect the emulsion from scratching and rough handling covers the emulsion layers.

The function of the gelatin is to keep the silver halide crystals evenly suspended over the base. The gelatin will not dissolve in cold water, but swells, thus exposing the silver halide crystals to the chemicals in the developing solution. The gelatin shrinks as it dries, leaving a smooth surface that becomes the radiograph.

This emulsion is sensitive to light, radiation, heat, chemical fumes, and bending. Great care must be taken not to expose the film accidentally to radiation, extreme heat, chemical fumes, or light. Minor bending can crack the surface of the emulsion, and major bending may loosen the protective wrapping and let in moisture or light.

Latent Image Formation

During radiation exposure the x-rays strike and ionize some of the silver halide crystals forming a **latent image** (latent means **invisible**). The image does not become visible until the film has undergone processing procedures. Film processing is explained in Chapter 8.

Processing changes the silver halide crystals that have a latent image into black specks of silver. These are the black areas seen on a dental radiograph. The amount of black silver specks varies depending on the structures radiographed. Thin structures that permit the passage of x-rays appear black (radiolucent). Thick, dense structures that absorb x-rays do not allow the x-rays to form a latent image on the film. These structures appear white (radiopaque) on the radiograph.

Film Packets and Packaging

The film manufacturer cuts the films to the sizes required in dentistry. Small films suitable for **intraoral** (inside the mouth) radiography are made into what is called a **film packet.** The terms "film packet" and "film" are often used interchangeably. Figure 7–2 is a picture of two film packets showing the tube side (above) and back side (below).

Film Packet

All intraoral **film packets** are assembled similarly. The film is first surrounded by black, lightproof paper. Next, a thin sheet of lead foil to shield the film from "backscatter" radiation is placed on the side of the film that will be away from the radiation source. An outer wrapping of moisture-resistant paper or plastic completes the assembly (see Figures 7–3 to 7–5). In most dental offices the film packet is referred to simply as the film.

The **film packet** consists of:

1. Film
2. Black paper wrapping
3. Lead foil
4. Cover wrapping

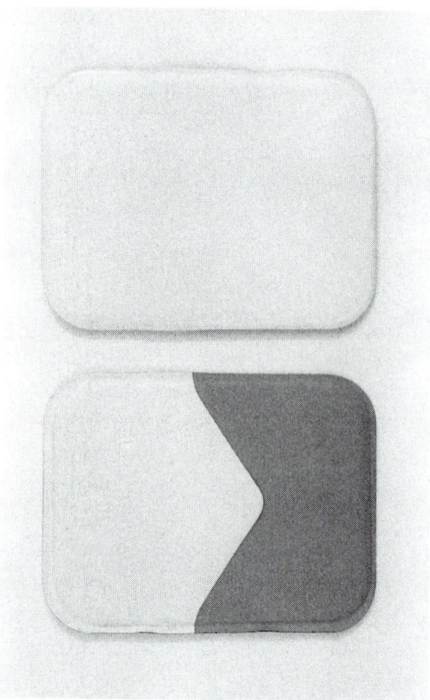

FIGURE 7–2. **Dental x-ray packets** showing the solid white tube side above and the color-coded back side below.

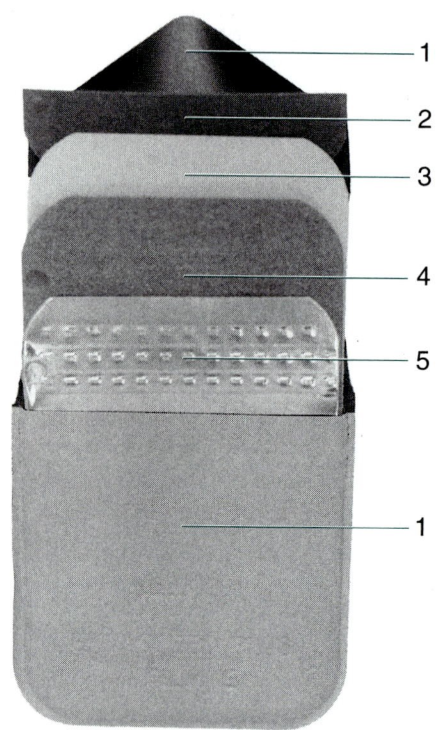

FIGURE 7–4. **Photograph of the back of an open film packet.** (**1**) Waterproof outer package. (**2**) Black paper. (**3**) Film. (**4**) Black paper. (**5**) Lead foil backing.

Film

Film packets may contain one or two **films.** When a packet containing two x-ray films is exposed, duplicate radiographs result. This is useful whenever a radiograph is needed for legal evidence or when a radiograph is to be sent to another practitioner to whom the patient is referred. Because several court rulings and a California law concerning the "patient's right of access to dental records" require the dentist to furnish records (including x-ray films) to the patient on demand, the use of the two-film packets has increased.

A small raised **identification dot** is located in one corner of the film. The raised dot is used to determine film orientation and is used to distinguish the right radiographs from the left radiographs.

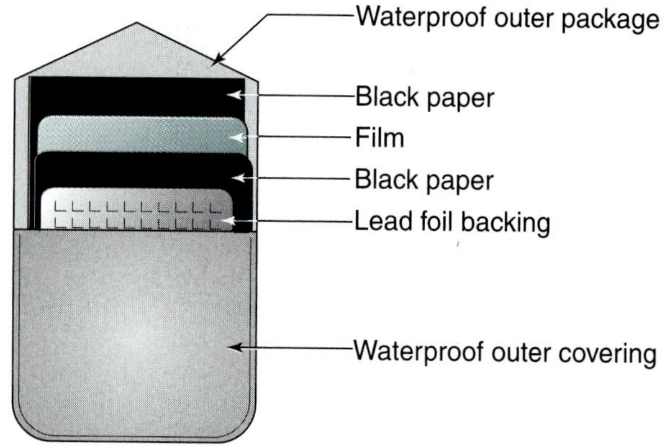

FIGURE 7–3. **Drawing of the back of an open film packet.**

Black Paper Wrapping

Black paper is wrapped around the film. The purpose of the black paper wrapping is to protect the film from light.

Lead Foil

A sheet of **lead foil** is located behind the film wrapped in black paper. The purpose of the lead foil backing is to absorb scattered radiation, thereby preventing scattered x-rays from striking the film emulsion from the back side of the film (the side away from the tube), thus fogging

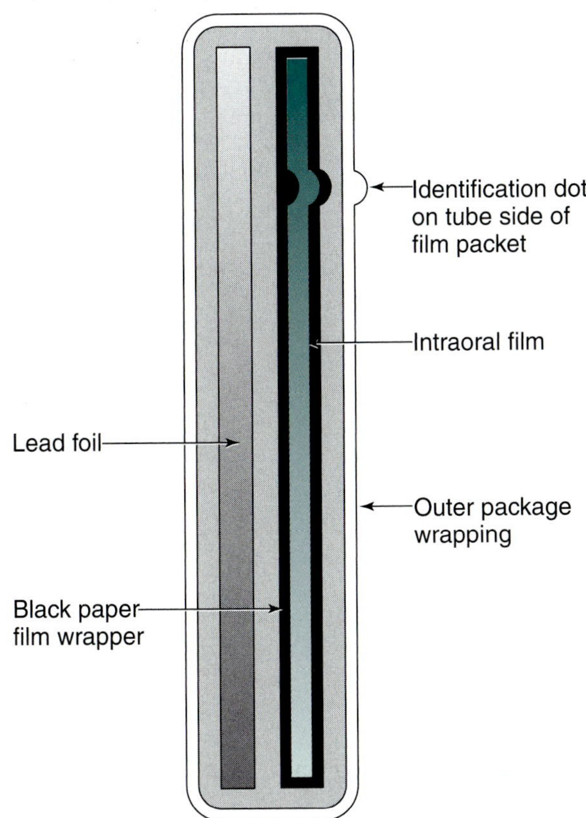

FIGURE 7–5. **Cross section of a film packet.**

the film. The lead is embossed with a pattern that becomes visible on the developed x-ray film in the event that the packet is accidentally positioned backwards during the exposure.

Packet Covering

The **packet covering** is an outer wrapping of moisture-resistant paper or soft vinyl plastic. The purpose of the wrapping is to hold the packet contents and to protect the film from light and moisture. Each film packet has two sides, a **tube side** that faces the tube (radiation source) and a **back side** away from the source of radiation (see Figure 7–2).

TUBE SIDE. The **tube side** is solid white (either paper or plastic) that is either smooth or slightly pebbly to prevent slippage. There is a small embossed dot near one of the corners that corresponds to the identification dot on the film. In intraoral radiography, the tube side of the film faces the lingual surfaces of the teeth to be x-rayed. The dot is also embossed on each film and aids in positioning it on a film mount and in identification of the patient's right and left side.

BACK SIDE. The **back side** containing the tab is white or may be color coded (see Table 7–1). This makes it easy to identify the back side. The following information is printed on the back side:

- Manufacturer's name
- Film speed
- Number of films in the packet (one or two).
- Circle or mark indicating the location of the identifying dot.
- The legend "opposite side toward tube."

Packaging

Film packets are packaged in cardboard boxes or plastic trays. Depending on the size, intraoral films are usually packaged 25, 50, or 150 to a box, the most popular being the 150-film packages. A layer of lead foil surrounds the films inside the container to protect them from damage by stray radiation or chemical fumes during storage.

Film Emulsion Speeds (Sensitivity)

Film speed (sensitivity) refers to the amount of radiation required to produce a radiograph of standard density. The faster the film speed, the less radiation required to get a standard density radiograph.

Factors that Determine Film Speed

Factors that determine film speed are:

- **Size of silver halide crystal.** The larger the crystal, the faster the film speed.
- **Thickness of emulsion.** Emulsion is coated on both sides of the film base to increase film speed.
- **Special radiosensitive dyes.** Manufacturers add special dyes that increase the film speed.

TABLE 7–1. **Kodak Film Packet Color Codes**

	One-film packet	Two-film packet
Ultra-speed (D)	Green	Gray
Ektaspeed (E)	Blue	Pink
Insight (F)	Lavender	Tan

The main factor that determines the film speed (film sensitivity) is the **size of the silver halide crystals** in the emulsion. The larger the crystals, the faster the film speed. Image sharpness is more distinct when the crystals are small. The larger crystals used in high-speed (fast) film results in a "graininess" that reduces the sharpness of the radiographic image. The loss of image sharpness is compensated for by the reduction in patient exposure.

Speed Groups

Trademark names like *super, ultra,* or *ekta* tell little or nothing about the actual film speed. The American National Standards Institute (ANSI) groups film speed using letters of the alphabet; speed group A for the slowest through F for the fastest. At the present time, F-speed is the fastest film available. Film speed is printed on the back side of each film packet.

Currently only **D-speed** (Kodak Ultra-Speed), **E-speed** (Kodak Ektaspeed), and **F-speed** (Kodak Insight) films are available. Kodak introduced their F-speed film in 2000 and subsequently stopped manufacturing E-speed film in late 2001. Although the F-speed film requires less exposure time than D-speed, many dentists still hesitate to use F-speed film in situations where a maximum of diagnostic interpretation is required because their eyes are accustomed to viewing the D-speed film. Similar problems with image definition occurred when the D films were first introduced.

The American Dental Association recommends that film speeds slower than D should not be used. The use of high-speed film has made it possible to reduce exposures to a fraction of the time formerly deemed necessary. This has contributed more to radiation safety than any other factor.

Types of Dental X-ray Film

There are two basic types of dental x-ray films:

1. **Screen film** (indirect-exposure film) is exposed primarily by a fluorescent type of light given off by special emulsion-coated intensifying screens that are positioned between the film and the x-ray source. The great intensity of the fluorescent light permits a significant reduction in the required exposure time.

   A **cassette,** generally made of metal and plastic, is required to protect and hold screen film in position during exposure. This is explained in greater detail later in this chapter.

2. **Nonscreen film** (direct-exposure film) is exposed when *x*-radiation comes into direct contact with the film emulsion.

Depending on where the film is to be used—inside or outside the mouth—the film is classified as **intraoral** or **extraoral.** Unfortunately, space limitations seldom permit the use of a cassette inside the mouth. Therefore, the small intraoral films are direct-exposure films. With few exceptions, the majority of extraoral films are screen films, hence, indirect-exposure films.

Intraoral Films

Intraoral films are designed principally for use inside the mouth. However, an intraoral film may be used to make an extraoral exposure. One may use any film whenever it can bring about the desired result.

There are five sizes of intraoral film, number 0, 1, 2, 3, and 4. The larger the number, the larger the size of the film.

Three types of intraoral films, each named after its most common use, are the **periapical,** the **bitewing,** and the **occlusal** (see Figure 7–6).

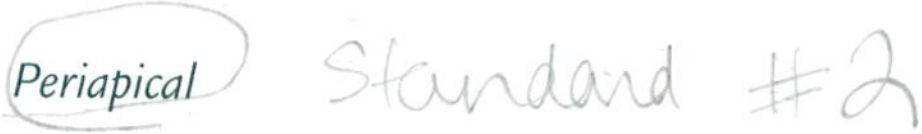

Periapical

Periapical films are used to make a detailed examination of the entire tooth, the periodontal membrane, and the surrounding bone tissues. Four sizes are manufactured (#0, #1, #2, and #3). The larger the number, the larger the film.

The #0 films are especially designed for small children and thus are often called **pedo** (from the Greek word *paidos,* child) or **pediatric** films. Both the #1 and #2 films are commonly used on larger children and adults. Use of the narrow #1 film is normally limited to exposing radiographs of the anterior teeth. Although it shows only two or three teeth, this film is ideal for areas where the mouth is narrow and curves a great deal. Its narrowness also makes it the best choice when film holders and the 16-in. (41-cm) target-film technique are used in the anterior areas or the mouth. The wider #2 film is generally referred to as the **standard film.** This film is used in at least 75% of all intraoral radiography. The extra-long #3 film, also called the **long bitewing** film, is rarely used as a periapical film.

Bitewing

The **bitewing** films are used to examine the crowns of the teeth, the alveolar crests, and the surfaces of the teeth that touch each other. The exposures made with these films show the coronal portions of both the maxillary (upper) and mandibular (lower) teeth and crestal bone

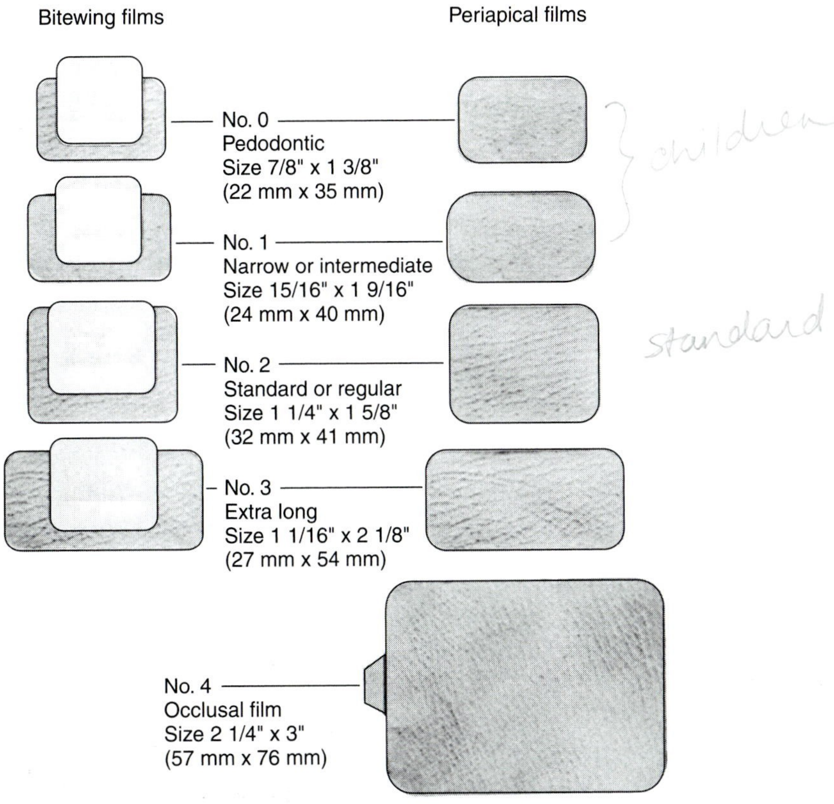

FIGURE 7–6. **Intraoral film.** With the exception of the large occlusal films that are used occlusally or extraorally on occasions, all intraoral films are available in two forms: plain for periapical use or with an attached bite tab for bitewing use. (Courtesy of Dentsply/Rinn Corporation)

on the same film. They are particularly valuable when the dentist is trying to determine the extent of proximal caries between the teeth.

All bitewing films are available in the same sizes as the periapical films and have the same film numbers (see Figure 7–6). The chief difference is that each film has a flap or tab attached to it on which the patient must bite to hold it in place between the occlusal surfaces of the maxillary and mandibular teeth. These films may be purchased with tabs. A periapical film can be converted to a bitewing film by being slipped into a commercially made cardboard film loop (see Figure 7–7). Also, there are commercial "sticky" tabs available to convert periapical film to bitewing film.

Occlusal

The **occlusal** films (#4) are the largest of the intraoral films. The patient normally holds them in position by

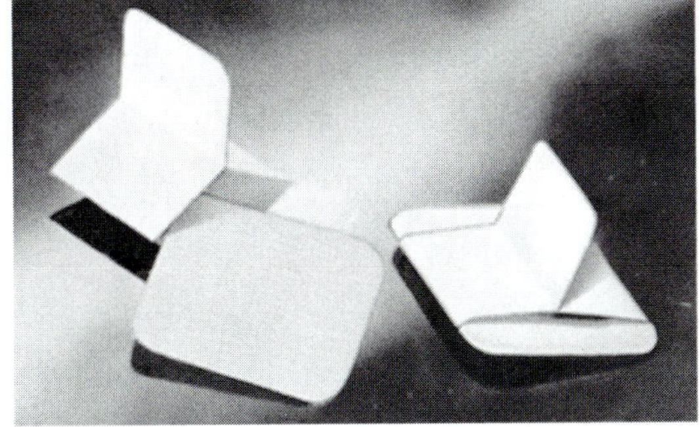

FIGURE 7–7. **Bite loops for bitewing films.** Bite loops offer an easy way to convert film from periapical to bitewing use. The loop is spread open, and the desired film is centered into the loop. The tube side of the film must face toward the bite tab and the source of radiation. Bite loops are available in various sizes. (Courtesy of Densply/Rinn Corporation)

biting directly on them. These films are ideal for making a rapid survey of a large area of the maxilla, mandible, and floor of the mouth. They can reveal gross pathological lesions, root fragments, bone and tooth fractures, and impacted or supernumerary teeth and many other conditions. Occlusal films may be used to make a rapid survey of an edentulous (without teeth) mouth.

The #4 occlusal film is the only one for which a cassette is available. Even though the cassette is quite thin, its extra bulk makes it difficult to position inside the mouth and limits its use. Few dental offices use the occlusal film cassette.

Occlusal films are sometimes used extraorally for radiographs of the third molar areas when it is not practical to place a film far back in the mouth or when the patient's face is swollen and opening the mouth is difficult. This versatile film has many other uses that are considered later in the text. Although only the #4 film is called the occlusal film, periapical films of any size can be used to make occlusal radiographs. Size #2 film is commonly used for occlusal exposures on the young child.

Extraoral Films

Extraoral films are designed for use outside the mouth.

Packaging

The larger extraoral films are generally packaged 25, 50, or 100 to a box. With the exception of films sold in Ready-Pack envelopes, films are sometimes sandwiched between two pieces of protective paper, and the entire group is wrapped in lead foil for protection. Because these films are designed for extraoral use, they require neither individual lead backing nor moistureproof wrappings.

Size

The films vary in size depending on what area is to be radiographed. The most common sizes are:

- 5 × 7-in. (13 × 18 cm), used mainly for lateral views of the jaw
- 8 × 10-in. (21 × 26 cm), used for profiles and posteroanterior views
- 5 or 6-in. × 12-in. (13 or 15 cm × 30 cm), used for panoramic radiographs of the entire dentition

Use

Extraoral films are used to examine structures of the skull, the maxilla and mandible, facial bones, and the temporomandibular joint. They can show the extent of a fracture, growth, or malignancy and can be used to study jaw development, tooth eruption, or any of a long list of normal and abnormal conditions.

Except for the panoramic radiographs, extraoral films are not frequently used by general practitioners. Major users are orthodontists, prosthodontists, and oral surgeons.

Orthodontists use facial profile radiographs, cephalometric headplates (*cephalometric*, meaning "measuring the head") periodically to record, measure, and compare changes in growth of the bones and the teeth.

Prosthodontists use facial profile radiographs to record the contour of the lips and face and the relationship of the teeth before removal. This helps them to construct prosthetic appliances that look natural.

Oral surgeons use extraoral radiographs extensively to determine the location and extent of fractures and to locate impacted teeth, abnormalities, malignancies, and injuries to the temporomandibular joint.

Classification

The large extraoral films are **classified** as **screen** and **nonscreen films.**

Screen Film

Screen film is a type of extraoral film used in a cassette sandwiched between two intensifying screens. Screen film is so called because they must be used with intensifying screens. Most of the exposure to screen film is from light given off by the crystals in the screens.

All screen films are more sensitive to blue and green fluorescent light—formed inside the cassette by the action of the x-rays on the crystals of the emulsion that coats the intensifying screens—than to x-radiation. This fluorescence increases enormously the amount of illumination inside the tightly closed cassette, thus drastically reducing the exposure time.

Screen film is sensitive to the fluorescent light given off by the crystals. Care must be taken to use proper screen-film combinations. Blue sensitive films must be used with screens that produce blue light and green sensitive films must be used with screens that produce green light.

Nonscreen Film

The **nonscreen film,** by way of contrast, is exposed directly to x-rays. It can be placed within a cardboard exposure holder or a cassette without intensifying screens. It is also available in a packaged form (Ready-Pack) that does not require loading under darkroom conditions. The use of nonscreen film should be discouraged because of the long exposure times required. Very little nonscreen film is being used today.

> NOTE: Advances in emulsion and processing technology are so rapid that the user must be extremely alert to use the correct combination of extraoral film, intensifying screen, darkroom illumination, and processing technique. Failure to do this will lead to very inferior results.

Cassettes

Cassettes hold and protect the film. Most are rigid and flat, but the ones used to make panoramic radiographs may be rigid or flexible, flat or curved. Cassettes are available in a variety of sizes. Most cephalometric exposures use a cassette measuring 8 × 10 in. (20 × 25 cm) whereas a cassette measuring 5 × 12 in. (13 × 30 cm) is commonly used for panoramic exposures.

A typical rigid cassette has a front and back cover joined together with a hinge. The front cover is constructed of plastic to permit the passage of the x-ray beam. The back cover is constructed of heavy metal to absorb x-rays (see Figure 7–8). Intensifying screens line the inside of the front and back covers. The film is placed between the two intensifying screens (see Figure 7–9). A spring-type clasp is used to close the cassette and prevent light leaks.

The protective paper surrounding the film must be removed when the screen film is placed in the cassette; otherwise the blue or green light rays emanating from the screens cannot reach the film surface. Closing the cassette tightly is important to obtain screen-to-film contact. When the cassette is not tightly closed, it causes the radiograph to be blurry. It is also important to remember that the tube side of the cassette must face toward the head or face of the patient because in all extraoral procedures, the film is outside the mouth and the x-rays enter the patient from the opposite side.

Cassettes must be marked with lead letters *L* and *R* to identify the patient's left and right side.

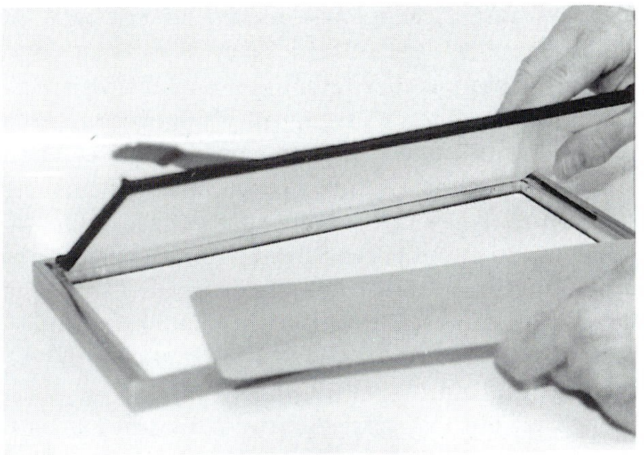

FIGURE 7–9. **View of open extraoral cassette.** The film is placed between the intensifying screens. The film must be loaded or unloaded in the darkroom with special subdued light.

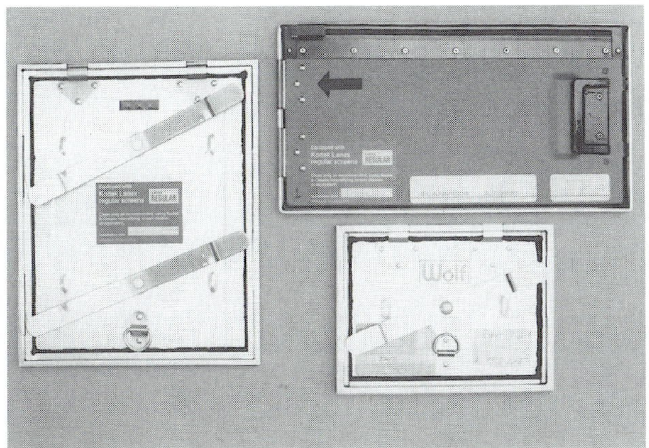

FIGURE 7–8. **The back side of three rigid cassettes of various sizes.**

Intensifying Screens

An **intensifying screen** transfers x-ray energy into visible light. The visible light, in turn, exposes the screen film. As the name implies, these screens "intensify" the effect of x-rays on film. The purpose of using intensifying screens is to reduce the radiation required to expose the film so the patient is exposed to less radiation.

An intensifying screen is a smooth cardboard or plastic sheet coated with minute fluorescent crystals mixed into a suitable binding medium. It produces the desired image in a shorter exposure time than is possible with nonscreen film.

Intensifying screens are based on the principle that crystals of certain salts—in this case, calcium tungstate, barium strontium sulfate, or rare-earth phosphors [lanthanum (La) and gadolinium (Gd)]—will fluoresce and emit energy in the form of blue or green light when they absorb x-rays. Each of these fluorescent crystals, also called **phosphors,** gives off blue or green radiations that vary in intensity according to the x-rays in that part of the image. As already mentioned, screen film is more sensitive to this type of light than to radiation. When the film is sandwiched tightly between two intensifying screens, the x-rays cause the crystals on the screens to fluoresce and return the emitted light to the emulsion to intensify the radiographic image (see Figure 7–10). The difference in the sensitivity of intensifying screens depends on:

- The size of the crystals
- The type of phosphor used
- The thickness of the emulsion

The conventional calcium tungstate screens give off a blue to violet fluorescent light, whereas the new rare-earth phosphor screens give off a green light when energized by x-rays. Several speeds of screens are available. One must be extremely careful to combine the correct film and screen. Some films are sensitive to blue light, whereas others produce best results when exposed to green fluorescent light.

Duplicating Film

emulsion side is dull
nonemulsion is shiny

A **duplicate radiograph** is identical to the original radiograph. Duplicate radiographs are useful for insurance claims and may be sent to another practitioner to whom the patient is referred. Special duplicating film is required to make a duplicate radiograph.

Duplicating film is a type of photographic film that appears similar to x-ray film but is exposed by the action of infrared and ultraviolet light rather than x-rays. Only one side of the film is coated with emulsion. The emulsion side appears dull, whereas the non-emulsion side is shiny. During the printing process, the duplicating film is superimposed with its emulsion side toward the radiograph that is to be copied. The duplication process is explained in Chapter 8.

Duplication film, boxed in quantities of 50, 100, or 150 sheets, is available in periapical sizes and in 5 or 6 × 12 in. (13 or 15 × 30 cm) and 8 × 10 in. (20 × 26 cm) sheets.

Film Storage and Protection

All dental films are extremely sensitive to heat, humidity, pressure and stray radiation. Precautions for storing and protecting films must be followed. **Film fogging** is

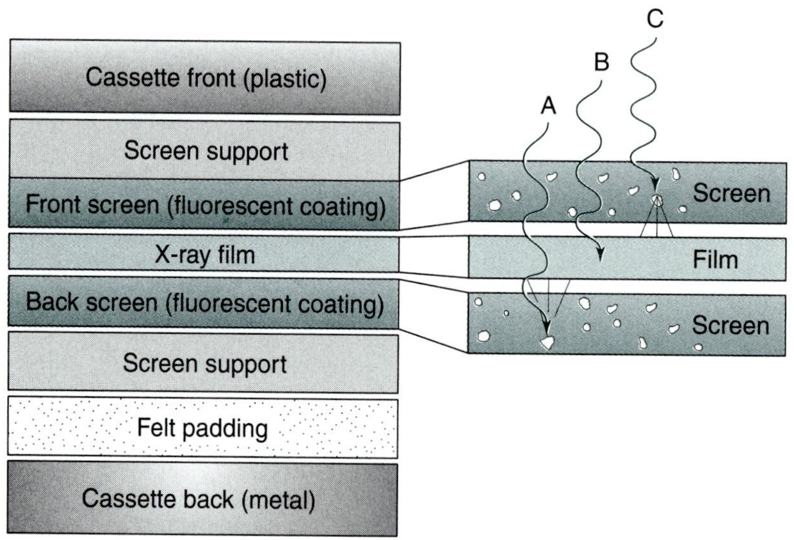

FIGURE 7–10. **Cross section of cassette and diagram showing the effect of x-ray and fluorescent light on the film. X-ray A** strikes a crystal in the screen behind the film producing light that then forms latent images in the silver bromide crystal of the film. **X-ray B** strikes a silver bromide crystal in the film forming a latent image. **X-ray C** strikes a crystal in the screen in front of the film producing light, which then forms latent images in the silver bromide crystals of the film.

the darkening of the finished radiograph caused by one of several factors, such as old or contaminated solutions, exposure to chemical fumes, pressure, faulty safelight, or scatter radiation.

Heat and Humidity

To prevent fogging, film should be **stored in a cool, dry place.** Ideally, all unexposed film should be stored at 50 to 70° Fahrenheit (10 to 21° Celsius) and 30 to 50% relative humidity.

Pressure

Pressure can fog film. Do not stack film too high. Do not place heavy objects on top of film.

Radiation

Stray **radiation** can fog film. Film should be stored in areas shielded from radiation.

Shelf Life

Dental x-ray film has a limited **shelf life.** The **expiration date** is printed on the film container (see Figure 7–11).

FIGURE 7–11. **Film container showing expiration date.**

All intraoral film should be placed so that the expiration date can be seen. The oldest film should be used first. All film must be used before the expiration date.

CHAPTER SUMMARY

X-ray film serves as an image receptor by recording the image. The film used in dental radiography is photographic film that has been especially adapted in size, emulsion, film speed, and packaging for dental uses. All x-ray film has a polyester base that is coated with a gelatin emulsion containing silver bromide (halide) crystals.

During radiation exposure, the x-rays strike and ionize some of the silver halide crystals forming a **latent image.** The image does not become visible until the film has undergone processing procedures.

The **film packet** consists of film, black paper wrapping, lead foil, and a cover wrapping.

Film speed (sensitivity) refers to the amount of radiation required to produce a radiograph of standard density. Film speed groups range from A for the slowest through F for the fastest. Currently only D-, E-, and F-speed films are available in the United States.

Intraoral films vary in size. Five sizes are available: 0, 1, 2, 3, and 4. Three types of intraoral film are used: **periapical,** to examine the entire tooth and surrounding tissues; **bitewing,** to disclose proximal tooth surfaces; and **occlusal,** to survey larger areas.

Extraoral films are designed for use outside the mouth. They are much larger than intraoral films. Extraoral films are used for panoramic, cephalometric, and lateral jaw exposures. The large extraoral films are classified as **screen** and **nonscreen films. Cassettes** hold and protect the film. Cassettes contain two intensifying screens that are coated with an emulsion containing phosphors that glow when energized by x-rays and produce a blue or green fluorescent light.

Duplicating film is a special type of photographic film that is used to duplicate dental radiographs.

All x-ray films are sensitive to heat, humidity, pressure, and radiation. Care must be exercised in storing and in handling the film during and after exposure.

REVIEW QUESTIONS

1. Which of these is contained in the film emulsion used for dental radiographs?
   (a) Barium sulfate
   (b) Calcium tungstate
   (c) Silver halide
   (d) Silver nitrate
2. As silver halide crystals in the film emulsion increase in size, image sharpness:
   (a) Increases.
   (b) Decreases.
   (c) Stays the same.
   (d) None of the above.
3. As silver halide crystals in the film emulsion increase in size, film speed:
   (a) Increases.
   (b) Decreases.
   (c) Stays the same.
   (d) None of the above.
4. The term meaning "hidden" or "invisible" image is:
   (a) Cassette.
   (b) Screen.
   (c) Latent.
   (d) None of the above.
5. What is the function of the lead foil in the x-ray packet?
   (a) Moisture protection
   (b) Absorb the backscatter radiation
   (c) To give rigidity to the packet
   (d) Protection against fluorescence
6. Which of these films has the greatest sensitivity to radiation?
   (a) B-speed
   (b) C-speed
   (c) D-speed
   (d) F-speed
7. Which of these films is the largest?
   (a) Periapical film
   (b) Bitewing film
   (c) Occlusal film
   (d) Pedodontic film

8. Which of these films is best suited when the dentist requests a radiograph of a specific tooth and its surrounding structures?
   (a) Panoramic
   (b) Occlusal
   (c) Cephalometric
   (d) Periapical

9. What term describes the crystals used in the emulsion on intensifying screens?
   (a) Halides
   (b) Phosphors
   (c) Sulfates
   (d) Bromides

10. Intensifying screens are used to:
    (a) Reduce exposure time.
    (b) Increase exposure time.
    (c) Improve radiographic detail.
    (d) Speed processing time.

11. A film that is placed outside the mouth during a x-ray exposure is called:
    (a) Occlusal film.
    (b) Periapical film.
    (c) Intraoral film.
    (d) Extraoral film.

12. What is the ideal storage temperature for x-ray films?
    (a) Under 32°F (0°C)
    (b) From 32 to 50°F (0 to 10°C)
    (c) From 50 to 70°F (10 to 21°C)
    (d) From 70 to 80°F (21 to 26.5°C)

13. Which of these is a screen film?
    (a) Occlusal
    (b) Bitewing
    (c) Panoramic
    (d) Periapical

14. Which of these films can produce an image with the greatest degree of definition?
    (a) Duplicating film
    (b) D-speed film
    (c) Pediatric film
    (d) E-speed film

15. The three types of intraoral films are the ____________, the ____________, and the ____________.

16. Which of these films use the shortest exposure time?
    (a) Nonscreen film
    (b) Screen film

17. Which type of film is used to copy a radiograph?
    (a) Duplicating film
    (b) Screen film
    (c) Nonscreen film
    (d) X-ray film

BIBLIOGRAPHY

Eastman Kodak. *Exposure and Processing for Dental Radiography*. Rochester, NY: Eastman Kodak, 1998.

Manny, E. F., Carlson, K. C., & McClean, P. M. et al. *An Overview of Dental Radiology*. Washington, DC: National Center for Health Care Technology (FDA/BRH), 1980.

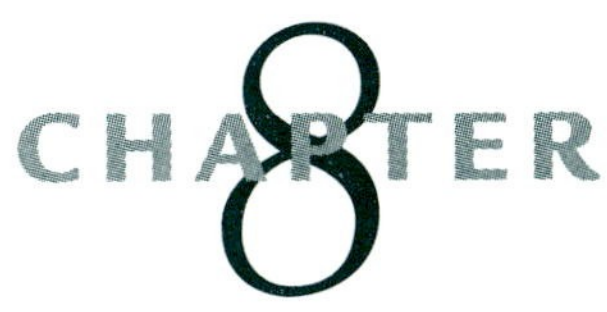

Dental X-ray Film Processing

OBJECTIVES

By the end of this chapter the student should be able to:

- Define the key words.
- Explain how a latent image becomes a visible image.
- List in sequence the steps in processing dental films.
- List and describe the four chemicals in the developer solution and explain the function of each ingredient.
- List and describe the four chemicals in the fixer solution and explain the function of each ingredient.
- List the necessary equipment items in the darkroom for film processing.
- Discuss safelights and safelight filters.
- List and discuss the step-by-step procedures for manual film processing.
- Discuss rapid film processing procedures.
- Discuss the advantages and disadvantages of automatic film processing.
- Discuss the disposal of radiographic processing chemicals and film wastes.

KEY WORDS

Acidifier
Activator
Cutting reducer
Developer
Developing Agent
Fixer
Fixing Agent
Halide
Hardening Agent
Latent Image
Light-tight
Oxidation
Preservative
Processing Tank
Radiolucent
Radiopaque
Replenisher
Restrainer
Rinsing
Safelight
Safelight filter
Selective reduction
Viewbox
Wetting agent

Introduction

Film processing is a series of steps that converts the invisible latent image on the dental x-ray film into a visible permanent image called a radiograph. A sequence of steps involving developing and fixing chemicals must be rigidly followed. Most processing is accomplished in a darkroom equipped with special lights.

At present three methods are used to process dental x-ray films:

- Traditional **manual processing**
- Chair-side **rapid processing**
- **Automatic processing**

The purpose of this chapter is to explain the fundamentals of film processing and processing solutions, to discuss the darkroom and equipment, and to describe the step-by-step procedures for manual and automatic processing. In addition, this chapter describes film duplication procedures and the disposal of radiographic processing chemicals and film wastes.

Fundamentals of Film Processing

Processing transforms the **latent image** (latent means "hidden"), which is produced when the x-ray photons are absorbed by the silver **halide** crystals in the emulsion, into a visible, stable image by means of chemicals. During the chemical processing a **selective reduction** of the exposed silver halide crystals takes place. Selective reduction means that the nonmetallic elements, the halides, are removed. Only the exposed silver remains (Figure 8–1).

The exposed silver halide crystals on the film are reduced to black metallic silver when immersed in the **developer** solution. The unexposed halide crystals (in film areas opposite metallic or dense structures that absorb and prevent the passage of x-rays) are unaffected at this time. After brief **rinsing** to remove any developer remaining on the film, the film is immersed in the **fixer** solution. The fixer removes the unexposed and undeveloped halide crystals, leaving behind only the black metallic silver. After the film is completely fixed, it is washed in running water to remove any remaining traces of the chemicals of the fixer and then is allowed to dry.

Thus, the images on the radiograph are made up of microscopic grains of black metallic silver. The amount of silver deposited will vary with the thickness of the tissues penetrated. Where only soft tissues were between the source of the radiation and the emulsion, the film will be black. Where passage of x-rays was blocked by metal fillings or restorations, the radiograph will be white.

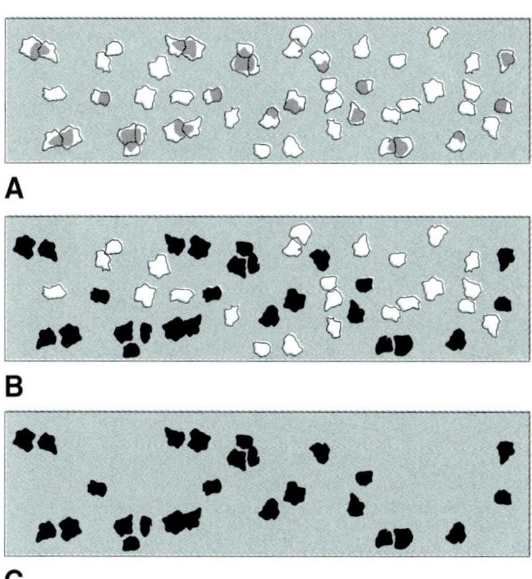

FIGURE 8–1. **Cross section of dental x-ray film emulsion.** (**A**) X-rays strike silver bromide crystals forming latent image sites (shown in gray). (**B**) After development, crystals struck by x-rays (latent image sites) reduced to black metallic silver. (**C**) Fixer removes unexposed, undeveloped crystals leaving the black metallic silver.

As we have already seen in Chapter 4, the amount of light transmitted through the film varies according to the thickness of tissues penetrated by the radiation and accounts for the shades of black, gray, and white. Dark areas are spoken of as **radiolucent** and light areas as **radiopaque.**

Processing

The steps in processing dental x-ray film are:

1. Development
2. Rinsing
3. Fixation
4. Washing
5. Drying

Development

The initial step in the processing sequence is the **development** of the film. The purpose of the developer solution is to reduce the exposed silver halide crystals into black metallic silver. The developing solution softens the gelatin emulsion, causing the emulsion to swell, exposing the silver halide crystals to the chemicals of the developer.

Rinsing

The second step in processing is **rinsing** the film in water. The purpose of the rinsing is to remove as much of the alkaline developer as possible before placing the film in the fixer. Rinsing preserves the acidity of the fixer and prolongs its useful life.

Fixation

The third step is the **fixation** of the film. The purpose of the fixer solution is to remove the undeveloped silver halide crystals from the film emulsion.

Washing

The fourth step in processing is **washing** the film in water to remove all chemicals left on the radiograph.

Drying

The final step is the **drying** the film. Films may be air-dried at room temperature or they may be dried in a heated cabinet.

The **processed films** are now called **radiographs.**

X-Ray Processing Solutions

The chemicals used in processing may be obtained in three forms:

- Powder
- Ready-to-use liquid
- Liquid concentrate

The concentrate form (see Figure 8–2) is used in most offices. It is easy to store, is fresh, and can be prepared in a few minutes. In many cities, regular tank cleaning and solution-changing services are available.

The processing chemicals are in the **developer,** which is slightly alkaline, and in the **fixer,** which is slightly acidic. Both the developer and fixer contain four constituents. The preferred vehicle for mixing these ingredients is distilled water; however, tap water is often used, provided it is known to contain no interfering chemicals, especially when run through filters.

Developer

The main purpose of the **developer** is to convert the exposed silver halide crystals into metallic silver grains.

There are four chemicals in the developer (see Table 8–1).

1. Developing agent (also called a reducing agent).
2. Preservative
3. Activator (also called an alkalizer)
4. Restrainer

The **developing agent** reduces the exposed silver halide crystals to metallic silver but has no effect on the unexposed crystals at recommended time-temperatures. It contains two chemicals, hydroquinone and elon. The hydroquinone works slowly but steadily to build up density and contrast in the film. The elon works fast to bring out the gray shades (contrast) of the image. Although both chemicals are more active at higher rather than lower temperatures, the hydroquinone becomes extremely active when the temperature of the solution is raised and is inactive at lower temperatures. Therefore the temperature of the developer is critical. Thus, the higher the temperature, the less time is required to develop the film.

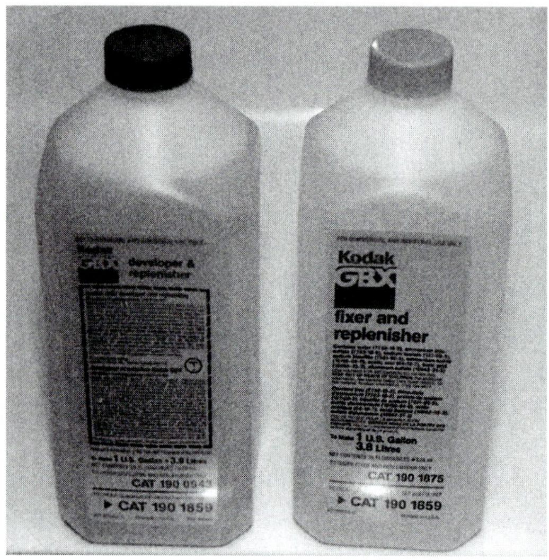

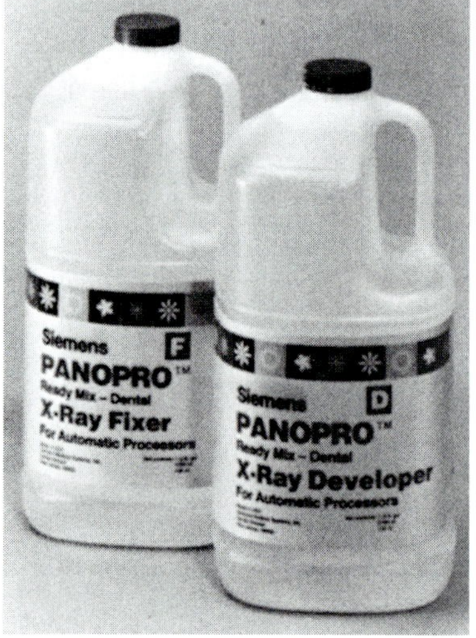

FIGURE 8–2. **Processing chemicals.** (**A**) Typical concentrate forms of developer and fixer for manual processing. Each bottle is mixed with sufficient water to make 1 gal (3.8 L) of solution, which is the normal capacity of an insert tank. (**B**) Panopro ready-mix developer and fixer for automatic processors. (Courtesy of Siemens Medical Systems, Dental Division, Iselin, NJ)

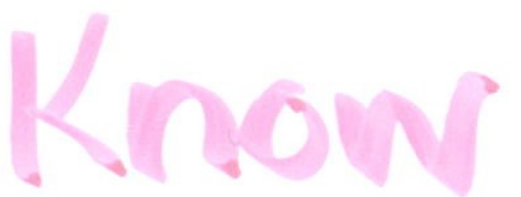

TABLE 8–1. Composition of Developer

Ingredient	Chemical	Action
Developing agents (reducing agents)	Hydroquinone	Reduces (converts) exposed silver halide crystals to black metallic silver. Slowly builds up black tones and contrast.
	Elon	Reduces (converts) exposed silver halide crystals to black metallic silver. Quickly builds up gray tones.
Preservative	Sodium sulfite	Prevents rapid oxidation of the developing agents.
Activator	Sodium carbonate	Activates developing agents by providing required alkalinity.
Restrainer	Potassium bromide	Restrains the developing agents from developing the unexposed silver halide crystals, which produce fog.

The **preservative,** sodium sulfite, protects the developing agents by slowing down the rapid oxidation rate of the developer.

The **activator,** usually sodium carbonate, provides the necessary alkaline medium required by the developing agents. It also softens and swells the gelatin, letting more of the exposed silver bromide crystals come into contact with the developing agents.

The **restrainer,** potassium bromide, restrains the developing agents from developing the unexposed silver halide crystals and therefore inhibits the tendency of the solution to chemically fog the film.

Fixer

The purpose of the **fixer** is to (1) **stop further development**—thereby establishing the image permanently on the film; (2) **remove (dissolve) the undeveloped silver halide crystals** (those that were not exposed to x-rays), and (3) **harden (fix) the emulsion.**

There are four chemicals in the fixer (see Table 8–2).

1. Fixing agent
2. Preservative
3. Hardening agent
4. Acidifier

The **fixing (clearing) agent,** ammonium thiosulfate or sodium thiosulfate, also known as "hypo" or hyposulfate of sodium, removes all unexposed and any remaining undeveloped silver halide crystals from the emulsion.

The **preservative,** sodium sulfite (the same chemical as used in the developer), slows the rate of oxidation and prevents the deterioration of the hypo and the precipitation of sulfur.

TABLE 8–2. Composition of Fixer

Ingredient	Chemical	Action
Fixing agent (clearing agent)	Ammonium thiosulfate or Sodium thiosulfate	Removes the unexposed and any remaining undeveloped silver halide crystals.
Preservative	Sodium sulfite	Slows the rate of oxidation and prevents deterioration of the fixing agent.
Hardening agent	Potassium alum	Shrinks and hardens the gelatin emulsion.
Acidifier	Acetic acid	Stops further development by neutralizing the alkali of the developer.

The **hardening agent,** potassium alum, shrinks and hardens the gelatin emulsion. This hardening continues until the film is dry, thus protecting it from abrasion.

The **acidifier,** acetic acid, provides the acid medium to stop further development by neutralizing the alkali of the developer.

Two other chemicals are sometimes used in processing radiographs—a **wetting agent** and a **cutting reducer.**

A **wetting agent** (a form of detergent) reduces the surface tension of the film. A teaspoon of wetting agent added to the developer will hasten film development. Moreover, the fully processed film will dry much faster if, after being properly washed, it is immersed for one minute in a pan of water to which a few drops of wetting agent have been added.

A **cutting reducer** is a combination of potassium ferrocyanide and fixer. It can be used in an emergency to lighten films that have been accidentally overexposed or overdeveloped. The use of a cutting reducer is indicated only when the film is too dark to diagnose and it is impossible or inadvisable to retake the film. Because much of the film density is lost when a reducer is used, this procedure should be attempted only as a last resort. The procedure varies slightly with the brand. Instructions should be carefully checked.

Changing Solutions

The processing solutions should be changed every 4 weeks or more often if the workload is extremely heavy. The useful life of the solution is determined by:

1. The original quality or concentration of the solution, determined by how carefully the proportions are measured and how the solution is stirred.
2. The freshness of the solution.
3. The number of films that are processed.
4. Contamination of the chemicals.

A small but significant amount of developer is lost daily through evaporation and by drops of developer adhering to the film surfaces and the film hanger as they are transferred to the rinse compartment. The loss in the fixer is smaller; actually, some dilution takes place by rinse water clinging to the film and hanger when they are transferred to the fixer and since some fixer is lost when the film hanger is subsequently removed, these factors about balance. The main loss of the fixer is from evaporation. The gradual dilution weakens the fixer solution.

Replenisher

Replenisher is a superconcentrated solution of developer or fixer. It is added to the developer or fixer in the processing tank to compensate for the loss of volume and strength from oxidation.

The first sign of developer exhaustion is a light film with a thin image. Fixer exhaustion can be recognized when the film has not cleared in two minutes and still shows a milky coating.

One hazard of permitting the solution levels to drop is that there may not be sufficient developer or fixer to cover all of the films attached to the uppermost clips of the film hanger. This may go unnoticed in the dim light of the darkroom and result in a partial image on the radiograph. This will not happen if the inserts are topped off daily.

Sometimes technicians overexpose or overdevelop the film when the solutions become weak. They should not, because overexposure subjects everyone to more radiation than necessary. Overdevelopment is inaccurate and results in a loss of diagnostic film quality.

Hardening Agents

Depending on whether the chemicals are primarily intended for use in manual, rapid, or automatic processors, special **hardening agents** may have been added to facilitate the transportation of the films through the roller systems of the automatic units.

Darkroom and Equipment

Until recently, a darkroom was absolutely necessary for processing films. Now one can do "chair-side processing" in normal light with certain rapid-processing units and daylight loader-equipped automatic processors. However, a darkroom is still required to load and unload the cassettes, to process certain films, and to do manual processing if the automatic processing equipment malfunctions.

Darkroom

The purpose of the darkroom is to provide a dark area where x-ray films can be safely handled and processed. In some offices, the **darkroom** is a large, well-equipped room; in others, it is just an afterthought. A well-equipped room makes processing much easier.

Cleanliness

Cleanliness and orderliness are essential. Because the films are handled in almost complete darkness, usually with just a very dim safelight, all needed materials must be within easy reach. The person doing the processing must know where each item is kept. The workbench must be absolutely free of water, dust, chemicals, or any other substance that can come in contact with unwrapped film. Particular care must be taken not to splash chemical solutions or water on the bench when moving films from one insert of the processing tank to the other. A messy darkroom is not only unpleasant to work in but can stain and damage clothes. More seriously dirty darkrooms can produce worthless radiographs.

Darkroom Requirements

The ideal darkroom is the result of good planning. It is large enough to meet the requirements of the office and is arranged with ample work space. The darkroom should be equipped with correct lighting, be well ventilated, and have adequate storage space for films and radiographic supplies. The darkroom should be located an adequate distance from the nearest x-ray machine. It should not be used as a general storage area for materials that produce dust or give off chemical fumes.

The darkroom door should have a lock to use when processing films to prevent anyone from entering and inadvertently spoiling the films through exposure to light.

Equipment

Special **equipment** is required in the darkroom for film processing. The following items are necessary in the darkroom.

1. Overhead white light
2. Darkroom safelight
3. Viewbox
4. Processing tank
5. Utility sink
6. Stirring paddles
7. Timer
8. Thermometer
9. Film hangers, drying racks, and drip pans
10. Electric fan
11. Film dryer
12. Wastebasket, lead foil container, and biohazard container
13. Ample storage facilities for radiographic supplies

Lighting

The control of darkroom **lighting** is important. Darkrooms should be light-tight. A light-tight room is one that is completely dark and excludes all light. X-ray film is very sensitive to white light. Any white light in the darkroom can blacken the film or cause film fog.

Although many darkrooms are painted black, if they are completely sealed to white light, a lighter-colored paint should be used. It will reflect more usable safelight than black paint. Felt strips may have to be installed around the door or any other area where a light leak is discovered. Fluorescent overhead lighting should not be used because of its afterglow. Two forms of illumination are desirable in the darkroom:

1. **White ceiling light**
2. **Safelight**

WHITE CEILING LIGHT. An overhead white ceiling light should provide adequate illumination for the size of the room to perform tasks such as cleaning tanks, filling them with chemicals, and performing darkroom housekeeping chores.

SAFELIGHT. A **safelight** is a special type of filtered light that can illuminate the darkroom while films are being processed. The safelight provides enough light in the darkroom to perform the minimum essential activities without exposing or damaging the film.

Safelights have filters to protect the film from light. A **safelight filter** removes the short wavelengths in the blue-green region of the visible light spectrum. The longer wavelength red-orange light is allowed to pass through the filter illuminating the darkroom. A variety of safelights with different types of filters are available. Some are designed to work best with intraoral films, others with extraoral films, and others are universal and can be used for both. An example of a universal filter is the Kodak GBX-2 safelight filter, which can be used when processing both intraoral film and extraoral screen films (see Figure 8–3).

Darkroom users must be aware that the emulsion can be damaged by prolonged exposure even to filtered light. Film handling should be limited to 2 1/2 minutes under safelight conditions or fogging (film darkening) may occur. The type of safelight required is indicated in the film processing instructions which comes inside the film package or printed in bold type on the outside of the film package. Safelight factors to consider which may fog unwrapped film are:

1. **Wattage** of the bulb (use 7 1/2 or 15 watts).
2. The **distance** between the lamp and the film. The rule is 2 1/4 watts per foot (0.3 m) and a 4-ft (1.2 m) minimum distance.

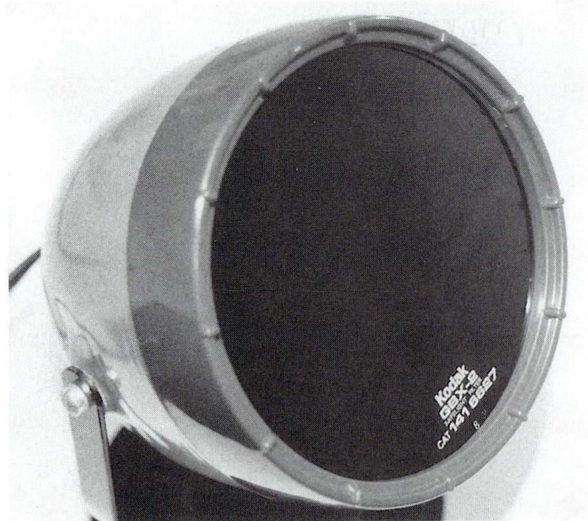

FIGURE 8-3. **This bracket-type lamp can provide either direct or indirect illumination.** It can be equipped with either a MORLITE 2 or a GBX 2 Safelight Filter, depending on the types of x-ray film to be handled. The safelight lamp should be located at least 4 ft (1.2 m) from the nearest working surface and equipped with a bulb wattage of either 15 or 7 1/2 watts depending on the speed of film emulsion.

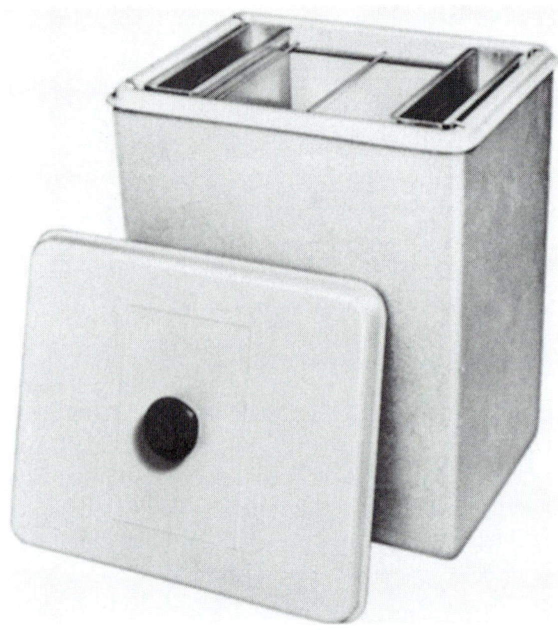

FIGURE 8-4. **Processing tank with removable inserts.** The central compartment holds the rinse water. The insert on the left is filled with the developer solution, and the insert on the right is filled with the fixer solution.

3. **Color** of the filter.
4. **Condition** of the filter. It must be free of scratches and not cracked.
5. **Length of time** that the film is subjected to safelight exposure. Any exposure over 2 1/2 minutes is likely to fog the radiograph.

Viewboxes

A **viewbox** is a light source (generally a lamp behind an opaque glass) used for viewing radiographs. Some darkrooms are equipped with wall-mounted viewboxes or illuminators. These emit considerable light, and care must be taken not to unwrap packets or leave the cover of the processing tank off when they are turned on.

Processing Tanks

A **processing tank** is a receptacle divided into compartments (for developer solution, water rinse, and fixer solution) used to process radiographs. The processing tank has two insert tanks placed inside the master tank (see Figure 8–4). The insert tanks hold the developer and fixer solutions. Traditionally, the left insert tank holds the developer solution, and the right insert tank contains the fixer solution. The area between the insert tanks holds water for rinsing and washing the films.

Most tanks are made of stainless steel, which does not react with processing chemicals. Insert tanks are large enough to accept an 8 × 10 in. (20 × 25 cm) extraoral film. The capacity of an insert tank is 1 gal (3.8 L).

The insert tanks are removable to facilitate cleaning. A small hole at the bottom of the insert tank lets the solution drain into the master tank when a small rubber plug is pulled out. The master tank is connected to the water intake and to the drain. When in use, fresh water circulates constantly. An overflow pipe keeps the level of the water constant when the tank is full. Some tanks are equipped with a temperature control device, a water-mixing valve that mixes the hot and cold water in the pipes to any desired temperature. A close-fitting light-proof cover completes the tank assembly (see Figure 8–5).

Utility Sink

A **sink** large enough to wash the processing insert tanks should be available in the darkroom.

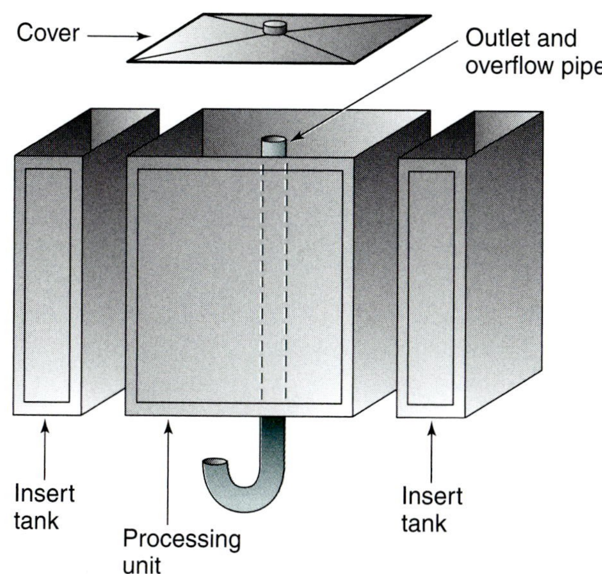

FIGURE 8-5. **Drawing showing the processing tank assembly.**

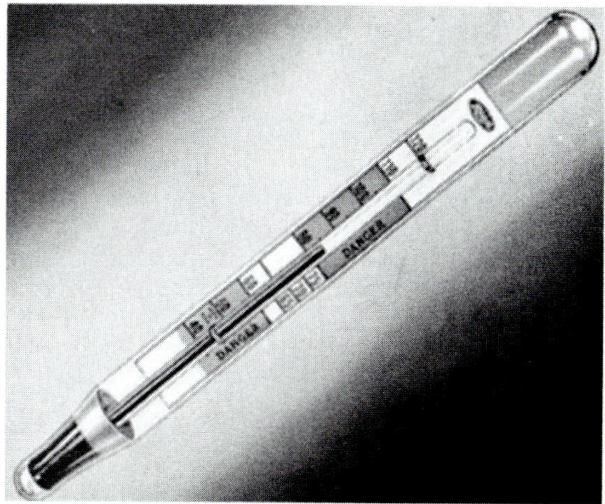

FIGURE 8-6. **Floating thermometer** for use in the developer solution or water compartment. When using the time-temperature method, the ideal temperature is 68°F (20°C). (Courtesy of Dentsply/Rinn Corporation)

Stirring Paddles

Two **stirring paddles,** or rods, must be available for mixing and stirring the chemicals. To avoid contamination, the developer and the fixer, each need their own stirring paddle. The paddles should be made of stainless steel or other material that does not react with the processing chemicals.

Thermometer

A **thermometer** is necessary to determine the temperature of the developing solution for time-temperature manual processing. Both clip type and floating thermometers are available. Floating thermometers are preferred because they can be left floating in the developing tank and easily picked up for reading (see Figure 8–6). Thermometers clipped to the side of the developing tank are more difficult to remove to read.

Timer

An accurate interval **timer** is necessary for time-temperature manual processing. The timer is used to indicate how long the film was placed in the developing solution, the fixing solution, and the wash water. The timer has an audible alarm to alert the radiographer to remove the films from the appropriate solutions.

Film Hangers, Drying Racks, and Drip Pans

A **film hanger** is a stainless steel device with clips used to attach films during processing (see Figure 8–7). Film hangers have an identification tag near the curved handle on which the patient's name can be written. Various sizes are available holding up to 20 films. Hangers should be washed after use. Only clean, dry hangers should be used. On a convenient wall several **drying racks** (towel racks) can be mounted for hanging film hangers. **Drip pans** should be placed underneath the drying racks to catch the water that may run off the wet films.

Electric Fan

An **electric fan,** placed to blow air on the drying racks, can be used to hasten film drying. Also, a fan helps circulate darkroom air.

Film Dryer

Commercial **film dryers** that circulate warm air around the films to reduce drying time are available.

Wastebasket, Lead Foil Container, and Biohazard Container

A **wastebasket** should be available in the darkroom for the disposal of waste items. Currently, suggested protocol is for lead foil to be separated from other film wrappings

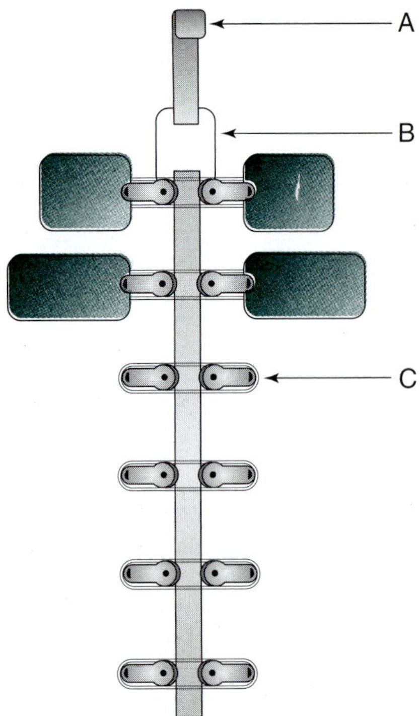

FIGURE 8–7. **Intraoral film hanger with 12 clips.** Various hangers ranging in capacity from a single film to 16 films are available. (**A**) Curved portion at the top of the hanger rests on upper rim of tank insert when films are immersed. (**B**) White plastic identification tag on which the patient's name can be written in pencil and later erased. (**C**) Clamps with three-point positive grip hold the firm securely in place and parallel to the film base. (Courtesy of Densply/Rinn Corporation)

and placed in appropriate container and the remainder of the film packet placed in a biohazard container.

Care of Tanks and Processing Solutions

The operator should always wear protective eyewear, mask, utility gloves, and a plastic or rubber apron when cleaning the tank or changing the solutions. The tank and its inserts should be scrubbed each time the solutions are changed. A solution made up of 1.5 oz (45 mL) of commercial hydrochloric acid, 1 qt (0.95 L) of cold water, and 3 qt (2.85 L) of warm water is sufficient to remove the deposits that frequently form on the walls of 1 gal (3.8 L) inserts. Commercial solutions for cleaning are available.

Cleaning the Processing Tank

To **clean the processing tank,** first pull the plug and drain the inserts, then thoroughly scrub all portions of the tank, inserts, and cover. Never use cleansing powders, as they will leave a residue that contaminates the processing chemicals. If the inserts appear to be coated, fill them with acid-cleaning solution and let them soak for 30 min; then drain out the cleaning solution and rinse them with plenty of water. All parts of the tank, including the cover, should be wiped clean before the plugs are replaced and the inserts filled.

Changing Solutions

Processing solutions should be changed at least every 4 weeks or as recommended by the manufacturer. The developer and the fixer are poured into the inserts until the level of the solutions reaches a mark on the side of the insert that indicates the full level (about 1 in. from the top). The central compartment must be filled with water. When that is done, the processing tank is ready for use. Most operators drain the central water compartment at the end of each working day.

Oxidation

Oxidation is the union of a substance—in this case, the developer—with the oxygen in the air. The developer especially is subject to oxidation in the presence of air and loses some of its effectiveness. Whenever possible, the processing tank should remain covered to prevent the possibility of oxidation and evaporation. The cover should be removed only when adding solutions to the proper level, when checking the temperature of the developer, and when inserting, removing, or changing the film hangers from one compartment or insert to another. The cover should be replaced immediately after any of these steps is completed.

Chemical Contamination

Chemical contamination is the mixing of the alkali developer with the acid fixer, an ever-present threat in film processing. Stirring paddles and thermometers must be cleaned after each use. Never use the same stirring paddle in both the developer and fixer without first cleaning it thoroughly. If the paddles are made of wood, separate ones must be used for each solution to prevent cross-contamination. Film hangers must be thoroughly rinsed to prevent chemicals from sticking to the clips for attaching the film.

Make sure that the part of the cover over the developer is always placed there. Care must be taken not to rotate the cover when it is removed, thereby causing a drop or two of condensed developer to fall into the fixer or vice versa. The operator can minimize this threat by labeling the inserts and the cover.

Manual Processing Procedures

Manual processing is a method used to process films in a series of steps performed by hand (see Table 8–3). First a word of caution concerning cross contamination. One should assume any patient could be the carrier of an infectious disease. See Chapter 22 on specific infection control procedures that pertain to manual processing.

The completion of the radiograph involves **preparation for processing, film processing,** and **final procedures.** Each of these involves a number of steps.

Preparation for Processing

The key to processing dental radiographs is adequate preparation. Preparation procedures are:

1. **Check the levels of the solution** to be sure the developer and fixer will cover the films on the top clips of the film hanger. The tanks are full when the solution levels are about one inch from the top. Add fresh solutions if necessary.
2. **Stir the developer and fixer** thoroughly to prevent the heavier chemicals from settling to the bottom and to equalize the temperature of the solutions.
3. **Determine the temperature of the developing solution.** A **floating thermometer** should be kept in the developer insert for frequent temperature reading. The temperature of the developer should be read after stirring.

   When developing dental x-ray film, always use a **time-temperature** development chart (see Table 8–4). The ideal (optimum) temperature for manual processing is 68°F (20°C) with a development time of 5 min. Following the time-temperature chart, one can see how much more time is required if the water and the developer are colder and how much less if they are warmer. Temperature variations from the ideal of 68°F (20°C) are acceptable as long as the developing time is correspondingly adjusted. Lower temperatures make the chemical reaction sluggish, and with higher temperatures the danger of fogging the film increases.

   The water should be allowed to circulate in the tank long enough before the films are processed to evenly adjust the temperature in all three compartments of the tank. Failure to do so may cause **reticulation**—a cracking of the film emulsion, producing a netlike pattern. Reticulation results when the film is removed from a warm solution (where the gelatin softens) and placed in a cold solution (cracking the gelatin).
4. **Select the proper film hanger** and write the name of the patient on the identification tag.

   Extraoral films are best identified by fastening an identification plate to one of the lower corners of the

TABLE 8–3. **Checklist for Processing Film Manually**

1. Check levels of developer and fixer
2. Stir processing solutions
3. Check temperature of developer
4. Label film hanger
5. Close and lock darkroom door
6. Unwrap film packets
7. Clip film to hangers
8. Set timer
9. Immerse films into developer solution and activate timer
10. Remove films from developer
11. Rinse films
12. Immerse films into fixer solution
13. Set and activate timer
14. Remove films from fixer
15. Wash films for minimum 20 min
16. Dry films
17. Mount films or place in labeled envelope

TABLE 8–4. **Time-Temperture Chart**

Temperature		Development Time (min)
60°F (15.5°C)		9
65°F (18.3°C)		7
68°F (20°C)	**optimum**	5
70°F (21.1°C)		4.5
75°F (23.9°C)		4
80°F (26.7°C)		3

face of the cassette. Special lettering sets, made of lead, are available. Minimum identification is the patient's name and the letters R (for right) and L (for left). These identifications become visible on the processed radiograph. Offices that handle a volume of the large extraoral film may use a film identification printer (see Figure 8–8).

5. **Close and lock the darkroom door.**
6. **Turn on the safelights and then turn off the overhead white light.**
7. **Unwrap each exposed film packet** on a clean working surface (use proper infection control procedures as explained in Chapter 22).
8. **Secure each unwrapped film to a clip on the hanger.** Check each film to make sure it is securely attached. Loose films may be lost at the bottom of an insert tank.

   Extraoral films are placed in special hangers that have channels into which the film fits or are attached to spring clips. To place the film in the hanger, hold the film in the right hand and grasp the hanger with the left. Next, guide the film into the channels until it is all the way into the hanger and the hinged retaining channel over the open end of the hangar can be closed.
9. **Set the timer.** Preset the interval timer to the time indicated for the solution temperature (see Table 8–2). The optimum developing time-temperature is 5 min at 68°F (20°C).

Film Processing

The **film processing** sequence consists of five steps: development, rinsing, fixation, washing, and drying.

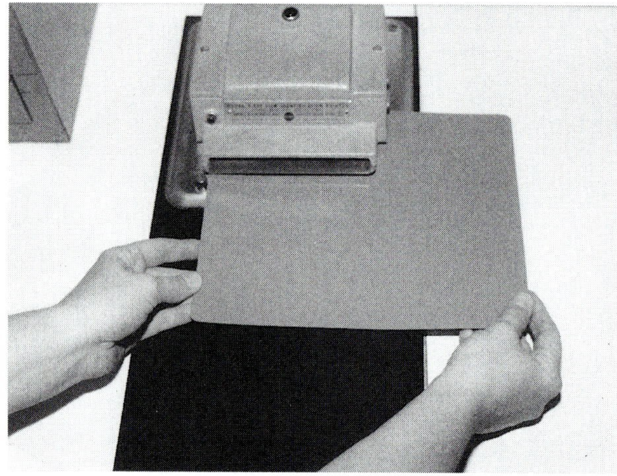

FIGURE 8–8. **Photographic printer** for including typed identification information on x-ray sheet film.

1. **Development.** Slowly and completely immerse the film hanger into the developing solution. Gently agitate the hanger up and down a few times—taking care not to splash—to eliminate air bubbles from clinging to the film. Allow the developer to make contact with all areas of the film. Hang the handle of the film hanger on the edge of the insert tank. Activate the timer and place the cover on the processing tank.
2. **Rinsing.** The purpose of the rinsing is to remove as much of the alkaline developer as possible before placing the film in the fixer. After the timer goes off, uncover the processing tank and lift the film hanger above the developing solution a few seconds to drain. Immerse the hanger into the rinse water for 20 to 30 sec. Gently agitate so that the water can touch all the film. Before transferring to the fixer, hold the hanger above the rinse water and allow to drain for a few seconds to prevent carrying too much water into the fixer.
3. **Fixation.** Immerse the hanger into the fixing solution and gently agitate to prevent air bubbles from clinging to the film. Hang the film hanger on the edge of the fixing solution insert tank. Set the timer and activate. A minimum fixation time of ten minutes is recommended. Place the cover on the processing tank.

Although the fixing time is not as critical as the developing time, and a film may occasionally remain in the fixer longer than necessary, the recommended time of 10 min should be followed. When the fixing time is too short, the result can be slow drying, poor hardening of the emulsion, a possible partial loss of detail, and the radiograph will darken. When the fixing time is excessively long, the image will lighten.

Quick Reading

When the radiograph is needed immediately for a **quick reading** of the x-ray image, the film may be read while it is still wet (wet reading). The film may be removed from the fixer as soon as it clears (usually after two or three minutes). It should then be rinsed in water for a short interval and taken into the operatory for viewing.

The film must be returned to the fixer as soon as possible to complete the fixation and permit further shrinking of the emulsion. If this is not done, some of the unexposed silver bromide grains may be left in the film, giving it a fogged and discolored appearance. Also, the emulsion may not completely harden.

4. **Washing.** Washing the film removes all chemicals left on the radiograph. After the timer goes off, remove the cover from the processing tank. Hold the film hanger above the fixing solution a few seconds to drain. Place the films in the circulating water. Set timer for a minimum of 20 min and activate. Replace processing cover. Longer washing is permissible, but the film should always be removed not later than the end of the working day.
5. **Drying.** After the timer goes off, remove the cover from the processing tank. Hold the film hanger above the water and gently shake to remove excess water. Allow the films to dry by one of the following methods.

   - Suspend the hanger from a drying rack. Take care that the film does not contact other films on adjacent racks or brush up against the wall.
   - Follow the same procedure but use a fan or blower to expedite the drying.
   - Place the film in a heated drying cabinet.

> **NOTE: Always use a drip pan when moving the film hangers from the processing tank to the drying area and leave the pan under the film hanger until the film is dry.**

Final Procedures

The steps in the **final procedures** include:

1. Check to see that none of the films have loosened from the clip and dropped on the floor or the bottom of the tank.
2. Clean up the work area. Wipe up any moisture caused by dripping or accidental splashing of the water or solutions.
3. Remove the dry films from the hangers and place them in properly identified protective envelopes or on film mounts with identifying data (film mounting techniques are discussed in Chapter 12).
4. Remove or erase identification markings from the hangers. Clean and replace hangers, and any equipment used.

At the end of the working day, turn off the water to the tank, drain the water compartment, and turn off all lights in the darkroom.

Rapid Processing Procedures

As already mentioned, one technique for obtaining a diagnostic radiograph in minimal time during an emergency situation is to remove it from the fixer as soon as it is cleared enough to wet-read the film. A newer technique, made possible by faster-acting chemicals and the introduction of the compact "chair-side darkroom" (see Figure 8–9), makes it possible to process the small intraoral films in normal light within 30 sec.

Rapid processing is most valuable in endodontic and oral surgery practices. A significant amount of chair time can be saved when it is necessary to expose a series of single films to check the progress in reaming out a root canal during endodontic treatment. Rapid processing enables the oral surgeon to instantly determine the extent or location of a fractured root. The general practitioner occasionally requires rapid confirmation of the success or failure of an operation performed. However, rapid processing has definite limitations and is never intended to replace conventional processing.

Since temperatures as high as 92°F (33.3°C) are used, the developing time must be kept short (as brief as 5 sec). Short developing and fixing times, combined with minimal washing, result in a substandard radiograph. It must be recognized that while rapid processing fulfills the dentist's need to receive rapid information, it is at the expense of image quality. Such films are frequently fogged, have poor image density and contrast, eventually discolor, and are seldom suitable for filing with the patient's permanent record.

The "chair-side darkroom" has two lighttight openings through which the hands can enter the working compartment when the lid is closed. The transparent plastic filtered top permits the operator to see while unwrapping the film packet and transferring it through the four cups filled with developer, rinse water, fixer, and wash water. For best results the solutions are heated to 85°F (29.4°C) by a calibrated heater in the unit. If normal radiographic density is desired, develop for 15 sec and fix for 30 sec. In the event that the film is to be retained with the permanent record, it should be refixed for 4 min and washed for 20 min at normal conventional darkroom temperatures and conditions.

Three **precautions** should be taken.

1. Change the water and solutions daily.
2. Clean drips or spills after each use to avoid contamination.
3. Close the light filtering top securely before processing the film.

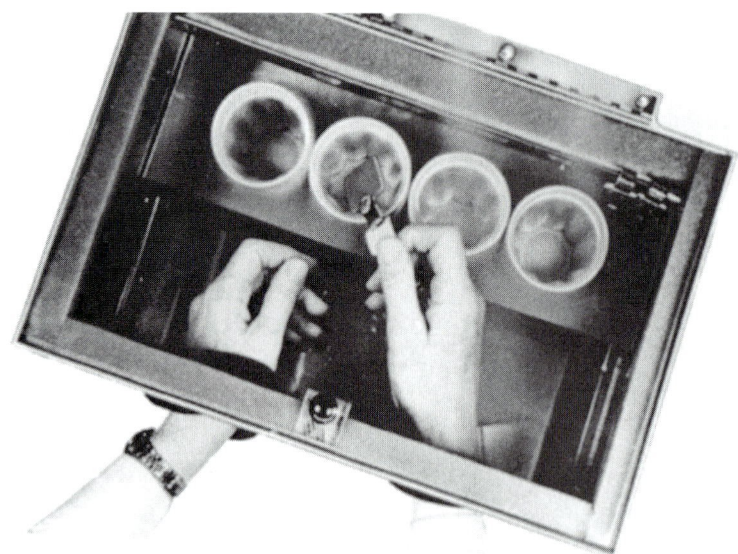

FIGURE 8–9. **Chair-side darkroom unit shown with view through plastic filtered top.** First cup is filled with developer concentrate mixed 1:1 with water, second cup with rinse water, third cup with fixer concentrate mixed 1:1 with water, and fourth cup with wash water. A heater with a thermostat keeps the solutions at optimum temperature for rapid processing. (Courtesy of Densply/Rinn Corporation)

Automatic Processing

Automatic processing is a simple method of processing dental x-ray film. It is often preferred over manual processing for the following reasons:

- **Less processing time.** Automatic processors produce a dry radiograph in about 5 minutes, whereas manual processing requires about one hour.
- **Time and temperature are automatically controlled,** providing less chance for operator error.

Although a large number of dentists have switched to automated processors, many continue to use manual processing. Because automated equipment can, and does, break down occasionally, and because the processor may only handle one or two types of film, the dental office continues to need a manually equipped darkroom.

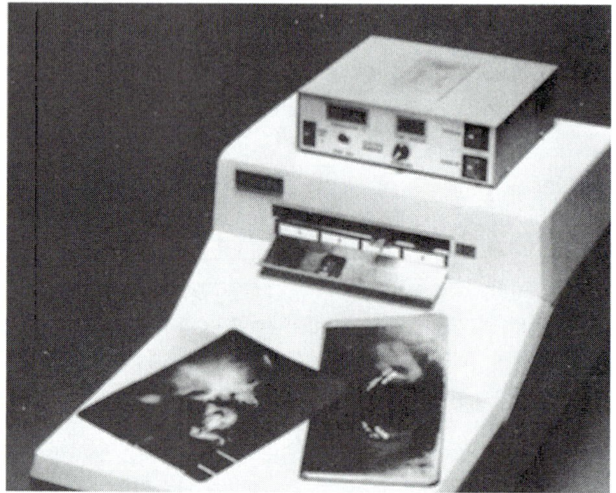

FIGURE 8–10. **Automatic processor,** equipped with solid-state time and temperature control, accommodates all films up to 8 in. × 10 in. (20 cm × 25 cm). It is capable of providing damp films for wet reading in just 50 seconds and films of archival quality in 4.5 minutes. (Courtesy of Philips Dental Systems)

Automatic Processing Unit

Automatic processing units vary in size and complexity (see Figure 8–10). Some have a limited capacity and process only intraoral or certain sizes of extraoral films. Others can handle any dental film regardless of size. Most are intended for use in the dark-room under safelight conditions. Automatic processors equipped with **daylight**

loaders have a light-tight baffle for inserting the hands while unwrapping the film and can be used right in the operatory.

Parts of the Automatic Processor

The automatic processor uses a roller transport system to move the film through the processing cycle.

The typical automatic processor consists of three compartments and a drying chamber (see Figure 8–11).

1. The **developer compartment** holds the developing solution.
2. The **fixing compartment** holds the fixing solution.
3. The **water compartment** holds the circulating water.
4. The **drying chamber** contains heated air that dries the wet film.

Unwrapped film is fed into the **film feed slot** on the outside of the processor. The **roller transport system** moves the film through the developer, fixer, water, and drying compartments. Motor-driven gears or belts propel the roller transport system. The film emerges from the processor in an opening on the outside of the processor called the **film recovery slot.**

All automatic processors require water. Some can be connected to plumbing system, whereas in others the water is self-contained. A heating unit warms the processing chemicals to the required temperature. As a rule, a 20-min warming-up period is required before the unit is operational. On most units, the processing cycle is set at approximately 5 min for intraoral film.

Processing Chemicals

The **processing chemicals** differ from those used in manual procedures by being supersaturated and having more hardener in the developer. The chemical solutions in automatic processors are heated to temperatures much higher than those used in manual processing—as high as 125°F (52°C) in some units. Fortunately, advanced film technology has produced emulsions that can withstand these temperatures for the short times required in automated processing without excessive softening or melting.

A recirculation system keeps the solutions agitated and distributed evenly. Some units automatically replenish the solutions; others depend on the operator to keep them at the correct level.

Procedures for Automatic Processing

Use the following step-by-step procedures for automatic processing.

1. Close and lock the darkroom door.
2. Turn on safelights and turn off overhead white light.
3. Unwrap film packets over a clean working surface using infection control procedures (see Chapter 22). Always handle the film by the edges.
4. Insert the film into the film feed slot one at a time. Make sure the film is straight when inserted to prevent overlapping.
5. Allow about 10 seconds between the insertion of each film.

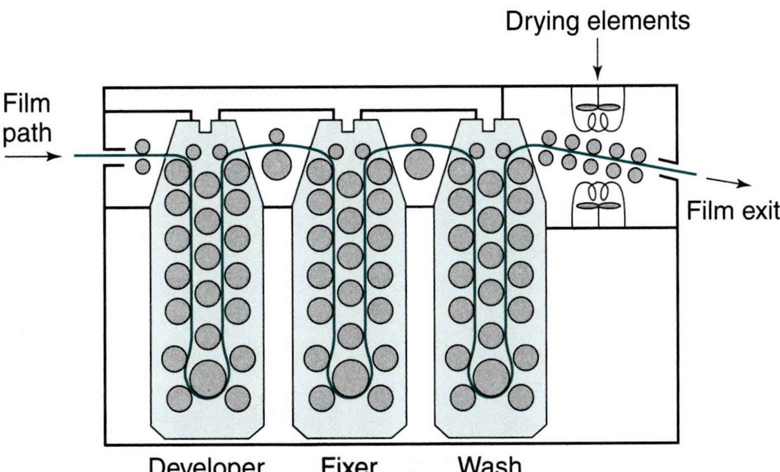

FIGURE 8–11. **Schematic illustration of automatic film processor.** Film is transported by roller assemblies.

6. If multiple feed slots are available, alternate slots when possible. Do not insert films too rapidly or overlapping may occur.
7. After all the films have been inserted, allow processing to occur (usually about 5 minutes).
8. Collect the processed radiographs from the film recovery slot.
9. Mount radiographs or place in labeled envelope.

Automatic processors equipped with daylight loaders do not need to use a darkroom.

Maintenance

Automatic processors can do an excellent job but only if the instructions for **maintenance** are scrupulously followed. Few pieces of equipment in the dental office require such diligent and regular care. Depending upon the workload, automatic processors require daily or weekly cleaning. For best results, a time should be set aside for regular cleaning and maintenance. If the rollers are not kept clean, the radiographs emerge streaked. An extraoral size film is used to clean the rollers. Each morning, the extraoral cleaning film should be run through the processor to remove any dirt and residual gelatin from the rollers. At least weekly, the roller assembly must be removed and cleaned in warm, running water and then soaked for 15 to 20 min. Read and follow manufacturer's instructions concerning care and maintenance.

Besides being difficult to clean and maintain other **disadvantages** of automatic processing are:

1. Artifacts occasionally occur on the radiographs (usually caused by excessive pressure of the rollers on the emulsion).
2. Film may become stuck between the rollers and cause jamming.
3. Problems with failure to identify the film.
4. Increased film fog because of high temperatures used.

Film Duplicating Procedures

A **duplicate radiograph** is an identical copy of the original radiograph. Radiographs should never leave the dental office unless they have been duplicated. There are increasing requirements for duplicating radiographs on the part of insurance companies and governmental agencies because of third-party payment plans. Also, duplicate radiographs are needed when referring patients to specialists or when the patient moves and changes dentists.

The necessity for film duplication has long been recognized. Some dentists solve the problem by using two-film packets. Others duplicate radiographs using a film duplicator.

Advantages of film duplication are:

- Film can be duplicated as often as necessary without additional patient exposure.
- Density of the radiograph can be varied for improved diagnostic quality by changing the time it is exposed to light in the duplicator.

Equipment

Duplicating radiographs requires **duplicating film** and a **duplicator.**

Duplicating Film

Duplicating film is available in sheet form in a variety of sizes. The film is emulsion-coated on one side only. Under a safelight, the emulsion side looks dull, while the noncoated side looks shiny. It is possible to duplicate either a single radiograph or a full-mouth series at a single printing.

Film Duplicator

A **film duplicator** is a device that provides a diffused light source (preferably ultraviolet) that evenly exposes the duplicating film. The film duplicator may be a commercial model (see Figure 8–12) or it may be a photographic printing frame and a light source. Large duplicators accommodate all film sizes, whereas small duplicators may only use #2 film and smaller (see Figure 8–13).

Procedures for Film Duplication

The process of film duplication is simple and rapidly learned. All duplication must be done in the darkroom under a safelight.

1. The original radiograph to be duplicated is placed with viewing side up on the light screen of the duplicator.
2. Under safelight conditions, the duplicating film is positioned on the original radiograph with the emulsion side away from the operator and in contact with the top of the original radiograph.
3. The cover is then closed to keep both radiograph and duplicating film in tight contact during the exposure.

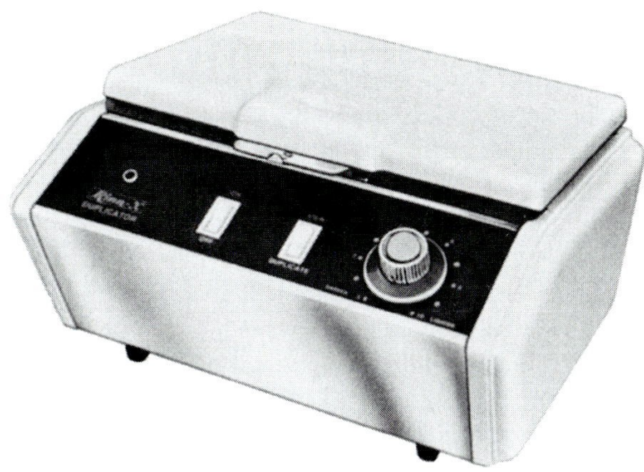

FIGURE 8-12. **Contact printer type of x-ray duplicating unit** containing a built-in fluorescent light source and a timer that turns on the lamp for a preset time to permit variations in density. This x-ray duplicator provides a convenient means for exposing duplicating film with dental radiographs. (Courtesy of Densply/Rinn Corporation)

If the contact is not tight, the duplicate radiograph will be fuzzy.

4. Select the proper exposure time (see manufacturer's instructions), set the timer, and activate the light source to expose the film.

Exposure time affects the density of the radiograph that is to be duplicated. A shorter exposure will increase the density (darkness) of the duplicate; a longer exposure will decrease (lighten) the duplicate. This fact can be taken advantage of to lighten an overexposed film or to darken one that was underexposed.

5. After the exposure is complete, the film is removed from the frame and processed in the same manner as a radiograph—manually or automatically.
6. Label the processed duplicate radiograph with the patient's name and date of exposure using a radiographic marking pencil. Also, be sure to label the patient's right and left sides.

Removal of Processing Stains from Uniform

Despite all precautions, uniforms will occasionally become soiled with developer or fixer stains. Of the two, the developer is more difficult to remove. Never launder a uniform before trying to remove the spot.

The best procedure is to rub a saturated soap solution into the spot as soon as possible, before it becomes permanently set into the fabric. Uniform shops and dental supply houses carry a number of very effective commercial spot removers, such as Fix Off™. If such a remover is not available, the spot may be soaked for 5 to 10 min in a solution of 1/2 oz (15 mL) of household bleach and 1/2 oz (15 mL) of vinegar to 1 gal (3.8 L) of warm water. Then rinse in plain water. Stubborn stains may require longer soaking. After the spot is removed, the uniform should be laundered as soon as possible.

Disposal of Radiographic Wastes

Today's dental office team should make every effort to **recycle** or **properly dispose of wastes** that may be harmful to the environment. Radiographic wastes include x-ray processing chemicals, intraoral film packets, and discarded radiographs.

The Federal Resource Conservation and Recovery Act (RCRA) of 1976 was enacted to "promote the protection of human health and the environment and to conserve valuable material and energy resources." In the past, the management of radiographic wastes was to discard them with the trash or pour them down the drain. This is no longer appropriate for materials listed by RCRA as hazardous.

In areas that have a municipal sewer system with a secondary biological wastewater treatment plant, x-ray processing solutions may be disposed into the system and considered to be effectively treated. However, the disposal of x-ray processing solutions into a septic tank

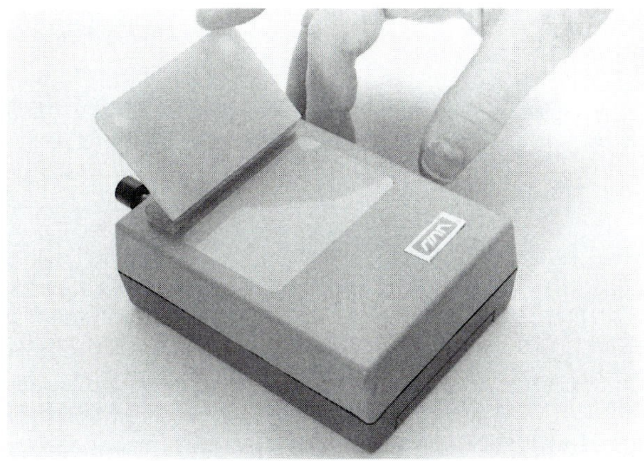

FIGURE 8-13. **Small film duplicator** accommodates film sizes #0, #1, and #2.

system could require state regulatory approval. One must be aware that some state and local waste management regulations are more stringent than the federal regulation. Be sure to check with your state Hazardous Waste Management Agency for regulations that exist in your area.

It may be convenient to have processing chemicals removed by a commercial waste disposal company. Contact your state Hazardous Waste Management Agency for a list of licensed companies in your area.

Silver, a metal regulated by most control agencies, is present in the fixing solution and in wash water. The amount of silver will depend upon the number of films processed. Some control agencies may require the removal of silver from the fixing solution before disposal. Silver recovery methods, such as the Kodak Chemical Recovery Cartridge, arc available (see bibliography).

Scrap film or discarded radiographs also contain silver and should be collected and recycled. Check with your local health department for a list of silver refiners and buyers.

Intraoral film packers contain plastic and lead foil that should be separated and properly disposed. The plastic components should be recycled. Lead is considered a hazardous waste under RCRA regulations dental film manufacturers and local scrap metal dealers are possible sources for recycling lead foil.

Every dental office should properly dispose of wastes, for today's actions will surely affect the quality of tomorrow's environment.

CHAPTER SUMMARY

Film processing is a series of steps that converts the invisible latent image on the dental x-ray film into a visible permanent image called a radiograph. The sequence of steps followed in all processing is developing, rinsing, fixing, washing, and drying.

Two processing chemicals are used—an alkaline developer and a slightly acid fixer. There are four chemicals in the **developer:** a developing agent, a preservative, an activator, and a restrainer. The developing solution reduces the exposed silver halide crystals to black metallic silver.

The film is **rinsed** thoroughly to remove the developer before the film is inserted in the fixer.

There are four chemicals in the **fixer:** a fixing agent, a preservative, a hardening agent, and an acidifier. The fixing solution removes the undeveloped silver halide crystals and hardens the emulsion.

The films are **washed** thoroughly to remove all chemicals.

The final step is drying the film. The processed film is now called a radiograph.

A darkroom is a completely darkened room used to process x-ray film. With the exception of automatic processors equipped with daylight loaders, all processing must be done in the darkroom under safelight conditions. Using the proper safelight is important because radiographic films vary in their sensitivity to light.

Dental offices process x-ray film by conventional **manual processing** and/or by **automatic processing.** Step-by-step procedure for manual and automatic processing are presented in this chapter.

Compared to manual processing, the chemicals used in automatic processing are more concentrated and contain more hardener. Also, automatic processing uses higher temperatures and shorter processing time.

A radiograph can be copied on duplicating film whenever it is necessary to send one out of the office to another dentist, insurance company, law firm, and so forth.

Every dental office should properly dispose of radiographic film wastes.

REVIEW QUESTIONS

1. Which term best describes the process by which the latent image becomes visible?
   (a) Reticulation
   (b) Reduction
   (c) Sensitivity
   (d) Preservation
2. What happens to the radiograph when a film is exposed to a safelight too long?
   (a) Radiograph appears white.
   (b) Radiograph becomes fogged.
   (c) Radiograph becomes reticulated.
   (d) Radiograph becomes attenuated.
3. How far above the work area in the darkroom should the safelight be located?
   (a) 6 to 8 in. (15 to 20 cm)
   (b) 1 1/2 ft (46 cm)
   (c) 2 1/2 ft (76cm)
   (d) 4 ft (1.2 m)
4. The Kodak GBX-2 safelight filter is recommended for:
   (a) Intraoral films only.
   (b) Extraoral films only.
   (c) Both intraoral and extraoral films.
   (d) None of the above.
5. Which of these is the correct processing sequence?
   (a) Rinse, fix, wash, develop, dry
   (b) Fix, rinse, develop, wash, dry
   (c) Develop, rinse, fix, wash, dry
   (d) Rinse, develop, wash, fix, dry
6. The basic constituents of the developer solution are:
   (a) Clearing agent, activator, preservative, restrainer.
   (b) Reducing agent, activator, preservative, restrainer.
   (c) Reducing agent, acidifier, preservative, restrainer.
   (d) Clearing agent, preservative, hardener, acidifier.
7. Which of the following reduces the exposed silver bromide crystals?
   (a) Developer
   (b) Wetting agent
   (c) Fixer
   (d) Cutting reducer
8. Which developing chemical becomes extremely active when the temperature is raised?
   (a) Sodium sulfite
   (b) Potassium bromide
   (c) Elon
   (d) Hydroquinone

9. Which ingredient of the developer is alkaline and causes the emulsion to soften and swell?

   (a) The developing agent
   (b) The preservative
   (c) The activator
   (d) The restrainer

10. Which ingredient of the fixer removes all unexposed and any remaining undeveloped silver halide crystals?

    (a) The fixing agent
    (b) The preservative
    (c) The activator
    (d) The restrainer

11. The film emulsion is hardened during:

    (a) Development.
    (b) Rinsing.
    (c) Fixation.
    (d) Washing.

12. The floating thermometer for manual processing should be placed in the:

    (a) Developing solution.
    (b) Water compartment.
    (c) Fixing solution.
    (d) Both b and c.

13. Light leaks in the darkroom will cause:

    (a) Lightening of the film.
    (b) Film fog.
    (c) Underdeveloped film.
    (d) Under exposed film.

14. The processing tank should be cleaned:

    (a) Every day.
    (b) Once a week.
    (c) Every two weeks.
    (d) Whenever the solutions are changed.

15. What is the ideal temperature when film is processed manually?

    (a) 60°F (15.5°C)
    (b) 68°F (20°C)
    (c) 75°F (23.9°C)
    (d) 83°F (28.3°C)

16. Chemically, what is the major difference between solutions used for manual processing and those used for rapid and automatic processing?

    (a) There is more acid in rapid processing solutions.
    (b) Manual processing solutions contain more preservative.
    (c) Rapid and automatic processing solutions contain more hardener.
    (d) Manual processing solutions are more alkaline.

17. Which term describes a fully processed radiograph that shows a network of cracks on its surface?
    (a) Fogged
    (b) Reticulated
    (c) Restrained
    (d) Proliferated
18. Replenisher is added to the developing solution to:
    (a) Compensate for oxidation.
    (b) Compensate for loss of volume.
    (c) Compensate for loss of solution strength.
    (d) All of the above.
19. If a dried radiograph were processed a second time, its appearance would show:
    (a) Increased contrast and density.
    (b) Decreased contrast and density.
    (c) Increased contrast only.
    (d) Increased density only.
    (e) No change in contrast or density.
20. What is the major problem encountered with automatic processors?
    (a) Overdevelopment of films
    (b) Underdevelopment of films
    (c) Amount of maintenance required
    (d) Films getting stuck between the rollers
21. What is the appearance of duplicating film when viewed under safelight conditions?
    (a) The nonemulsion side appears dull.
    (b) The nonemulsion side appears pebbly.
    (c) The emulsion side appears shiny.
    (d) The emulsion side appears dull.
22. Radiographic wastes include ____________, ______________, and __________.

BIBLIOGRAPHY

Eastman Kodak. *Exposure and Processing for Dental Radiography*. Rochester, NY: Eastman Kodak, 1998

Eastman Kodak. *Management of Photographic Wastes in the Dental Office*. Rochester, NY: Eastman Kodak, 1991.

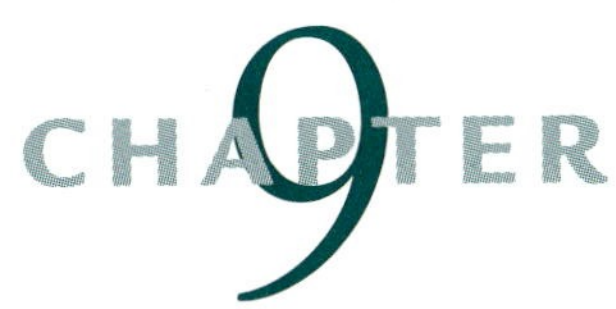

Identifying and Correcting Faulty Radiographs

OBJECTIVES

By the end of this chapter the student should be able to:

- Define the key words.
- Identify the types of radiographic errors caused by faulty exposure techniques.
- Identify the types of radiographic errors caused by incorrect film positioning and angulation of the central ray.
- Identify the types of radiographic errors caused by faulty processing techniques.
- Identify the types of radiographic errors caused by chemical contamination.
- Identify the types of radiographic errors caused by film handling.
- Identify problems caused by outdated film.
- Identify problems caused by faulty safelight conditions.

KEY WORDS

Cone cut
Distomesial projection
Elongation
Fog
Foreshortening
Horizontal angulation
Mesiodistal projection
Overlapping
Pressure mark
Reticulation
Vertical angulation

Introduction

It is important to be able to tell when a radiograph is inadequate and to understand why. Only clear, properly processed radiographs with minimal distortion of the image have diagnostic value to the dentist. Radiographs that fail to meet these standards must often be retaken. However, good common sense should be used in determining when a retake is absolutely needed. For example, a radiograph may show a major cone cut or artifact and yet show excellent quality of image at the root where an abcess is suspected. Such a radiograph, especially if it is a part of a full-mouth series in which the damaged film area is probably shown correctly on the neighboring film areas, should not be retaken. To do so would expose the patient to unnecessary radiation.

The purpose of this chapter is to help the student recognize the appearance of faulty radiographs, identify possible causes of such errors, and to know what steps are necessary to correct them.

Problems Caused by Faulty Exposure Techniques

Many **faulty radiographs** are caused by **errors in exposure technique,** such as incorrect positioning of the film packet, incorrect positioning of the **position indicating device (PID),** or incorrect exposure factors. Of course, position errors may also mean that the patient's head moved after the film, tube head, and PID were positioned or that the patient allowed the film to slip. The radiographer must always caution patients not to move their head and to hold the film firmly.

Incorrect Positioning of the Film

Absence of the Apical Structures (see Figure 9–1)

- ***Probable cause:*** Film was not placed high enough (maxillary) or low enough (mandibular) in the patient's mouth. Ideally, there should be approximately a 1/4-in. (6.4-mm) margin above or below the crown of

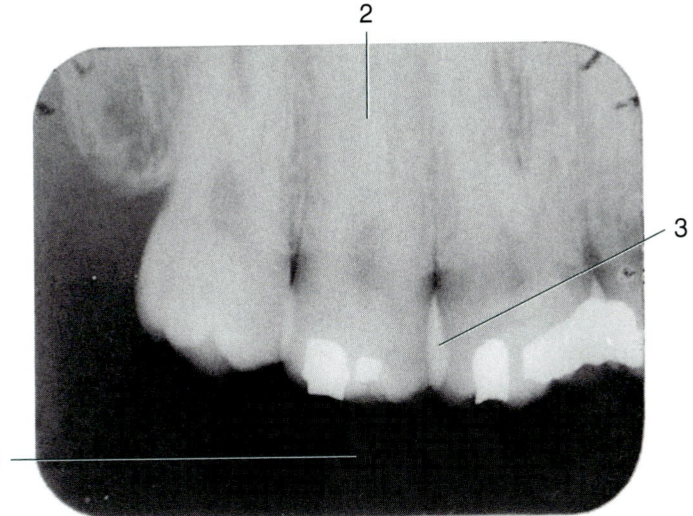

FIGURE 9–1. **Radiograph of maxillary molar.** (**1**) Excessive occlusal margin with resultant absence of the complete apical structures is caused by film being placed too low in mouth. (**2**) Tooth structures are elongated because the vertical angulation was insufficiently steep (too low). (**3**) Overlapping in the proximal areas is seen because in horizontal angulation the central beam was not directed through the interproximal spaces.

the tooth. When the paralleling technique is used, this error may also be caused by the film not being parallel to the long axes of the teeth.

- ***Correction:*** In the maxillary areas, raise the film in the patient's mouth. In the mandibular areas, lower the film in the patient's mouth. When paralleling, verify that the film and long axes are parallel.

Absence of Coronal Structures (see Figure 9–2)

- ***Probable cause:*** Film not placed high enough or low enough in the patient's mouth. Ideally there should be a 1/4-in. (6.4-mm) margin above or below the crown of the tooth. When the paralleling technique is used, this error may also be caused by the film not being parallel to the long axes of the teeth.
- ***Correction:*** In the maxillary areas, lower the film in the patient's mouth. In mandibular areas, raise the film in the patient's mouth. When paralleling, verify that the film and the long axes are parallel.

Absence of Mesial Structures

- ***Probable cause:*** Film was placed too far back in the patient's mouth.
- ***Correction:*** Move the film mesially (toward the front of the mouth).

Absence of Distal Structures

- ***Probable cause:*** Film was placed too far forward in the patient's mouth.
- ***Correction:*** Move the film distally (toward the back of the mouth).

Slanting or Diagonal Instead of Straight Occlusal Plane (see Figure 9–3)

- ***Probable cause:*** Edge of the film was not parallel with the incisal or occlusal plane of the teeth, or the film holder was not placed flush against the occlusal surfaces. When this error occurs in bitewing radiographs, it is usually caused by the top edge of the film contacting the lingual gingiva or the curvature of the palate.
- ***Correction:*** Straighten the film packet. The use of a cotton roll between the film and the tooth may make this easier.

NOTE: The cotton roll should be on the side of the bite block away from the film so that it is not included in the exposure.

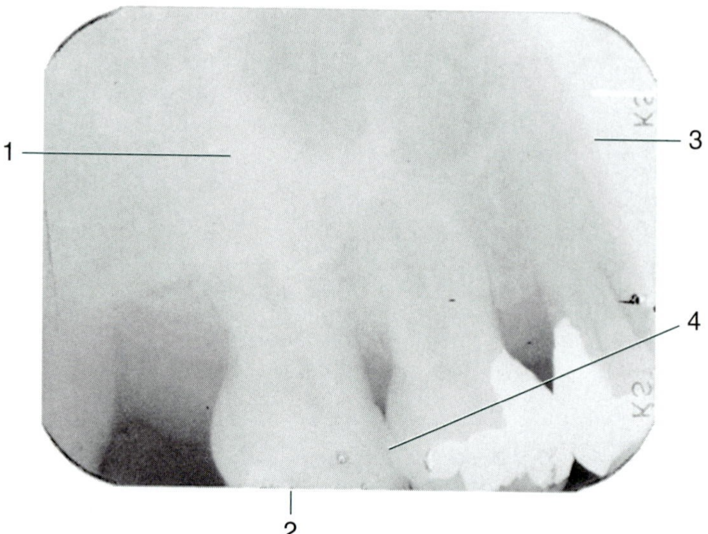

FIGURE 9–2. **Radiograph of maxillary molar area.** (**1**) Light image caused by underexposure or underdevelopment. (**2**) Absence of occlusal margin or all coronal structures is seen as the film was placed too high in mouth, not parallel to long axis of the teeth, and vertical angulation was too steep (too high). (**3**) Cone cut, an unexposed area caused by faulty centering of the PID. (**4**) Overlap in interproximal area is traceable to faulty horizontal angulation.

Vertical Instead of Horizontal Film Placement in the Posterior Areas

- ***Probable cause:*** Film was placed with its longest dimension vertically. This is seldom desirable in posterior areas.
- ***Correction:*** Rotate the film so that the widest dimension is placed horizontally and the film edge is parallel with the occlusal plane.

Horizontal Instead of Vertical Film Placement in the Anterior Areas

- ***Probable cause:*** Film was placed with its widest dimension horizontally. Such placement is undesirable and produces major dimensional distortion of the image; furthermore, these anterior teeth are sometimes longer than the narrow dimension of the film.
- ***Correction:*** Rotate the film so that the longest dimension is placed vertically. The short edge of the film should be placed parallel to the incisal edges of the anterior teeth.

Bent Film Packet (see Figure 9–4)

- ***Probable cause:*** Corner of film bent by radiographer to prevent discomfort to the patient.
- ***Correction:*** Handle film carefully. Do not bend film.

Diamond or Herringbone Pattern (see Figure 9–5)

- ***Probable cause:*** Film was reversed and the back side was facing the teeth and the radiation source.
- ***Correction:*** Turn the film so that the tube side faces toward the teeth and the radiation source.

Incorrect Position of Identification Dot

- ***Probable cause:*** Dot positioned in apical area.
- ***Correction:*** Position the dot in incisal or occlusal area.

> **NOTE: When placing films into film holders always put the dot in the slot.**

Incorrect Positioning of the Tube Head or PID

Elongation of the Image

Elongation or stretching of an image can occur when using the bisecting angle technique.

- ***Probable cause:*** Insufficient **vertical angulation** of the central beam (PID).
- ***Correction:*** Increase the vertical angulation. Also check the position of the film and the patient's head.

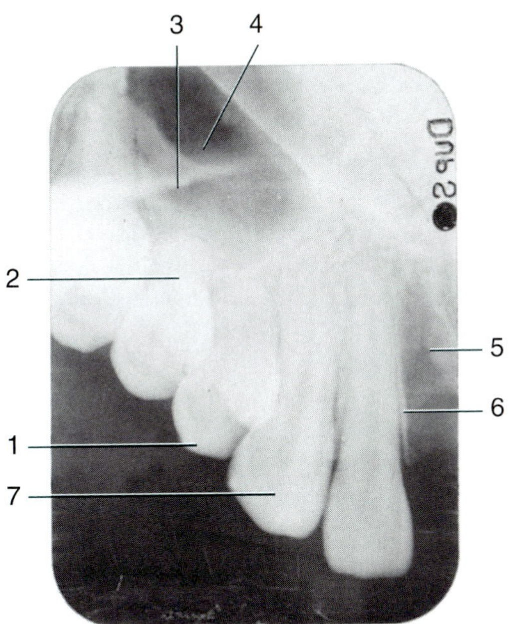

FIGURE 9–3. **Radiograph of maxillary canine area.** (**1**) Slanting or diagonal occlusal plane is caused by improper positioning of the film packet. (**2**) Extreme foreshortening is caused by a combination of excessive vertical angulation and faulty film position. (**3**) Distortion of image is caused by film bending. (**4**) Maxillary sinus, (**5**) recent extraction site, (**6**) lamina dura, and (**7**) canine is not properly centered in film.

Foreshortening of the Image

Foreshortening can occur when using the bisecting angle technique.

- ***Probable cause:*** Excessive vertical angulation of the central beam (PID).
- ***Correction:*** Decrease the vertical angulation. Also check the position of the film and the patient's head.

Overlapping of the Image (see Figures 9–1, 9–2, and 9–6)

- ***Probable cause:*** Incorrect rotation of the tube head and PID in the horizontal plane. Superimposition of the images of proximal surfaces occurs when the central beam is not directed perpendicularly toward the film through the interproximal spaces. The two common errors are **mesiodistal** and **distomesial** projections. When the angle of projection in the horizontal plane is from mesial to distal (mesiodistal projection), the mesiobuccal root of maxillary molars appears to be superimposed over the lingual root, and the areas of **overlapping contacts** are larger in the posterior part of the radiograph. Conversely, when the angle of projection is from distal to mesial (distomesial projection), the distobuccal root of maxillary molars appears to be superimposed over the lingual root, and the areas of overlapping contacts are larger in the anterior part of the radiograph.

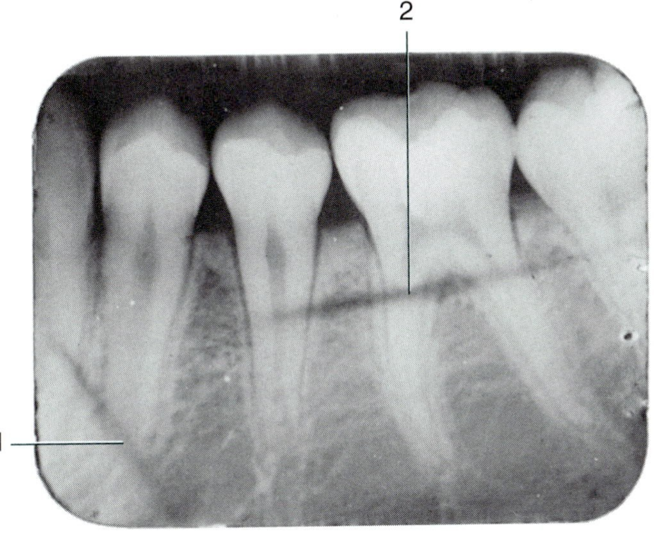

FIGURE 9–4. **Radiograph of mandibular posterior area.** (**1**) Distortion caused by bending the lower left film corner and pressure mark (thin radiolucent line). (**2**) Long radiolucent streak is a pressure mark caused by bending or by careless handling with excessive force.

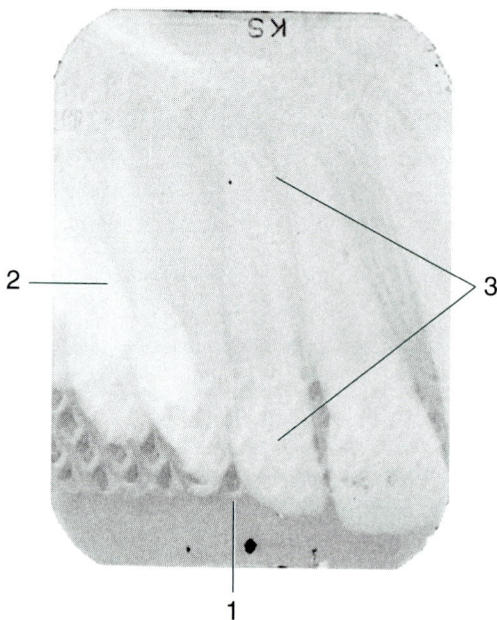

FIGURE 9-5. **Radiograph of maxillary anterior area.** (**1**) Film is not correctly centered and occlusal plane is not straight. (**2**) Foreshortening of images of the premolar and canine caused by a combination of excessive vertical angulation and faulty film placement. (**3**) Light image and two bars of herringbone (diamond) pattern showing that the film was accidentally reversed during placement in the mouth. The image is light because the lead foil absorbed some of the x-rays.

- ***Correction:*** Unless there is also elongation or foreshortening, maintain the vertical angulation. To compensate for mesiodistal angulation, change the direction of the PID so that the central ray is projected more to the distal; to compensate for distomesial angulation, change the direction of the PID so that the central ray is projected more to the mesial.

Cone Cut (see Figures 9–2, 9–7, and 9–8)

- ***Probable cause:*** The primary beam of radiation was not directed toward the center of the film and did not completely expose all parts of the film. The XCP instrument was assembled incorrectly.
- ***Correction:*** Maintain **horizontal** and **vertical angulation** and move the tube head either up, down, mesially, or distally, depending on which area of the radiograph shows a clear unexposed area. Check to see that the XCP instrument is assembled correctly.

Exposure Factors

Light (Thin) Image (see Figures 9–2, 9–5, and 9–9)

- ***Probable cause:*** Insufficient exposure time in relation to milliamperage, kilovoltage, and distance selected. Also timer inaccuracy or faulty switch. May also be caused by insufficient time in the developer, weak or oxidized developer, or reversed film.
- ***Correction:*** Increase the exposure time, the milliamperage, the kilovoltage, or a combination of these factors. If the problem persists, check the accuracy of the timer or switch for possible malfunction. Always use the proper time and temperature in development.

Dark Image (see Figure 9–10)

- ***Probable cause:*** Overexposure (excessive mAs, kVp, or time). Alternate cause: too long in the developer or temperature too high.
- ***Correction:*** Decrease the exposure time, the milliamperage, the kilovoltage, or a combination of these factors. Properly process film.

Absence of Image

- ***Probable cause:*** Failure to turn on the line switch or to maintain firm pressure on the activator button during the exposure. Alternate causes: electrical failure, malfunction of the x-ray machine or processing errors (placing the film in fixer first or having the emulsion dissolve in warm rinse water).
- ***Correction:*** Turn on the x-ray machine and maintain firm pressure on the activator button during the entire exposure period. On newer machines, listen for the audible tone that indicates that x-rays are being produced.

Miscellaneous Errors in Exposure Technique

Poor Definition

- ***Probable cause:*** Movement during exposure. Caused by patient movement, film slippage, or vibration of the tube head.
- ***Correction:*** Steady the tube head before starting exposure. Ask the patient to maintain steady pressure on the film holder and not to move.

Double Image

- ***Probable cause:*** Accidentally exposing the same film twice.
- ***Correction:*** Always develop or place the exposed film in the film safe immediately after exposure.

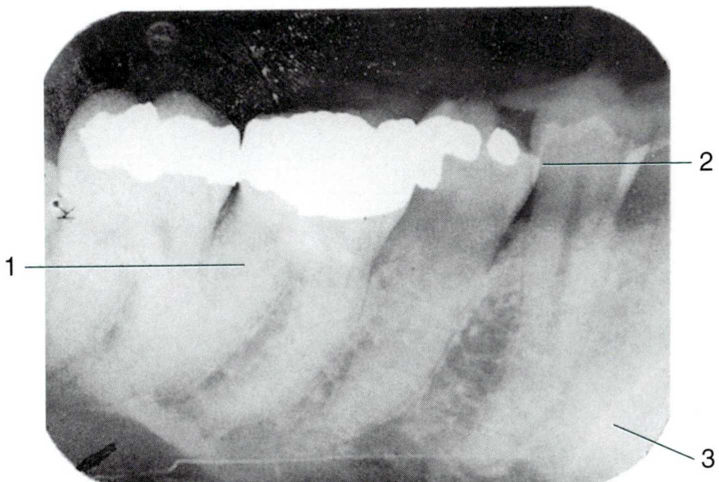

FIGURE 9-6. **Radiograph of mandibular premolar area.** (**1**) Distorted image and poor definition is caused by movement of the patient, the film, or the tube head during the time of exposure. (**2**) Overlapping of adjacent tooth structures is caused by error in horizontal angulation. (**3**) Distortion of image is caused by bending of the film packet during placement in the mouth.

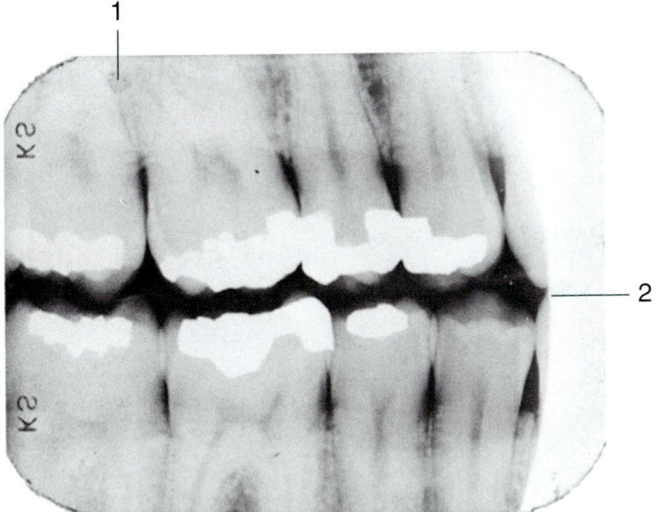

FIGURE 9-7. **Premolar bitewing film.** (**1**) Identification dot. (**2**) Cone cut is caused by not directing the central ray toward the middle of the film. The white circular area was beyond the range of the x-ray beam and was not exposed.

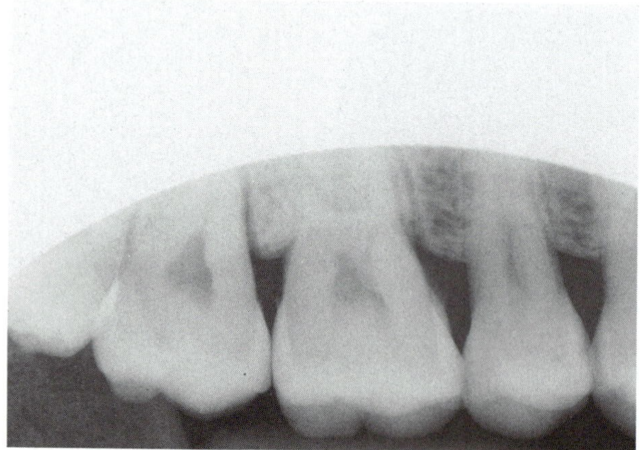

FIGURE 9–8. **Radiograph of maxillary posterior area showing cone cut** due to posterior XCP instrument assembled incorrectly.

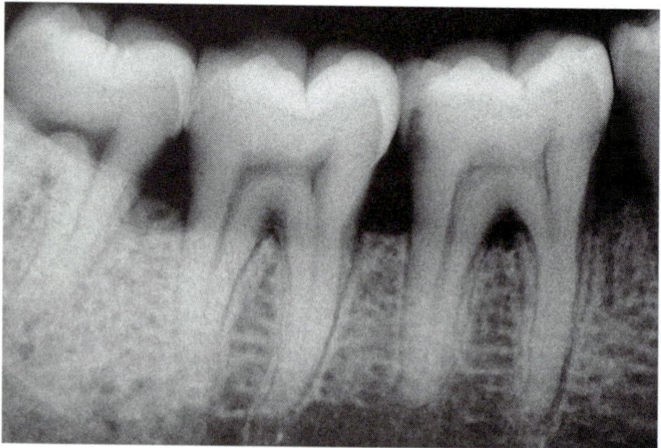

FIGURE 9–10. **Radiograph of mandibular molar area.** Overexposed radiograph results in dark radiograph.

Superimposed Image

- *Probable cause:* Failure to first examine the mouth and remove any appliances such as removable bridges, partial or full dentures, and space maintainers.
- *Correction:* Look in the patient's mouth and remove any appliance.

Pressure Marks (Black Streaks) (see Figure 9–4)

- *Probable cause:* Bending or excessive pressure that causes the film emulsion to crack.

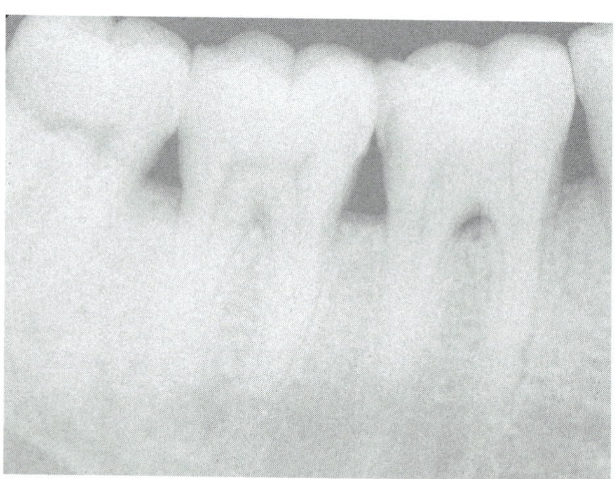

FIGURE 9–9. **Radiograph of mandibular molar area.** Underexposed radiograph results in a light image.

- *Correction:* Avoid excess pressure on the film. Do not bend the film except for minimal softening of corners to avoid hurting the patient with the sharp edges of the film packet.

Wrapping Paper Stuck to Film

- *Probable cause:* Break in wrapping by rough handling enabled saliva to penetrate to the emulsion. Moisture softened the emulsion, causing the black paper to stick to the film.
- *Correction:* Careful handling prevents a break in the seal of the film packet. Always blot moisture from the film packet after removing it from the mouth.

Problems Caused by Faulty Processing Techniques

Another major cause of faulty radiographs can be traced to **errors in the processing technique.** Many of these, such as misreading the temperature on the thermometer, forgetting to wind or set the timer, setting the timer incorrectly, failure to remove the film from the developer when the timer rings, and damage to the emulsion by handling or by chemical contamination, can be blamed on haste and carelessness.

Failure to Follow the Suggested Time-Temperture Cycle

Light Image (see Figures 9–2 and 9–9)

- *Probable cause:* Underdevelopment—film not left in developer for long enough time. The colder the developer, the longer the time required. Alternate causes: weakened developer, underexposure, or fixer contamination of the developer.

- ***Correction:*** Check the temperature of the developer and consult the time-temperature chart before placing the film in developer. If necessary, fill the inserts of manual tanks with fresh solution.

NOTE: Always allow automatic processors to fully reach operating temperature before developing films.

Dark Image

- ***Probable cause:*** Overdevelopment—film left in developer for too long a time. The warmer the developer, the less time is required. Alternate cause: overexposure to radiation.
- ***Correction:*** Check the temperature of the developer and consult the time—temperature chart before placing the film in developer.

Absence of Image

- ***Probable cause:*** Film was placed in fixer before being placed in developer, or emulsion may have dissolved in warm rinse water. Alternate cause: Film may not have been exposed.
- ***Correction:*** Place the film in developer first and promptly remove the film at the end of the washing period.

Faulty Handling of the Film

Smudged Film (see Figure 9–11)

- ***Probable cause:*** Fingermarks on the dry film or on the soft wet emulsion.
- ***Correction:*** Avoid contact with the surface of the radiograph. Handle films carefully and by the edges only. Hands should be clean and free of moisture.

Thin Black Lines

- ***Probable cause:*** Static electricity was produced when the film was pulled out of the wrapping too fast.
- ***Correction:*** Pull the film out of the wrapping slowly.

White Lines or Marks (see Figure 9–12)

- ***Probable cause:*** Soft film or emulsion was scratched by a sharp object such as a film clip or film hanger. Scratching removes the emulsion from the base.

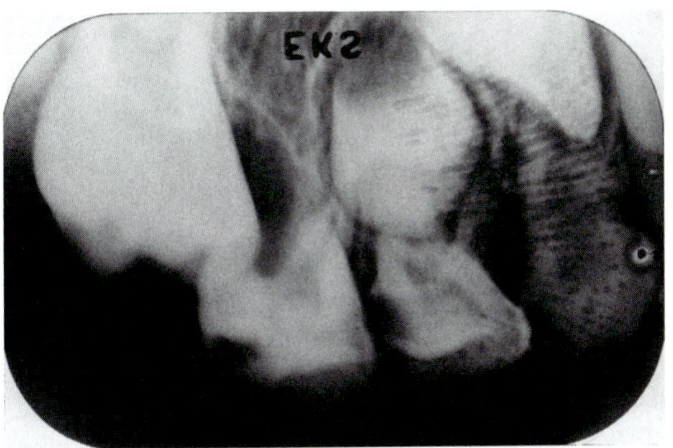

FIGURE 9–11. **Radiograph of deciduous molar area showing fingerprint.**

- ***Correction:*** Be careful when inserting a second film hanger into an insert. Avoid contact with other films or hangers.

Black Image

- ***Probable cause:*** Film was accidentally exposed to white light or exposed for a long period in warm developer.
- ***Correction:*** Turn off all light in the darkroom except the proper safelight before unwrapping the film. Lock the door or warn others to stay out by turning on the "in-use" sign.

Partial Image

- ***Probable cause:*** Level of the developer was too low to cover the entire film.
- ***Correction:*** Replenish the processing solutions to the proper level or fasten the films to lower clips on the hanger.

Clear Areas on Film

- ***Probable cause:*** Films stuck together in developer, so developer was not able to act on both sides of the film emulsion. Alternate cause: attaching two films to a clip through failure to separate films in double-film packets.
- ***Correction:*** Agitate films gently when inserting into the developer; make certain that films do not touch those on other hangers.

Dark Areas on Film

- ***Probable cause:*** Films stuck together in fixer. The fixer was not able to remove the undeveloped silver halide crystals or to neutralize the developer in those areas, and development continues partially.

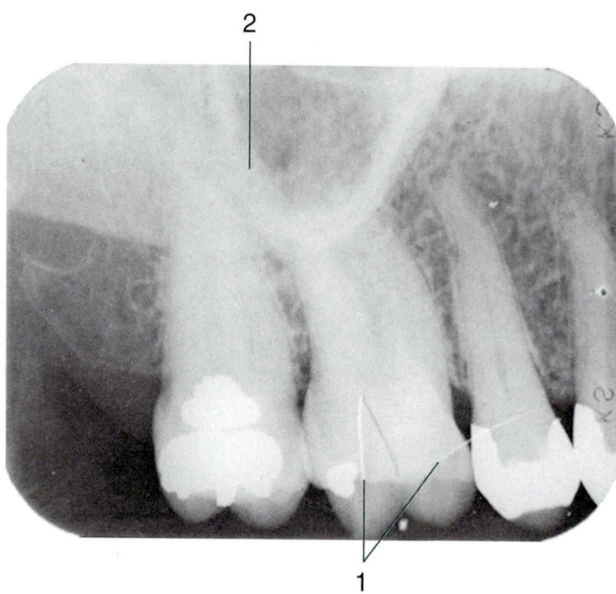

FIGURE 9–12. **Radiograph of maxillary posterior area.** (**1**) White streak marks show where the softened emulsion was scratched off the film during processing. (**2**) U-shaped radiopaque band of dense bone shows the outline of the zygoma.

- ***Correction:*** Agitate films gently when inserting into the fixer; make certain the films do not come in contact with those on other hangers. Feed films into automatic processors slowly and one at a time.

Reticulation (see Figure 9–13)

- ***Probable cause:*** Temperature of processing solutions is too hot, or there is too great a difference between the temperature of the processing solutions and the rinse water. Temperature differences of 10°F may cause the film to become pitted and reticulated through the softening and melting of the emulsion.
- ***Correction:*** Determine that the temperature in the processing solutions is approximately the same as that of the rinse water. Do not begin to process the film until the circulating water has cooled or warmed the developer and fixer. In manual processing, temperatures in excess of 80°F (26.7°C) should be avoided.

Curled Films

- ***Probable cause:*** Too rapid drying of the film through the use of excessive heat.
- ***Correction:*** Slower, more gradual drying. Avoid prolonged drying in the electric dryer.

Scratched Film (see Figure 9–12)

- ***Probable cause:*** Failure to protect the dried radiograph.
- ***Correction:*** Careful handling of processed radiographs. Mount the radiographs promptly and enclose in a protective envelope.

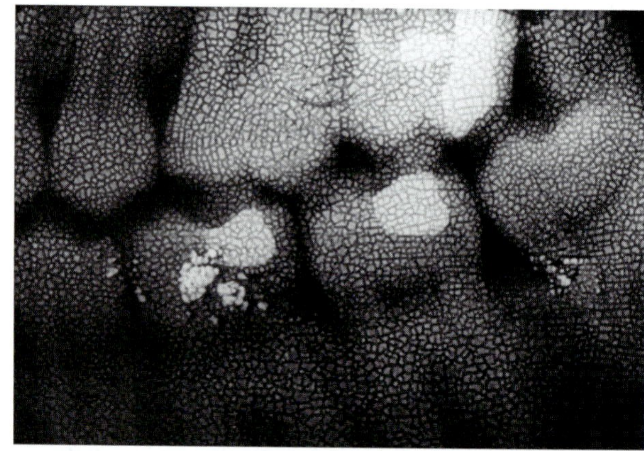

FIGURE 9–13. **Radiograph showing reticulation.**

Chemical Contamination

White Spots on Film

- ***Probable cause:*** Premature contact with fixer—drops of fixer have been splashed on the workbench
- ***Correction:*** Clean the workbench and place a clean towel on the work area before opening the film packet

Dark Spots on Film (see Figure 9–14)

- ***Probable cause:*** Premature contact with developer—drops of developer may have been splashed on the workbench.
- ***Correction:*** Clean the workbench and place a clean towel on the work area before opening the film packet.

Iridescent Stain

- ***Probable cause:*** Oxidation and exhaustion of developer.
- ***Correction:*** Replace the developer with fresh solution.

Dark Brown or Gray film

- ***Probable cause:*** Oxidation and exhaustion of fixer.
- ***Correction:*** Replace the fixer with fresh solution.

Brownish-Yellow Stains

- ***Probable cause:*** Insufficient or improper washing of the film.
- ***Correction:*** Rinse in circulating water for at least 20 min., preferably 30. Always return the film that was taken out for "wet-reading" for completion of fixing and washing.

Problems Caused by Fog on the Film

Still another cause of inadequate radiographs is the formation of a thin, cloudy layer that fogs the film surface. **Fog** diminishes contrast and makes it difficult and often impossible to interpret the radiograph. Fog on radiographs is produced in many ways and can occur before or after the film is exposed or during processing. Most fogged radiographs have a similar appearance, and it is difficult to determine the cause unless one knows, for example, that the film was outdated; in that case one would suspect it to be age fog.

Fog Caused during Storage

Age Fog (see Figure 9–15)

- ***Probable cause:*** Overage film was used.
- ***Correction:*** Watch the date on film boxes. Use the oldest film first. Rotate film stock so that the oldest film is used before newer film. Do not overstock film.

Storage Fog

- ***Probable cause:*** Film stored in warm, damp area or in vicinity of fume producing chemicals.
- ***Correction:*** Store in cool, dry, fume-free area.

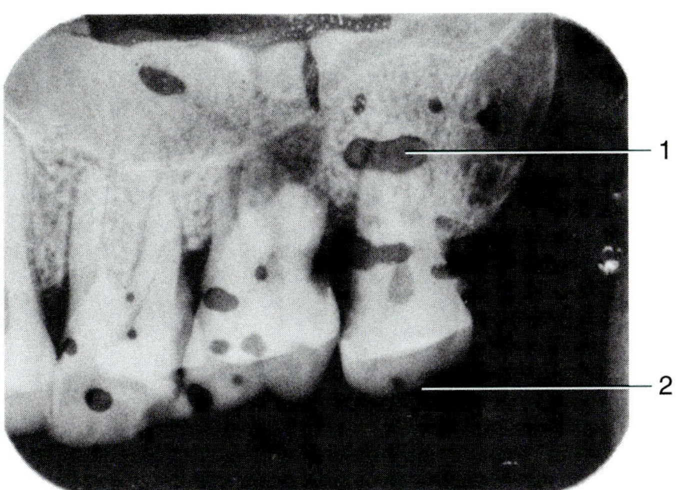

FIGURE 9–14. **Radiograph of maxillary molar area.** (**1**) Dark spots on radiograph are caused by premature contact of film surface with developer splashed on workbench (bench should always be clean). (**2**) Uneven occlusal margin caused by poor film positioning.

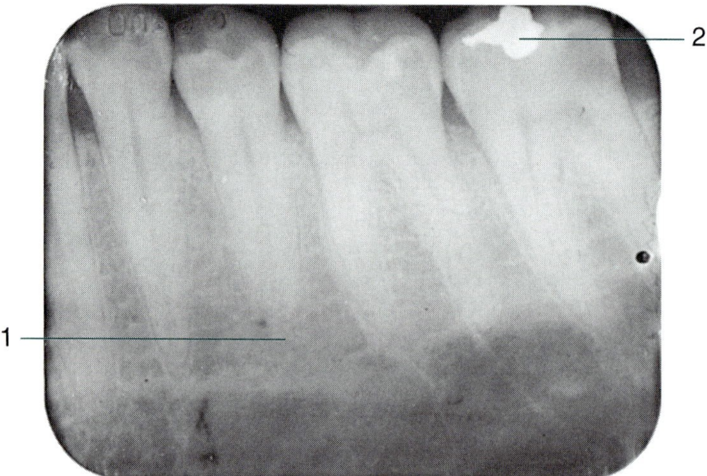

FIGURE 9–15. **Radiograph of mandibular premolar area.** (**1**) Entire radiograph is fogged, with a resultant lack of contrast. Fog may be caused by overage film (as in radiograph shown), storage, exposure to radiation or light, contaminated chemicals, or numerous other causes. (**2**) Metallic restoration.

Fog Caused before or after Exposure

Radiation Fog

- ***Probable cause:*** Film not properly protected before or after exposure.
- ***Correction:*** Store film at safe distance from the source of x-rays or protect it by placing it in a lead-lined dispenser. Never take more than one film out of the dispenser at a time, and place the film in the film safe (a lead lined box) after exposure is made.

Fog during Processing

Safelight Fog

- ***Probable cause:*** Incorrect size of safelight bulb or prolonged exposure to the safelight. Also scratched or cracked filter or the incorrect filter for type of film used.
- ***Correction:*** Check the size of the safelight bulb. Minimize exposure to the safelight. Replace scratched filter. Follow film manufacturer's recommendations on type of filter to use with type of film used.

White Light Fog

- ***Probable cause:*** Light leak around the door of the darkroom or a minute break in the wrapping of the film. Scratched or cracked safelight filter.
- ***Correction:*** Check the darkroom for white light leaks. Check the filter for cracks and scratches. Avoid rough handling or bending of the film packet.

Processing Contamination Fog

- ***Probable cause:*** Contamination of processing chemicals.
- ***Correction:*** Avoid contamination of processing chemicals. Always replace the tank cover in the same way and rinse the film to remove developer before moving the film hanger into the fixer insert.

Chemical Fog

- ***Probable cause:*** Development for too long a time or at too high a temperature.
- ***Correction:*** Develop at recommended time-temperature cycle.

Cigarette Fog

- ***Probable cause:*** Smoking in the darkroom. The glow of the cigarette is sufficient to fog the film.
- ***Correction:*** Do not smoke in the darkroom. Smoking in a dental facility is undesirable, as well as illegal in many states.

CHAPTER SUMMARY

The dental radiographer should be able to identify what type of error was made in handling, exposing, or processing any radiograph and should be aware of what must be done to avoid repetition of the same mistake.

Faulty radiographs are traceable to many causes. Frequently several different errors may cause similar-looking defects. The well-trained radiographer handles film carefully and develops neat work habits. The price of good diagnostic radiographs is expertise and meticulous attention to details in all stages.

Most unsatisfactory radiographs can be attributed to faulty film handling, using incorrect exposure factors, failure to project the central ray toward the center of the film in both the horizontal and vertical planes, failure of the film to remain where placed, and poor processing techniques. Only clear, properly processed radiographs with minimal distortion that show the entire intended areas have real diagnostic value.

Processing errors cause absence of image, partial image, light image, dark image, scratched film, curled film, reticulation, smudged areas, black lines, brown and opaque spots, and so forth. Each error can usually be attributed to one of several possibilities. Being aware of the cause helps the operator to prevent repeating the mistake. The goal should be to do it right the first time.

The majority of errors made at chair-side during exposure can be avoided if the operator is well-trained, skillful, and dedicated. Your goal should always be the production of radiographs of excellent quality with high diagnostic yield.

REVIEW QUESTIONS

1. What should be done with the film when a previous radiograph of the maxillary molar area did not show the third molar?
   (a) Raise in the mouth
   (b) Lower in the mouth
   (c) Move forward in the mouth
   (d) Move backward in the mouth
2. What does a diamond or herringbone pattern on the processed radiograph indicate?
   (a) Average film
   (b) Underexposed film
   (c) Reversed film
   (d) Overdeveloped film
3. Which of these conditions is caused by insufficient vertical angulation?
   (a) Elongation
   (b) Overlapping
   (c) Foreshortening
   (d) Cone cutting

4. A radiograph of the maxillary molar area shows that the mesiobuccal root is superimposed over the lingual root. What correction is needed?
   (a) Increase the vertical angulation
   (b) Change the direction of horizontal angulation toward the mesial
   (c) Decrease the vertical angulation
   (d) Change the direction of the horizontal angulation toward the distal

5. What error was made when the area of overlapped contacts is much larger in the second molar area than in the first premolar area?
   (a) Excessive vertical angulation
   (b) Insufficient vertical angulation
   (c) Mesiodistal projection of horizontal angulation
   (d) Distomesial projection of horizontal angulation

6. Which of these conditions results from a failure to direct the central ray toward the middle of the film packet?
   (a) Cone cut
   (b) Overlapping
   (c) Elongation
   (d) Foreshortening

7. Which of these indicates that the radiograph was overexposed?
   (a) Light image
   (b) Reticulation
   (c) Dark image
   (d) Thin black lines

8. Which of these indicates that the film was not properly washed?
   (a) Light image
   (b) Fogging
   (c) Brownish-yellow stains
   (d) White spots

9. Which of these conditions indicates that the level of the developer in the tank insert was too low?
   (a) Partial image
   (b) Cone cut film
   (c) Light image
   (d) Reticulation

10. Which of these is not a cause of fogging of the radiograph?
    (a) Exposure to scatter radiation
    (b) Use of overage film
    (c) Underexposure
    (d) Chemical-fume contamination of film

11. What is the probable cause of reticulation?
    (a) Overexposure
    (b) Underexposure
    (c) Differences in processing solution temperatures
    (d) Cracks in the safelight

12. How will static electricity appear radiographically?
    (a) As black lines
    (b) As brownish/yellow stain
    (c) As white lines
    (d) As fog
13. Give two reasons a film may appear blank.
14. Explain how cone cut occurs and how it appears on a processed film.

BIBLIOGRAPHY

Eastman Kodak. *Exposure and Processing for Dental Radiography*. Rochester, NY: Eastman Kodak, 1998.

Eastman Kodak. *Successful Intraoral Radiography*. Rochester, NY: Eastman Kodak, 1998.

White S. C. & Pharoah, M. J. *Oral Radiology Principles and Interpretation*, 4th ed. St. Louis: Mosby, 2000.

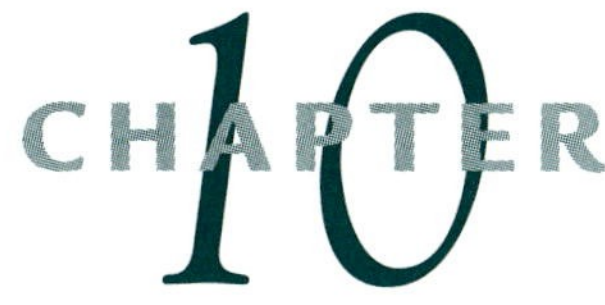

Quality Assurance in Dental Radiography

OBJECTIVES

By the end of this chapter the student should be able to:

- Define the key words.
- Differentiate between quality assurance and quality control.
- List the four objectives of quality control tests.
- Make a step wedge with cardboard and lead foil and demonstrate how to use it.
- Describe how to test for light leaks in the darkroom.
- Describe the safelight test.
- Describe two daily tests for the automatic processor.
- Discuss the test for developer solution strength using a step wedge device.
- Discuss three causes of light radiographs and correction measures.
- Discuss three causes of dark radiographs and correction measures.
- List five problems with film surface marks, their causes, and correction.
- Describe who benefits from quality assurance programs.

KEY WORDS

Output
Quality assurance
Quality control
Step wedge

Introduction

Quality assurance is defined as the planning and carrying out of procedures to assure high-quality radiographs with maximum diagnostic information (yield) while minimizing the exposure to dental patients and personnel. This takes the conservative view that the minimum of radiation should be used to get the job done. Remember the ALARA concept, where ALARA stands for "as low as reasonably achievable." Quality assurance includes both quality control techniques and quality administration procedures (see Table 10–1).

The purpose of this chapter is to present quality control tests that are used to monitor dental x-ray equipment and the x-ray processing system. In addition, quality administration procedures and operator competence are discussed.

Quality Control

Quality control is defined as a series of tests to assure that the radiographic system is functioning properly and that the radiographs produced are of an acceptable level of quality. These tests include the monitoring of x-ray equipment and the x-ray processing system. A log of all tests performed, including dates, results, and corrective actions should be made.

The **objectives** for these tests are to:

1. Identify any problems in the radiographic system before image quality is compromised.
2. Maintain a high standard of image quality within the dental office.
3. Keep patient and occupational exposures to a minimum.
4. Reduce the x-ray retake rate.

The **quality control tests** should be conducted for:

- X-ray machines
- The darkroom
- Processing equipment
- X-ray film
- Processing solutions

TABLE 10-1. **Quality Assurance Includes Both Quality Control and Quality Administration**

Quality Control	Quality Administration
X-ray machines	Written plan
Darkroom	Monitoring and maintenance schedule
Processing equipment	Assigned staff responsibilities
X-ray film	Record-keeping log and periodic evaluation

X-ray Machines

Periodic comprehensive **testing of the x-ray machine** is essential to a quality assurance program. These tests should include beam alignment, collimation, filtration (beam quality), output, timer accuracy, and tube head stability (see Table 10–2). A qualified health physicist should conduct most of these tests. State and local health departments may provide x-ray equipment testing as part of their registration or licensing programs. The dental office staff can perform some of these tests. A helpful free pamphlet entitled *Quality Control Tests for Dental Radiology* is available from Eastman Kodak (Kodak Publication No. ME-504a).

The office staff can **test** the consistency of the **output** of the x-ray machine by using a stepwedge device (see Figure 10–1). A **step wedge** is a device of layered metal steps used to determine film density and contrast. Such a step wedge can be obtained commercially or be made in the dental office by:

1. Dividing a piece of cardboard the size of a #2 x-ray film into thirds.
2. Leaving the first third uncovered and covering the remaining two thirds with two pieces of lead backing from a discarded film packet.
3. Covering the final third with three additional pieces of lead backing and taping them down.

TABLE 10-2. **Quality Control Tests for Dental X-ray Machines**

1. Beam alignment
2. Collimation
3. Filtration (beam quality)
4. Output
5. Timer accuracy
6. Tube head stability

The result is a step wedge device that can be used to measure the consistency of the x-ray machine and to check the quality of the developing solution (see developing solution test).

Output Consistency Test

Prepare a **step-wedge reference radiograph.**

1. Place the step wedge on top of a fresh x-ray film packet.
2. Expose the film using the same exposure factors used for a molar view of an adult patient.
3. Process the film using fresh chemicals at recommended time and temperature.

Keep this **reference radiograph.** Daily or periodically expose and process another radiograph under the same conditions.

Compare the densities on the **daily radiograph** with the **reference radiograph.**

1. View daily radiograph side-by-side to the reference radiograph on a viewbox.
2. If the densities match, the output of the x-ray machine is consistent.
3. If the densities do not match (check to make sure fresh chemicals and proper time and temperature were used for processing), a qualified health physicist should exam the x-ray machine.

Darkroom

Check the **darkroom** to determine that it is adequately ventilated, free from chemical fumes, within the prescribed temperature range, beyond the reach of stray radiation, and light tight. Also, check to see that the safelight and filter are not defective or giving off too much light.

Test for Light Leaks

Whether the darkroom is **light-tight** can be determined by closing the door and turning off all lights, including the safelight. Light leaks, if present, become visible after about five minutes when the eyes become accustomed to the dark. After the darkroom is determined to be light-tight, the safelight can be tested.

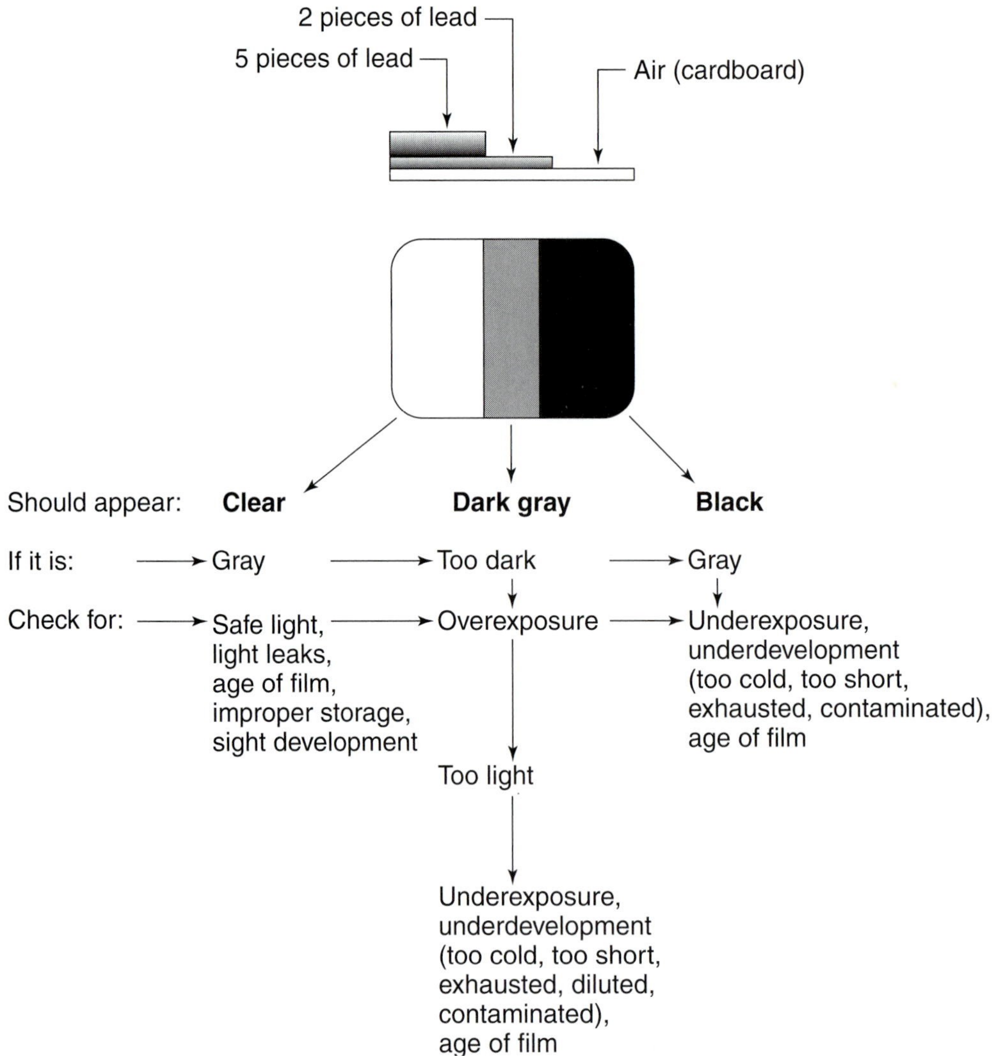

FIGURE 10-1. **Sketch of a step-wedge.** A step-wedge is useful in making visual comparisons for quality control. (Courtesy of Dr. A. Peter Fortier, Louisiana State University, School of Dentistry, and Department of Dental Diagnostic Science, School of Dentistry, University of Texas at San Antonio)

Safelight Test

Test to find out if the **safelight** is really safe:

1. Turn off all darkroom lights.
2. Unwrap an unexposed dental film.
3. Place a coin on the film emulsion surface.
4. Turn on the safelight for approximately the time you take to unwrap a full-mouth series of film (about 4 min).
5. Then process the film.

If the outline of the coin appears, the safelight is not safe for use with that type of film. The filter may be scratched, the wattage of the bulb may be too great, the light may be too close to the work area, or the film may not be designed for use with that particular light and filter combination.

Processing Equipment

All **processing equipment** including the automatic processor, manual processing equipment, cassettes, intensifying screens, and view box need to be checked on a periodic basis.

Automatic Processor

If an **automatic processor** is used, check to see if the water circulating system is working properly and that correct solution levels, replenishment, and temperatures are maintained. Follow the manufacturer's procedure and maintenance directions. When cleaning, be careful to keep oil and grease off the rollers.

Great care must be used when feeding films into automatic processors. Bent films tend to become stuck and jam up in the rollers. It is best to feed the films in slowly and make sure that they go in straight and in the right direction. Failure to insert the films into automatic units in the right sequence or order can result in serious problems in identification.

Two **daily tests** are helpful when using **automatic processors.**

1. Begin by processing an unexposed film. The film should come out of the return chute clear and dry. If it does not, check the solutions, the safelight, or look for possible light leaks. If the film is still moist, check the dryer temperature.
2. Then process a film that has been exposed to light. This film should be black and dry after processing. If not, check both the solutions and the temperature of the dryer.

Manual Processing

If **manual processing** is used, determine whether the thermometer and timer are accurate, whether wet or dry chemicals are adhering to the mixing paddles and film holders, and whether the work area is clean and free of dust. Monitor the temperature and levels of the processing solutions.

Cassettes and Intensifying Screens

Quality control procedures include periodically examining **cassettes** and **intensifying screens.**

CASSETTES. Extraoral **cassettes** should be checked for **warping, light leaks,** and **screen-film contact.** Warping and light leaks result in fogged radiographs. Poor screen contact results in a fuzzy image. Defective cassettes should be repaired or replaced.

INTENSIFYING SCREENS. **Intensifying screens** should be examined for **cleanliness** and **scratches.** Any specks of dirt, paper, or other material will absorb the light given off by the screen crystals. This results in white specks on the processed radiograph. Dirty screens should be cleaned monthly with solutions recommended by the screen manufacturer. Any scratched or damaged screen should be repaired or replaced.

Viewbox

If functioning properly the **viewbox** should give off a uniform, subdued light. Some viewers have fluorescent light tubes that will glow after the light is turned off. Film emulsions are sensitive to this afterglow and can be damaged.

X-ray Film

Only fresh **x-ray film** should be used for making dental radiographs. Film manufacturers use a series of quality control tests to assure dental x-ray film is of high quality and fresh. The dental office must make sure dental x-ray film is properly stored, protected, and used before its expiration date. Check the expiration date on the x-ray film box and always use the oldest film first.

Fresh Film Test

1. Use fresh processing chemicals.
2. Under darkroom conditions, unwrap one unexposed film.
3. Process film.
   - The film is fresh if it appears clear with a slight blue tint.
   - If the film appears fogged, it should not be used.

Processing Solutions

Quality control is extremely important in processing the dental x-ray films. As explained in Chapter 8, **processing solutions** should be changed every 4 weeks or as recommended by the manufacturer. However, to determine the freshness of the **developer** and **fixer solutions,** several simple tests can be made. Some should be performed daily, others as the occasion demands.

Developer Solution

The **developer solution** is the most critical of the processing solutions and demands careful attention. When the developer solution deteriorates and loses strength, the resulting radiographs lighten. A simple test can be made to make sure the strength of the developer solution is adequate.

One of two tests may be used. The test may be done using a step wedge device or with a commercial device such as the dental radiographic normalizing and monitoring device (see Figure 10–2).

Step-wedge Device

To test the developer solution strength using a step-wedge device:

1. Using a step wedge as described earlier in this chapter, place the step wedge on top of a fresh film packet.
2. Expose the packet using the same exposure factors used for a molar view of an adult patient.
3. Repeat this procedure 10 times to create a supply of exposed film packets for testing.
4. Process one exposed film in fresh chemicals to make a **reference radiograph.**
5. The nine remaining films become control films and should be stored in a cool, dry place protected from x-rays.
6. Daily, before processing patient's radiographs and after replenishing processing solutions, process one of the exposed step-wedge films.
7. Compare the densities of the step-wedge radiograph with the densities of the reference radiograph side by side on a viewbox.
   - If the densities match, the developer solution is adequate.
   - If the densities do not match, the developer solution has deteriorated and must be changed.

Dental Radiographic Normalizing and Monitoring Device

A **dental radiographic normalizing and monitoring device** is available commercially (see Figure 10–2). (It can be purchased from Dental Radiographic Devices, P.O. Box 9294, Silver Springs, MD 20906.) The device has a filmstrip with several density steps for comparison to a test film. Step-by-step instructions are printed on front of the device.

Fixer Solution

The **fixer solution** removes the undeveloped silver halide crystals from the film resulting in clear areas on the processed radiograph. With fresh fixer solution, clearing time is 2–3 min. As the fixer solution loses strength, the film takes a longer time to clear.

The following is a **test for clearing time.**

1. Under darkroom conditions, unwrap a fresh film and place it in the fixer solution.
2. Time the film for clearing.
   - If the film clears in 4 min or less, the fixer solution is adequate.
   - If the clearing time is over 4 min, the fixer should be replaced.

Guides to Common Problems

Three common problem areas are radiographic **density, film surface marks,** and **drying** problems.

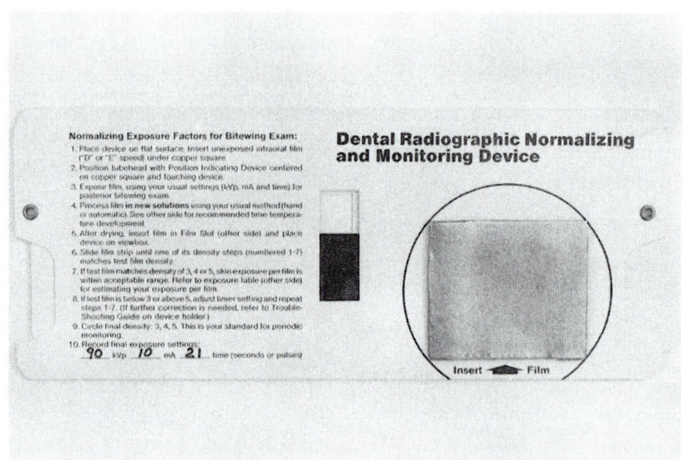

FIGURE 10–2. **Dental radiographic normalizing and monitoring device.**

1. A convenient checklist of problems with **density** is shown in Table 10–3.
2. Checklist of problems with **marks on the film surface** is presented in Table 10–4.
3. Table 10–5 is a checklist for **film drying** problems.

Study the three tables carefully. Know and understand the possible cause and correction for each problem.

Quality Administration Procedures

Quality administration refers to conducting a quality assurance program in the dental office. The **quality assurance program** should include:

- Written plan
- Monitoring and maintenance schedule
- Assigned staff responsibilities
- Record-keeping log and periodic evaluation

Written Plan

The dentist, with staff assistance, should develop a **written plan** that must be carried out to promote quality assurance. The plan should include, but not limited to, the following **quality assurance guidelines.**

1. The purpose of the quality assurance program.
2. Written assignment of duties and responsibilities.
3. Radiographic quality should be continuously monitored against a standard reference radiograph.
4. Processing chemicals should be evaluated daily.
5. On a monthly basis, the darkroom (including the safelight), all viewboxes, cassettes, and screens should be checked.
6. There should be comprehensive testing of the x-ray machine on a yearly basis or as state regulations require.
7. A daily log of all quality assurance tests and retake radiographs should be maintained.

TABLE 10-3. **A Guide to Film Density Problems**

Problem	Cause	Correction
1. Light films	a. Developer nearing exhaustion	a. Drain developer solution, clean tank, and fill with new developer solution.
	b. Developer contaminated	b. Same as above.
	c. Developer temperature too low	c. Be sure standby switch is on. Be sure heater pad is plugged in. Check thermostat—adjust or replace. Check heating pad and replace if defective.
	d. Processing speed too fast	d. Increase total processing time.
	e. Exposure time too short	e. Increase exposure time in 20% steps.
2. Dark films	a. Exposure time too long	a. Decrease exposure time in 20% steps.
	b. Fixer in developer	b. Change developer.
	c. Thermostat failure, causing solutions to overheat	c. Replace thermostat.
3. Fogged film	a. Incorrect safelight filter or bulb	a. Use a 6B filter with 15-watt bulb.
	b. Excessive light	b. Check that safelight bulb is of proper wattage. Be sure there are no light leaks in darkroom.
	c. Developer temperature too high	c. Check thermostat—adjust or replace.
	d. Light leak between processor and daylight loader	d. Block light leak with black tape.
4. Gray films	a. No water in wash section	a. Add water.

Courtesy of Dr. A. Peter Fortier, Louisiana State University, School of Dentistry, and Department of Dental Diagnostic Science, School of Dentistry, University of Texas at San Antonio.

TABLE 10-4. **A Guide to Problems with Film Surface Marks**

Problem	Cause	Correction
1. Pressure marks	a. Foreign material on roller	a. Clean rollers.
	b. Rough handling of film before processing	b. Due to sensitivity of film emulsions, gentle handling should be practiced.
2. Film with greenish-yellow hue	a. Depleted fixer	a. Replace fixer.
	b. Improper film	b. Use film made for automatic processing.
	c. Wrong fixer	c. Use rapid-process fixer.
	d. Processor speed too fast	d. Reduce processor speed.
3. Emulsion peeling	a. Deposits on developer roller	a. Clean roller.
	b. Solution temperature too high	b. Turn off standby switch. Check thermostat.
	c. Wash water temperature too high	c. Reduce wash water temperature.
	d. Improper film	d. Use film made for automatic processing.
4. Film scratches	a. Rough handling of film before processing	a. Gentle handling of films should be practiced.
	b. Sticking roller	b. Check racks, gears, and gear mesh.
	c. Foreign material on roller	c. Clean rollers.
	d. Burr on input slot	d. Remove burr.
5. White chalky film	a. Lack of wash water	a. Check water supply.
	b. Fixer precipitated	b. Replace fixer.

Courtesy of Dr. A. Peter Fortier, Louisiana State University, School of Dentistry,and Department of Dental Diagnostic Science, School of Dentistry, University of Texas at San Antonio.

8. Periodically, the entire staff should evaluate the quality assurance program.

It should be a matter of pride in each office that the radiographs are of high quality and that the exposure levels to radiation are held to the absolute minimum. The quality assurance program must have the support of the dentist and auxiliary personnel in order to be successful.

Monitoring and Maintenance Schedules

A **monitoring schedule** listing all the quality control tests, person responsible for each test, and the frequency of testing should be posted in the office. Some tests, such as determining the strength of the processing solutions, are carried out each work day. Other tests, such as determining the output of the x-ray machine, may be made annually.

TABLE 10-5. **A Guide to Film Drying Problems**

Problem	Cause	Correction
1. Films damp or wet	a. Processor speed too fast	a. Increase processing time.
	b. Defective dryer fan heater	b. Replace defective fan heater.
	c. Improper film	c. Use film mode for automatic processing.
	d. Wrong developer and/or fixer	d. Use only rapid-processing developer and fixer.

Courtesy of Dr. A. Peter Fortier, Louisiana State University, School of Dentistry, and Department of Dental Diagnostic Science, School of Dentistry, University of Texas at San Antonio.

A **maintenance schedule** for x-ray machines and processing equipment must be posted. Check-off lists can be used to record maintenance and inspections.

Staff Duties and Responsibilities

Specific duties and responsibilities should be assigned to staff members. Each member must be informed of how and why the tasks are to be performed. The duties of each individual must be clearly defined.

The dentist usually delegates most radiographic procedures to the dental assistant and/or dental hygienist. However, the final responsibility legally rests with the dentist.

Log and Periodic Evaluation

A **log** should be kept of all quality control tests. Include the date, the specific test, the results, action taken if any, and the person who conducted the test. Also, a log of all radiographs retaken should be recorded to identify recurring problems.

The entire office personnel should meet periodically to **evaluate** the logs and the quality assurance program.

Competent Operator

The operator must be competent in exposing, processing, and mounting dental radiographs. Even a trained and dedicated worker may have an occasional failure. Therefore personnel must be trained to recognize problems, their causes, and how to correct them. Such training generally works out best if done on a one-on-one basis in the dental office.

The dental radiographer must have patient cooperation. Failure to inform the patient about what is to be done is a frequent cause of retakes. This is especially true with young patients. The operator should take the time to explain the necessity of what is to be done, tell the patient how long the procedure lasts, and caution the patient against movement.

Operator errors may result in undiagnostic radiographs that must be retaken. Retakes result in unnecessary radiation to the patient and lost time for the operator and the patient. Retakes should not be made without knowing why. Always strive to keep retakes to a minimum.

Frequent **chair-side operator errors** include:

1. Failure to correctly center the film packet
2. Incorrect vertical or horizontal positioning of the position indicating device (PID)
3. Failure to place the identification dot on the film packet into the incisal or occlusal area
4. Using the wrong exposure factors
5. Positioning the film backwards

Operator errors and retakes should be logged to identify recurring problems. Ideally, each film exposed is recorded in a log and this log should be periodically reviewed and the cause of problems detected and corrected. To improve operator competency, training can be done on a one-on-one basis in the dental office. In many areas, continuing education courses are available.

Benefit of Quality Assurance Programs

Everyone concerned benefits from a well-organized program. Once the office personnel are trained properly, such programs take as little as 15 to 20 min/day. Quality assurance programs are cost-effective once initial expenditures have been made. The resulting improved image quality helps the dentist to see what otherwise might be missed or misinterpreted. Retakes can often be reduced as well as the radiation dose to the patient and operator.

Programs must be flexible and allow for change as new techniques come into being. There is a necessity for the dentist and the entire staff—assistants, hygienists, and clerical personnel—to meet on a regular basis to discuss the effectiveness of the programs and to evaluate them. The records or log of all unsatisfactory radiographs and the reason for the retakes should be examined. If such examination shows any pattern of one particular error being made repeatedly—or by the same person—corrective measures are in order.

CHAPTER SUMMARY

Quality assurance is defined as the planning and carrying out of procedures to assure high-quality radiographs with maximum diagnostic information (yield) while minimizing the exposure to dental patients and personnel.

Quality control is defined as a series of tests to assure that the radiographic system is functioning properly and that the radiographs produced are of an acceptable level of quality. These tests include the monitoring of x-ray equipment and the x-ray processing system.

The quality control tests should be conducted for x-ray machines, the darkroom, processing equipment, x-ray film, and processing solutions. All processing equipment including the automatic processor, manual processing equipment, cassettes, intensifying screens, and view box all need to be checked on a periodic basis. Only fresh x-ray film should be used for making dental radiographs.

The developer solution is the most critical of the processing solutions and demands careful attention. When the developer solution deteriorates and loses strength, the resulting radiographs lighten. A simple test can be made to make sure the strength of the developer solution is adequate.

Three common problem areas are radiographic density, film surface marks, and drying problems.

Quality administration refers to conducting a quality assurance program in the dental office. The quality assurance program should include a written plan, a monitoring and maintenance schedule, assigned staff responsibilities, a record-keeping log and periodic evaluation of the program. The majority of errors made at chair-side during exposure can be avoided if the operator is well trained, skillful, and dedicated. Everyone concerned benefits from a well-organized quality assurance program.

REVIEW QUESTIONS

1. The entire office staff should be dedicated to the concept of quality assurance.
   (a) True
   (b) False
2. The goal of quality assurance is to achieve maximum diagnostic yield from each radiograph.
   (a) True
   (b) False
3. Any radiograph that is less than perfect should be retaken immediately.
   (a) True
   (b) False
4. The output of the x-ray machine should be tested weekly.
   (a) True
   (b) False
5. The drifting of the tube head should be corrected by a trained repairperson.
   (a) True
   (b) False
6. Automatic processors require little or no servicing.
   (a) True
   (b) False

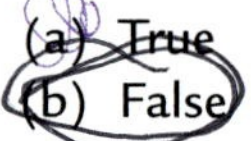

7. A step-wedge is a valuable tool to use in quality control tests.

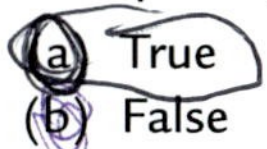

   (a) True
   (b) False

8. Regardless of who exposes and processes the radiographs, the final responsibility rests with the dentist.
   (a) True
   (b) False

9. In radiography, film blackening is called ______________.

10. Which testing device is used in quality control to compare the density of the radiographic image?
    (a) A safelight
    (b) A step wedge
    (c) A viewer
    (d) A photoreceptor

11. With fresh fixer solution, the clearing time should be:
    (a) 1–2 min.
    (b) 2–3 min.
    (c) 4–5 min
    (d) 6–7 min

12. Processing solutions should be changed about every:
    (a) Day.
    (b) Week.
    (c) 1–2 weeks.
    (d) 4 weeks.

13. The most critical quality control test that requires daily monitoring is testing the:
    (a) Darkroom for light leaks.
    (b) Strength of the developer solution.
    (c) Output of the x-ray machine.
    (d) Safelight.

BIBLIOGRAPHY

American Academy of Dental Radiology Quality Assurance Committee. Recommendations for quality assurance in dental radiography. *Oral. Surg.* 1983, 55:421–426.

Eastman Kodak. *Quality Assurance in Dental Radiography*. Rochester, NY: Eastman Kodak, 1998.

Farman, A. G., & Hines, V. G. Radiation safety and quality assurance in North American dental schools. *J. Dent. Educ.* 1986, 50:304–308.

Quality Assurance for Diagnostic Imaging Equipment: Recommendations of the National Council on Radiation Protection and Measurements. Bethesda, MD: NCRP publications; 1988. NCRP Report no. 99.

CHAPTER 11

Normal Radiographic Anatomy

OBJECTIVES

By the end of this chapter the student should be able to:

- Define the key words.
- Describe why it is important to recognize and identify normal anatomical landmarks of the face and head.
- Recognize and identify the facial and cranial bones.
- Name all of the anatomical landmarks of the maxilla and mandible.
- Differentiate between the terms radiopaque and radiolucent.
- Differentiate between cortical and cancellous bone.
- Recognize and describe the radiographic appearance of all structures of the teeth and the alveolus.
- Name and identify all landmarks or structures normally seen on radiographs of the maxillary and mandibular tooth areas.

KEY WORDS

Ala
Alveolar bone
Alveolar process
Alveolus
Angle of mandible
Anodontia
Apical foramen
Cancellous bone
Cementum
Condyle
Cortical bone
Deciduous teeth
Dentin
Enamel
External auditory meatus (foramen)
Foramen
Fossa
Genial tubercles
Glenoid fossa
Hamulus
Incisive foramen (anterior palatine foramen)
Inferior border of mandible
Inverted Y
Lamina dura
Lateral fossa
Lingual foramen
Mandibular canal
Maxilla
Maxillary sinus
Maxillary tuberosity
Median palatine suture
Mental foramen
Mental fossa
Mental ridge
Mylohyoid ridge
Nasal fossa (cavity)
Nasal septum
Nasal spine
Nutrient canal
Oblique ridge
Periodontal ligament
Permanent teeth
Process
Pulp chamber (cavity)
Radiolucent
Radiopaque
Ramus
Septum
Sinus (maxillary)
Submandibular fossa
Supernumerary teeth
Suture
Symphysis
Trabecular bone
Tragus
Tubercle
Tuberosity (maxillary)

Introduction

The dental radiographer must be able to recognize and identify normal anatomical landmarks that may be seen on radiographs of the teeth, the jaw structures, or the skull areas. There are three reasons for this:

1. To ensure that the film was positioned and exposed in such a manner that all the desired areas and anatomical structures are clearly visible so that the radiograph thus produced is of diagnostic value.
2. To assist in determining into which frame of the x-ray mount each radiograph is to be mounted.
3. To assist in interpreting radiographs.

It is assumed that most students using this text will be studying dental and cranial anatomy and have access to a skull and an anatomy text. The student should periodically review the major landmarks of the face and the structures surrounding the teeth until he or she is completely familiar with them and able to identify them positively on a skull, radiograph, or patient.

The purpose of this chapter is to review the anatomical landmarks of the face and skull and to describe the normal anatomical landmarks of the maxilla and mandible as seen on radiographs.

Significant Normal Anatomical Landmarks

Anatomical landmarks in this chapter are separated into the following groups:

1. Landmarks of the face
2. Landmarks of dental interest on the skull
3. Specific landmarks of the maxilla and mandible

Facial Landmarks

The surface **landmarks of the face** cannot be distinguished on a radiograph, but they help the radiographer to rapidly locate a number of important planes and structures. Such landmarks (see Figure 11–1) as the **tip of the nose,** the **ala (wing) of the nose,** the **inner canthus of the eye,** the **outer canthus of the eye,** the **tragus of the ear,** and the **symphysis of the chin** are often used in certain techniques of placing the film and directing the position indicating device (PID).

The positioning of the patient's head during intraoral radiographic procedures is often determined by aligning the midsagittal plane perpendicularly and the ala-tragus line parallel to the floor. Plane alignments and film positioning are explained in Chapters 13 and 14.

Bones and Anatomical Structures of the Cranium and Face

Although most anatomical landmarks that can be used to interpret or mount intraoral radiographs are located on the maxillae or the mandible, the radiographer should also be able to recognize and identify the major bones and anatomical structures of the cranium and face. Such

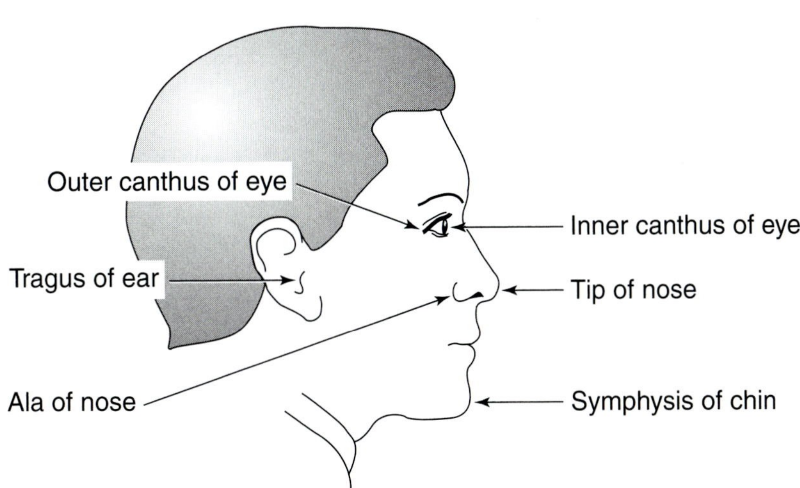

FIGURE 11–1. **Landmarks of the face.**

knowledge is useful when making cephalometric, temporomandibular joint, or panoramic exposures.

With some practice, skill in recognizing the names of the bones and anatomical structures can be achieved by comparing the labeling on the illustrations that follow with their appearance on a dry skull. To make it easier to locate these bones or structures, turn the skull so that it is oriented in the same direction as the illustration at which you are looking. Many structures can be seen readily; others may only be seen from one specific direction. You should be aware that not all of these can be identified on dental radiographs. For an in-depth study, an anatomy text is suggested.

One of the first steps is to become familiar with the names and locations of the cranial and facial bones that may be seen on dental radiographs. Using Figure 11–2 (**frontal view of the skull**), attempt to locate the following bones on the skull: the **frontal bone,** the right and left **parietal bones,** the right and left **zygomas** (**zygomatic bone,** also called **malar bone** or **cheekbone**), the **sphenoid bone,** the right and left **nasal bones,** the right and left **maxilla,** and the **mandible.** Figure 11–3 shows the **nasal septum** and the **nasal spine.**

Use Figure 11–4 (**lateral view of the skull**), to locate the following bones and structures: the **frontal bone,** the **parietal bone,** the **temporal bone,** the **occipital bone,** the **nasal bone,** the **zygoma** (**zygomatic bone, malar bone,** or **cheekbone**), the **maxilla,** the **mandible,** the **zygomatic arch,** which is made up of the temporal process of the zygoma and the zygomatic process of the temporal bone, the **external auditory meatus (foramen),** and the **styloid** and the **mastoid processes** of the temporal bone.

Landmarks of the Maxilla and Mandible

The teeth are located within the alveolar processes of the **maxillae** and the **mandible;** thus most dental radiographs include portions of these bones. The maxillae are two bones, a right and left maxilla, whereas the mandible is a single bone. Generally, but not always, the same structures appear on both right and left sides.

Maxilla

Compare the labeling on Figure 11–5. Locate the following structures on the **maxilla:** the **median palatine suture, maxillary tuberosity** area, and the **incisive (anterior palatine) foramen.** The **maxillary sinus** is an empty space within the maxilla.

Mandible

Next compare the labeling on Figures 11–6 and 11–7. Locate the following areas and structures on a mandible: **body, ramus, inferior border, alveolar process, angle of the mandible, condyle, coronoid process, sigmoid (mandibular) notch, mandibular foramen** (the **man-**

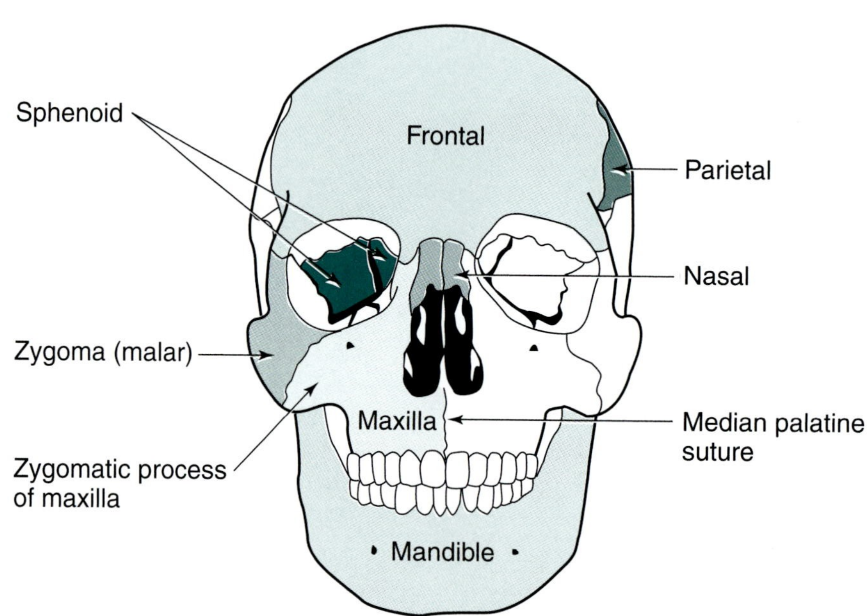

FIGURE 11–2. **Frontal view of the skull.**

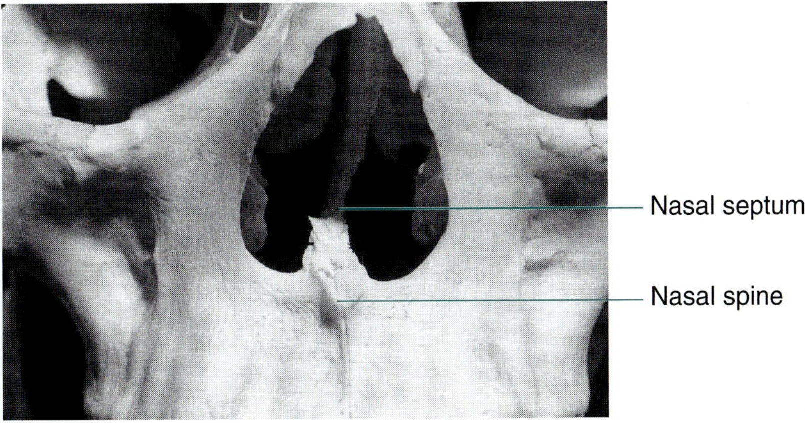

FIGURE 11-3. **Frontal view of the nose.**

dibular canal is located within the mandible between the **mandibular foramen** and the **mental foramen**), **mental foramen, mental ridge, symphysis, lingual foramen, genial tubercles, oblique ridge, mylohyoid ridge,** and the **submandibular fossa.**

The location of these structures of the maxilla and mandible should be memorized, and identification should be practiced frequently. Some of the landmarks listed are visible only in the larger occlusal and extraoral radiographs. The number shown on any radiograph depends on the size of the film and the area exposed

Radiographic Appearance of the Alveolar Bone and Tooth Area

As explained in Chapter 4, the terms **radiolucent** and **radiopaque** are used to describe the appearance of the black and white areas of any radiograph.

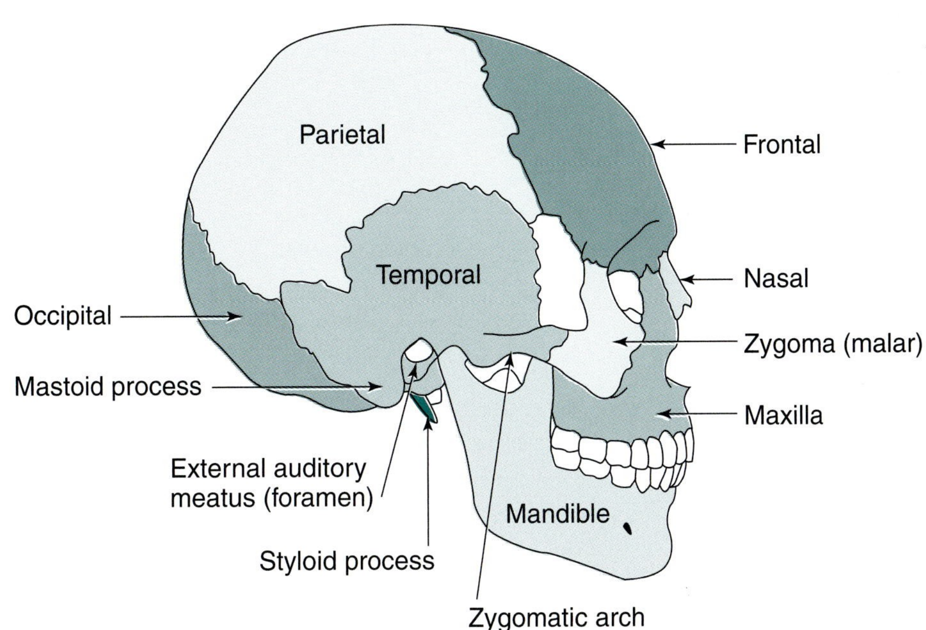

FIGURE 11-4. **Lateral view of the skull.**

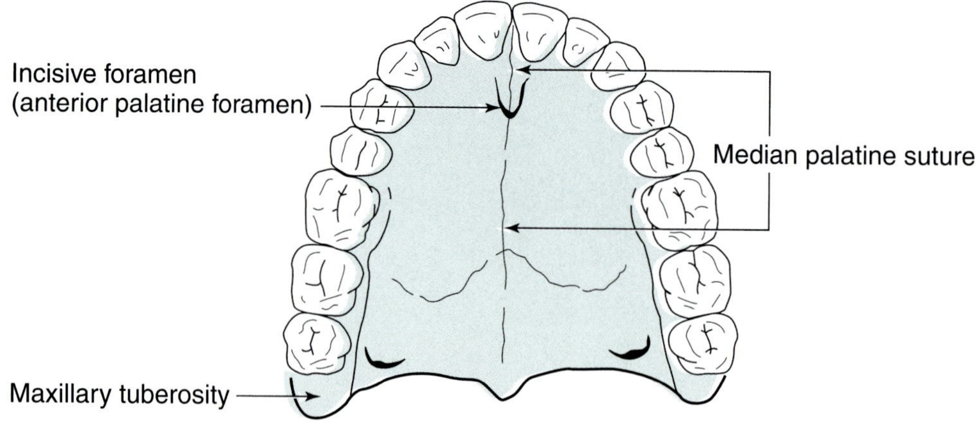

FIGURE 11-5. **Palatal view of maxilla.**

Radiolucent is defined as that portion of the processed radiograph that is **dark** because the exposed structures lack density; or refers to a substance that permits the passage of x-rays with little or no resistance. The opposite term is **radiopaque,** which is defined as that portion of the processed radiograph that appears **light** because the structures in the path of the x-rays are dense and absorb or resist the passage of the x-ray beam. Obviously, the majority of structures in the path of the x-rays are not of equal density; therefore most structures will appear as some shade of gray rather than just black or white.

Before considering the specific bones and structures visible in a full mouth series of radiographs, it is important to recognize and identify the normal appearance of **alveolar bone** and the **structures of the teeth.** Compare the drawing in Figure 11–8 with a radiograph of the same area shown in Figure 11–9.

Bone

Although **bones** appear solid, they are solid only on the outside and are honeycombed within. Bone is classified as **cortical bone,** a compact or dense form of bone, such as that which lines the outside layers of the maxillae and the mandible, and **cancellous** or **spongy bone,** which forms the bulk of the inner bone.

Small, interconnected **trabeculae** (bars or plates of bone) form a multitude of various-sized compartments

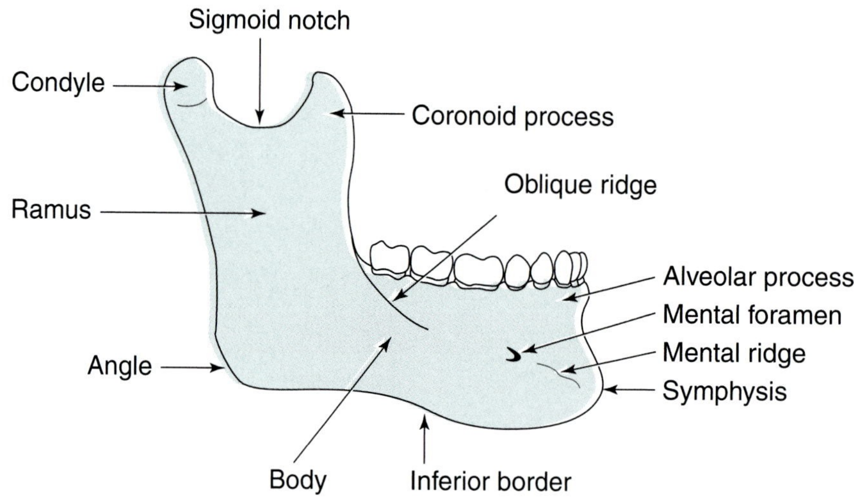

FIGURE 11-6. **Lateral view of detached mandible.**

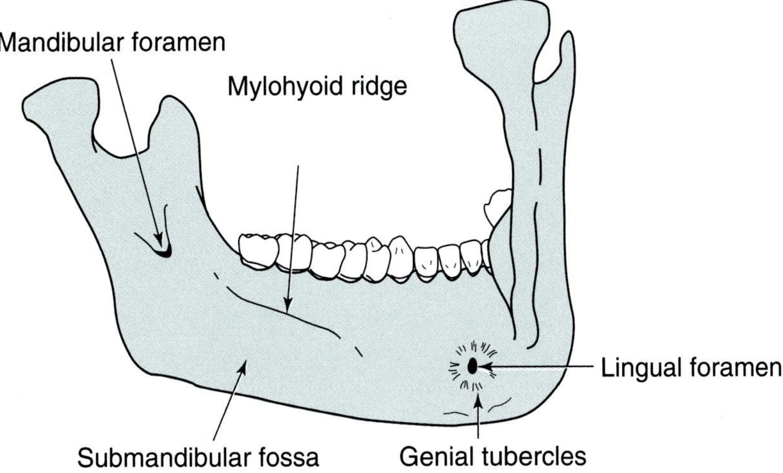

FIGURE 11–7. **Lingual view of detached mandible.**

that account for the honeycomb appearance. These trabecular spaces are usually filled with fat, blood, or bone cells, which accounts for the difference in the radiographic appearance of bone.

All bone tissues appear radiopaque. The compact or cortical outside layer appears extremely radiopaque (white), whereas the cancellous bone varies in radiopacity (shades of gray) according to the size and number of the trabecular spaces. The area may even appear almost radiolucent (black) if these spaces are very large or if the bone is thin, as is the case in the submandibular fossa.

By definition, the **alveolar process** is that portion of the maxilla or mandible that surrounds and supports the teeth. It is composed of the **lamina dura** and the **supporting bone.** The lamina dura is the hard, **cortical** bone that lines the **alveolus** (the tooth socket). On radiographs the **lamina dura** appears as a thin radiopaque (white) border that outlines the shape of the alveolus

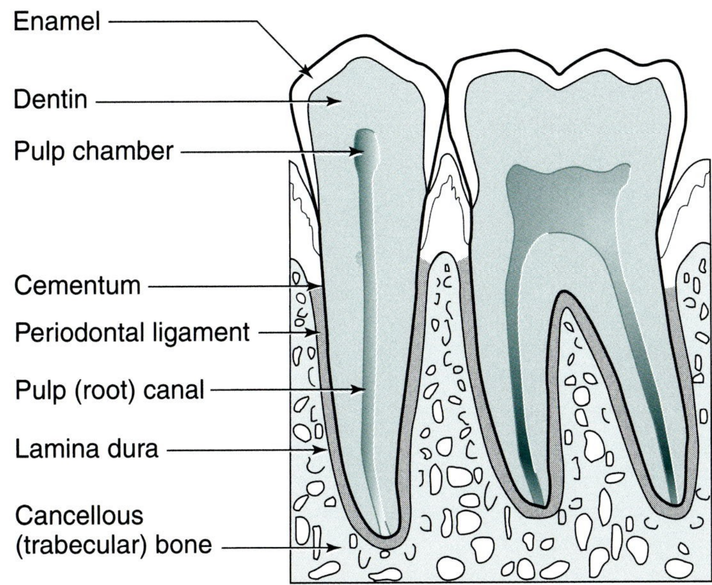

FIGURE 11–8. **Drawing of mandibular premolar (bicuspid) area.**

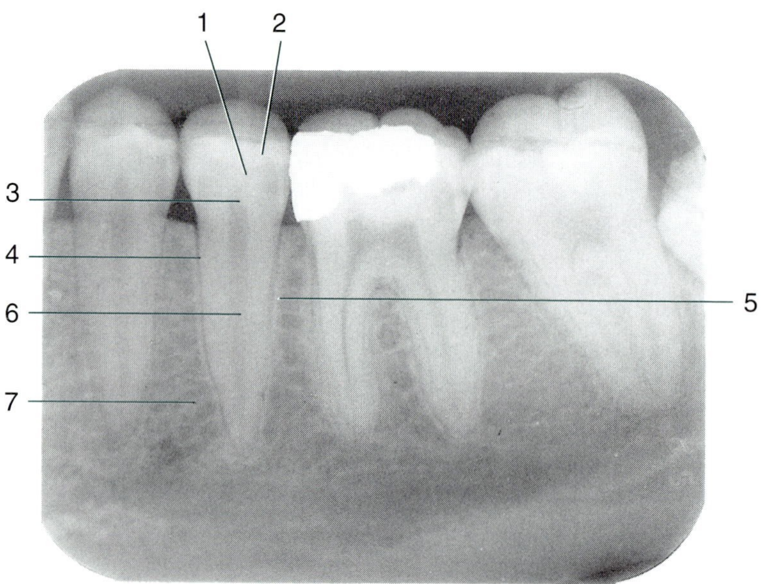

FIGURE 11-9. **Radiograph of mandibular premolar (bicuspid) area.** This radiograph shows (**1**) dentin, (**2**) enamel, (**3**) pulp chamber, (**4**) periodontal ligament, (**5**) lamina dura, (**6**) pulp (root) canal, and (**7**) cancellous (trabecular) bone. Note that because only a very thin layer of cementum covers the root, it is indistinguishable from the underlying dentin.

(the root of the tooth). The supporting bone is cancellous and varies in density in the different parts of the alveolar process.

Teeth

The **teeth** are attached to the **lamina dura** by the fibers of the **periodontal ligament,** which is so thin that sometimes it is not radiographically visible. When visible, it has the appearance of a thin radiolucent (dark) border between the lamina dura and the roots of the teeth.

The tooth structures are enamel, dentin, cementum, and pulp. **Enamel,** the hardest body structure, covers the crown and is very radiopaque. The underlying **dentin** is not as dense and appears less radiopaque. The **cementum** that covers the roots is even less dense. Because only a thin layer of cementum covers the root, it is generally indistinguishable from the underlying dentin. Although all three highly calcified tooth structures vary in radiopacity in direct proportion to the thickness of each structure in the path of the x-ray beam, for descriptive purposes enamel, dentin, and cementum are considered radiopaque.

The tooth **pulp** that occupies the **pulp chamber** and the **root canals** is the only noncalcified tooth tissue. As this soft tissue offers only minimal resistance to the passage of x-rays, it appears radiolucent. The end of the root canal is called the **apical foramen.** This foramen permits the passage of nerves and blood vessels that nourish the tooth structures.

Nutrient Canals

Nutrient canals are thin radiolucent lines of fairly uniform width that sometimes exhibit radiopaque borders. They contain blood vessels and nerves that supply the teeth, bone, and gingivae. Nutrient canals are most often visualized in the anterior of the mandible and in edentulous areas.

Dentition

To correctly identify and interpret the radiographs, one needs to understand the **dentition.** Young children have 20 **deciduous** (**baby** or **primary**) **teeth** that are gradually lost as they grow older. During the transition years they have a mixed dentition—that is, both deciduous and permanent teeth. A radiograph may show several deciduous teeth with partially resorbed roots, which are in a process of **exfoliation,** as well as permanent teeth, whose roots are not yet fully formed, which are in the process of eruption. This is a normal phenomenon and is to be expected in radiographs of children 10 to 12 years old and younger (see Figure 11–10). There are 32 **permanent** (**secondary** or **succedaneous**) **teeth,** provided that all four of the third molars (wisdom teeth) are formed. Third molars are frequently missing or malpositioned.

Occasionally, teeth form but are unable to erupt: these are described as **impacted** teeth. Some people have one or more extra teeth; these are called **supernumerary teeth.** Another deviation is the congenital absence of certain teeth, described as **anodontia.** These conditions occur so frequently that, although not desirable, they are not considered pathological (see Chapter 26).

Radiographic Appearance of Maxillary Landmarks

The normal landmarks visible in radiographs of the **maxilla** vary in radiopacity or radiolucency in direct proportion to the densities of the exposed tissues. Individual difference, the manner in which the film was positioned, and the angle at which the exposure was made, determines which landmarks may be visible on a radiograph of any given film placement area. Indeed, the expected landmark may not be visible at all, or perhaps on only a radiograph of the right or the left side.

Each normal structure is identified at least once on the drawings shown in Figures 11–11, 11–13, 11–15, and 11–17. Study the radiographs following each drawing to become proficient at recognizing and identifying normal maxillary anatomical landmarks Figures 11–12, 11–14, 11–16, 11–18, and 11–19.

Radiopaque Landmarks of the Maxilla

Beginning with a radiograph of the incisor area and progressing posteriorly toward the molar area, it is generally possible to observe several or all of the following **maxillary radiopaque** structures:

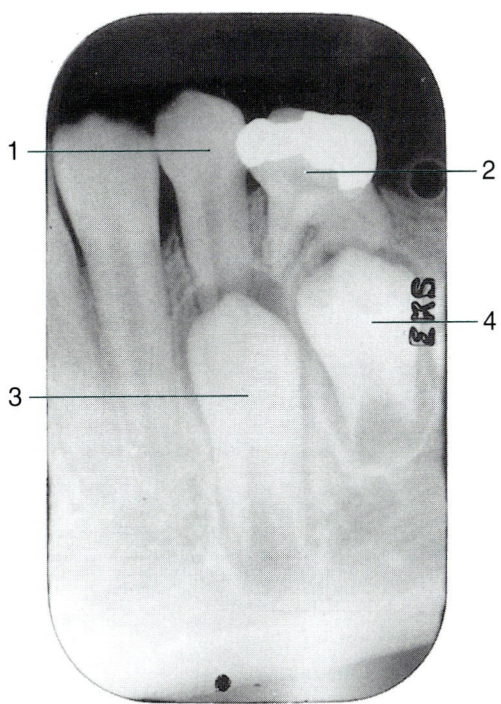

FIGURE 11–10. **Radiograph of mixed dentition in mandibular canine (cuspid) area.** This radiograph shows (**1**) deciduous canine (cuspid), (**2**) deciduous first molar with partially resorbed roots, (**3**) permanent canine (cuspid), and (**4**) permanent first premolar (bicuspid) with incomplete root formation.

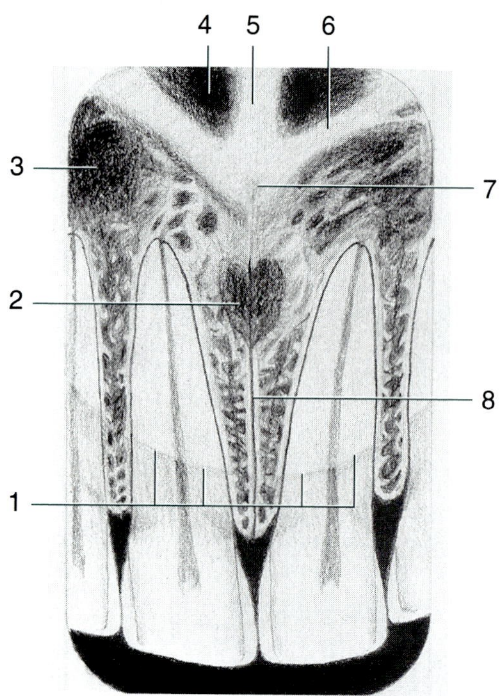

FIGURE 11–11. **Drawing of maxillary midline area.** Shown are the (**1**) outline of nose, (**2**) incisive foramen (anterior palatine foramen), (**3**) lateral fossa, (**4**) nasal fossa, (**5**) nasal septum, (**6**) border of nasal fossa, (**7**) nasal spine, and (**8**) median palatine suture.

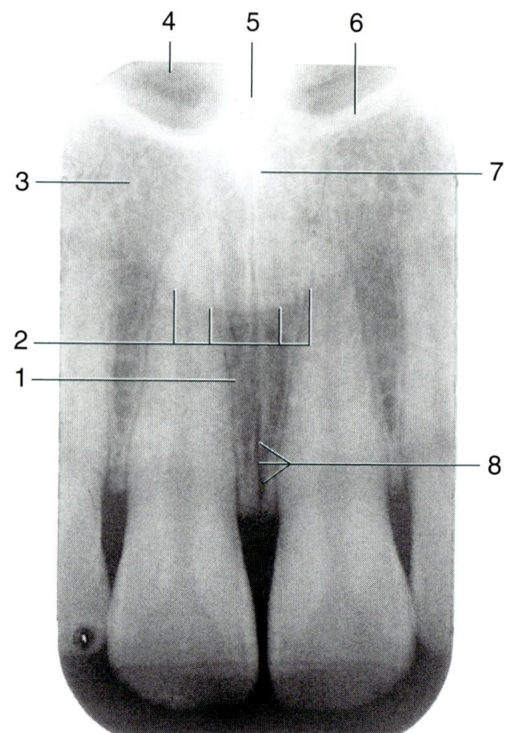

FIGURE 11–12. **Radiograph of maxillary incisor area.** This radiograph shows the (**1**) incisive (anterior palatine) foramen, indicated by an irregularly shaped, rounded radiolucent area. Also seen are the (**2**) outline of the nose, (**3**) lateral fossa, (**4**) nasal fossa (radiolucent), (**5**) nasal septum (radiopaque), (**6**) border of nasal fossa, (**7**) nasal spine, and (**8**) median palatine suture.

1. **Nasal septum.** A dense cartilage structure that separates the right nasal fossa from the left.
2. **Anterior nasal spine.** A V-shaped projection from the floor of the nasal fossa in the midline.
3. **Inverted Y.** An important landmark seen in the canine-premolar area, made up of the lateral wall of the nasal fossa and the anterior-medial wall of the maxillary sinus.
4. Thin dense bone forming the **floor** or **inferior border** of the sinuses.
5. **Septum.** A wall (or partition) may be seen separating the maxillary sinus into two or more compartments.
6. **Zygomatic process** of the maxilla. Appearing as a broad U-shaped band often seen above the roots of the first and second molars.
7. **Zygoma** (malar or cheekbone). Extends laterally and distally from the zygomatic process of the maxilla.
8. **Zygomatic arch.** Which is continuous with the zygoma and extends distally.
9. **Maxillary tuberosity.** The extension of the alveolar bone behind the molars and marks the posterior limits of the maxillary arch.
10. **Pterygoid plates** of the sphenoid.
11. **Hamulus (hamular process).** Which is a downward projection of the medial pterygoid plate. Appears as a hooklike structure that serves as a muscle attachment.
12. **Coronoid process** of the mandible can sometimes be seen overlapping the maxillary tuberosity.

Radiolucent Landmarks of the Maxilla

The following structures appear **radiolucent** on radiographs of the maxillary areas:

1. **Median palatine suture.** A thin line that delineates the midline of the palate and the junction of the right and left maxilla. Frequently seen between the central incisors.

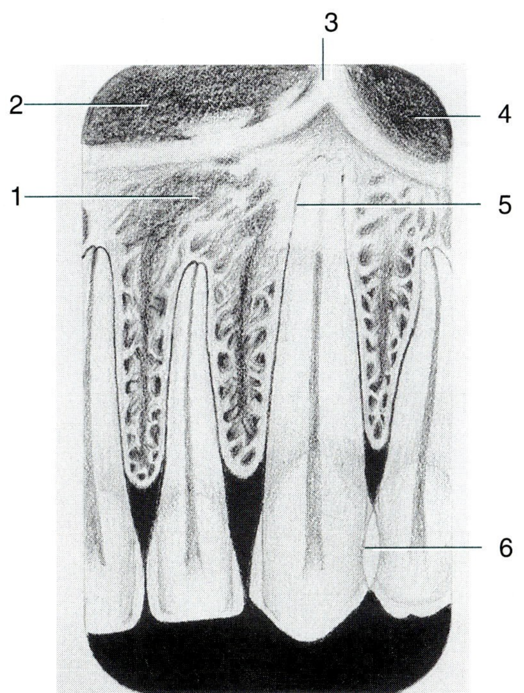

FIGURE 11–13. **Drawing of maxillary canine (cuspid) area.** The drawing shows the (**1**) lateral fossa, (**2**) nasal fossa, (**3**) inverted Y (border of nasal fossa and maxillary sinus), (**4**) maxillary sinus, (**5**) canine (cuspid) eminence, and (**6**) dense radiopaque area caused by overlapping of the mesial surface of the first premolar over the distal surface of the canine (cuspid).

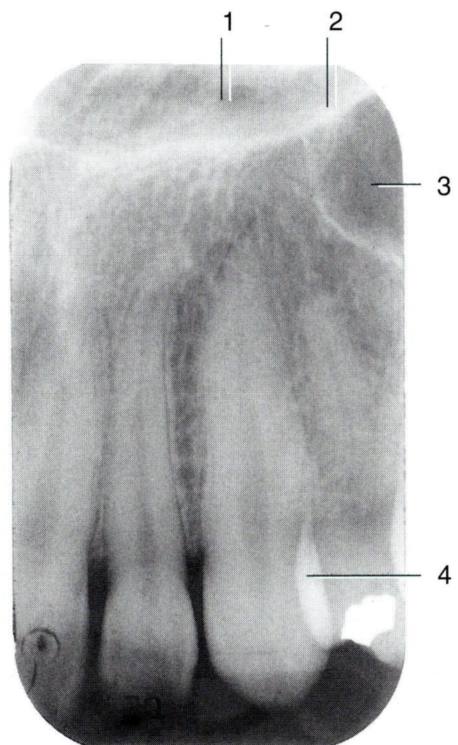

FIGURE 11–14. **Radiograph of maxillary canine (cuspid) area.** Shown are the (**1**) nasal fossa, (**2**) inverted Y (border of the nasal fossa and maxillary sinus), (**3**) maxillary sinus, and (**4**) dense radiopaque area caused by overlapping of the mesial surface of the first premolar over the distal surface of the canine (cuspid).

2. **Incisive foramen (anterior palatine foramen).** A round or pear-shaped opening that varies greatly in size, serves for the passage of nerves and blood vessels. It is often visible near or between the apices of the central incisors (this foramen can easily be mistaken for an abscess, cyst, or granuloma).
3. **Nasal fossa.** A large air space divided by the nasal septum, often visible above the roots of the incisors.
4. **Maxillary sinus.** A large air chamber inside the maxilla, visible in the areas from the canines (cuspids) to the molars.

Radiographic Appearance of Mandibular Landmarks

Each **mandibular landmark** is identified at least once on the drawings shown in Figures 11–20, 11–22, 11–24 and 11–27. Study the radiographs following each drawing in Figures 11–21, 11–23, 11–25, 11–26, 11–28, and 11–29 to become proficient at recognizing and identifying normal mandibular anatomical landmarks.

Radiopaque Landmarks of the Mandible

Continuing the method used to identify and mount the maxillary radiographs, it is generally possible to observe several or all of the **radiopaque** structures on radiographs of the **mandibular** tooth areas.

1. **Genial tubercles.** Four small bony crests on the lingual surface that serve for muscle attachments. Generally visible as a round radiopaque "doughnut" at the midline below the apices of the central incisors.
2. **Mental ridge.** Located on the lateral surface, the mental ridge appears as a radiopaque line extending from the premolar region to the symphysis.

(text continues on p. 178)

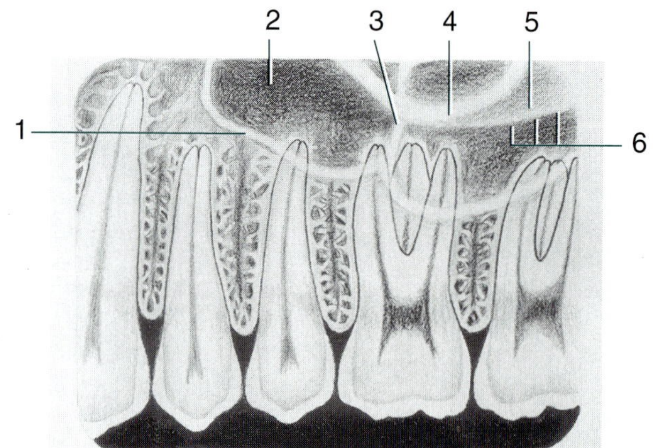

FIGURE 11-15. **Drawing of maxillary premolar (bicuspid) area.** Drawing shows the (**1**) border (floor) of maxillary sinus, (**2**) maxillary sinus, (**3**) septum in maxillary sinus dividing the sinus into two compartments, (**4**) zygomatic process of maxilla, (**5**) zygoma, and (**6**) lower border of zygomatic arch.

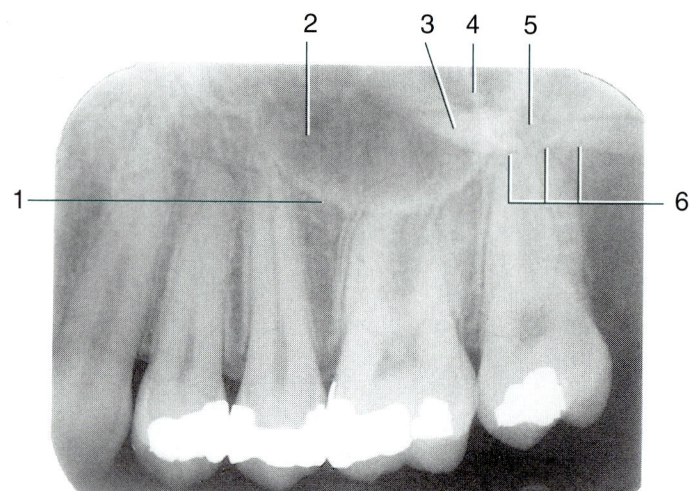

FIGURE 11-16. **Radiograph of maxillary premolar (bicuspid) area.** This radiograph shows the (**1**) border (floor) of maxillary sinus, (**2**) maxillary sinus, (**3**) zygomatic process of maxilla, (**4**) septum in maxillary sinus dividing the sinus into two compartments, (**5**) zygoma, and (**6**) lower border of zygomatic arch.

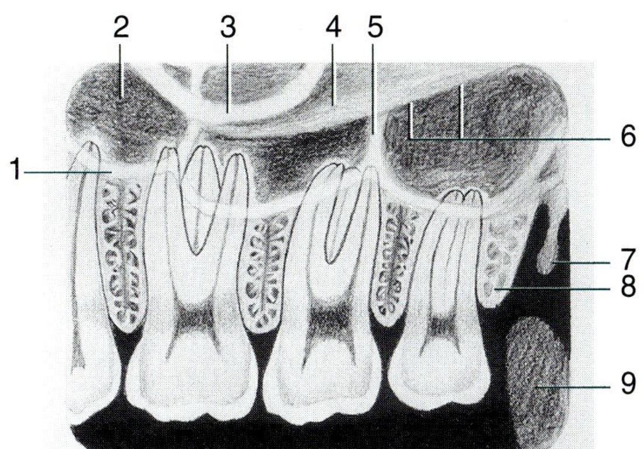

FIGURE 11-17. **Drawing of maxillary molar area.** Illustrated in the drawing are the (**1**) border (floor) of maxillary sinus, (**2**) maxillary sinus, (**3**) zygomatic process of maxilla, (**4**) zygoma, (**5**) septum in maxillary sinus, (**6**) lower border of zygomatic arch, (**7**) hamulus (hamular process), (**8**) maxillary tuberosity, and (**9**) coronoid process (mandible).

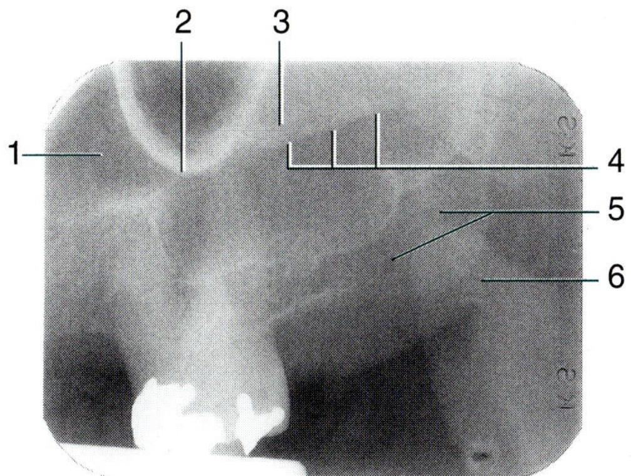

FIGURE 11-18. **Radiograph of maxillary molar area.** This radiograph shows (**1**) maxillary sinus, (**2**) zygomatic process of maxilla, (**3**) zygoma, (**4**) lower border of zygomatic arch, (**5**) maxillary tuberosity, and (**6**) coronoid process of the mandible.

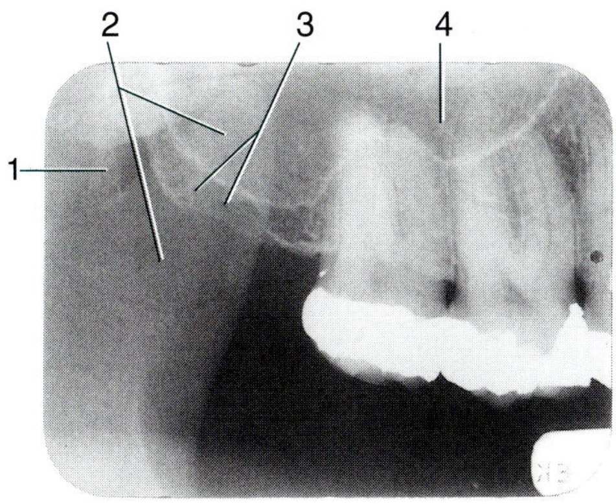

FIGURE 11-19. **Radiograph of maxillary molar area.** This radiograph shows (**1**) hamulus (hamular process), which is a downward projection of the medial pterygoid plate, (**2**) coronoid process of the mandible, (**3**) maxillary tuberosity, and (**4**) maxillary sinus.

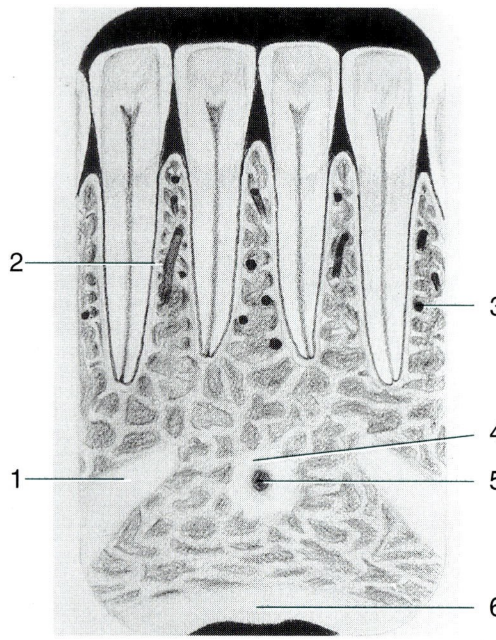

FIGURE 11-20. **Drawing of mandibular midline area.** The illustration shows (**1**) mental ridge, (**2**) nutrient canal, (**3**) nutrient foramen, (**4**) genial tubercles, (**5**) lingual foramen, and (**6**) inferior border of mandible.

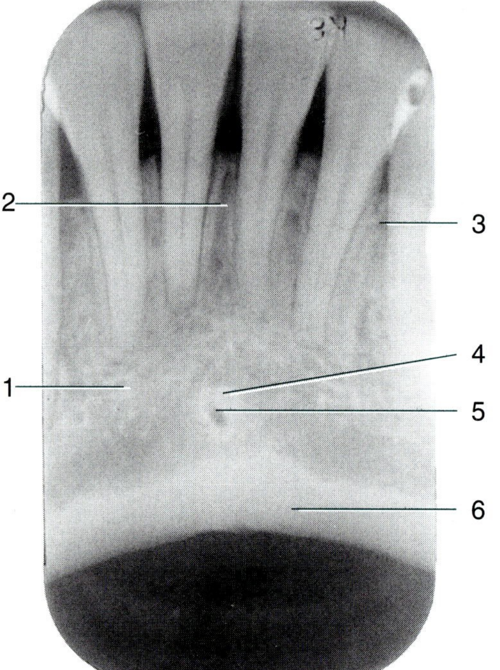

FIGURE 11-21. **Radiograph of the mandibular incisor area.** This radiograph shows the (**1**) mental ridge, (**2**) nutrient canal, (**3**) nutrient foramen, (**4**) genial tubercles surrounding the lingual foramen, (**5**) lingual foramen, and (**6**) inferior (lower) border of the mandible (radiopaque band of dense cortical bone).

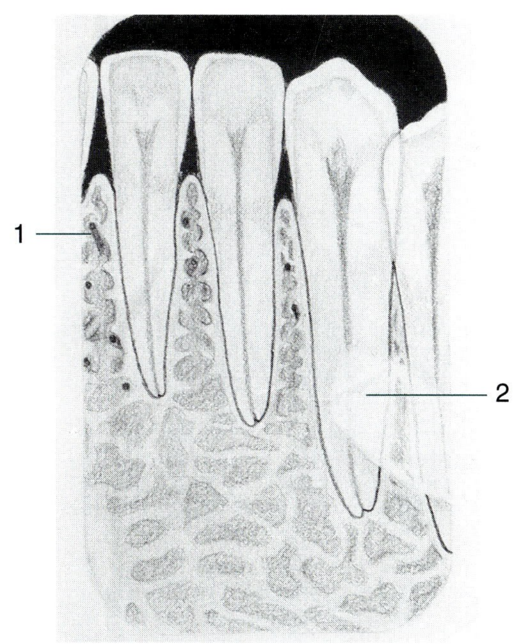

FIGURE 11-22. **Drawing of mandibular canine (cuspid) area.** Illustrated in the drawing are the (**1**) nutrient canal, and (**2**) torus mandibularis (lingual torus).

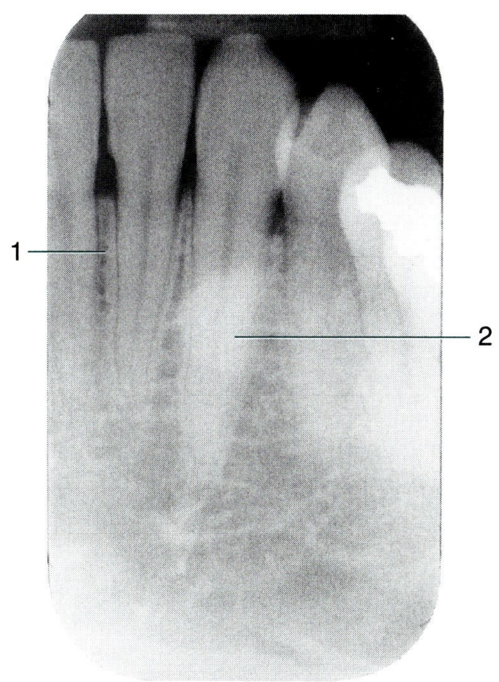

FIGURE 11-23. **Radiograph of mandibular canine (cuspid) area.** The (**1**) nutrient canal, and (**2**) torus mandibularis (lingual torus) are seen in this radiograph.

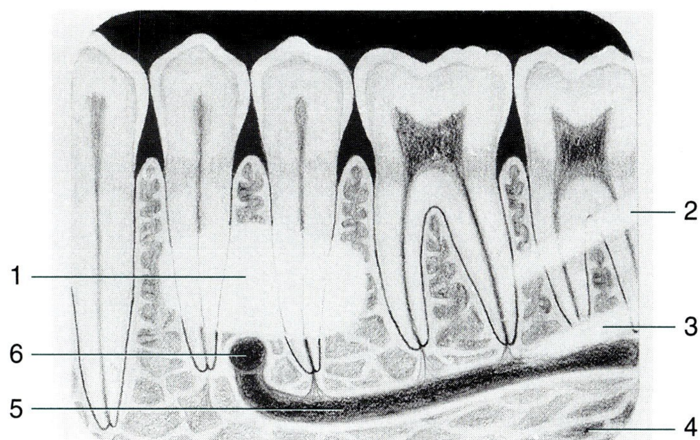

FIGURE 11-24. **Drawing of mandibular premolar (bicuspid) area.** This drawing shows the (**1**) torus mandibularis, (**2**) oblique ridge, (**3**) mylohyoid ridge, (**4**) submandibular fossa, and area where the bone of the mandible is extremely thin and offers little resistance to the passage of radiation and therefore appears radiolucent instead of radiopaque as denser bone does, (**5**) mandibular canal, and (**6**) mental foramen.

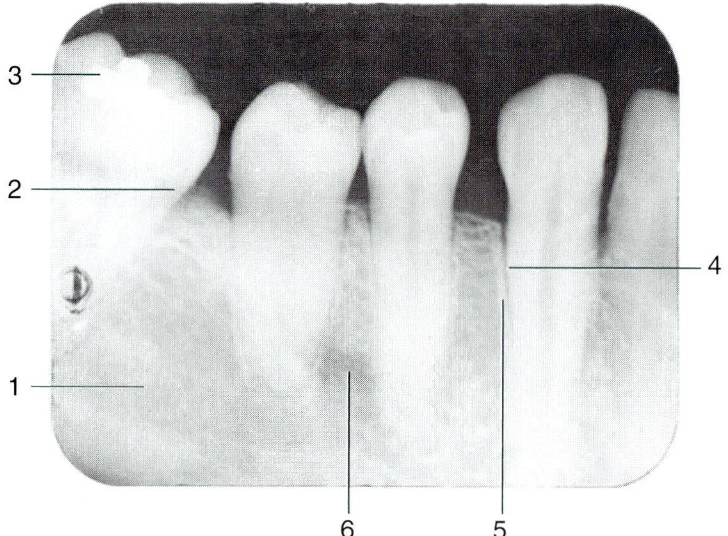

FIGURE 11-25. **Radiograph of mandibular premolar (bicuspid) area.** Radiograph shows (**1**) submandibular fossa, an area where the bone of the mandible is extremely thin and offers little resistance to the passage of radiation and therefore appears radiolucent instead of radiopaque as denser bone does, (**2**) cervical burnout at cemento-enamel junction (radiolucent), (**3**) metal restoration, (**4**) thin radiolucent line indicating periodontal ligament space, (**5**) thin radiopaque line as the lamina dura, and (**6**) small radiolucent circle as the mental foramen.

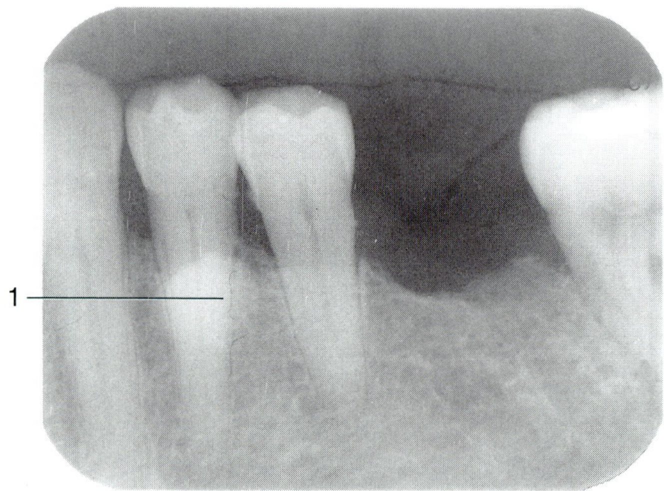

FIGURE 11-26. **Radiograph of mandibular premolar (bicuspid) area.** Shows the (**1**) torus mandibularis (lingual torus).

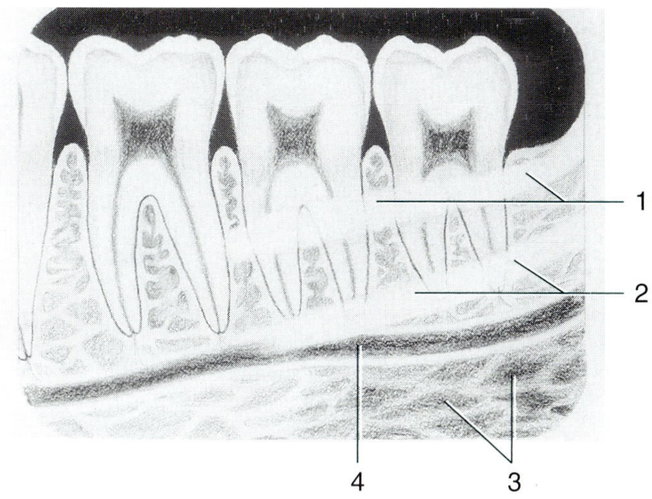

FIGURE 11-27. **Drawing of mandibular molar area.** Drawing illustrates the (**1**) oblique ridge, (**2**) mylohyoid ridge, (**3**) submandibular fossa, an area where the bone of the mandible is extremely thin and offers little resistance to the passage of radiation and therefore appears radiolucent instead of radiopaque as dense bone does, and (**4**) mandibular canal, a wide diagonal radiolucent area outlined above and below by a thin radiopaque line.

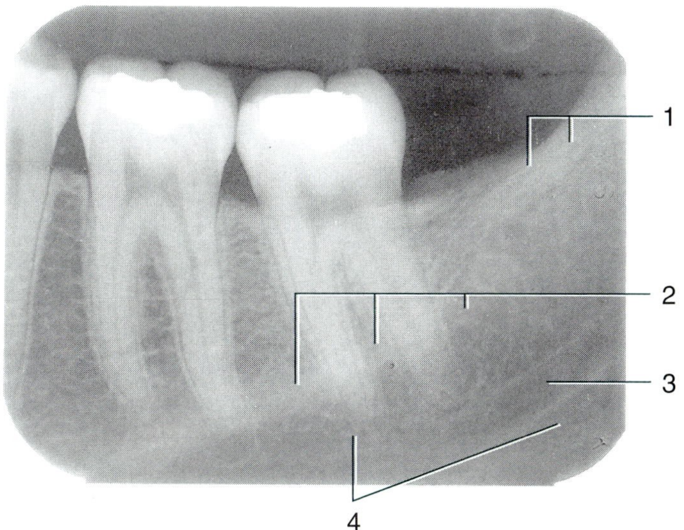

FIGURE 11-28. **Radiograph of mandibular molar area.** Shown are the (**1**) oblique ridge, (**2**) mylohyoid ridge, (**3**) mandibular canal, and (**4**) submandibular fossa, an area where the bone of the mandible is extremely thin and therefore appears somewhat radiolucent.

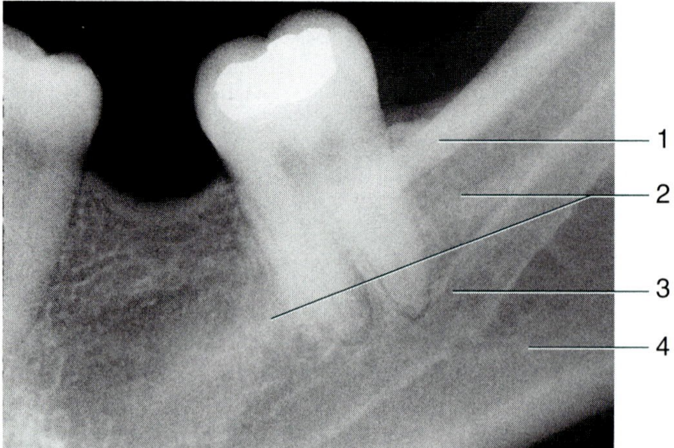

FIGURE 11–29. **Radiograph of mandibular molar area.** Shown are the (**1**) oblique ridge, (**2**) mylohyoid ridge, (**3**) mandibular canal, a wide diagonal radiolucent area outlined above and below by a very thin radiopaque line, and (**4**) submandibular fossa.

3. **Oblique ridge.** A continuation of the anterior border of the ramus that extends downward and forward on the lateral surface of the mandible. The oblique ridge appears as a radiopaque line of varied width across the molar region.
4. **Mylohyoid ridge** is an irregular crest of bone for muscle attachments on the lingual surface of the mandible in the molar region. The mylohyoid ridge appears as a radiopaque line parallel and always below the oblique ridge.
5. **Inferior border** of the mandible is a heavy layer of cortical bone, visible only if the radiograph is deeply depressed in the floor of the mouth.

Radiolucent Landmarks of the Mandible

The following structures appear **radiolucent** on radiographs of the **mandibular** areas.

1. **Lingual foramen.** A very small circular area surrounded by the genial tubercles. Occasionally seen in the central incisor area but often so small that it goes unnoticed.
2. **Mental foramen.** A small opening on the lateral side of the body of the mandible, often seen near the apices of the premolars (bicuspids).
3. **Mental fossa.** A depression on the labial aspect of the mandibular incisor area. Some consider the mental fossa to be an accentuated thinness of the mandible in the incisor area. On a mandibular incisor radiograph, the mental fossa appears as a generalized radiolucent area around the incisor apices.
4. **Submandibular fossa.** A large irregular-shaped area below the mylohyoid ridge and the roots of the mandibular molars, in which the bone is quite thin and can easily be mistaken for a lesion.
5. **Mandibular canal.** a canal for the passage of the mandibular nerve and blood vessels. Outlined by very thin layers of cortical bone, the mandibular canal can often be seen in the premolar-molar areas below the apices of the teeth.

CHAPTER SUMMARY

Knowledge of the anatomical landmarks of the face and skull is needed to properly position the film packet and direct the radiation through the proper point of entry. This can be acquired through practice and study by using a skull and a textbook and followed by clinical exercises. With this training and experience, dental radiographers can learn to identify most landmarks and structures of the maxillae and mandible. This is essential for interpreting and mounting the radiographs.

Dental anatomical landmarks are separated into the following groups: face, skull, maxilla and mandible. Although facial landmarks cannot be distinguished on a radiograph, they help the radiographer locate important planes and structures when placing the film and directing the PID. Knowledge of skull landmarks is useful when making cephalometric, temporomandibular joint, or panoramic exposures.

One must be familiar with all radiopaque and radiolucent landmarks of the maxilla and mandible in order to interpret or mount intraoral radiographs.

As experience is gained, the radiographer should be able to differentiate between normal and abnormal structures of the jaws, teeth, and periodontium and recognize most restorative materials.

REVIEW QUESTIONS

1. Which of these terms describes the ability to read a radiograph?
   (a) Case presentation
   (b) Prognosis
   (c) Dissertation
   (d) Interpretation
2. Which of these is a facial landmark?
   (a) Coronoid process
   (b) Glenoid fossa
   (c) Tragus
   (d) Mylohyoid ridge
3. Which of these is not a mandibular landmark?
   (a) Incisive foramen
   (b) Lingual foramen
   (c) Coronoid process
   (d) Mental foramen
4. Which of these structures appears radiolucent?
   (a) Enamel
   (b) Dental pulp
   (c) Dentin
   (d) Alveolar bone
5. Which of these structures appears radiopaque?
   (a) Maxillary sinus
   (b) Nasal fossa
   (c) Maxillary tuberosity
   (d) Mental foramen
6. Which of these appears most radiopaque?
   (a) Trabecular bone
   (b) Cementum
   (c) Dentin
   (d) Enamel

7. A bony projection that extends downward and slightly posterior in many maxillary molar radiographs is the _____________ process.
   - (a) Mastoid
   - (b) Styloid
   - (c) Condylar
   - (d) Hamular

8. In a radiograph of the maxillary molars, which of the following structures may obscure the roots of the teeth?
   - (a) Zygomatic process of the maxilla
   - (b) Maxillary tuberosity
   - (c) Mastoid process
   - (d) Mylohyoid ridge

9. When nutrient canals open at the surface of the bone, they often appear as:
   - (a) Small radiolucent lines.
   - (b) Large radiopaque lines.
   - (c) Small radiolucent dots.
   - (d) Small radiopaque dots.

10. The inverted-Y landmark is composed of which two structures?
    - (a) Junction of the right and left nasal cavity
    - (b) Inferior border of the nasal cavity and anterior border of the maxillary sinus
    - (c) Floor of the orbit and floor of the maxillary sinus
    - (d) Floor of the orbit and anterior border of the maxillary sinus

For questions 11–19, match each term with its definition.

a. cortical bone
b. cancellous bone
c. fossa
d. sinus
e. canal
f. foramen
g. septum
h. suture
i. ridge

_____ 11. An extended elevation or crest of bone
_____ 12. A dividing wall or partition
_____ 13. A depression or recess in bone
_____ 14. A tubular passageway through bone
_____ 15. Hard or compact bone
_____ 16. A cavity or hollow space in bone
_____ 17. A hole or opening in bone
_____ 18. Sponge-like bone
_____ 19. Immoveable joint found between bones

BIBLIOGRAPHY

Farman AG, Nortje CJ, & Wood RE. *Oral and Maxillofacial Diagnostic Imaging*. St Louis: Mosby, 1993.

White SC, & Pharoah MJ. *Oral Radiology Principles and Interpretation*, 4th ed. St. Louis: Mosby, 2000.

CHAPTER 12

Mounting and Viewing Dental Radiographs

OBJECTIVES

By the end of this chapter the student should be able to:

- Define the key words.
- List the five advantages of mounting radiographs.
- Discuss the use and importance of the identification dot.
- List the recommended order for mounting radiographs.
- List and describe the step-by-step procedures for mounting radiographs.
- List five items to be carefully checked after the radiographs are mounted.
- Describe the optimal conditions for viewing radiographs.
- Describe how to block out excess light during film viewing.

KEY WORDS

Anatomical order
Film mount
Film mounting
Identification dot
Mount
Viewbox
Viewer
Viewing

Introduction

Mounting radiographs is an important step in the interpretation of dental radiographs. Dental radiographs must be mounted in the correct anatomic order. The dental radiographer must have a thorough knowledge of the normal anatomy of the teeth and jaws (see Chapter 11) in order to mount radiographs correctly.

Optimal viewing is essential for interpreting dental radiographs. The dental radiographer must be knowledgeable about radiographic viewing conditions.

The purpose of this chapter is to describe basic step by step procedures for mounting and viewing dental radiographs.

Mounting the Radiographs

Mounting is the placement of radiographs in a holder arranged in **anatomical order** (see Figure 12–1). The **advantages of mounting** are:

- Intraoral radiographs are easier to view and interpret.
- Mounting decreases the chance of error caused by confusing radiographs of the patient's right and left side.
- Less handling of individual radiographs results in fewer scratches and finger marks.
- Mounts mask out distracting sidelight making radiographs easier to view and interpret.
- Mounted radiographs are easier to store.

Mounting generally refers only to intraoral films. The large extraoral radiographs are already identified through the use of metal lettering and are usually placed in a protective envelope. The patient's name and the date of the exposure are always written on the outside of these envelopes.

Film Mounts

Film mounts are celluloid, cardboard, or plastic holders with frames or windows for the radiographs (see Figure 12–2). Attaching the radiographs to the film mounts is called **mounting.** Film mounts are available in many sizes and with numerous combinations of windows or frames to fit films of different sizes. Most mounts are large enough to accommodate a full-mouth series of radiographs, although some hold only a few or even a single radiograph. Standard ready-made mounts are used in

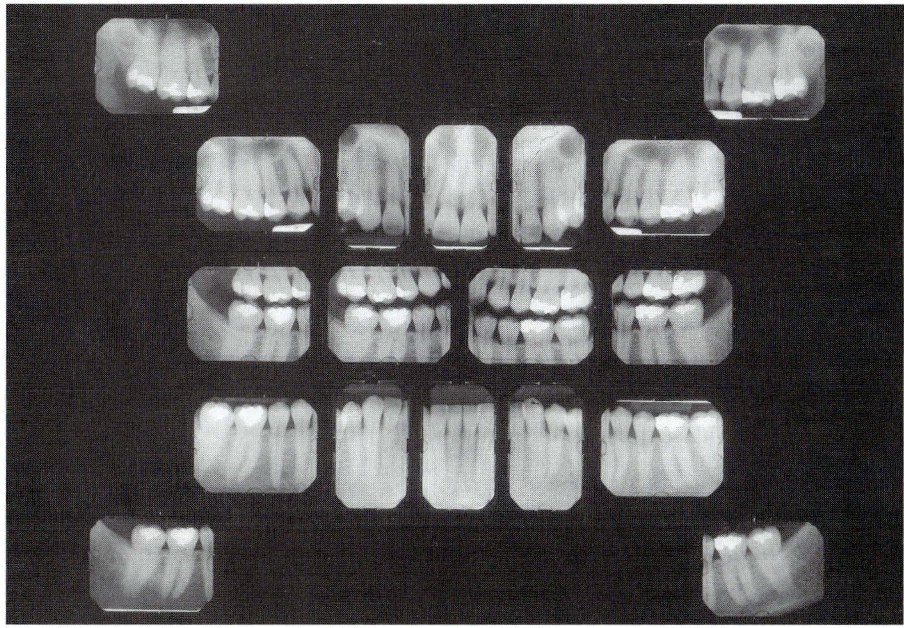

FIGURE 12–1. **Full-mouth series mounted in an opaque mount.**

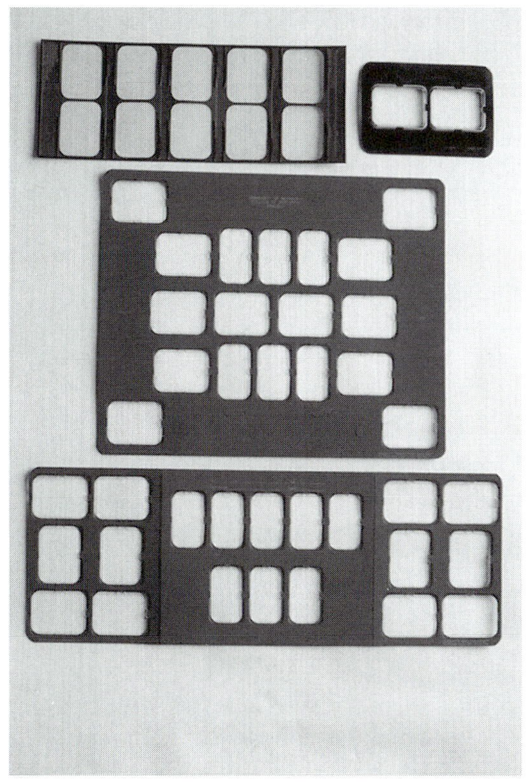

FIGURE 12–2. **Examples of various film mounts.** Film mounts are available in a variety of sizes and film combinations.

most dental offices; however, several firms will make custom mounts to suit special needs. Black mounts are often preferred because they can block out extraneous light from the viewbox.

Identification Dot

A little **identification dot** near the edge of the film appears convex or concave depending on the side from which the film is viewed. When the film is mounted with the convex dot toward you, the patient's left side is on your right (see Figure 12–3). The purpose of the identification dot is to distinguish the patient's right from the left side.

Methods

In the past, two methods of film mounting were commonly used. The first method, now obsolete but still used by some dentists, had the radiographs mounted so that they gave the effect of viewing the patient from behind. In this arrangement the concave part of the dot faces the viewer.

The second method, now taught by all dental colleges, mounts the radiographs so that they are viewed from the front of the patient. The **convex part of the dot faces the viewer.** All national organizations, including the American Dental Association, recommend and use the latter method.

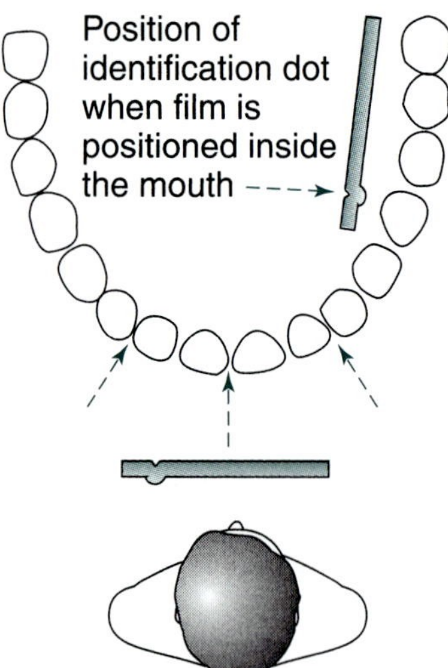

FIGURE 12–3. **Identification dot.** Regardless of the tooth area involved, whenever an x-ray film is positioned in the mouth, the raised portion of the identification dot (the convexity) must face the x-ray tube and the source of radiation. Therefore, when the film is viewed from outside the mouth or from in front of the patient, the convex part of the dot faces the person viewing the film.

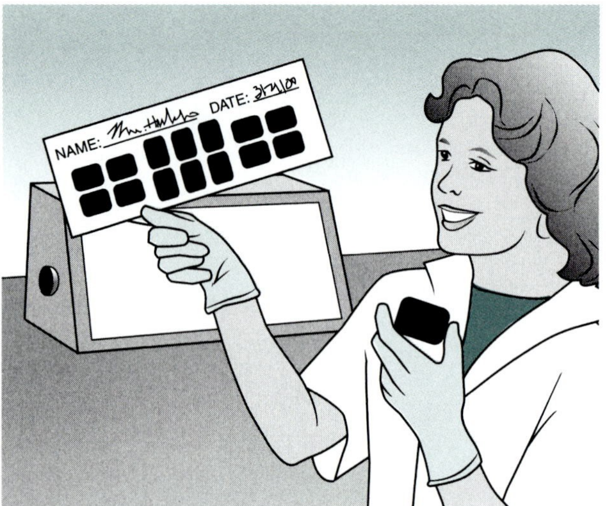

FIGURE 12–4. **Radiographer mounting radiographs.** When mounting radiographs, keep hands clean and dry to avoid scratching or marring the image. Some offices require the use of thin, light cloth gloves.

Occasionally, single intraoral radiographs are not mounted but are slipped into a coin envelope and attached to the record card. However, it is better to mount even a single or a small group of radiographs; a full-mouth series should always be mounted for easier and faster viewing.

Obviously, each film mount must be identified with at least the patient's name, case number if applicable, and the date. Few things are as useless in a dental office as unidentifiable radiographs.

Mounting Procedures

Radiographs should be mounted immediately after processing (see Figure 12–4).

The following step-by-step procedures are recommended for **mounting** a set of radiographs.

1. Write the patient's name, case number (if applicable), and date of exposure on the mount.
2. Lay a clean, light colored towel over the workbench in front of a viewbox.
3. Wash hands to prevent smudging the films.
4. Handle the radiographs by their edges to avoid smudging or scratching them (see Figure 12–5).
5. Arrange the radiographs so that all the identification dots face in the same direction, the convex side toward the viewer.

   Several distinctive tooth characteristics and bone structures make mounting easier.

   - Roots and crowns of the maxillary anterior teeth are larger than those of the mandibular teeth.
   - Maxillary molars generally have three roots and the mandibular molars only two roots.
   - Most roots curve toward the distal.
   - Large radiolucent areas denoting the nasal fossa or the maxillary sinus indicate that the radiograph is of a maxillary area.
   - The radiolucent mental foramen indicates that the film belongs in the mandibular premolar (bicuspid) area.
   - The body of the mandible has a distinct upward curve toward the ramus in the molar area.
6. With these characteristics firmly in mind, hold the radiographs up to the viewbox and separate them into three groups.
   - **Bitewing.** Crowns of both maxillary and mandibular teeth are seen on bitewing radiographs.

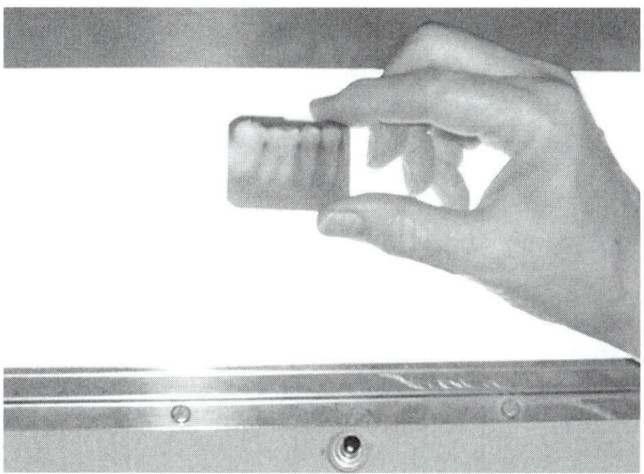

FIGURE 12-5. **Radiographs should be handled by the edges only.**

- **Anterior periapical.** Anterior periapical radiographs are oriented vertically.
- **Posterior periapical.** Posterior periapical radiographs are oriented horizontally.

7. The radiographs of each of these groups are then identified as maxillary or mandibular (study Table 12–1) and as right or left (the order of teeth is used to distinguish right from left).
8. Arrange the radiographs in anatomical order on the work surface (roots of maxillary teeth point up and roots of mandibular teeth point down).
9. Place each radiograph in the proper frame of the mount.

The recommended sequence for mounting radiographs is:

- Bitewings
- Maxillary anterior periapicals
- Mandibular anterior periapicals
- Maxillary posterior periapicals
- Mandibular posterior periapicals

The beginner should follow the recommended sequence. However, the sequence for mounting is usually a matter of preference. Many like to mount the bitewings first, so there is a base of reference for mounting periapicals by comparing restorations or carious lesions. Some like to mount the anterior periapicals first, then the bitewings, and last the posterior periapicals.

10. After the last radiograph has been mounted, the entire film mount should be carefully checked to see that:

TABLE 12-1. **Anatomical Landmarks Distinguishing Maxillary Radiographs from Mandibular Radiographs**

Area	Maxillary Anatomical Landmarks	Mandibular Anatomical Landmarks
Incisor	Incisive foramen	Lingual foramen
	Median palatine suture	Genial tubercles
	Nasal fossa	Nutrient canals
	Nasal septum	Mental ridge
	Anterior nasal spine	Mental fossa
Canine (cuspid)	Inverted Y	
	Lateral fossa	
Premolar (bicuspid)	Maxillary sinus	Mental foramen
Molar	Maxillary sinus	Mandibular canal
	Zygomatic process of maxilla	External oblique ridge
	Zygoma	Mylohyoid ridge (internal oblique ridge)
	Maxillary tuberosity	Submandibular fossa
	Hamulus	
	Coronoid process of mandible	

- Identification dots all face the same direction.
- All radiographs are arranged in proper anatomical order.
- No radiographs were reversed or mounted upside down.
- The radiographs are firmly attached to the mount.
- The patient's name and date are on the mount.

Viewing the Radiographs

Proper **viewing** is essential for the interpretation of dental radiographs. One must be familiar with and understand optimal viewing conditions and the proper sequence of viewing the radiographs.

Who Views the Radiographs?

Dental radiographs are viewed by any trained professional (dentist, dental hygienist, or dental assistant) with a knowledge of normal anatomic landmarks of the maxilla, mandible, and related structures. Radiographs may be interpreted by all members of the dental team, but the dentist is responsible for the final interpretation and diagnosis.

Viewing Equipment

A **viewbox** and a **magnifying glass** are required for optimal film viewing (see Figure 12–6). Many types of viewboxes are available, both built-ins and portables. The preferred type for dental office use has a dark nonreflective frame, a frosted glass panel, and a rheostat to vary the intensity of the light.

- **Viewbox.** The viewbox must have lighting of uniform intensity and evenly diffused. A variable light intensity viewbox is best. The viewing surface should be large enough to accommodate a full set of intraoral radiographs as well as uncounted extraoral radiographs. A cardboard template should be used to mask out distracting light around the mount.

  Blocking out excess sidelight reduces glare and facilitates viewing. The use of black cardboard or frosted film mounts also helps to reduce glare and enhances the detail of the images. Always use subdued room lighting to allow the eyes to adapt to the light level of the radiographs.
- **Magnifying glass.** A hand-held magnifying glass should be used to aid the viewer. Some viewers are equipped with a magnifying device (see Figure 12–7).

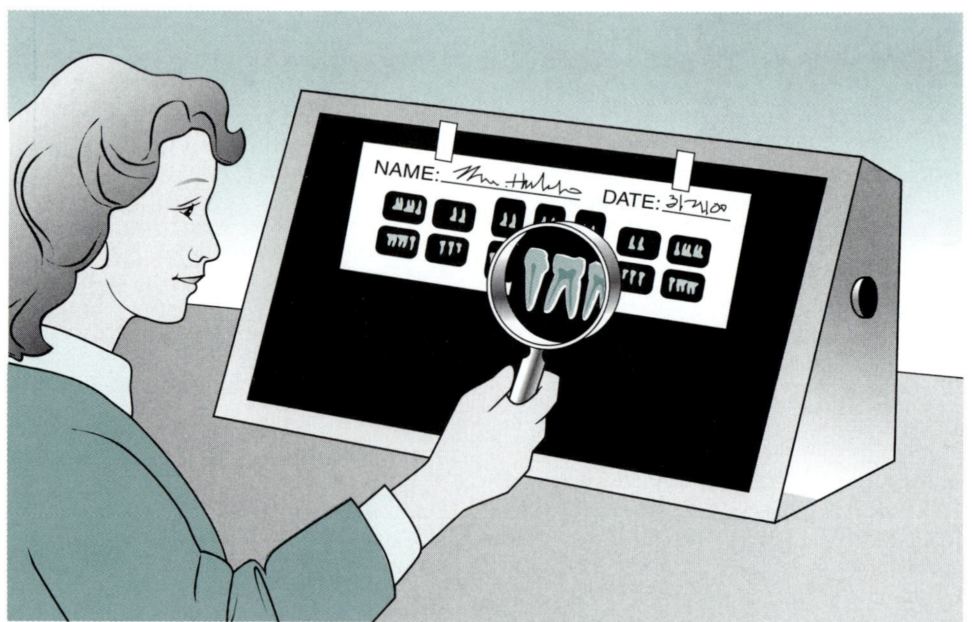

FIGURE 12–6. **Radiographer viewing radiographs.** Radiographs should be viewed in subdued room lighting, using a variable light-intensity viewbox, an opaque template on the viewbox to eliminate distracting light around the mount, and a magnifying glass.

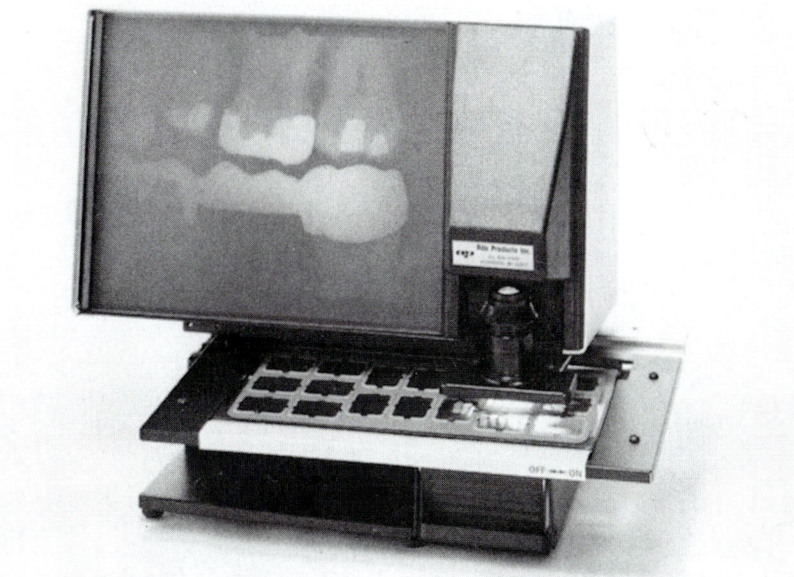

FIGURE 12-7. **Viewer-enlarger-projector.** Used as a viewer, the radiographs can be observed on a 9 x 12-in. (32 x 39-cm) screen. High-low light control gives the image the brightness needed for diagnosis. Used as an enlarger, the size of the radiograph is increased eight times. By removing the viewing screen, the unit can be converted into a projector. (Courtesy of Ada Products, Inc.)

Mounted radiographs show the relations between major tooth areas and reveal each tooth in its entirety. Depending on the radiographer's training and responsibility in the dental office, the individual may now proceed to make a preliminary interpretation and discuss it with the dentist.

Step-by-Step Procedures for Viewing Radiographs

The following step-by-step procedures should be followed meticulously to prevent errors in interpretation. Always use a systematic method and view mounted radiographs in sequential order (see Figure 12–8).

1. Start with the right maxillary molar radiograph in the upper-left side of the film mount.
2. Proceed horizontally to the left maxillary molar radiograph in the upper right side of the film mount. Examine each maxillary periapical radiograph carefully.
3. Next, move down to the left mandibular molar radiograph in the lower-right side of film mount.
4. Proceed horizontally to the right mandibular radiograph in the lower-left side of the mount. Examine each mandibular periapical radiograph carefully.
5. Move up to the bitewing radiographs starting with the right molar bitewing radiograph on the left side of the film mount. Proceed horizontally, examining each bitewing radiograph until you finish with the left molar bitewing radiograph on the right side of the film mount.

A thorough examination is best accomplished when a specific sequence of analysis is used. The mounted radiographs must be viewed in a systematic order to prevent errors in interpretation. The radiographs must be examined three times. During the first exam, look only for caries, the second exam for periodontal disease, and the third exam for all other abnormalities.

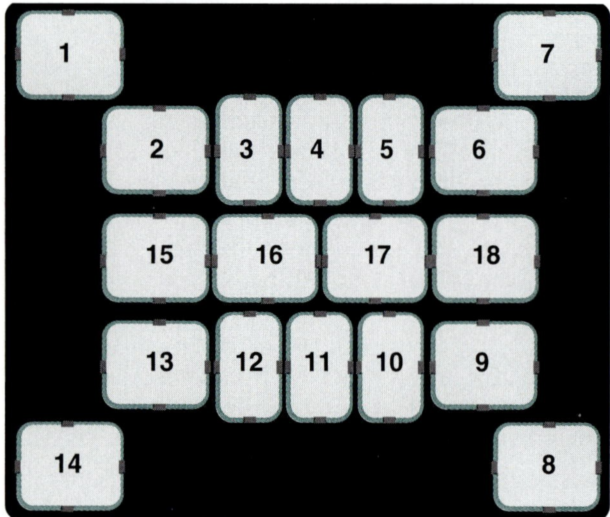

FIGURE 12–8. **Proper sequence for viewing radiographs.** The radiographer should view the radiographs in the sequence illustrated. Start with number 1 and proceed clockwise through number 18.

First Exam: Concentrate on Caries

The radiographer should first view the radiographs looking only for caries (see Chapter 28). Pay close attention to the interproximal areas at or below the contact points. Check restorations carefully for recurrent caries. Often caries found on one view cannot be detected on another because of superimposition of the restoration.

Second Exam: Concentrate on Periodontal Disease

The radiographer should repeat the examination sequence, concentrating on periodontal disease (see Chapter 27). Make a second visual circuit through each radiograph, examining the bone of the alveolar process. Note the presence of calculus. Examine all regions of the alveolar process to determine the extent and severity of alveolar bone loss.

Third Exam: Concentrate on All Other Abnormalities

The radiographer should make a third visual circuit through each radiograph looking for all other diseases and abnormalities (see Chapter 26). Look for unerupted, missing, and impacted teeth. Examine all surfaces of the teeth and supporting structures for evidence of disease and abnormalities.

All findings must be noted in the patient's record. Although all professionals may record findings, it is the responsibility of the dentist for final interpretation and diagnosis.

Filing and Storing Dental Radiographs

After the radiographs are mounted, they should be placed in a protective envelope and given to the dentist to examine before they are discussed with the patient. The radiographs should be in the operatory room along with other records each time the patient visits the office.

After the appointment, the radiographs should be **filed** until needed again. They may be **stored** along with the record folder or in a separate x-ray filing cabinet. The radiographs may be filed by either name or case number, as long as they can be located rapidly when needed. The need for an orderly filing system cannot be overstressed; missing radiographs can be a source of much annoyance. Some dentists store current radiographs in one file and older ones in another. When new radiographs are exposed, the old ones are often removed from the mounts and placed into smaller envelopes, identified and dated, to conserve space.

All radiographs should be **handled with care** to prevent smudging or scratching. Radiographs should be protected from heat damage by storage in cool, well-ventilated areas.

Although radiographs are seldom used after more than 6 months or 1 year because oral conditions change constantly in most patients, they are valuable for comparing present with previous conditions. Sometimes they are needed in a court of law. Therefore, dentists should preserve them until they are certain that the statute of limitations for their state has expired.

Helpful Hints

- Always use a viewbox to examine radiographs.
- Block out all distracting side light from the viewbox.
- Do NOT hold radiographs up to the light to view.
- Always use a magnifying glass.
- Record all radiographic findings in the patient's record.

CHAPTER SUMMARY

It is customary to arrange the radiographs of a full-mouth series in anatomical order on some form of film mount. These mounts vary in size and number of frames, but all have space for identifying information: patient's name and date of exposure. Each film has an identification dot in one of the corners by which it is possible to determine on which side of the face it was exposed. When the radiograph is mounted with the convex portion of the dot toward the viewer, the radiographs of the patient's left side are on the right side of the mount as seen by the viewer.

Viewing radiographs is facilitated if a viewbox with magnification and a variable light intensity is used. The mounted radiographs must be viewed in a systematic order to prevent errors in interpretation. The radiographs must be examined three times. The first exam looking only for caries, the second exam for periodontal disease and the third exam for all other abnormalities.

Radiographs should be filed or stored until needed.

REVIEW QUESTIONS

1. All dental schools now teach that for viewing, radiographs should be mounted as though:
   (a) You are seated on the tongue looking out.
   (b) You are facing the patient.
   (c) You are viewing the patient from behind.
   (d) You are viewing the patient from the side.
2. Which of these helps to determine whether the radiograph is of the patient's right or left side?
   (a) Lamina dura
   (b) Film emulsion
   (c) Location of the septum
   (d) Identification dot
3. When mounting dental radiographs, the buccal or labial aspect is determined by:
   (a) Position of the teeth on the film
   (b) Convexity of the dot toward the operator
   (c) Concavity of the dot toward the operator
   (d) None of the above
4. Mounting is the placement of radiographs in a holder arranged in anatomical order.
   (a) True
   (b) False
5. All radiographs should be handled with care to prevent smudging or scratching.
   (a) True
   (b) False

6. Mounted radiographs should be viewed by holding the mount up to room light.
   (a) True
   (b) False
7. The mounted radiographs must be viewed in a systematic sequence to prevent errors in interpretation.
   (a) True
   (b) False
8. When new radiographs are exposed, the old ones are often removed from the mounts and discarded.
   (a) True
   (b) False
9. A desirable film mount should be:
   (a) Always made of cardboard.
   (b) Always made of plastic.
   (c) Translucent to allow light to reach the film.
   (d) Black to block out light transmission and prevent glare.
10. Who has the final responsibility to diagnose the radiograph?
    (a) The dental assistant
    (b) The dental technician
    (c) the dental hygienist
    (d) The dentist
11. List the step-by-step procedures for mounting a set of dental radiographs.
12. List the step-by-step procedures for viewing dental radiographs.

BIBLIOGRAPHY

Langland, O. E. & Langlais, R. P. *Principles of Dental Imaging*. Philadelphia: Williams & Wilkins, 1997.

White, S. C. & Pharoah, M. J. *Oral Radiology Principles and Interpretation*, 4th ed. St. Louis: Mosby, 2000.

PART V: Intraoral Techniques

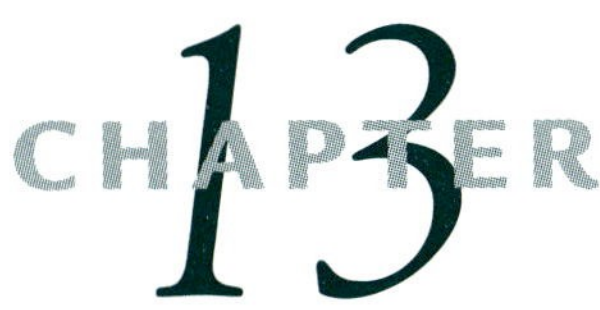

Intraoral Radiographic Procedures

OBJECTIVES

By the end of this chapter the student should be able to:

- Define the key words.
- Identify the three intraoral x-ray examinations.
- List the five rules for shadow casting.
- Discuss the principles of the paralleling technique.
- Discuss the principles of the bisecting technique.
- Compare the paralleling and bisecting techniques.
- Locate the points of entry on the face.
- Explain the proper patient seating position.
- Explain horizontal and vertical angulation.

KEY WORDS

Angulation
Bisecting technique
Bisector
Biteblock
Bitewing radiograph
Film holder
Horizontal angulation
Intraoral
Negative angulation
Occlusal radiograph
Paralleling technique
Penumbra
Periapical radiograph
Point of entry
Positive angulation
Vertical angulation
Zero angulation

Introduction

Intraoral radiography consists of methods of exposing dental x-ray films within the oral cavity. It includes:

- Positioning the patient in the chair.
- Selecting a film packet of suitable size.
- Determining how the film is to be positioned and held in place while the exposure is made.
- Aiming the position indicating device (PID).
- Setting the control devices correctly to make the exposure.

All these steps need careful planning. Techniques described in this chapter will help the dental radiographer make good radiographs.

The purpose of this chapter is to describe the fundamentals of shadow casting, and to explain the principles of the paralleling and bisecting technique.

Intraoral Procedures

The three common types of intraoral radiographic examinations each use a slightly different film and technique, and each has a different objective.

1. **Periapical examination.** The fundamental purpose of which is to show the apices of the teeth and the surrounding bone.
2. **Bitewing examination.** This shows the coronal portions of the teeth and the alveolar crests of bone of both the maxilla and mandible of a given area on one film.

3. **Occlusal examination.** Its purpose is to show the entire maxillary or mandibular arch, or a portion thereof, on a single film.

Techniques

There are two basic **techniques** employed in intraoral radiography, **bisecting** and **paralleling**. Either technique can be modified to meet special conditions and requirements. Each gives good results if one exercises care and remembers the fundamental principles of the technique. Paralleling is the technique of choice.

The first and earliest technique is called the **bisecting, bisecting-angle,** or the **short-cone technique.** The second and newer technique, now taught in all dental schools, is referred to as the **paralleling, right-angle, extension-cone,** or **long-cone technique.** To avoid confusion, these techniques are described as the **bisecting** and **paralleling** techniques in this text.

In 1904, Dr. W. A. Price suggested the basics of both the bisecting and paralleling methods. As others were working on the same problems and were unaware of Price's contributions, the credit for developing angulation techniques went to others.

The concept of the **bisecting technique** originated in 1907 through the application of a geometric principle known as the **rule of isometry.** This theorem states that "two triangles having equal angles and a common side are equal triangles" (see Figure 13–1). Because this theory was first suggested by A. Cieszynski, a Polish engineer, it became known as **Cieszynski's rule of isometry.**

The bisecting technique was the only method used for many years. However, since many radiographers experienced difficulties and obtained unsatisfactory results, the search for a less complicated technique that would produce better radiographs more consistently resulted in the development of the paralleling technique by Franklin McCormack in 1920.

Fundamentals of Shadow Casting

It is important to understand the **fundamentals of shadow casting** because they apply to creating a radiograph. Remember:

1. The radiograph is a film with a shadow image.
2. The source of the x-ray photons is the focal spot on the target of the x-ray tube.
3. The function of the film is to record the shadow image.

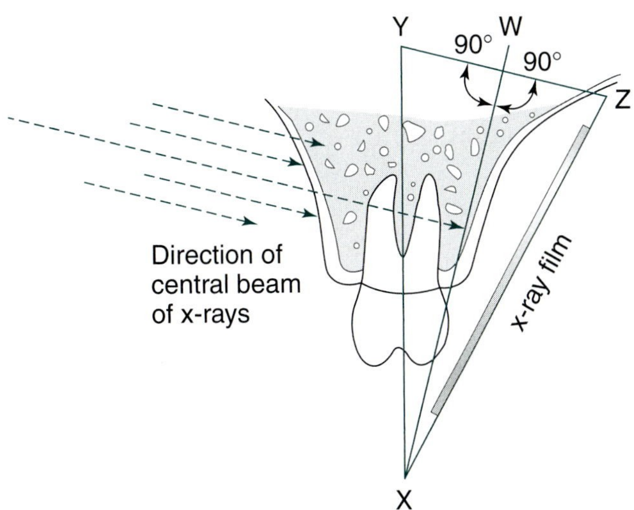

FIGURE 13–1. **Rule of isometry applied to the bisecting technique.** Line XY passes through the long axis of a maxillary first premolar while the film is positioned along line XZ. The central beam of radiation is directed perpendicularly through the apical area of the tooth toward the bisector XW. Because triangles WXY and WXZ are equal, the shadow image cast of the film will be approximately equal to the length of the film provided that the bisector line is correctly estimated. Most errors in foreshortening and elongation are traceable to incorrectly estimating the location of the bisector line.

When a hand is placed between a nearby light source such as an electric bulb and a flat object such as a tabletop, the shadow of the hand is seen on the tabletop. The same happens in dental radiography, where x-rays cast a shadow of the tooth on the film.

There are five basic rules for casting a shadow image (see Chapter 4).

1. Use the smallest possible source **(focal spot)** of radiation.
2. The **object** (tooth) should be as **far** as practical from the source.
3. The **object** (tooth) and the **recording plane** (film) should be as **close** to each other as possible.
4. The **object** (tooth) and the **recording plane** (film) should be **parallel** to each other.
5. The **radiation** (central ray) must **strike both the object** (tooth) and the **recording plane** (film) at right angles.

Neither of the intraoral techniques completely meets all five requirements for accurate shadow casting. In the **bisecting technique,** the object and film are not parallel to each other and the radiation does not strike the object and the film at right angles. In the **paralleling technique,** the distance between the object and the film is greater than ideal in most film placement areas.

Princlples of the Paralleling Technique

The basic principles of the **paralleling technique** are:

- The film is placed parallel to the long axes of the teeth being radiographed.
- The central ray is directed at right angles to both the teeth and film (see Figure 13–2).

Oral structures, particularly the curvature of the palate, make it difficult to place the film parallel to the long axes of the teeth. The paralleling technique achieves parallelism by placing the film away from the crowns of the teeth. To compensate for the **increased object-film distance,** the **target-film distance** is also **increased.** Normally, the target-film distance used in paralleling is 16 in. (41 cm). The accepted rule is that the target-film distance should be as long as is practical with the equipment used.

Paralleling is accomplished by using a **film holder.** Advanced and sophisticated film holders have made the paralleling technique easy. The newest film holders vary from simple disposable biteblocks that require no sterilization to complex devices that indicate the correct angle for directing the x-ray beam in relation to the teeth and film (see Figures 13–3, 13–4, and 13–5). Little trouble should arise in choosing a suitable holder to produce good results.

Advantages of the paralleling technique include:

- The image has only **minimal dimensional distortion** when compared with the bisecting technique.
- The paralleling technique is **simple** and **easy to learn.**
- It takes **less time** to direct the rays perpendicular to the tooth than at a hard-to-locate bisector.

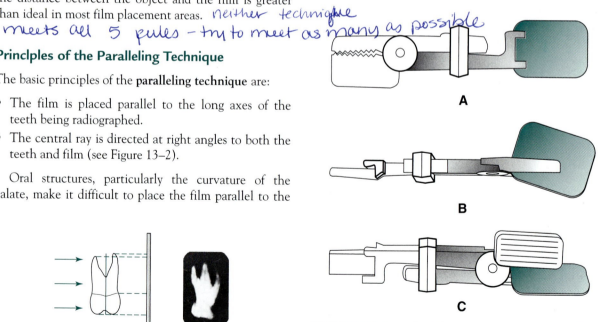

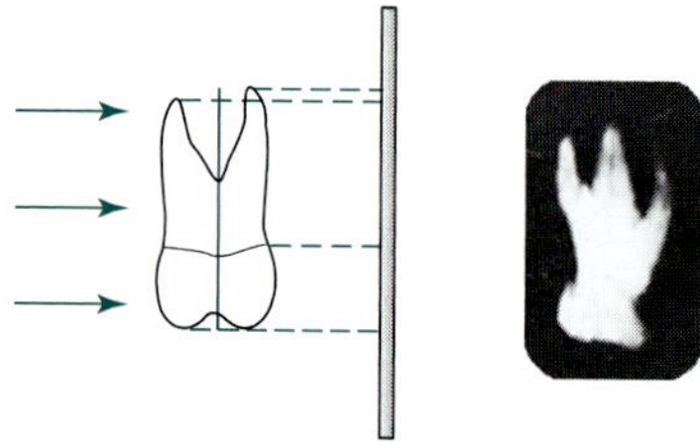

FIGURE 13–2. **Principle of the paralleling technique.** The x-ray beam is directed perpendicular to the recording plane of the film, which has been positioned parallel to the long axis of the tooth. (Courtesy of Dentsply/Rinn Corporation)

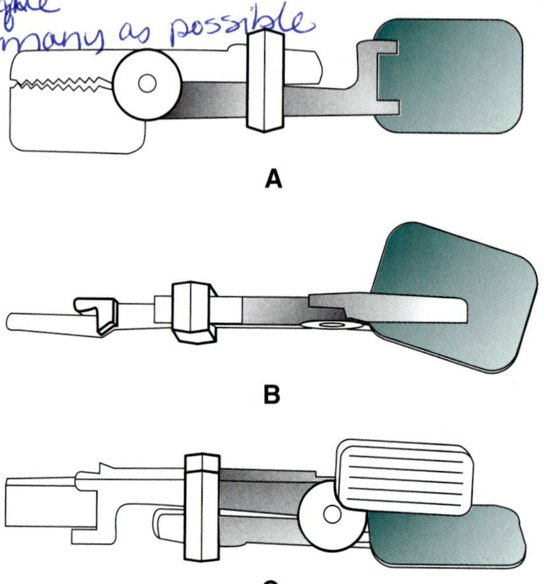

FIGURE 13–3. The **Rinn EEZEE-GRIP film holder.** This versatile film holder provides an excellent and simple method of standardizing the technique for intraoral radiography. The film is positioned to x-ray (**A**) the anterior areas, (**B**) the mandibular third molar area, and (**C**) the posterior areas. (Courtesy of Dentsply/Rinn Corporation)

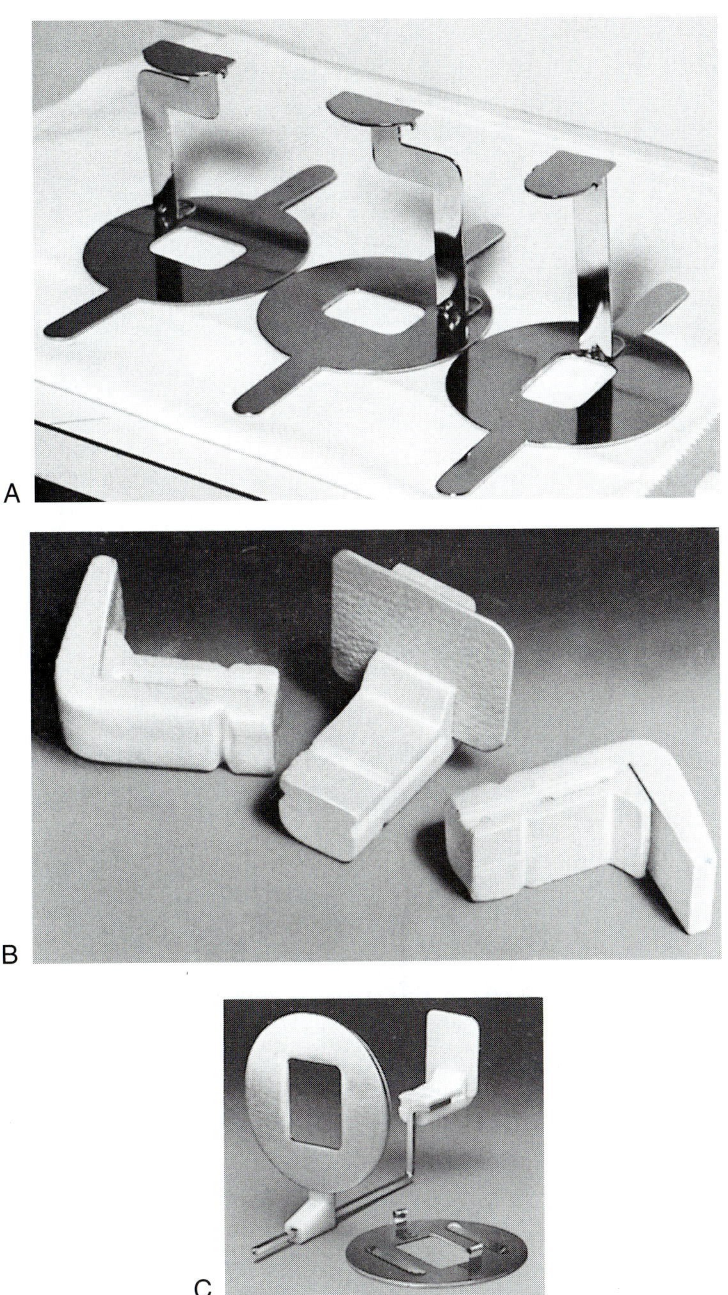

FIGURE 13–4. **Film Holders.** (**A**) Set of **"precision" instruments** featuring metal collimating shield that restricts the x-ray beam to the size of the opening, providing just enough radiation to expose the film properly (Courtesy of Isaac Masel company). (**B**) **Disposable XCP bite blocks.** (**C**) A **stainless-steel collimation device** that can be substituted for the plastic aiming device used in the BAI and XCP instruments. This reduces the amount of radiation the patient receives. (Courtesy of Dentsply/Rinn Corporation)

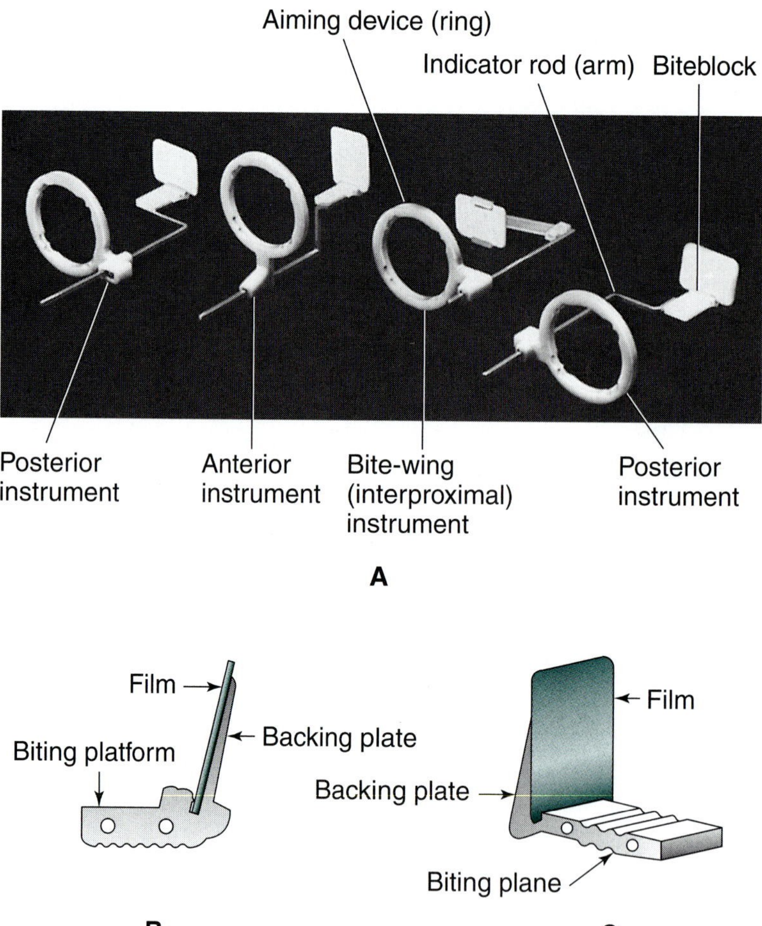

FIGURE 13–5. **Film Holders.** (**A**) **XCP (extension cone paralleling) instruments** for aligning and holding x-ray film packets. The instruments automatically indicate the correct horizontal and vertical angle. The complete kit includes one anterior instrument, right and left posterior instruments, and a bitewing instrument. The difference between the XCP and the BAI (bisecting angle) instruments is the periapical biteblocks. (**B**) **Anterior biteblock of BAI.** The raised platform on which the patient bites is close to the backing plate. The 105-degree angle of the backing plate keeps the film close to the lingual surface of the tooth. (**C**) **Anterior biteblock of XCP.** The biting plane is at a right angle (90 degrees) with the backing plate. The patient bites down far enough back on the biting plane to keep film and teeth parallel. (Courtesy of Dentsply/Rinn Corporation.)

Disadvantages of the paralleling technique include:

- **Difficulty in film placement.** Children and patients with small mouths and low palatal vaults may present some problems.
- **Patient discomfort** caused by the film holder impinging on oral tissues.

Principles of the Bisecting Technique

The **bisecting technique** is based on the geometric principle called the **rule of isometry.** The rule of isometry theorem states "that two triangles having two equal angles and a common side are equal triangles."

When the **bisecting principle** is applied to casting a shadow of a tooth on a film, the angle formed by the long axis of the tooth and the plane of the film must be bisected. The beam must be directed perpendicularly through the apex of the tooth toward the bisecting line (see Figure 13–1).

One must first imagine a line, called the **bisector,** and direct the radiation beam to it instead of to the long axis of the tooth or the film plane. This procedure is necessary because the irregularities of the oral tissues and the curvature of the palate seldom allow the film to lie parallel to the tooth.

Theoretically, two isometric triangles (triangles having equal measurements) are formed when the central ray is directed perpendicularly toward the bisector, and the film image that results should be the same size as the tooth. However, in practice this does not always happen. The image is usually satisfactory for diagnostic purposes, but some dimensional distortion is inherent in the bisecting technique.

An **advantage** of the bisecting technique is:

- It can be used when it is impossible to place the film parallel to the teeth. Examples are patients with small mouths, children, patients with low palatal vaults, and patients with cleft palate.

Disadvantages of the bisecting technique are:

- Operators have trouble **estimating the location of the bisector.** Thus, they may misdirect the central rays and cause the resulting image to be either elongated or foreshortened.
- The **degree of magnification** on the radiograph is **unequal** because all teeth and surrounding bone structures have depth besides length and width. For example, the buccal roots of a maxillary molar show more magnification than the lingual root, which is located closer to the film.
- **Dimensional distortion** occurs when the three-dimensional tooth and bone structures are projected on the two-dimensional recording plane of the film. This means that structures farther from the film appear more elongated than those closer to the film (see Figure 13–6).
- The **steeper vertical angle** of projection of the beam necessitated by directing the rays perpendicularly to the bisector instead of the tooth causes a **shadow of the zygomatic process of the maxilla** to be **superimposed over the molar roots** in the maxillary areas.

Comparing the Paralleling and Bisecting Techniques

The dental radiographer should **compare the paralleling and bisecting techniques** to fully understand them. Important differences include the **distances** used, the **angles** one selects, and the **film-holding** method (see Figure 13–7).

Distances

As we have seen, **target-film** and **object-film distances** differ in the two techniques.

Target-Film Distance

The shorter 8-in. (20.5-cm) target-film distance is generally, but not necessarily, used in the bisecting method. In the paralleling method, a longer target-film distance is preferred to compensate for the greater object-film distance. The use of a 16-in. (41-cm) target-film distance with the bisecting technique will improve the quality of the image. The 8-in. (20.5-cm) target-film distance is the minimum distance one should use with the paralleling technique.

Object-Film Distance

A shorter object-film distance is used in bisecting procedures, with the exception of the mandibular molar areas, where film placement is almost identical with both techniques. The film is placed as close to the teeth as possible thus forming an angle between the long axes of the teeth and film. In the paralleling technique the film must be placed farther from the teeth in order to get the film and teeth parallel.

Angle of Beam to Object and Film

Another difference is in the **angle at which the x-ray beam strikes the tooth** structures and the **film plane.** In the bisecting method, the central rays are aimed perpendicularly to the bisector and therefore do not strike either

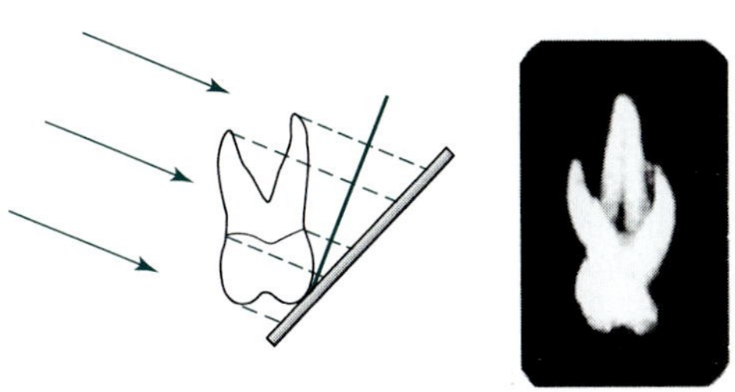

FIGURE 13-6. **Principle of the bisecting technique.** The x-ray beam is directed perpendicular to the imaginary line that bisects the angle formed by the recording plane of the dental x-ray film and the long axis of the tooth. (Courtesy of Dentsply/Rinn Corporation)

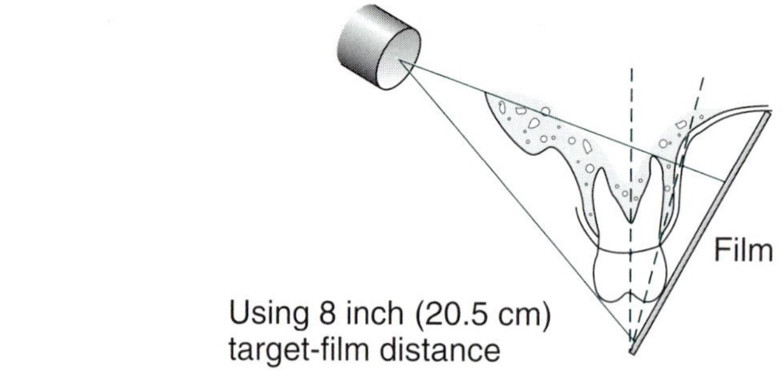

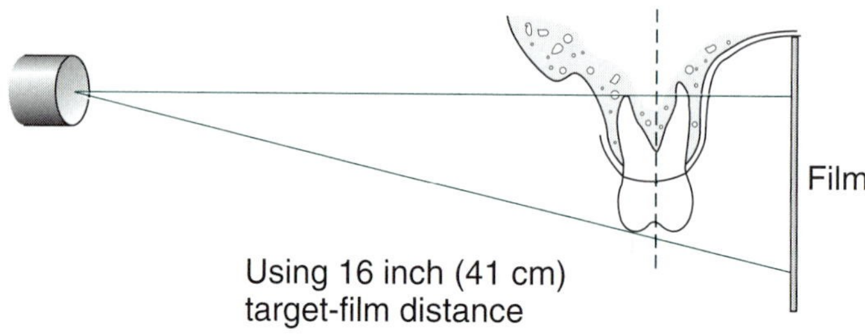

FIGURE 13-7. **Comparison of the bisecting and paralleling methods.** In the bisecting angle method, the film is positioned adjacent to the tooth, and the target-film distance is approximately 8 in. (20.5 cm). In the paralleling method, the film is positioned near the center of the oral cavity where it must be retained in a position parallel to the long axes of the teeth, and the target-film distance is approximately 16 in. (41 cm). (Courtesy of Dentsply/Rinn Corporation)

the tooth or the film at a right angle. In the paralleling method, they are directed at a right angle (perpendicularly) to both the long axes of the teeth and to the film plane. Thus, the bisecting method produces more dimensional distortion (see Figure 13–8).

Bisecting images are not **anatomically accurate** because dimensional distortion is inherent in the bisecting technique. The paralleling technique uses a parallel relationship between the film and the tooth structures for a more accurate image (see Figure 13–9).

Film-Holding Method

Film holders are used to hold the film in both the bisecting method and the paralleling method.

Unless special holders that indicate x-ray beam positions are used in the bisecting technique, patients are usually seated upright with their head straight. This position is necessary for consistent results in determining the best horizontal and vertical angulations of the x-ray beam. Head positions and angulations are described in the next section.

In the paralleling technique, the patient's head can be in any position, so the patient can easily be placed horizontally in a contour chair. The horizontal angulation is determined in the same manner in both techniques. The vertical angulation necessarily differs because the rays are directed at the bisector instead of at the long axes of the teeth.

Proficiency should be developed in both techniques. An operator using the paralleling technique may change to the bisecting method for one or two exposures during a full-mouth series because of anatomical limitations such as heavy muscle attachments or the shape of the palate. The paralleling technique is the preferred method.

Points of Entry

The **point of entry** is the spot on the surface of the face at which the central ray is directed (see Figure 13–10). Points of entry are most helpful when using the snap-a-ray or other such film holding devices. With most film-holding instruments, the aiming ring will determine the

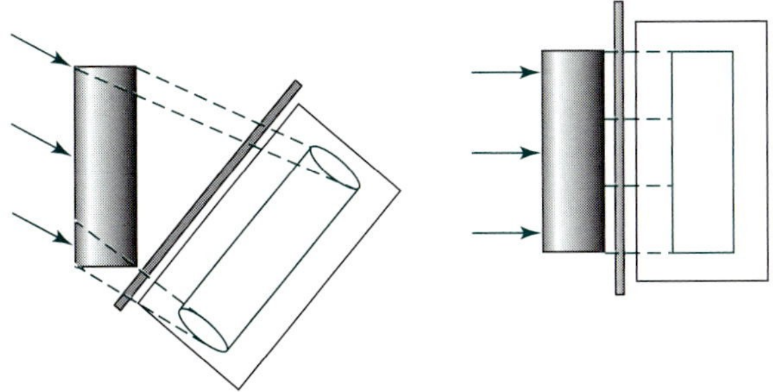

FIGURE 13–8. **Dimensional distortion.** The figure on the left shows dimensional distortion such as found in the bisecting technique. It occurs when a three-dimensional object is projected on a two-dimensional surface, creating an angular relationship between the object and the film. The part of the object farthest from the film is projected in an incorrect relationship to the parts closest to the film. Such distortion is eliminated in the paralleling technique, shown in the figure on the right. The film is positioned parallel to the object, so that all parts of the object are in their true relationship to one another. (Courtesy of Dentsply/Rinn Corporation)

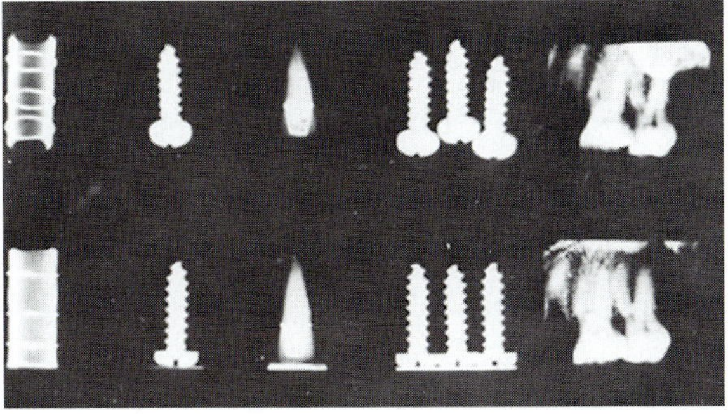

FIGURE 13–9. **Paralleling technique.** The superior radiographic quality of the paralleling technique is readily demonstrated when results are compared. Radiographs produced by the **bisecting technique (top)** are not anatomically accurate in most instances, since obvious dimensional distortion is inherent in this technique. This kind of distortion does not occur with the **paralleling technique (bottom)** in which objects are reproduced in their normal size and relationship. (Courtesy of Dentsply/Rinn Corporation)

point of entry by its predetermined relationship to the film packet.

Points of entry are located at the level of the apices of the teeth. Chapter 11 referred to anatomical landmarks that can be used to determine the location of the apices of the teeth. When the patient is seated in the conventional position, the apices of the maxillary teeth are located along an imaginary line drawn from the ala of the nose to the tragus of the ear.

The following **landmarks** are helpful in **determining** the **point of entry.** For **maxillary** teeth these are located along an extension of the ala-tragus line as follows:

1. The tip of the nose for the incisors.
2. The depression formed by the ala of the nose for the canines.
3. A point below the pupil of the eye for the premolars.
4. A point below the outer canthus of the eye for the molars.

A point directly below the same landmarks and approximately 1/2 inch (13 cm) above an imaginary line parallel to the lower border of the **mandible** is used to locate the point of entry for the corresponding mandibular teeth. These points of entry are only approximations. With a little practice, the point of entry for each maxillary and mandibular tooth position can be determined at a glance.

The truest image is produced when the central rays are directed through the point of entry toward the apices of the roots. However, the increased use of smaller beam diameters and film holders with collimating devices that limit the size of the beam makes it preferable to direct the central rays through the middle of the teeth instead of through the apices. The end of the PID should almost touch the face with its midpoint centered over the point of entry. Failure to project the central ray through this point and toward the middle of the film packet results in cone cutting.

Patient Seating Position

The **conventional position** is to **seat the patient upright** and adjust the headrest so that the plane of occlusion for the jaw being examined is parallel to the floor. The midsagittal plane that divides the patient's head into a right and left side is perpendicular to the floor (see Figure 13–11). Although an experienced radiographer can expose radiographs with the patient either upright or supine, the use of predetermined head positions is recom-

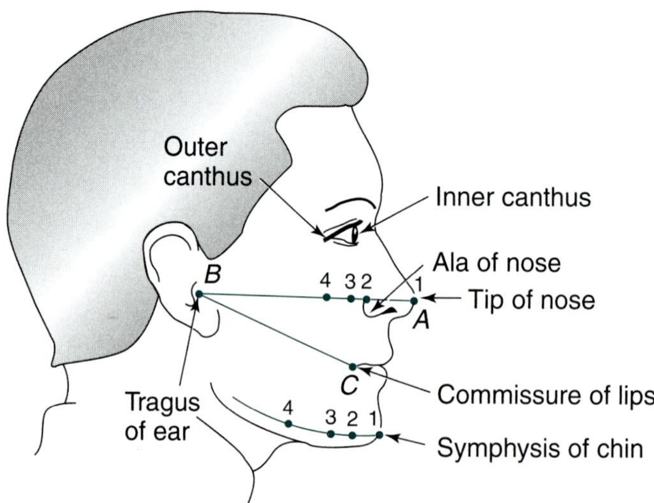

FIGURE 13–10. **Points of entry.** The facial landmarks that provide the radiographer with a quick reference for the positioning of the PID and the directing of the central beam of radiation. Unless special film holders are used that eliminate the need for positioning, the patient is seated upright with the midsagittal plane perpendicular to the floor.

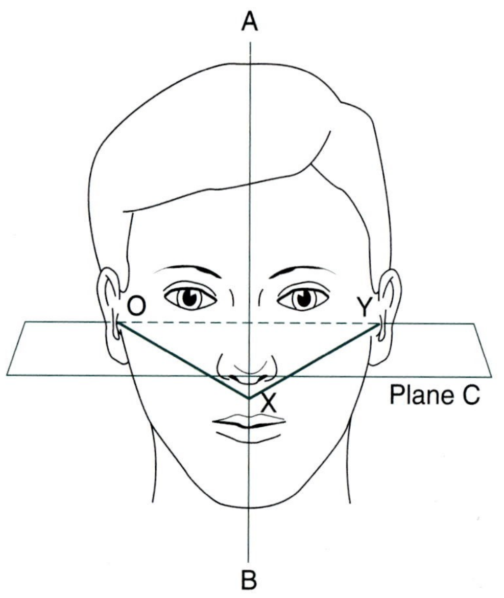

FIGURE 13–11. **Head divided by midsagittal plane and occlusal plane.** The midsagittal plane (**A-B**) must always be perpendicular to the floor, and the occlusal plane (**C**) must be parallel with the floor unless special film-holding devices are used. The O-X is the line of orientation for the maxillary teeth. It is also known as the **ala-tragus** line. The apices of the roots of the maxillary teeth are located close to this line.

mended for the beginner. This makes it possible to standardize the procedure.

Horizontal and Vertical Angulation Procedures

Angulation is defined as the procedure by which the tube head and PID are aligned to obtain the optimum angle at which the radiation is to be directed toward the film. Angulation is changed by rotating the tube head horizontally and vertically. The x-ray machine is constructed with three swivel joints to support the yoke and tube head. One of these, located at the top and center of the yoke where it attaches to the extension arm, permits horizontal movement of the tube head to control the antero-posterior dimensions. The other two swivel joints are located at either side of the yoke. These permit the tube head to be rotated up or down in a vertical direction to control the longitudinal dimensions of the resulting image. One of the most difficult procedures for the beginner to learn is how to determine the correct direction of the central beam in the **horizontal** and **vertical** planes.

Horizontal Angulation

Horizontal angulation may be explained as a procedure used to direct the central rays perpendicularly (at a right

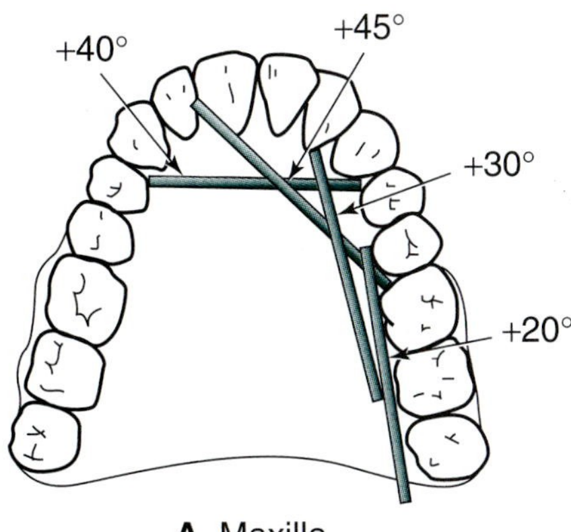

A Maxilla

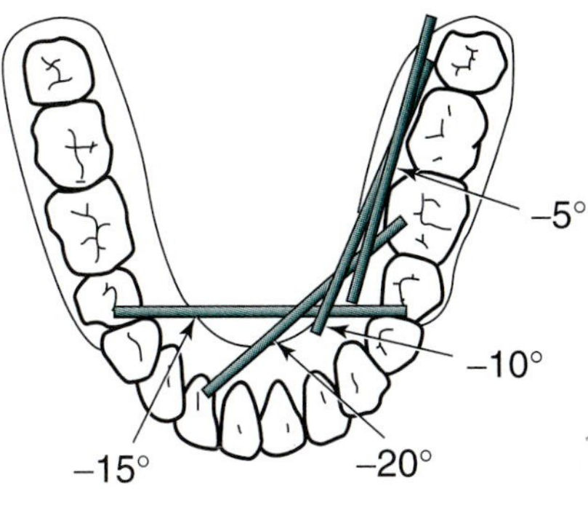

B Mandible

FIGURE 13–12. **Horizontal angulation.** Horizontal angulation is determined by directing the x-ray beam perpendicularly to the mean tangent of the teeth being radiographed, which is also the corresponding position of the film. The beam passes directly through the interproximal spaces. Standard #2 film is shown; however, the narrow #1 film is recommended for the incisor and canine region. The average vertical angulation is also shown on (**A**) the **maxilla,** in positive (+) degrees and (**B**) the **mandible,** in negative (−) degrees.

angle) toward the film surface in a horizontal plane (see Figure 13–12). Identical steps are followed in the bisecting and paralleling methods. To change direction, swivel the tube head from side-to-side. The objective is to permit the central rays to pass directly through the interproximal spaces. Incorrect alignment in the horizontal plane through deviation of the angulation toward the mesial or the distal results in an overlapping of the tooth structures shown on the radiograph.

Vertical Angulation

Vertical angulation may be described as a procedure used to direct the central rays perpendicularly toward the film surface in a vertical plane. Because the film position, with the exception of the mandibular molar area, is not the same in bisecting and paralleling the technique procedures differ. The direction of the central ray is changed by swiveling the tube head vertically so that the tip of the PID is raised or lowered (see Figure 13–13).

Vertical angulation is customarily described in degrees. On most x-ray machines the vertical angles are scaled in intervals of 5 degrees on both sides of the yoke where the tube head is connected. The vertical angulation of the tube head and the PID begins at zero. In that position the PID is parallel to the plane of the floor. All deviations from zero in which the tip of the PID is tilted toward the floor are called **positive** (plus) **angulations.** Those in which the PID is tipped upward toward the ceiling are called **negative** (minus) **angulations.**

Average Vertical Angles for the Bisecting Technique

When the **bisecting technique** is used, the central ray—in the vertical plane—must be directed through the roots of the teeth perpendicularly toward the bisector (see Figure 13–1). When the patient's head is in the conventional position, predetermined vertical angulations can often be used. Obviously, such angulations will vary from patient to patient. The **average vertical angulations** listed in Table 13–1 are intended only as a guide and should not replace good judgment. Many prefer to mini-

TABLE 13–1. Average Vertical Angulations

Maxillary incisors	+ 40 degrees
Maxillary canines	+ 45 degrees
Maxillary premolars	+ 30 degrees
Maxillary molars	+ 20 degrees
Mandibular incisors	− 15 degrees
Mandibular canines	− 20 degrees
Mandibular premolars	− 10 degrees
Mandibular molars	− 5 degrees

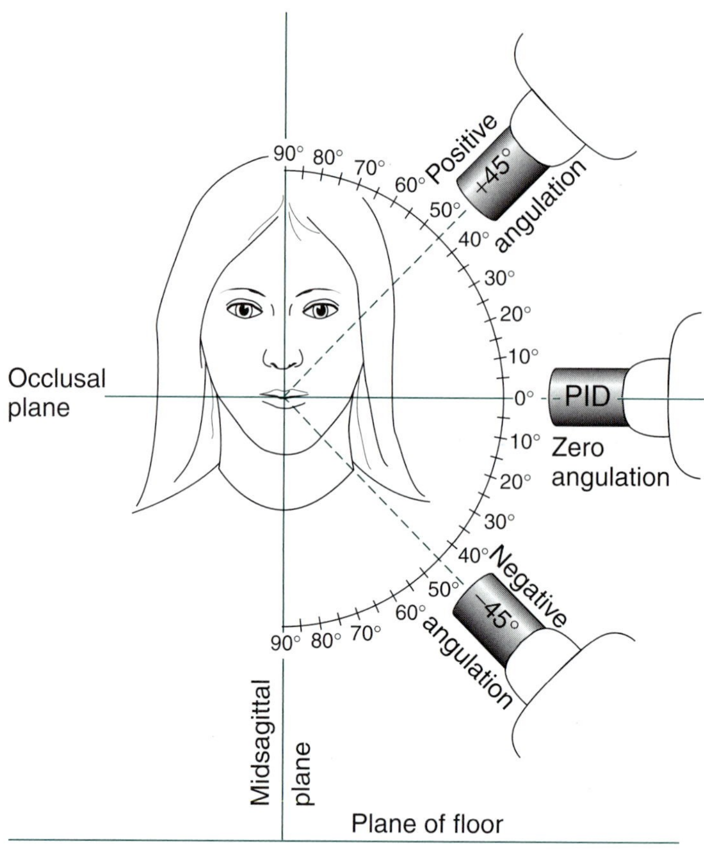

FIGURE 13–13. **Vertical angulation.** Diagram showing patient sitting in the preferred position upright in dental chair with midsagittal line perpendicular and occlusal plane parallel with the floor. Zero angulation is achieved when the long axis of the PID is directed parallel to the floor. All vertical angulations above the occlusal plane are called positive or plus (+) angulations. These are used for all maxillary and bitewing exposures. Vertical angulations below the occlusal plane are negative or minus (−) angulations. These are used for all mandibular exposures. Average vertical angulations are used when the film is held by the patient, as in the bisecting technique. Film holders can be used that automatically indicate the correct horizontal and vertical angulations, eliminating the necessity for numerically setting the angulations and for placing the patient's head in a predetermined position.

mize guesswork by using some form of film holder, as shown in Figure 13–5.

Sometimes it may be necessary to **increase** or to **decrease** the vertical angulation. For example, a change from +40 to +50 degrees or from −10 to −20 degrees is called an increase in vertical angulation; the reverse, a change from +50 to +40 degrees or from −20 to −10 degrees is called a decrease in vertical angulation.

The operator should be alert to observe anatomical variations and to understand what change in angulation is required in each instance. For example, the table of average angulations (see Table 13–1) suggests that the average vertical angulation for the maxillary molars is about +20 degrees. Changes are indicated when the patient's vault (palate) is high or low; depending on the degree of the deviation from normal, a change of at least 5 degrees is called for. Therefore when the vault is high, the angulation is decreased to +15 degrees or less because the film packet now lies in a more vertical plane in the mouth. Conversely, when the vault is low, an increase to

+25 degrees or more should be made, since the film packet now assumes a more horizontal position. In the mandibular region, if the floor of the mouth is shallow or the teeth are facially inclined, the vertical angulation should be increased by 5 to 10 degrees. It should be decreased by 5 to 10 degrees when the floor of the mouth is very deep or the teeth incline lingually.

When the vertical angle is correctly estimated and the rays are directed perpendicularly to the bisector, no appreciable distortion results. **Excessive vertical angulation** foreshortens the image. **Insufficient vertical angulation** elongates the image.

When the **paralleling technique** is employed, the central ray in the vertical plane must be directed perpendicularly (at right angle) through the roots of the teeth toward the film packet (see Figure 13–2). **Excessive vertical angulation** may result in the loss of the crown and **insufficient vertical angulation** may result in the loss of the apex.

CHAPTER SUMMARY

The three common types of intraoral radiographic procedures are the periapical, bitewing, and occlusal surveys. Each of these examinations differs in purpose, and a variety of film sizes may be used to achieve the desired result.

Both the paralleling and bisecting techniques are used to produce a shadow image of the tooth on the exposed radiograph. The paralleling technique produces superior results. Neither of these completely satisfies all the requirements for accurate, shadow casting. Each technique has its advantages and disadvantages. The skilled operator, within the limits of the equipment available, must select the technique that fits the occasion. All schools are now teaching the paralleling method.

Horizontal angulation is achieved in the same manner in both techniques. The central ray is directed perpendicularly to the film in the horizontal plane.

The technique for vertical angulation differs in that, in bisecting, the central ray is aimed perpendicularly in the vertical plane at the bisector rather than at the film. The method of positioning and holding the film also differs. In bisecting, the film is positioned closer to the teeth and is sometimes held by digital pressure; in paralleling, the film is farther from the teeth, and the use of a film holder is mandatory.

Unless special film-holding devices that indicate the correct angulation are used, care must be taken to seat the patient so that the occlusal plane is parallel with the floor and the median line perpendicular to it.

REVIEW QUESTIONS

1. Which of these is not an intraoral survey?
   (a) Bitewing
   (b) Occlusal
   (c) Panoramic
   (d) Periapical
2. Who first described the rules of the bisecting technique?
   (a) Roentgen
   (b) Coolidge
   (c) Updegrave
   (d) Cieszynski

3. What term describes the imaginary line between the long axis of the tooth and the film plane?
   (a) Tangent
   (b) Median
   (c) Bisector
   (d) Midsagittal

4. Which of these target-film distances is generally used in the paralleling technique?
   (a) 7 in. (18 cm)
   (b) 8 in. (20.5 cm)
   (c) 12 in. (30 cm)
   (d) 16 in. (41 cm)

5. Which term describes the formation of a fuzzy shadow around the outline of the image on the radiograph?
   (a) Penumbra
   (b) Delineation
   (c) Definition
   (d) Reticulation

6. With the bisecting technique, what is the effect on the radiographic image if the vertical angulation is 15 degrees greater than necessary?
   (a) Overlapping
   (b) Cone cutting
   (c) Elongation
   (d) Foreshortening

7. In the bisecting technique, the film is placed:
   (a) Parallel to the tooth.
   (b) As close as possible to the tooth.
   (c) Parallel to the bisector.
   (d) Perpendicular to the bisector.

8. In the paralleling technique, a long target-film distance is required to:
   (a) Compensate for the greater object-film distance.
   (b) Avoid image magnification.
   (c) Both a and b.
   (d) None of the above.

9. What is the result of incorrect horizontal angulation?
   (a) Adumbration
   (b) Cone cutting
   (c) Reticulation
   (d) Overlapping

10. What change in angulation should be made when a patient has an unusually low vault?
    (a) Horizontal angulation is shifted mesially
    (b) Horizontal angulation is shifted distally
    (c) Vertical angulation is increased
    (d) Vertical angulation is decreased

11. **In the paralleling technique, the tooth and the** film **must be parallel to each other.**
12. **The** paralleling **technique produces superior radiographs.**

BIBLIOGRAPHY

Eastman Kodak. *Successful Intraoral Radiography*. Rochester, NY: Eastman Kodak, 1998.

Rinn Corporation. *Intraoral Radiography with Rinn XCP/BAI Instruments*. Elgin, IL: Dentsply/Rinn Corporation, 1983.

White, S. C. & Pharoah, M. J. *Oral Radiology Principles and Interpretation*, 4th ed. St. Louis: Mosby, 2000.

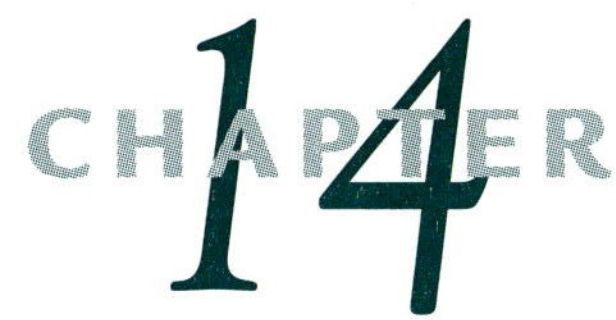

The Periapical Examination

OBJECTIVES

By the end of this chapter the student should be able to:

- Define the key words.
- Select the type and number of films required to make a complete periapical survey.
- Identify and be able to assemble and position film holders for the paralleling and bisecting techniques.
- Discuss film retention for paralleling procedures.
- State the four rules for using the XCP instruments.
- Describe patient preparation for the paralleling technique.
- State the method of positioning the film packet for maxillary and mandibular periapical exposures when using the paralleling technique.
- Discuss film retention for bisecting procedures.
- State the method of positioning the film packet for maxillary and mandibular periapical exposures when using the bisecting technique.
- Differentiate between conventional periapical film placement and endodontic film placement techniques.

KEY WORDS

Aiming ring
Bisector
Biteblocks
Endodontia
Film holder
Full-mouth survey
Horizontal placement
Mean tangent
Periapical radiograph
Vertical placement

Introduction

The purpose of the **periapical examination** is to view the entire tooth and surrounding bone. The word **periapical** is derived from the Greek word ***peri*** (means around) and the Latin word ***apex*** (means highest point). Therefore, as the word suggests, the **periapical radiograph** shows the entire tooth including the root end and surrounding bone.

The purpose of this chapter is to present the step-by-step procedures for exposing a full-mouth series of periapical radiographs using both the paralleling and bisecting techniques and to describe endodontic radiographic techniques.

Film Requirements

The **periapical examination,** frequently called the **full-mouth survey** (see Figure 14–1), can be made with any of the three periapical film sizes (#0, #1, #2) or any combination of these films. **Film size** depends on:

- The age of the patient
- The size of the mouth opening
- The shape of the dental arches
- The presence or absence of unusual conditions or anatomical limitations
- The film holder and technique used
- The patient's ability to tolerate the film.

Normally, a minimum of 14 films (see Figure 14–2) is used to cover the following tooth areas:

- One film each for the maxillary and mandibular incisor area
- One film in each of the four canine (cuspid) areas (two in the maxillary and two in the mandibular arches)
- One film in each of the four premolar (bicuspid) areas (two in the maxillary and two in the mandibular arches)

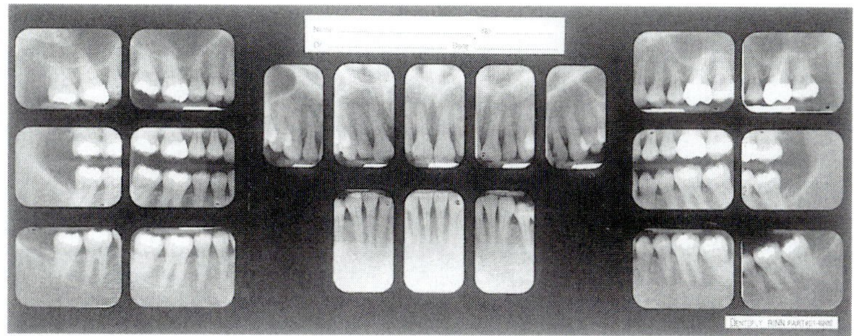

FIGURE 14–1. **Full-mouth radiographic survey.** The 20-film radiographic series shown includes 4 bitewing films in addition to the 8 anterior and 8 posterior periapical films.

- One film in each of the molar areas (two in the maxillary and two in the mandibular arches)

More films may be required for unusual conditions or for narrow arches requiring small films. The general rule is to use the largest film that can readily be positioned. Doing so minimizes the number of exposures.

Some dentists choose to use the narrow #1 film instead of the #2 film for exposures of the anterior teeth. Three film combinations are often used when the narrow #1 film is employed.

The **first method** uses five films for the maxillary anterior teeth (see Figure 14–3A). One film centered at the midline over the central incisors, one each for the later-

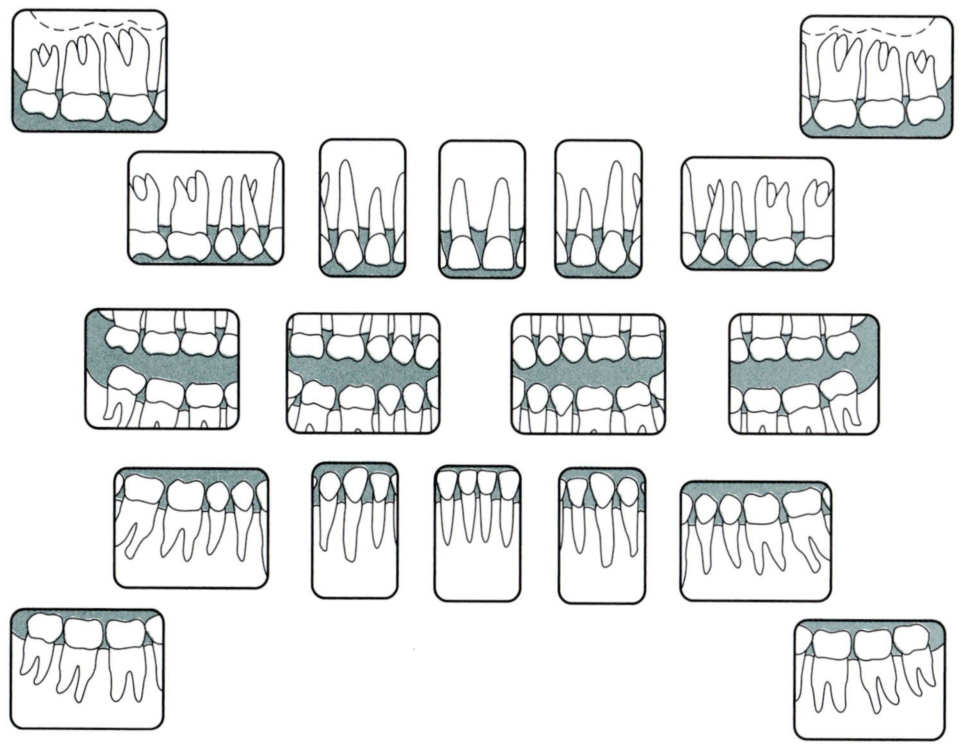

FIGURE 14–2. **Full-mouth survey.** Drawing of 18-film **full-mouth survey** using 14 periapical and 4 bitewing films.

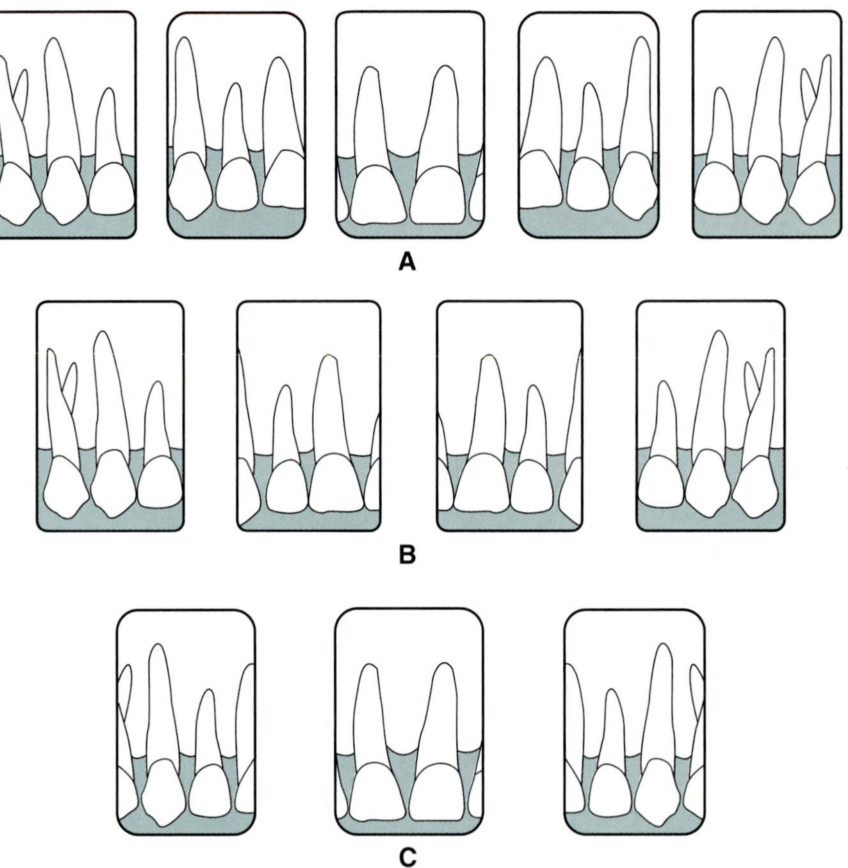

FIGURE 14–3. **Maxillary anterior film placement.** (**A**) Five film survey. (**B**) Four film survey. (**C**) Three film survey.

als, and one each for the canines (cuspids). Three films are used for the mandibular arch where the teeth are smaller. One film centered over the incisors and one film centered on each of the canines.

The **second method** uses four films for the maxillary anterior teeth (see Figure 14–3B) and four for the mandibular anterior teeth. The films centered over each of the central-lateral incisor regions and each of the canines (cuspids).

The **third method** uses three films for the maxillary anterior teeth (see Figure 14–3C). One film centered at the midline over the central incisors and one film centered over each of the lateral-canines. Three films are used for the mandibular arch. One film centered over the incisors and one film centered on each of the canines.

Usually the standard #2 film is used to make the posterior periapical exposures.

Placement of the Film Packet

Regardless of which technique is used or how the film is held in place, correct **placement of the film packet** is important to prevent the film from bending or moving during exposure, thus causing distortion.

With few exceptions, all films for the anterior areas are placed with the longest dimension of the film vertically (described as **vertical placement**). Films for the posterior areas are placed with the widest dimension horizontally (described as **horizontal placement**).

Regardless of which technique is used, the edge of the film packet is placed in a parallel relationship with the incisal/occlusal line of the teeth. Place films gently to prevent tissue irritation or gagging. Slight rolling of the film corners toward the lingual makes it easier to place the film and increases the patient's comfort. However, excessive bending of the film results in creases, streaks, and distortion.

The **identification dot** is always positioned toward the occlusal or incisal edges where it is least likely to interfere with diagnostic information.

It is always best to keep the film surface as flat as possible. A film holder with a backing plate on the biteblock makes this almost automatic.

Sequence of Film Positioning

A definite **sequence of film positioning** should be followed to prevent omitting an area or exposing an area twice. Develop a set **routine** to prevent errors and save time.

Opinions differ as to which region should be exposed first in making a full-mouth survey. Some operators prefer to make the first exposure in the right maxillary molar region and continue in sequence to the left maxillary molar region, then drop down to the left mandibular molar region, finishing in the right mandibular molar region.

Others begin with the anterior exposures, on the theory that the patient is less liable to gag when a film is placed in this region than when it is placed in the upper-molar region where the tissues are more sensitive. Gagging is frequently psychological (see Chapter 24). If the first few films produce no discomfort, the patient will become used to the feel of the film and will accept it.

With an experienced operator who can place the film skillfully and rapidly, it probably makes little difference which area is exposed first. But the same order of film placement should always be followed to make sure that all regions are exposed. The following sequence of film positioning is recommended for the beginning student.

- Maxillary anterior
- Mandibular anterior
- Maxillary posteriors
- Mandibular posteriors
- Bitewings

Anterior film placements are more comfortable and allow the patient to be accustomed to the procedure. Also the patient is less likely to gag on anterior film placements. The bitewing examination (see Chapter 15) is suggested to be last because the patient tolerates them well and the radiographic procedure ends pleasantly.

Because the paralleling technique produces superior radiographs, schools now begin by teaching the paralleling methods first and devote minimal time to bisecting procedures. Because of this trend, the paralleling technique is described first. Also, this text will describe the five maxillary anterior film positions.

Paralleling Technique

As described in Chapter 13, the basic principles of the **paralleling technique** are:

- The **film** is placed **parallel** to the **long axes of the teeth** being radiographed.
- The **central ray** is directed **at right angles** to both the **teeth and film** (see Figure 13–2).

Oral structures, particularly the curvature of the palate, make it difficult to place the film parallel to the long axes of the teeth. The paralleling technique achieves parallelism by placing the film away from the crowns of the teeth. Paralleling is accomplished by using a **film holder.** To compensate for the increased **object-film distance,** the **target-film distance** is also increased.

Film Retention for Paralleling Procedures

Film holders are required with the paralleling technique to make sure the film is parallel to the teeth. The simplest holders are wood, plastic, or styrofoam **biteblocks** with a backing plate and slot for film retention. The film can be inserted either vertically for the anteriors or horizontally for the posteriors.

Slightly more complex is the **EEZEE-GRIP** (formerly the Snap-A-Ray) holder shown in Figure 13–3, a double-ended instrument that holds the film between two plastic jaws that are locked in place. The plastic jaw serves as a bite plane in the posterior areas. The other end of the instrument is a backing plate with a slot that holds the film during anterior exposures.

The metal **precision** film holders (see Figure 14–4) have a metal facial shield attached to an arm on which the patient bites. At the end of the arm a backing plate supports the film and holds it parallel to the shield.

The **XCP instruments** (see Figure 14–5) and the rectangular collimated instruments (see Figure 14–6) function in a similar manner. These instruments must be assembled prior to use and have separate components for anterior and posterior positioning. The XCP instruments were developed in an attempt to simplify paralleling procedures and minimize dimensional distortion. These instruments are simple to position, and highly adaptable in that the patient may be in any position.

Because it is not practical to describe the technique for the use of each of the many available film holders, the

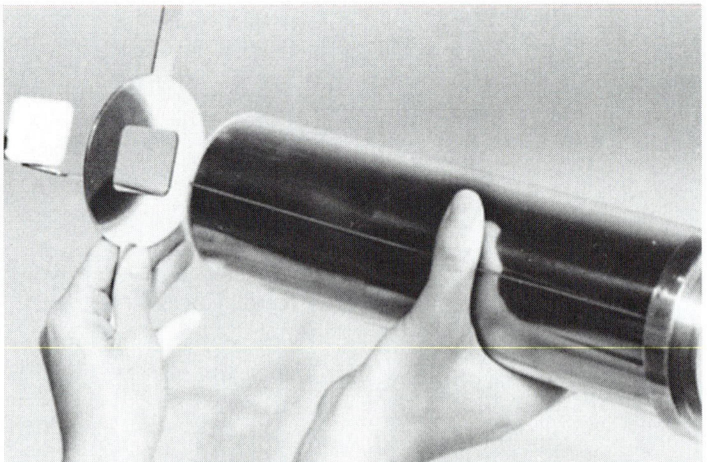

FIGURE 14–4. **Metal "precision" posterior x-ray film holder for use with long, round, metal-type PID.** The metal collimating shield, combined with the lead-lined cone, restricts the size of the x-ray beam and reduces tissue radiation. Precision instruments are available for anterior, posterior, and bitewing radiography in adult and child sizes. (Courtesy of Isaac Masel Company)

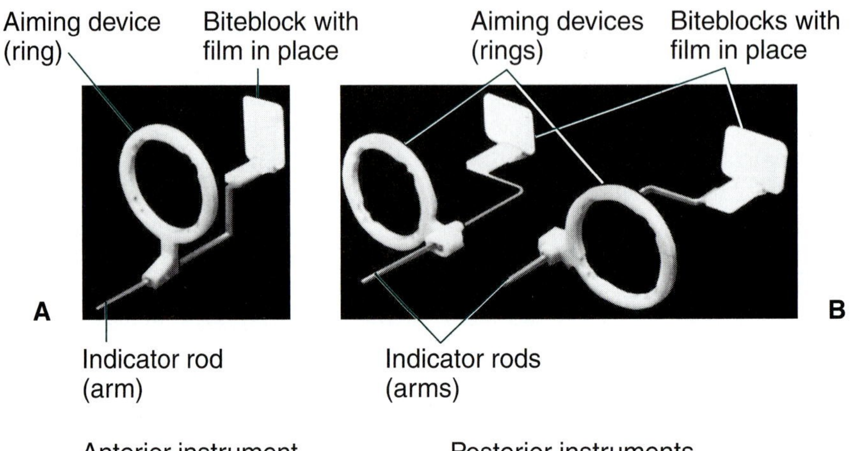

FIGURE 14–5. **XCP instruments.** The assembled Rinn XCP instruments are intended for use with the paralleling technique using the 16-in. (41-cm) target-film distance. Each instrument consists of an indicator rod (arm), and aiming device (ring), and a biteblock. By substituting a 105-degree biteblock for the 90-degree biteblock shown here, these instruments become the BAI instruments suitable for use with the bisecting technique. (**A**) The assembled anterior XCP instrument with film positioned vertically in the biteblock. (**B**) The posterior instruments with the films positioned horizontally in the biteblocks. One instrument is used for exposure on the maxillary right and the mandibular left, while the other is used for exposure on the maxillary left and on the mandibular right. (Courtesy of Dentsply/Rinn Corporation)

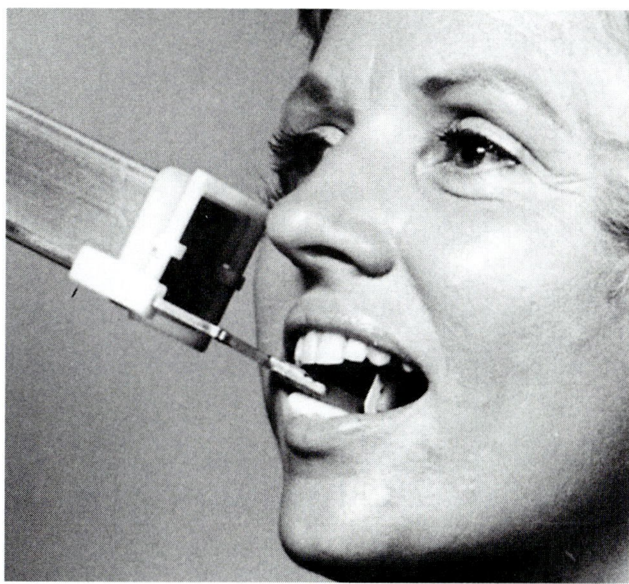

FIGURE 14–6. **Rectangular instrumentation for reduced tissue exposure.** Lead-lined rectangular PID limits the size of x-ray beam. Slots on the PID align with studs on the placement holder. Both the XCP and the BAI instruments can be modified by substituting the rectangular aiming device for the circular one. The use of a lead-lined collimating device makes possible reductions of 50 percent or more in tissue exposure area. (Courtesy of Dentsply/Rinn Corporation)

descriptions and illustrations for the following sequence of tooth regions are based on the use of the XCP instruments. Other instruments require slight changes in technique.

Rules for XCP Instuments

There are **four basic rules** for using the Rinn XCP instrument.

1. **Film placement.** Place the film to cover the area of the teeth to be examined. This insures the proper teeth are seen in the radiograph.
2. **Bite on end of biteblock.** Position the film as far away from the teeth as possible by using the entire horizontal length of the biteblock (except in the mandibular premolar and molar regions where the film can be close to the teeth and be parallel). This ensures the film is parallel to the long axis of the tooth.
3. **Bite firmly on biteblock.** Have the patient bite firm (not hard) on the biteblock. This assures the biteblock is flat against the teeth and not rotated. Use of sterilized cotton rolls placed on the biteblock opposite side of film provides stablization and comfort to the patient. Then the patient doesn't have to bite as tight or firm.
4. **Align the PID to the aiming ring.** The PID should be parallel to the indicator rod and the end of the PID should be parallel to the aiming ring. This assures correct vertical and horizontal angulation.

Patient Preparation for Paralleling Technique

After completing the infection control procedures described in Chapter 22, proceed by:

1. Seating the patient.
2. Explaining the radiographic procedures to the patient.
3. Adjusting chair to comfortable working level.
4. Adjusting headrest to position patient's head so that the occlusal plane is parallel to the floor and the midsagittal plane (midline) is perpendicular to the floor.
5. Placing lead apron and thyroid collar on the patient.

6. Removing eyeglasses and objects from the mouth that may interfere with the procedure.

Maxillary Periapical Exposures

Maxillary Central Incisor Exposure

To make the **maxillary central incisor exposure** (see Figure 14–7), use the following steps.

1. Insert the film vertically into the film holder with the identification dot into the slot.
2. Center the film holder and film packet at the midline on the contact of the central incisors.
3. Position the film as far away from the teeth as possible by using the entire horizontal length of the biteblock.
4. Rest the biteblock on the incisal edges of the teeth to be radiographed and ask the patient to slowly close firmly on the biteblock. A cotton roll may be inserted between the mandibular teeth and the biteblock for stability and comfort.

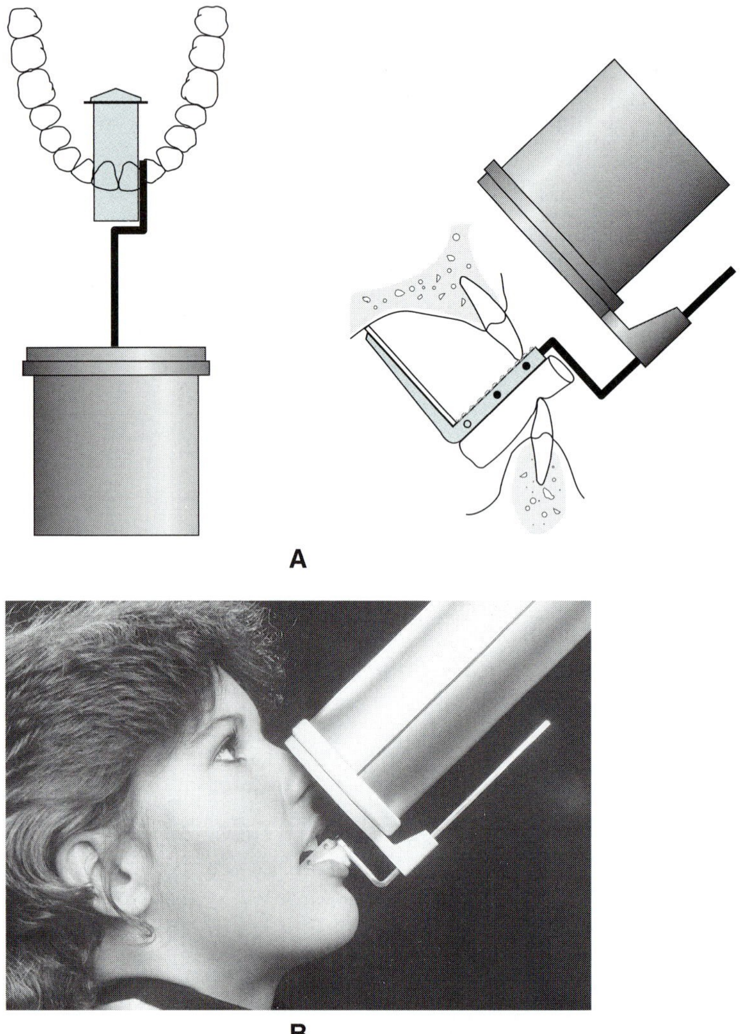

FIGURE 14–7. **Maxillary central incisor exposure.** (**A**) Diagram shows relationship of film, teeth, XCP instrument, and PID. As in all anterior areas, film is positioned with longest dimension vertically. Film is parallel to teeth with the block inserted to its full length to position the film back toward the region of the first molars. (**B**) Photograph of patient showing position of XCP instrument and long circular PID. (Courtesy of Dentsply/Rinn Corporation.)

5. Slide the aiming ring down the indicator rod to close approximation to the skin surface.
6. Align the PID parallel to the indicator rod and the end of the PID parallel to the aiming ring.
7. Make the exposure.

Maxillary Lateral Incisor Exposure

To make the **maxillary lateral incisor exposure** (see Figure 14–8), use the following steps.

1. Insert the film vertically into the film holder with the identification dot into the slot.
2. Center the film holder and film packet on the lateral incisor.
3. Position the film as far away from the teeth as possible by using the entire horizontal length of the biteblock.
4. Rest the biteblock on the incisal edges of the teeth to be radiographed and ask the patient to slowly close firmly on the biteblock. A cotton roll may be in-

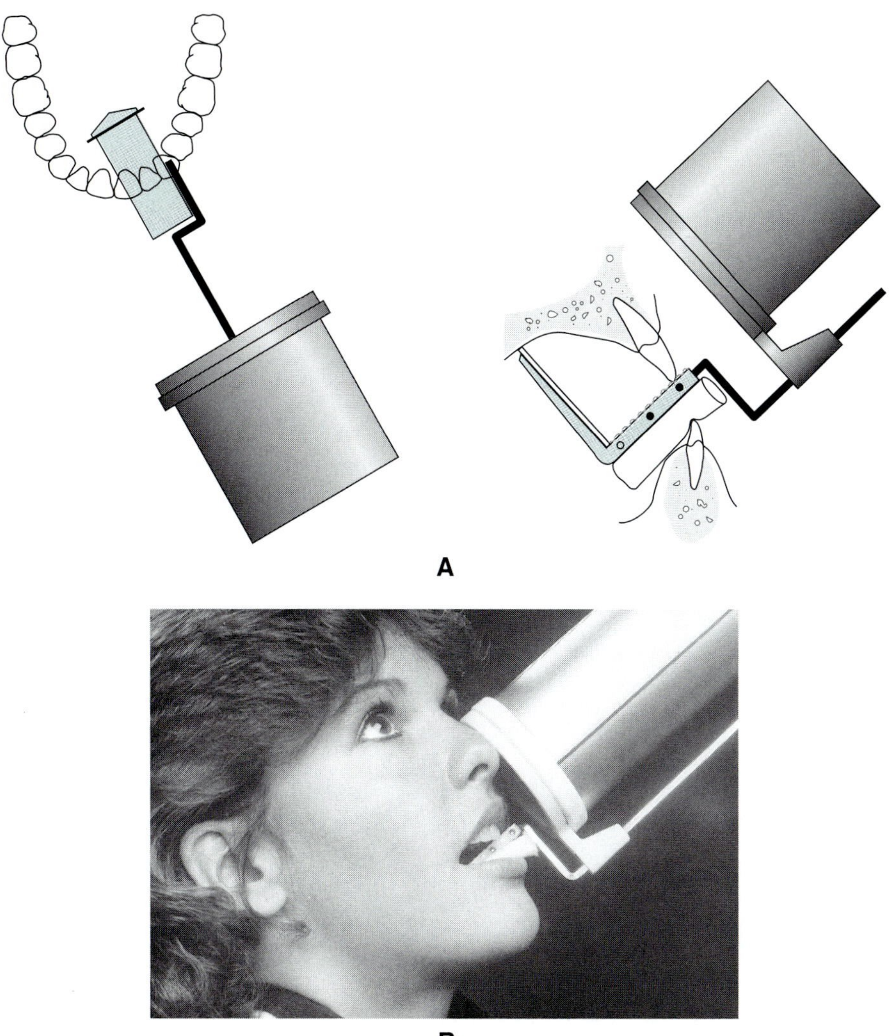

FIGURE 14–8. **Maxillary lateral incisor exposure.** (**A**) Diagram shows relationship of film, teeth, XCP instrument, and PID. As in all anterior areas, film is positioned with longest dimension vertically. Film is parallel to teeth with the block inserted to its full length to position the film as far away as possible from the teeth to be radiographed. (**B**) Photograph of patient showing position of XCP instrument and long circular PID. (Courtesy of Dentsply/Rinn Corporation)

serted between the mandibular teeth and the bite-block for stability and comfort.

5. Slide the aiming ring down the indicator rod to close approximation to the skin surface.
6. Align the PID parallel to the indicator rod and the end of the PID parallel to the aiming ring.
7. Make the exposure.

Maxillary Canine (Cuspid) Exposure

To make the **maxillary canine (cuspid) exposure** (see Figure 14–9), use the following steps.

1. Insert the film vertically into the film holder with the identification dot into the slot.
2. Center the film holder and film packet on the maxillary canine (cuspid).
3. Position the film as far away from the teeth as possible by using the entire horizontal length of the biteblock.
4. Rest the biteblock on the incisal edges of the teeth to be radiographed and ask the patient to slowly close firmly on the biteblock. A cotton roll may be inserted between the mandibular teeth and the bite-block for stability and comfort.

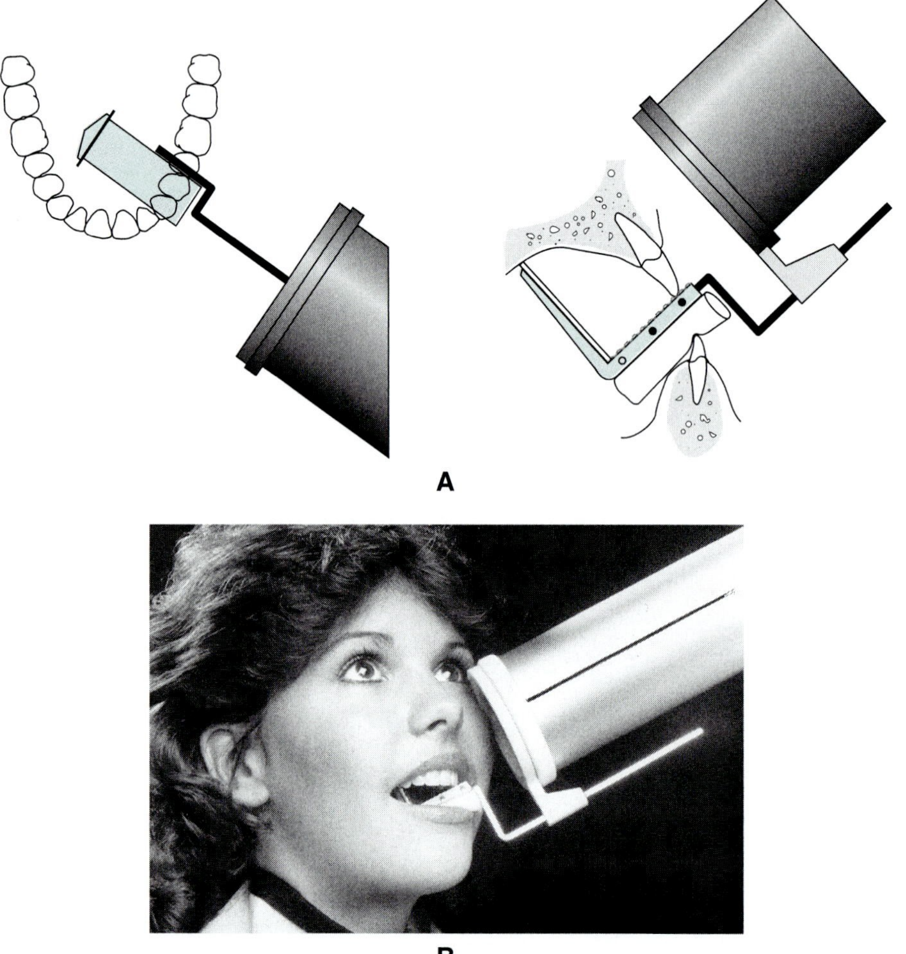

FIGURE 14–9. **Maxillary canine (cuspid) exposure.** (**A**) Diagram shows relationship of film, teeth, XCP instrument, and PID. As in all anterior areas, film is positioned with longest dimension vertically. Film is parallel to teeth with the block inserted to its full length to position the film as far away as possible from the teeth to be radiographed. (**B**) Photograph of patient showing position of XCP instrument and long circular PID. (Courtesy of Dentsply/Rinn Corporation.)

5. Slide the aiming ring down the indicator rod to close approximation to the skin surface.
6. Align the PID parallel to the indicator rod and the end of the PID parallel to the aiming ring.
7. Make the exposure.

Maxillary Premolar (Bicuspid) Exposure

To make the **maxillary premolar (bicuspid) exposure** (see Figure 14–10), use the following steps.

1. Use the larger #2 film and place it with its widest dimension horizontally into the film holder with the identification dot into the slot.
2. Center the film holder and film packet over the second premolar (bicuspid) so that the anterior edge of the film covers the distal half of the canine (cuspid).
3. Position the film as far away from the teeth as possible by using the entire horizontal length of the biteblock.
4. Rest the biteblock on the occlusal edges of the teeth to be radiographed and ask the patient to slowly close firmly on the biteblock. A cotton roll may be inserted between the mandibular teeth and the biteblock for stability and comfort.
5. Slide the aiming ring down the indicator rod to close approximation to the skin surface.

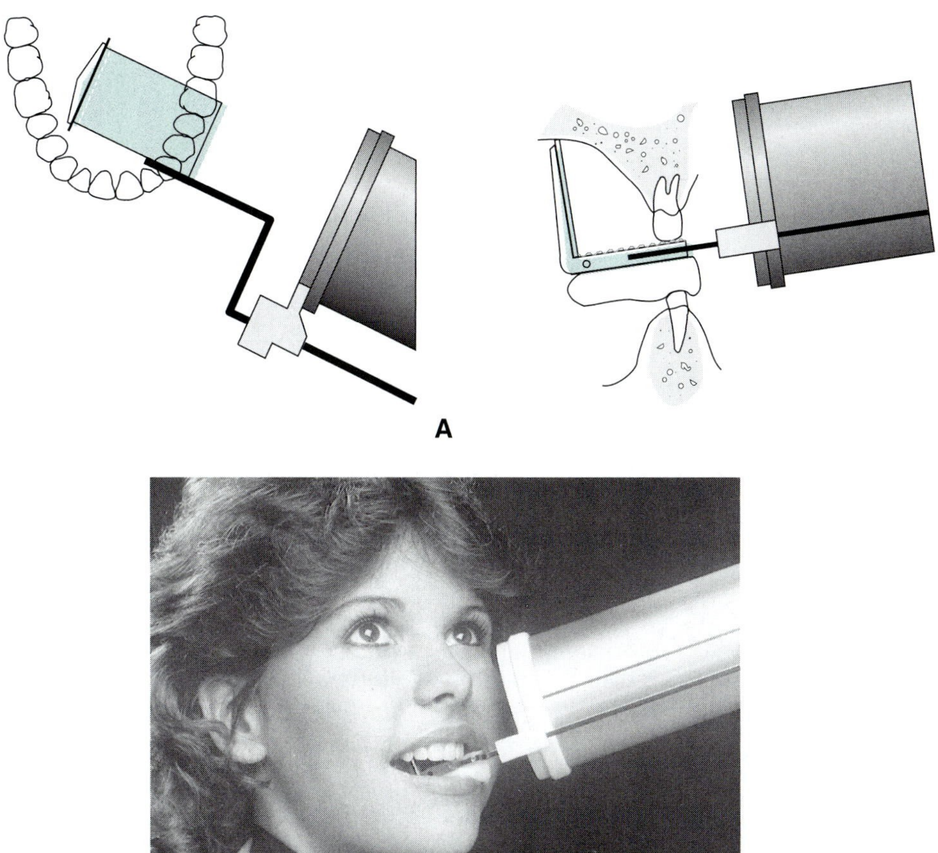

FIGURE 14–10. **Maxillary premolar (bicuspid) exposure.** (**A**) Diagram shows relationship of film, teeth, XCP instrument, and PID. As in all posterior areas, film is positioned with longest dimension horizontally. Film is parallel to teeth with the block inserted to its full length to position the film as far away as possible from the teeth to be radiographed. (**B**) Photograph of patient showing position of XCP instrument and long circular PID. (Courtesy of Dentsply/Rinn Corporation)

6. Align the PID parallel to the indicator rod and the end of the PID parallel to the aiming ring.
7. Make the exposure.

Maxillary Molar Exposure

To make the **maxillary molar exposure** (see Figure 14–11), use the following steps.

1. Use the larger #2 film and place it with its widest dimension horizontally into the film holder with the identification dot into the slot.
2. Center the film holder and film packet over the embrasure between the first and second molars so that the anterior edge of the film covers the distal half of the second premolar.
3. Position the film as far away from the teeth as possible by using the entire horizontal length of the biteblock.
4. Rest the biteblock on the occlusal edges of the teeth to be radiographed and ask the patient to slowly close firmly on the biteblock. A cotton roll may be inserted between the mandibular teeth and the biteblock for stability and comfort.
5. Slide the aiming ring down the indicator rod to close approximation to the skin surface.
6. Align the PID parallel to the indicator rod and the end of the PID parallel to the aiming ring.
7. Make the exposure.

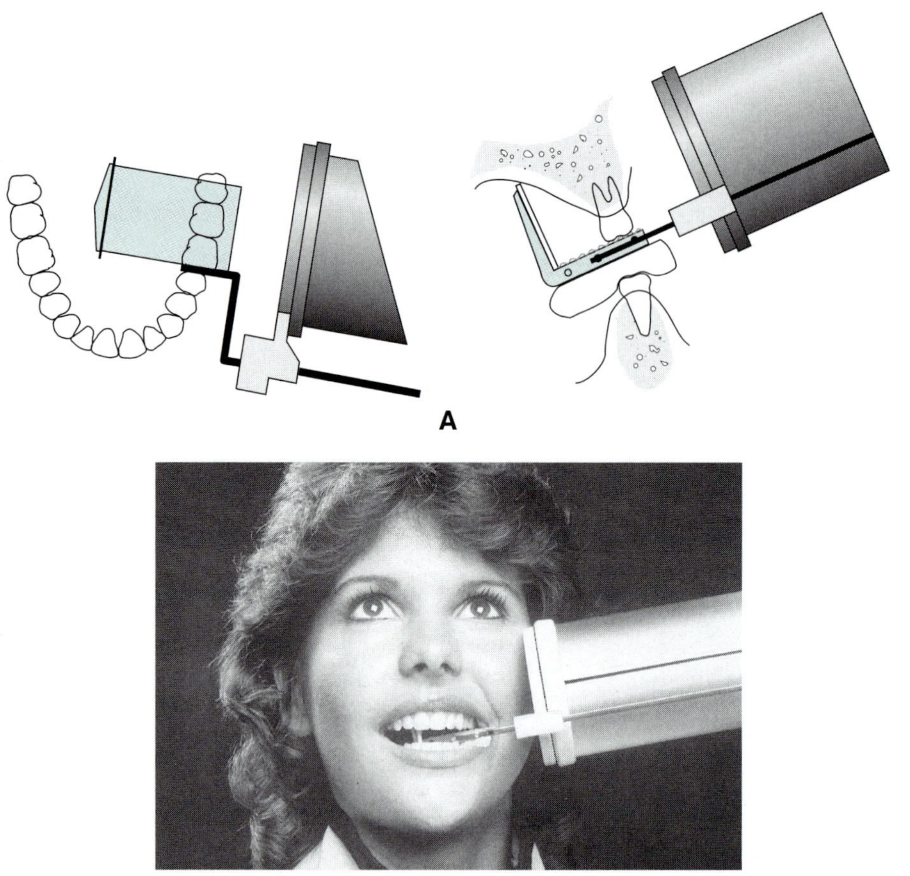

FIGURE 14–11. **Maxillary molar exposure.** (**A**) Diagram shows relationship of film, teeth, XCP instrument, and PID. As in all posterior areas, film is positioned with longest dimension horizontally. Film is parallel to teeth with the block inserted to its full length to position the film as far away as possible from the teeth to be radiographed. (**B**) Photograph of patient showing position of XCP instrument and long circular PID. (Courtesy of Dentsply/Rinn Corporation)

Mandibular Periapical Exposures

Mandibular Incisor Exposure

To make the **mandibular incisor exposure** (see Figure 14–12), use the following steps.

1. Insert the film vertically into the film holder with the identification dot into the slot.
2. Insert the film holder and film packet by directing the lower edge of the film toward the floor of the mouth and against the frenum of the tongue. Do this by first turning the film holder so that the film is parallel with the floor and then gradually raising the holder so that the film assumes a vertical position in the mouth. If resistance is encountered, ask the patient to first raise and then relax the tongue.
3. Center film holder and film packet on the contact between the central incisors.
4. Position the film as far away from the teeth as possible by using the entire horizontal length of the biteblock.
5. Rest the biteblock on the incisal edges of the teeth to be radiographed and ask the patient to slowly close firmly on the biteblock. A cotton roll may be in-

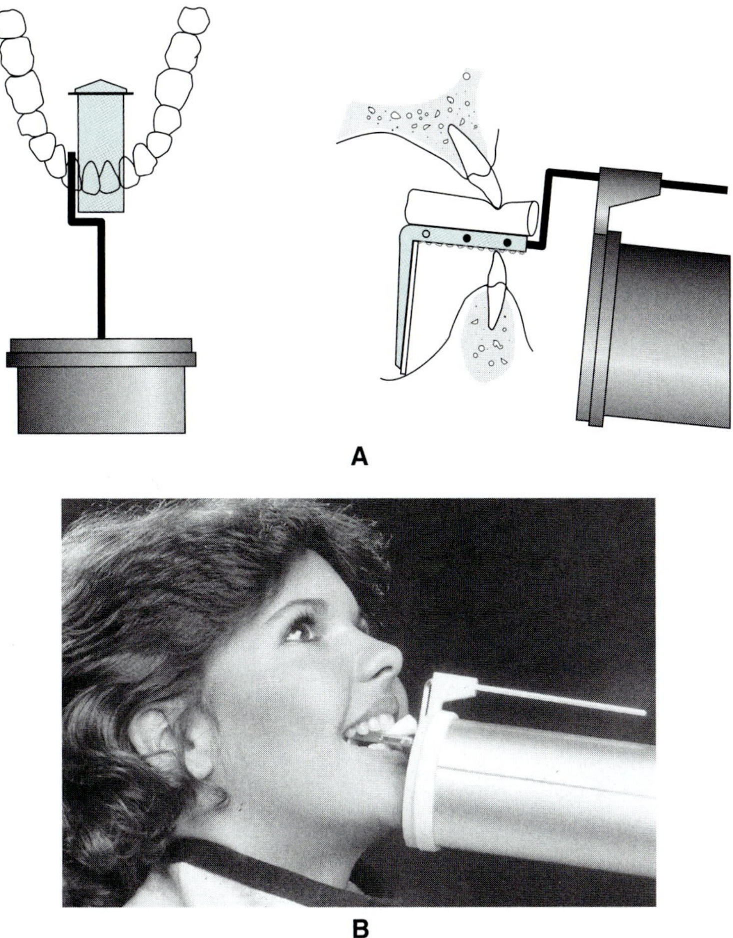

FIGURE 14–12. **Mandibular incisor exposure.** (**A**) Diagram shows the relationship of film, XCP instrument, and PID. Film is positioned with widest dimension vertically in anterior areas and parallel to teeth. A cotton roll may be used between the opposing teeth and the biteblock, causing the opposing teeth to force the biteblock firmly against the biting surfaces of the teeth to be x-rayed. (**B**) Photograph of patient showing position of XCP instrument and long circular PID. (Courtesy of Dentsply/Rinn Corporation)

serted between the maxillary teeth and the biteblock for stability and comfort.

6. Slide the aiming ring down the indicator rod to close approximation to the skin surface.
7. Align the PID parallel to the indicator rod and the end of the PID parallel to the aiming ring.
8. Make the exposure.

Mandibular Canine (Cuspid) Exposure

To make the **mandibular canine (cuspid) exposure** (see Figure 14–13), use the following steps.

1. Insert the film vertically into the film holder with the identification dot into the slot.
2. Insert the film holder and film packet by directing the lower edge of the film toward the floor of the mouth.
3. Center film holder and film packet on the canine (cuspid).
4. Position the film as far away from the teeth as possible by using the entire horizontal length of the biteblock.
5. Rest the biteblock on the incisal edges of the teeth to be radiographed and ask the patient to slowly close firmly on the biteblock. A cotton roll may be inserted between the maxillary teeth and the biteblock for stability and comfort.
6. Slide the aiming ring down the indicator rod to close approximation to the skin surface.

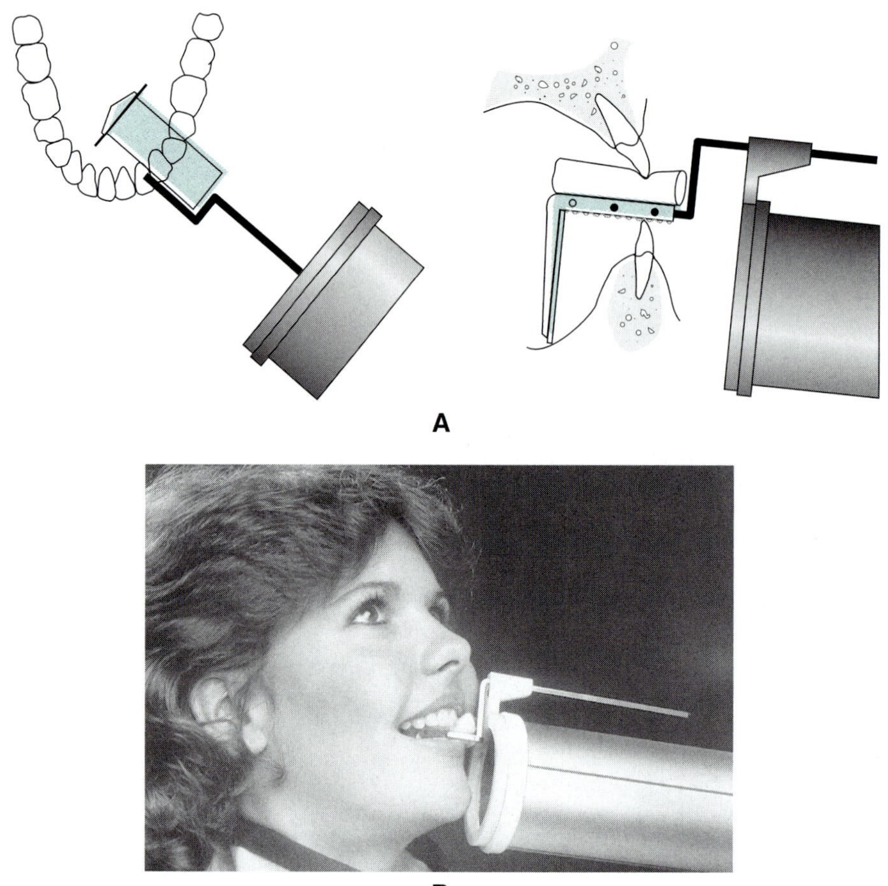

FIGURE 14–13. **Mandibular canine (cuspid).** (**A**) Diagram shows the relationship of film, XCP instrument, and PID. Film is positioned with widest dimension vertically in anterior areas and parallel to teeth. A cotton roll may be placed between the opposing teeth and the biteblock, causing the opposing teeth to force the biteblock firmly against the biting surfaces of the teeth to be x-rayed. (**B**) Photograph of patient showing position of XCP instrument and long circular PID. (Courtesy of Dentsply/Rinn Corporation)

7. Align the PID parallel to the indicator rod and the end of the PID parallel to the aiming ring.
8. Make the exposure.

Mandibular Premolar (Bicuspid) Exposure

To make the **mandibular premolar (bicuspid) exposure** (see Figure 14–14), use the following steps.

1. Use the larger #2 film and place it with its widest dimension horizontally into the film holder with the identification dot into the slot.
2. Insert and center the film holder and film packet over the second premolar (bicuspid). The anterior edge of the film should include the distal half of the canine (cuspid).
3. Rest the biteblock on the occlusal edges of the teeth to be radiographed and ask the patient to slowly close firmly on the biteblock. A cotton roll may be inserted between the maxillary teeth and the biteblock for stability and comfort.
4. Slide the aiming ring down the indicator rod to close approximation to the skin surface.
5. Align the PID parallel to the indicator rod and the end of the PID parallel to the aiming ring.
6. Make the exposure.

Mandibular Molar Exposure

To make the **mandibular molar exposure** (see Figure 14–15), use the following steps.

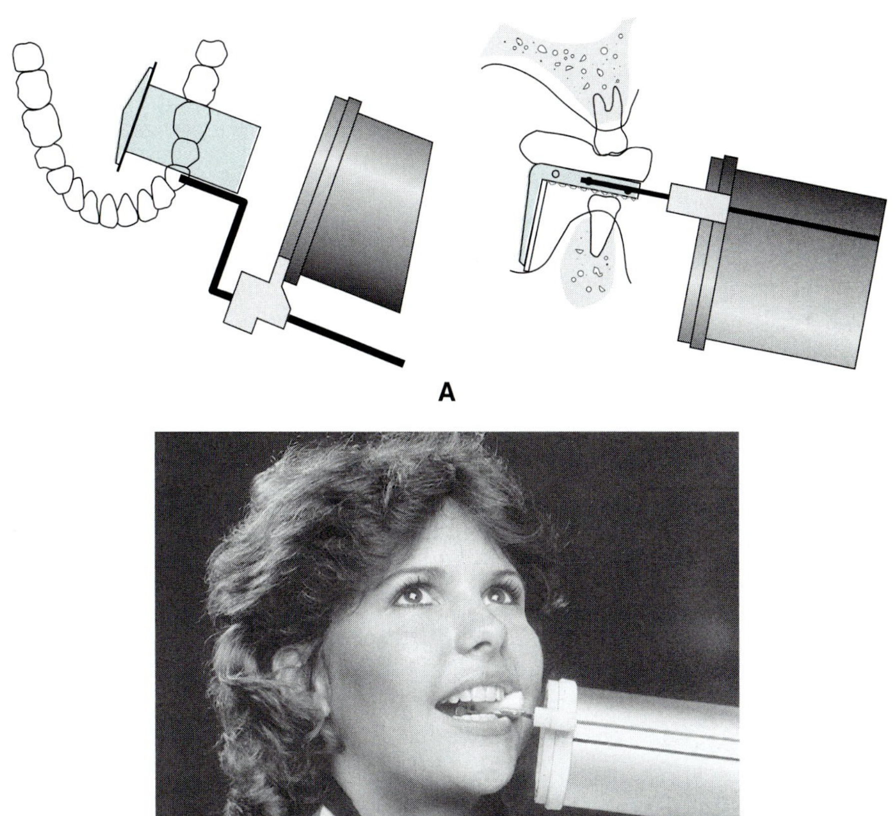

FIGURE 14–14. **Mandibular premolar (bicuspid) exposure.** (**A**) Diagram shows the relationship of film, XCP instrument, and PID. Film is positioned with widest dimension horizontally in posterior areas and parallel to teeth. A cotton roll may be placed between the opposing teeth and the biteblock, causing the opposing teeth to force the biteblock firmly against the biting surfaces of the teeth to be x-rayed. (**B**) Photograph of patient showing position of XCP instrument and long circular PID. (Courtesy of Dentsply/Rinn Corporation)

1. Use the larger #2 film and place it with its widest dimension horizontally into the film holder with the identification dot into the slot.
2. Insert and center the film holder and film packet over the second molar. The anterior edge of the film should include the distal half of the second premolar (bicuspid). In this region the film slides into the sulcus between the teeth and the tongue and close to the teeth.
3. Rest the biteblock on the occlusal edges of the teeth to be radiographed and ask the patient to slowly close firmly on the biteblock. A cotton roll may be inserted between the maxillary teeth and the biteblock for stability and comfort.
4. Slide the aiming ring down the indicator rod to close approximation to the skin surface.
5. Align the PID parallel to the indicator rod and the end of the PID parallel to the aiming ring.
6. Make the exposure.

Bisecting Technique

As explained in Chapter 13, the **bisecting technique** is based on the geometric principle called the **rule of isometry.** The rule of isometry theorem states that two triangles having two equal angles and a common side are equal triangles.

When the **bisecting principle** is applied to casting a shadow of a tooth on a film, the angle formed by the long axis of the tooth and the plane of the film must be bisected. The beam must be directed perpendicularly through the apex of the tooth toward the bisecting line

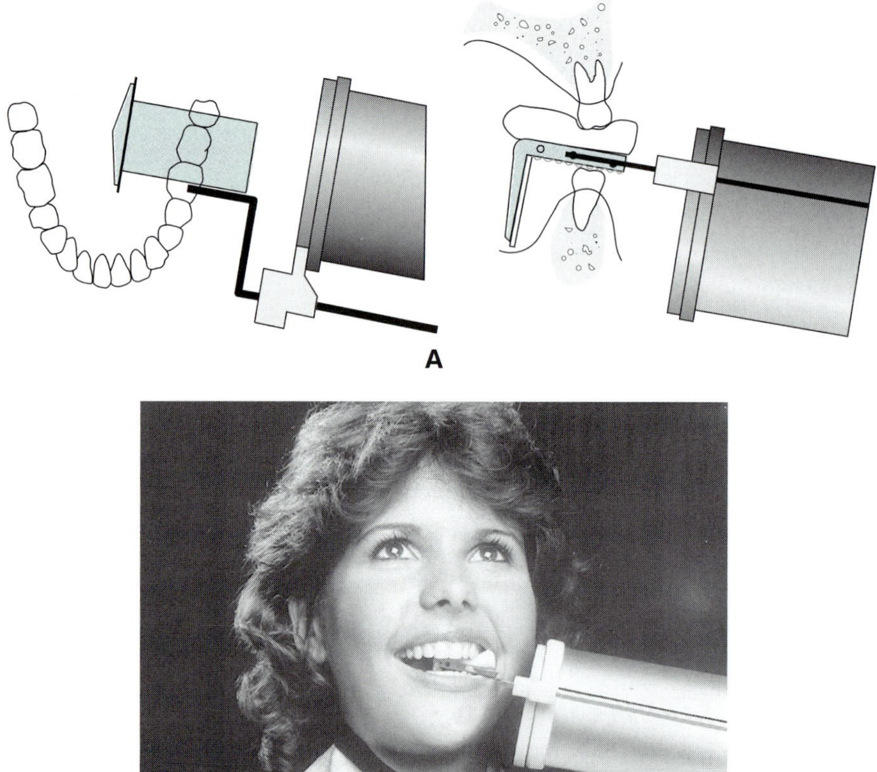

FIGURE 14-15. **Mandibular molar exposure.** (**A**) Diagram shows the relationship of film, XCP instrument, and PID. Film is positioned with widest dimension horizontally in posterior areas and parallel to teeth. A cotton roll may be placed between the opposing teeth and the biteblock, causing the opposing teeth to force the biteblock firmly against the biting surfaces of the teeth to be x-rayed. (**B**) Photograph of patient showing position of XCP instrument and long circular PID. (Courtesy of Dentsply/Rinn Corporation)

(see Figure 13–1). One must first imagine a line, called the **bisector,** and direct the radiation beam to it instead of to the long axis of the tooth or the film plane. This procedure is necessary because the irregularities of the oral tissues and the curvature of the palate seldom allow the film to lie parallel to the tooth.

Theoretically, two isometric triangles (triangles having equal measurements) are formed when the central ray is directed perpendicularly toward the bisector, and the film image that results should be the same size as the tooth. However, in practice this does not always happen. The image is usually satisfactory for diagnostic purposes, but some dimensional distortion is inherent in the bisecting technique. The bisecting technique is a good method to know but is not recommended except when anatomical irregularities require its use.

Film Retention for Bisecting Procedures

Film retention can be accomplished by either the **digital method** or **film holders.** It is highly recommended that film holders, such as the Dentsply/Rinn BAI instruments, be used. In fact, the digital method should not be used because the finger and hand used to support the film are exposed to unnecessary primary radiation. Also, the patient may exert too much pressure and bend the film or allow the film to slip resulting in an inadequate radiograph. The digital method is included here only for completeness.

Whenever the **digital method** is used, the film is positioned and the patient is instructed to use the thumb to hold the film in all maxillary areas and to use the index finger in all mandibular areas. The left hand holds the film on the right side and vice versa. All fingers except the one holding the film must be kept out of the path of the x-ray beam.

A variety of **holders,** ranging in complexity from plastic biteblocks to the **bisecting-angle instruments (BAI),** may be selected. The BAIs are assembled and used in the same manner as the XCP instruments, the only difference being that the biting platform is set at a 105-degree angle. When correctly used, these instruments reduce errors of judgment by automatically indicating correct horizontal and vertical angulation.

To avoid repetition of instructions for each of the eight usual areas of film placement, it will be assumed that, unless a special film holder is used, the digital method is described. This should not be mistaken for a recommendation to use the digital method.

NOTE: Always use film holders.

Patient Preparation for Bisecting Technique

Use the same patient preparation as for the paralleling technique with the patient's head in the conventional position (see Figure 13–11).

Maxillary Periapical Exposures

Maxillary Incisor Exposure

The **maxillary incisor exposure** (see Figure 14–16), if the #2 film is used, it is centered at the midline, and both central and lateral incisors are shown on the same film. If the exposure is made with the narrower #1 film, less of the lateral incisors will be shown. Many operators prefer to center the narrower film between the central and lateral incisors. This requires a film for the right and left sides. To make this exposure, the following steps are used.

1. Position the film vertical and allow about 1/8 in. (3 mm) to extend below incisal edges.
2. Instruct the patient to hold the film with the thumb by exerting a slight pressure against the lower middle part of the film. Either thumb may be used if the film is centered at the midline; otherwise, ask the patient to use the hand opposite to the side on which the film is placed.
3. Establish the horizontal angulation by directing the central rays through the embrasure either between the central incisors or between the central and lateral incisors perpendicularly toward the film.
4. Establish the vertical angulation by determining the location of the bisector. In most instances this will be between +40 and +45 degrees.
5. Center the PID over the point of entry near the tip of the nose. Adjust the PID so its end almost touches the patient's skin.
6. Make the exposure.

Maxillary Canine (Cuspid) Exposure

To make the **maxillary canine (cuspid) exposure** (see Figure 14–17), follow these steps.

1. Use essentially the same procedures for film placement as for the central incisors. Position the film vertically so that the canine is in the center and the lateral is included. Allow an incisal margin of about 1/8 in. (3 mm).
2. Change the horizontal angulation so that the central ray passes through the distal of the canine, perpendicularly to the **mean tangent** of the film.
3. Change the vertical angulation to about +45 degrees.

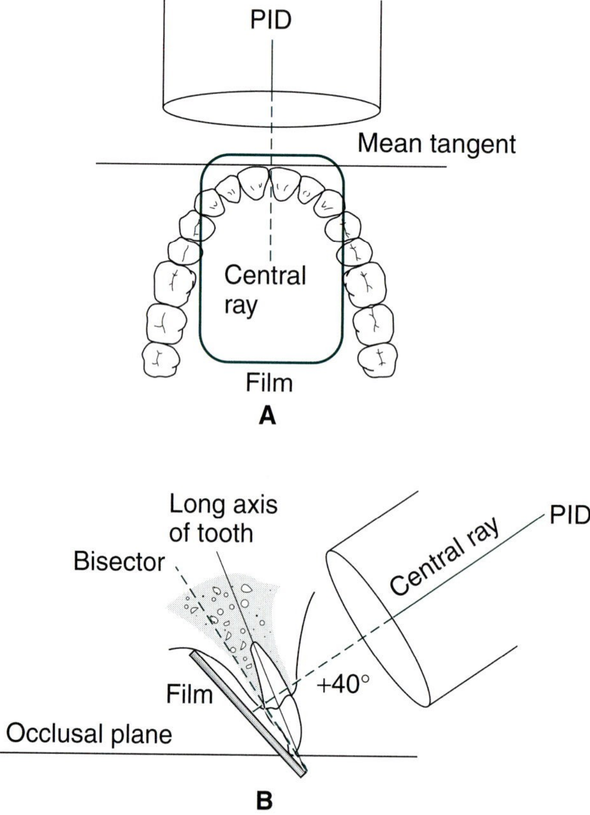

FIGURE 14–16. **Maxillary incisors, film packet, and PID position.** (**A**) Horizontal projection is through midline embrasure and perpendicular to mean tangent. (**B**) Vertical projection is directed perpendicular to bisector at approximately +40 degrees with PID tilted downward.

4. Center the PID over the point of entry near the center of the root of the canine, at the ala of the nose.
5. Make the exposure.

Maxillary Premolar (Bicuspid) Exposure

To make the **maxillary premolar (bicuspid) exposure** (see Figure 14–18), follow the same basic procedures, but make the following changes.

1. Grasp the film at the center and insert it horizontally. Use the thumb of the opposite hand to press the film toward the palate. If necessary, slightly soften the upper film corners to conform with the shape of the palate. Center the film over the premolar area and position it so the distal half of the canine is included. Allow a 1/8-in. (3 mm) occlusal margin.
2. Change the horizontal angulations so that the central ray passes through the embrasure between the premolars.
3. Change the vertical angulation to about +30 degrees.
4. Center the PID over the point of entry, located on the ala-tragus line directly below the pupil of the eye.
5. Make the exposure.

Maxillary Molar Exposure

To make the **maxillary molar exposure** (see Figure 14–19), follow these steps.

1. Adjust the headrest as necessary to parallel the occlusal plane with the floor. Center the film horizontally over the molar area and let the front edge of the film cover the distal half of the second premolar. Oc-

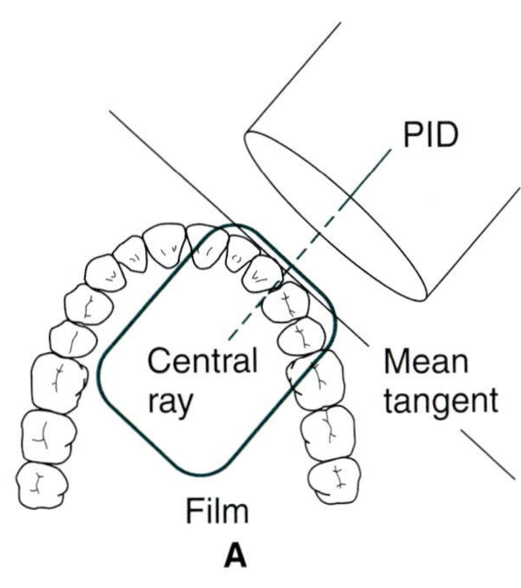

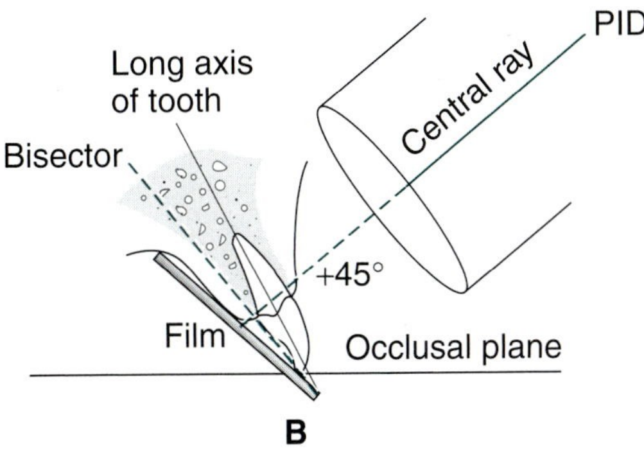

FIGURE 14–17. **Maxillary canine (cuspid), film packet, and PID position.** (**A**) Horizontal projection is through canine and perpendicular to mean tangent. (**B**) Vertical projection is directed perpendicular to bisector at approximately +45 degrees with PID tilted downward.

casionally, it may be desirable to position the film farther back to include erupting third molars.

2. Change the horizontal angulation so that the central ray passes through the embrasure between the first and second molars.
3. Change the vertical angulation as needed, usually to between +20 and +25 degrees. Depending on whether third molars are impacted or not, the vertical angulation required may be as steep as +55 degrees. Direct the central rays horizontally through the embrasure between the first and second molars perpendicularly toward the film.
4. Center the PID over the point of entry on the ala-tragus line, directly below the outer canthus of the eye. When unerupted or impacted third molars are suspected, direct the center of the PID about 1/2 in. (12 mm) farther back and higher.
5. Make the exposure.

Mandibular Periapical Exposures

Mandibular Incisor Exposure

The **mandibular incisor exposure** is shown in Figure 14–20. If the #2 film is used, it is centered at the midline, and all four incisors will be shown on the radiograph. Number 1 film may either be centered at the midline or to the right or left of the midline, so that the center of the film is between the central and lateral incisors. To make this exposure, the following steps are used.

1. Check the patient's head position and make a mental note of abnormal occlusion or other irregularities.
2. Grasp the film packet along the narrow edge between the index finger and the thumb. Position the film vertically and allow it to extend about 1/4 in. (6 mm) above the incisal edges. If resistance is encountered, ask the patient to first raise and then relax the tongue.
3. Instruct the patient to hold the film with the index finger of either hand by exerting a slight pressure against the upper middle of the film. A cotton roll may be placed between the film and the tooth to avoid bending the film and shaping it to the arch.
4. Establish the horizontal angulation by directing the central rays through the embrasures either between the central incisors or between the central and lateral incisors perpendicularly toward the film.
5. Establish the vertical angulation by determining the location of the bisector (halfway between the long axis of the tooth and the film plane). In most instances this will be between −15 and −20 degrees.
6. Center the PID over the point of entry, a point on the chin about 1 in. (2.5 cm) above the lower border of the mandible. Adjust the end of the PID so that it almost touches against the skin.
7. Make the exposure.

Mandibular Canine (Cuspid) Exposure

To make the **mandibular canine (cuspid) exposure** (see Figure 14–21), follow the same basic procedures but make the following changes.

1. Place the film as for the preceding exposure but center it vertically over the canine. Allow 1/4 in. (6 mm) to protrude over the incisal edges.

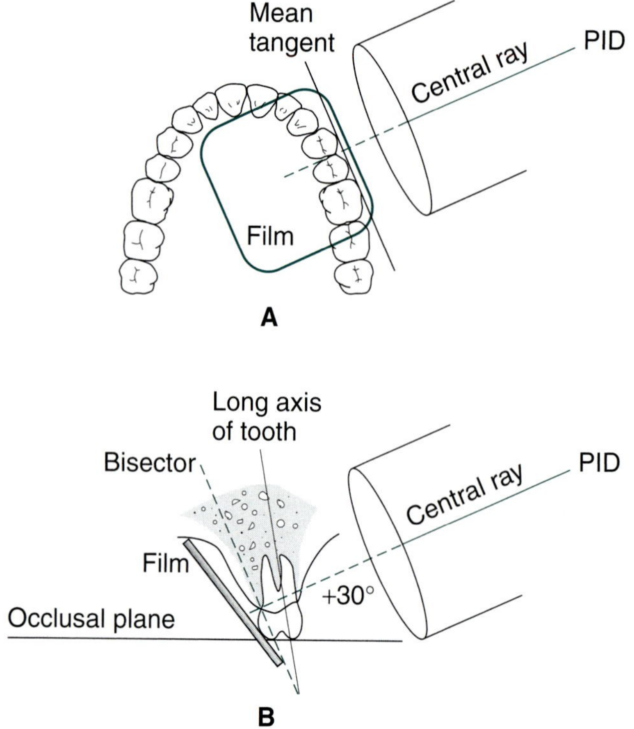

FIGURE 14–18. **Maxillary premolars (bicuspids), film packet, and PID position** (**A**) Horizontal projection is through embrasure between premolars and perpendicular to mean tangent. (**B**) Vertical projection is directed perpendicular to bisector at approximately +30 degrees with PID tilted downward.

2. Change the horizontal angulation so that the central ray passes through the embrasure between the canine and the first premolar.
3. Change the vertical angulation to about –20 degrees.
4. Change the point of entry to the center of the root of the canine about 1 in. (2.5 cm) above the inferior border of the mandible.
5. Make the exposure.

Mandibular Premolar (Bicuspid) Exposure

To make the **mandibular premolar (bicuspid) exposure** (see Figure 14–22), follow the same basic procedures but make the following changes.

1. Place the film as before with minor modifications. Grasp the film at the corner and insert it horizontally. Use the index finger of the opposite hand to press the film against the lingual. Center the film over the premolar area and move the film forward enough so that the front edge covers the distal half of the canine. Allow about 1/8 in. (3 mm) of the film to protrude above the occlusal surfaces of the teeth.
2. Change the horizontal angulation so that the central ray passes through the embrasure between the second premolar and first molar.
3. Change the vertical angulation as needed, usually between –10 to –15 degrees.
4. Center the PID over the point of entry slightly below the pupil of the eye and about 1/2 in. (12 mm) above the lower border of the mandible.
5. Make the exposure.

Mandibular Molar Exposure

To make the **mandibular molar exposure** (see Figure 14–23), follow the same basic procedures but with the following changes.

1. Make adjustments in the occlusal plane because this often curves in the molar area. Place the film in the same manner as before but center the film between the

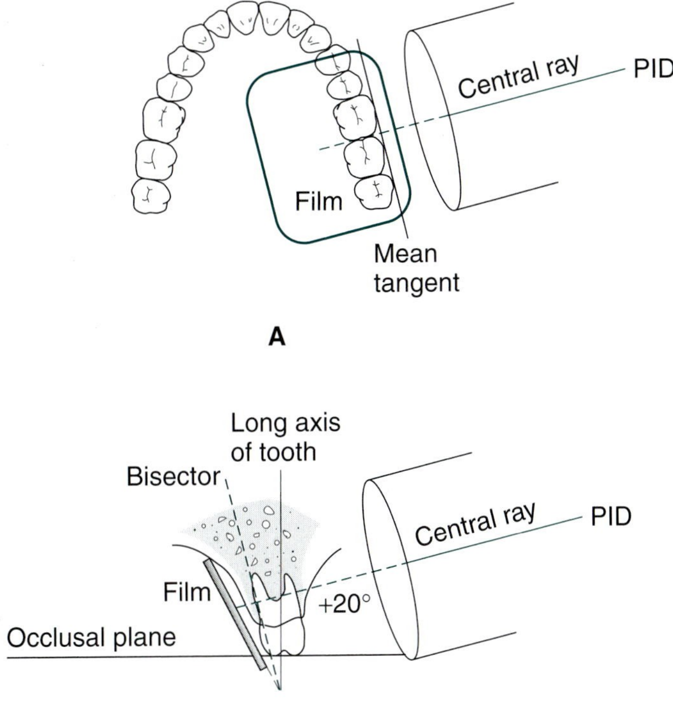

FIGURE 14–19. **Maxillary molars, film packet, and PID position.** (**A**) Horizontal projection is through embrasure between first and second molars and perpendicular to mean tangent. (**B**) Vertical projection is directed perpendicular to bisector at approximately +20 degrees with PID tilted downward.

first and second molars. Unless the main interest is in the third molar area, place the film forward far enough to cover the distal half of the second premolar. Allow a 1/8-in. (3 mm) margin above the occlusal edge.

2. Change the horizontal angulation so that the central ray passes through the embrasure between the first and second molar.
3. Change the vertical angulation to about −5 degrees.
4. Center the PID over the point of entry slightly below the outer canthus of the eye and about 1/2 in. (12 mm) above the lower border of the mandible (farther back for third molar exposures).
5. Take the exposure.

Variations

Because of anatomical limitations, rotation of the teeth, variations in the height of the palate, the presence of unerupted third molars, or excessive root lengths, one must occasionally depart from the usual procedures. Such changes include horizontal or vertical angulation and film placement.

1. Frequently the embrasures between the molars are not at right angles to the plane of a film that is parallel to the mean tangent of the buccal surfaces of the teeth. Consequently, overlapping of the contact areas results. One can overcome this by a slight alteration of the film placement so that the anterior border of the film is closer to the lingual than the posterior.
2. Often a conventionally positioned film that shows the tuberosity region reveals a coronal portion of a third molar to be at the level of apices of the second molar. In this case, one places the film as far back as anatomy and patient comfort permit. Drastic changes in both vertical and horizontal angulations may be required. This varies according to the location of the embedded tooth.
3. Absolute parallelism between the film and the long axes of the teeth is difficult to accomplish in patients with low palatal vaults. If the discrepancy from

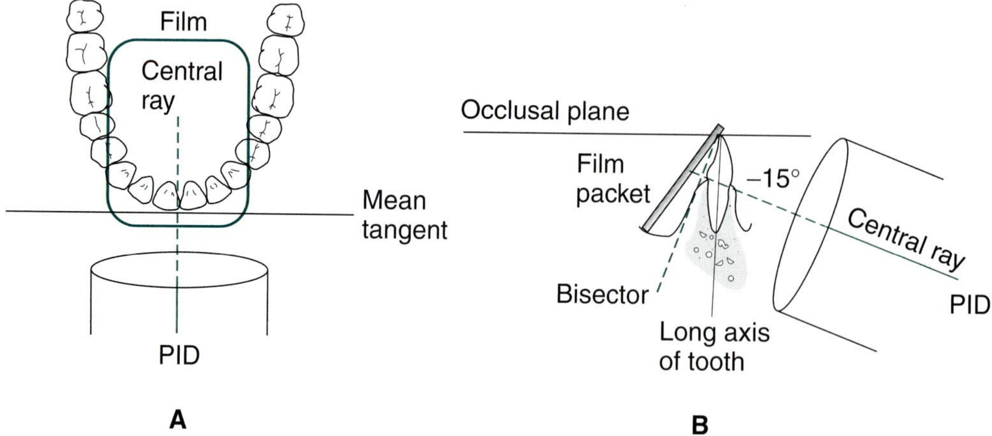

FIGURE 14–20. **Mandibular incisors, film packet, and PID position.** (**A**) Horizontal projection is through midline embrasure and perpendicular to mean tangent; (**B**) vertical projection is directed perpendicular to bisector at approximately −15 degrees with PID tilted upward.

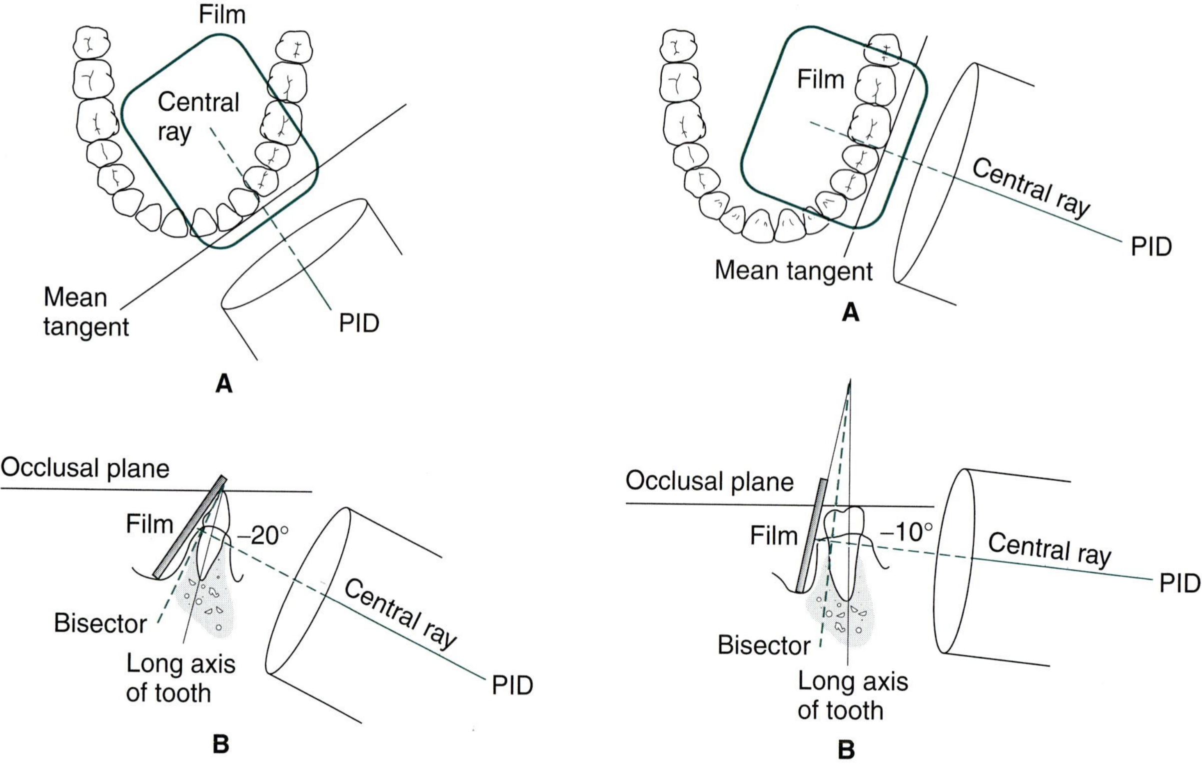

FIGURE 14–21. **Mandibular canine (cuspid), film packet, and PID position.** (**A**) Horizontal projection is through embrasure between canine and first premolar and perpendicular to mean tangent. (**B**) Vertical projection is directed perpendicular to bisector at approximately −20 degrees with PID tilted upward.

FIGURE 14–22. **Mandibular premolar (bicuspid), film packet, and PID position.** (**A**) Horizontal projection is through embrasure between the premolars and perpendicular to mean tangent. (**B**) Vertical projection is directed perpendicular to bisector at approximately −10 degrees with PID tilted upward.

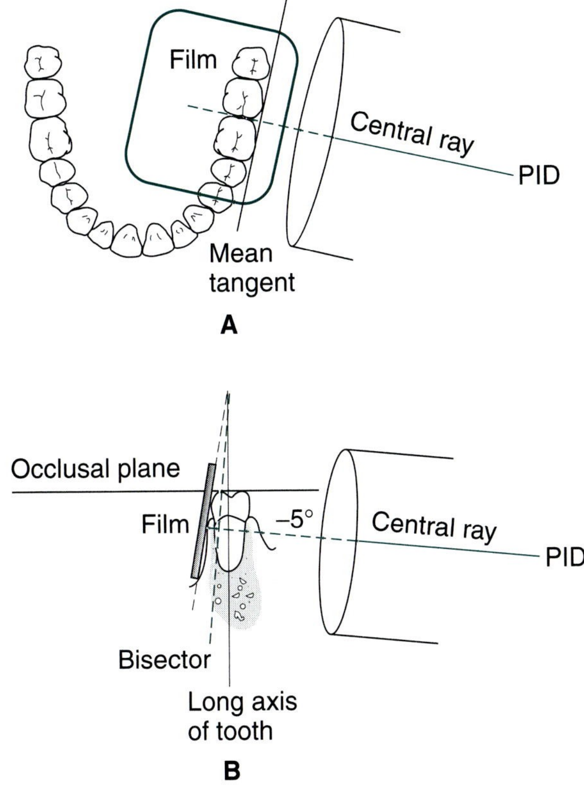

FIGURE 14–23. **Mandibular molars, film packet, and PID position.** (**A**) Horizontal projection is through embrasure between first and second molar and perpendicular to mean tangent. (**B**) Vertical projection is directed perpendicular to bisector at approximately −5 degrees with slight upward tilt of PID.

parallelism does not exceed 15 degrees, the radiograph is generally acceptable. In many instances, one can solve the problem of low vault by using two cotton rolls, one on each side of the biteblock. These may parallel the film with the long axes adequately but will reduce periapical coverage. Occasionally, especially when the roots are longer than average, one can increase periapical coverage by making the vertical angulation 5 to 15 degrees greater than indicated.

Bone and tissue density vary with the age and physical structure of the patient. Moreover, in most persons the bone structures are thinnest in the mandibular incisor region and densest in the maxillary molar region. Thus, for the best radiographs, it may be desirable to make minor changes in exposure time or milliamperage to vary the film density. Obviously, exposure time must be decreased for children and edentulous patients. As experience is gained, most operators learn to make variations based on age, size, and estimated density of the bone structures.

Endodontic Radiography Technique

Endodontia (from the Greek words endon, meaning "within," and odontos, meaning "tooth") is best defined as that branch of dentistry that deals with the cause, diagnosis, prevention, and treatment of diseases of the dental pulp. Treatment is generally accomplished by removing the nerves and tissues of the pulp cavity and replacing them with some form of filling material. The technique is often described as **pulp canal** or **root canal treatment.**

Although most of the periapical procedures described can be applied in endodontic radiographic exposures, there are some differences. These differences add to the difficulty of obtaining radiographs of high quality. Many of the exposures, particularly those made in the posterior areas of the mouth, are made under poor visual conditions. The placement of the film and holder is further complicated by the coverage of the area with a rubber dam and by the reamers, broaches, files, or the silver or

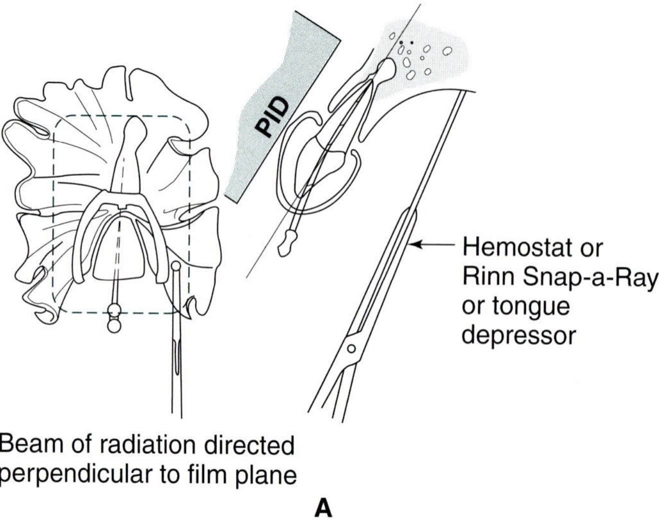

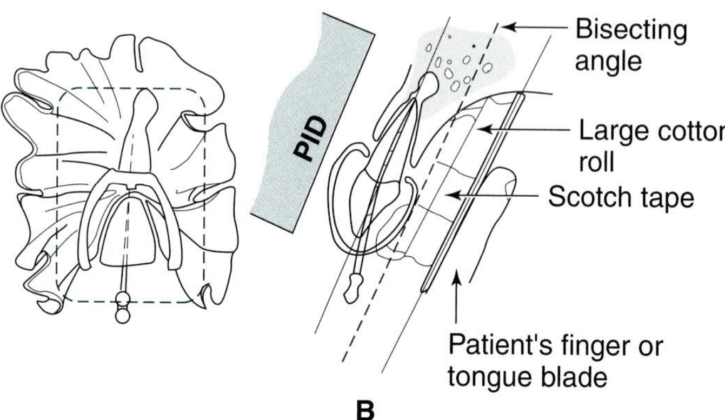

FIGURE 14–24. **Endodontic technique for maxillary anterior region.** (**A**) Preferred paralleling method. (**B**) Modified bisecting and angle method. (Courtesy of John W. Preece, DDS, Department of Dental Diagnostic Science, School of Dentistry, University of Texas at San Antonio)

gutta-percha points, which of necessity must be left in place while the film is exposed.

A series of films on the same tooth is needed for the dentist to evaluate various stages of endodontic treatment. The initial film is exposed to determine the preoperative condition and to make a diagnosis. Additional radiographs are made as the work progresses to determine the length of the root; the position of a reamer, broach, or file in the canal; or the position of the sealer and point or points (the tooth may have several canals). And finally a posttreatment radiograph is needed to make sure that the canal or canals are closed satisfactorily. Periodic follow-up radiographs may be needed.

The avoidance of distortion or magnification of the image is a major concern in endodontic treatment because the length of each canal must be accurately measured. Therefore the paralleling technique, which consistently produces the least distortion, should be used whenever possible. Although preoperative and postoperative radiographs are made in the usual manner, some technique modifications are required for the "working" radiographs that are exposed with the rubber dam and instruments in place.

The XCP or the disposable biteblocks should be used where possible. However, compromises must often be made when exposing working films. It may become necessary to use methods that rely heavily on visual alignment of the PID with the film while it is held in place either by the patient's finger (least satisfactory), the hemostat, the tongue depressor with cotton rolls attached, or the "EEZEE-GRIP" holder.

The preferred method for radiographing the anterior regions of the mouth is the paralleling principle (see Figure 14–24A). The next best procedure is to scotch-tape two large cotton rolls to a film and tape both to a tongue depressor or have the patient hold the film-cotton roll combination against the area of interest. The cotton rolls position the film farther away from the crown of the tooth and permit, at least partially, placing the film more nearly parallel to the long axis of the tooth. The beam of radiation is then directed perpendicularly to the film plane, or perpendicularly to a plane bisecting the long axis of tooth and film (see Figure 14–24B).

Obviously, severe space restrictions may occasionally require some experimentation with less acceptable methods. With minor changes, the technique for exposing the mandibular anterior regions is the same.

If true paralleling is not possible when exposing the posterior teeth (maxillary or mandibular), a 20-degree compromise technique often produces good or acceptable results. Film-holding methods similar to those described for the anterior regions can be used, but the film is placed as parallel as possible (within 20 degrees) to the long axis of the tooth, and the beam of radiation is directed perpendicularly to the film.

It often happens that when multirooted teeth, such as the maxillary first premolar, are radiographed, the buccal and lingual roots appear superimposed. This can be remedied by a shift of the tube head and PID. (Refer to the buccal-object rule in Chapter 26.) For example, the buccal root can be separated from the lingual root if a second exposure is made and the tube head is moved toward the mesial. If that is done, the lingual root canal will appear to move in the direction of the tube shift (mesial position in relation to the buccal canal), and the buccal canal will appear to move in a direction opposite to the tube shift.

Helpful Hints

- Explain the radiographic procedures to be performed to the patient.
- Set the exposure factors (kVp, mA, and time) before placing the film in the patient's mouth.
- Place each film packet in the biteblock with the "dot in the slot."
- Position the film to cover the area of interest.
- Be sure the patient bites firm on the biteblock.
- Be gentle, but firm.
- Use the word "uncomfortable" in place of "hurt."
- Praise the patient for "helping" you.

CHAPTER SUMMARY

The full-mouth radiographic survey of an adult patient is normally made with a minimum of 14 standard-sized films—more if narrow films are used in the anterior areas or if bitewing films are included. Exposures are made in the incisor, canine, premolar, and molar areas of the mandible and maxilla. Every effort should be made to center the film over the area of interest, and to make a final check to determine that the horizontal and vertical angulations are correct in relation to the film and the teeth.

When the bisecting technique is used, the film may be held in position by the patient's finger or by a film-holding device. Because the film is positioned farther from the teeth in the paralleling technique, some form of film-holding device is always required. Modifications or variations in film placement or exposure techniques may be required when the mouth is small, when anatomical abnormalities exist or when the patient is uncooperative. Some technique modifications may be necessary when taking endodontic radiographs.

The paralleling technique produces radiographs with the least dimensional distortion and is the technique of choice.

REVIEW QUESTIONS

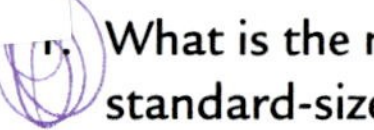

1. What is the normal film requirement for the adult periapical survey when standard-sized film packets are used?
   (a) 12
   (b) 14
   (c) 16
   (d) 18

2. Which of these factors does not need to be considered when deciding which film size to use when making the full-mouth survey?
   (a) Age of the patient
   (b) Shape of the dental arches
   (c) Previous accumulated exposure
   (d) Patient's ability to tolerate the film packet

3. How wide should the margin above or below the occlusal edge be on posterior radiographs?
   (a) 1/16 in. (1.5 mm)
   (b) 1/8 in. (3 mm)
   (c) 1/4 in. (6 mm)
   (d) 3/8 in. (9 mm)

4. Which part of the film packet should face the lingual surface of the teeth and the source of radiation?
   (a) The narrow edge
   (b) The printed side
   (c) The widest edge
   (d) The tube side

5. In what location should the identification dot be on a correctly placed film?
   (a) Toward the midline
   (b) Toward the incisal or occlusal
   (c) Toward the palate or floor of the mouth
   (d) Toward the distal

6. Anterior films are placed vertically in the mouth.
   (a) True
   (b) False

7. Posterior films are placed vertically in the mouth.
   (a) True
   (b) False

8. Why is a film holder necessary when using the paralleling technique?
   (a) To stabilize the film in a position parallel to the teeth
   (b) To make sure the film is at a right angle to the teeth
   (c) To make sure the film is perpendicular to the teeth
   (d) None of the above

9. State the four rules for using the XCP instruments. p. 215
10. Describe all 16 periapical film placements using the paralleling technique.
11. Which of these is not a part of the assembled XCP holder?
    (a) Aiming ring
    (b) Biteblock
    (c) Extension tube
    (d) Indicator rod
12. In which of these tooth areas is it often necessary to make a large deviation from average vertical angulation?
    (a) Mandibular premolar
    (b) Mandibular molar
    (c) Maxillary third molars
    (d) Maxillary premolar
13. In which of these areas is it occasionally advisable to position the film vertically instead of horizontally?
    (a) Mandibular premolars
    (b) Mandibular third molar
    (c) Maxillary premolars
    (d) Maxillary third molars
14. The avoidance of radiographic distortion or magnification is a major concern in endodontic treatment because:
    (a) The tooth is to be extracted.
    (b) The length of the canal must be accurately measured.
    (c) The canal may already be filled.
    (d) The canal may be too large.

BIBLIOGRAPHY

Del Rio, C. E., Canales, M. L., & Preece, J. W. *Radiographic Technique for Endodontics*. San Antonio: University of Texas Dental School at San Antonio, 1982.

Eastman Kodak. *Successful Intraoral Radiography*. Rochester, NY: Eastman Kodak, 1998.

Rinn Corporation. *Intraoral Radiography with Rinn XCP/BAI Instruments*. Elgin, IL: Dentsply/Rinn Corporation, 1983.

White, S. C., & Pharoah, M. J. *Oral Radiology Principles and Interpretation*, 4th ed. St. Louis: Mosby, 2000.

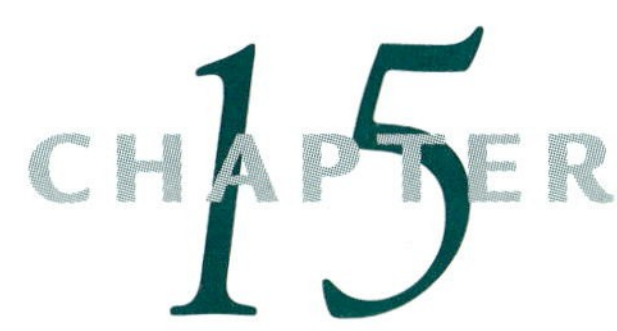

The Bitewing Examination

OBJECTIVES

By the end of this chapter the student should be able to:

- Define the key words.
- State the purpose of the bitewing examination.
- Compare the difference between periapical and bitewing radiographs.
- List the four sizes of film that can be used for bitewing surveys.
- Identify the size and number of films required to make an adult bitewing survey.
- Explain horizontal angulation.
- Explain positive and negative vertical angulation.
- State the recommended vertical angulation for bitewing exposures.
- Compare the methods of holding the bitewing film in position.
- Describe the film placements for the posterior bitewing examination.
- Describe the film placements for the anterior bitewing examination.

KEY WORDS

Bitetab
Bitewing radiograph
Contact areas
Embrasures
Film loop
Horizontal angulation
Interproximal radiograph
Negative angulation
Overlap
Point of entry
Positive angulation
Vertical angulation

Introduction

The purpose of the **bitewing examination** is to view the crowns and alveolar bone of both the maxillary and mandibular teeth on a single radiograph. Bitewing films are exposed more often than any other type of dental film. Bitewing radiographs are especially useful to detect **caries** in posterior teeth. They are also used to examine crestal bone of patients with **periodontal disease.**

The **bitewing film** has a **wing,** or **tab** attached to the film. The patient **bites** on the **wing** to hold the film in place. The bitewing examination is sometimes referred to as the interproximal examination.

The purpose of this chapter is to explain the bitewing examination and to describe the step-by-step procedures for conducting bitewing examinations.

Fundamentals of Bitewing Radiography

The **bitewing (interproximal) examination** is made either in conjunction with the complete periapical examination or alone at the time of regular checkups. Bitewing radiographs showing the crowns and alveolar crests of both the maxillary and mandibular teeth on the same film are ideal for examining dental caries that begin in the interproximal areas of the teeth and periodontal bone loss near the gingival line.

An **advantage** of the bitewing over the periapical film is that it can be positioned near and almost parallel to the teeth of both arches when the patient's jaws are closed. This often makes it possible to see decay and the height of the alveolar crests better than on periapical films of the same area, because the film is closer to the teeth and the central ray can be directed at a more ideal angle.

One of the great values of the **bitewing radiograph** is that it reveals caries in the earliest stages. This is particularly important in the premolar and molar regions, where small carious lesions are often concealed by the wide bucco-lingual diameters of these teeth. Such lesions are frequently unnoticed in a visual inspection.

A **disadvantage** of the bitewing radiograph is that it does not show apical conditions or lesions.

Film

The bitewing survey can be made with two to eight films, using size #0, #1, #2, or #3. Several factors must be considered when deciding what size film to select. The length and curvature of the posterior arches vary in all individuals. A single small film placed on each side of the mouth often provides adequate coverage in a small child or young adult. The preferred size for the deciduous and mixed dentition bitewing survey is the standard #2 film, but often tissue sensitivity or anatomical limitations make it advisable to select a smaller film. On most adults, four #2 films (two on each side) are generally preferred.

Some dentists routinely make the posterior bitewing survey with one #3 (extra-long) film on each side. The advantage is only one film is exposed on each side. When compared with the standard #2 film, the longer film has two serious disadvantages. One is that in most dental arches there are two slightly divergent pathways of the posterior teeth, one for the premolars and the other for the molars. As the central rays pass through these divergent embrasures, some of the interproximal structures **overlap** on the radiograph. The other disadvantage is that the long film is too narrow to reveal all of the periodontal crestal bone level. A good rule to remember is to use the largest-sized film that will do the job without causing discomfort to the patient.

Manufacturers package most film sizes with **bitetabs** attached to them. If such special films are not stocked in the office, it is easy to paste a bitetab to the tube side of the selected periapical film or to slide the film into a bite **loop,** thus converting it into a bitewing film. For **posterior** use, fasten the tab or slide the film into the loop so that the film can be positioned in the mouth with its longest dimension horizontal. The film is positioned in the mouth with its longest dimension vertically for **anterior** bitewing projections.

Angulations

The correct **horizontal** and **vertical angulations** are critical to produce a useful bitewing radiograph.

Horizontal Angulation

Horizontal angulation is the positioning of the central ray (PID) in a horizontal (side-by-side) plane. The horizontal angulation for bitewing exposures is the same as that used for periapical radiographs of the same area. The central ray (PID) should be directed perpendicular to the curvature of the arch, through the contact points of the teeth. The contact points should appear open. Incorrect horizontal angulation results in closed (overlapped) contact points and the radiograph is useless for diagnostic purposes.

Vertical Angulation

Vertical angulation is the positioning of the central ray (PID) in a vertical (up and down) plane. Vertical angulation is measured in degrees as seen on the side of the tube head. **Positive** (+) **angulation** is the positioning of the central ray (PID) **downward** toward the floor. **Negative** (–) **angulation** is the positioning of the central ray (PID) **upward** toward the ceiling.

The **correct vertical angulation is +10 degrees** because the maxillary posterior teeth have a slight buccal inclination and the mandibular posterior teeth have a slight lingual inclination. Incorrect vertical angulation results in a distorted image and the radiograph may be useless for diagnostic purposes.

Point of Entry

The **point of entry** for the central ray for all bitewing exposures is on the level of the incisal or occlusal plane (near the lip line) at a point opposite the center of the film and through the interproximal spaces of the teeth being x-rayed.

Methods of Holding the Bitewing Film Packet in Position

Several methods are used to stabilize the film; all of them make use of some type of **bitetab, film loop,** or **film holder.** Because anterior films must be placed vertically in the mouth, bitetabs that can be fastened to the tube side with adhesive are easiest to use. The film loop, into which the film can be slid with the tube side facing the tab, is most often used for posterior exposures.

The Rinn bitewing instrument (see Figure 15–1) is similar in appearance to the XCP instruments described in Chapters 13 and 14. It differs in that the indicator rod is straight and short and the plastic block has two slots between which the film is inserted with the exposure side (tube side) facing the thin biting plane of the block. Either the conventional round aiming ring or the newer rectangular aiming device can be used with the long or short position indicating device (PID) to align the central beam vertically and horizontally.

The metal or metal-and-plastic film holders are easy to autoclave, assemble, and position. By eliminating the necessity for numerical angulation or specific head positioning, many of the common errors such as cone cutting, closed interproximal spaces, overlapping crowns, and diagonal occlusal planes can be reduced when film holders are used. Specific instructions are available from the various manufacturers.

The exposure techniques that follow are based on the use of bitetabs or film loops. Because the overwhelming majority of bitewing films are exposed in the premolar and molar regions, the techniques for the posterior exposures are described first.

Posterior Bitewing Examination

If two radiographs are to be made on each side, position one film in the premolar (bicuspid) and the other in the molar region. If only one radiograph is to be taken on each side, center a single film behind the molars and premolars (Figure 15–2). Keep in mind that all contacts in the premolar (bicuspid) and molar region **must be open** including the distal contacts of both the maxillary and mandibular canines (cuspids).

Although vertical angulations may vary slightly from patient to patient, the average vertical angulation used is +10 degrees.

Regardless of the technique used, the horizontal angulation is directed perpendicularly through the **embrasures** toward the film. Extreme care must be exercised when positioning the PID in the horizontal plane. If the central ray is not directed through the interproximal spaces, or is projected mesiodistally or distomesially instead of at right angles (perpendicularly), the tooth structures in the **contact areas** will be overlapped. Then it will be difficult or even impossible to locate small cavities or decay under restorations, thus defeating the purpose of the bitewing radiograph (Figure 15–3).

As a rule, the film packet is placed horizontally in the posterior areas and vertically in the anterior areas. Two exceptions are:

1. When the posterior portion of the dental arch is very curved or irregular and it is difficult or impossible to find a common angle of projection through the embrasures.
2. When the patient has severe bone loss, horizontal film placement will not show the extent of periodon-

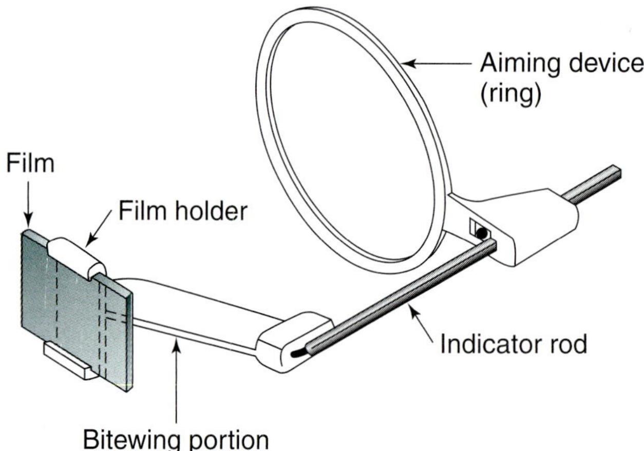

FIGURE 15-1. **The Rinn bitewing instrument.** This instrument consists of a plastic biteblock with a thin biting portion that supports the film-holding device at one end and a receptacle for insertion of the metal indicator rad at the other end. A ring slides over the rod. The instrument is also available with a rectangular aiming device for use with the collimated rectangular PID. (Courtesy of Dentsply/Rinn Corporation)

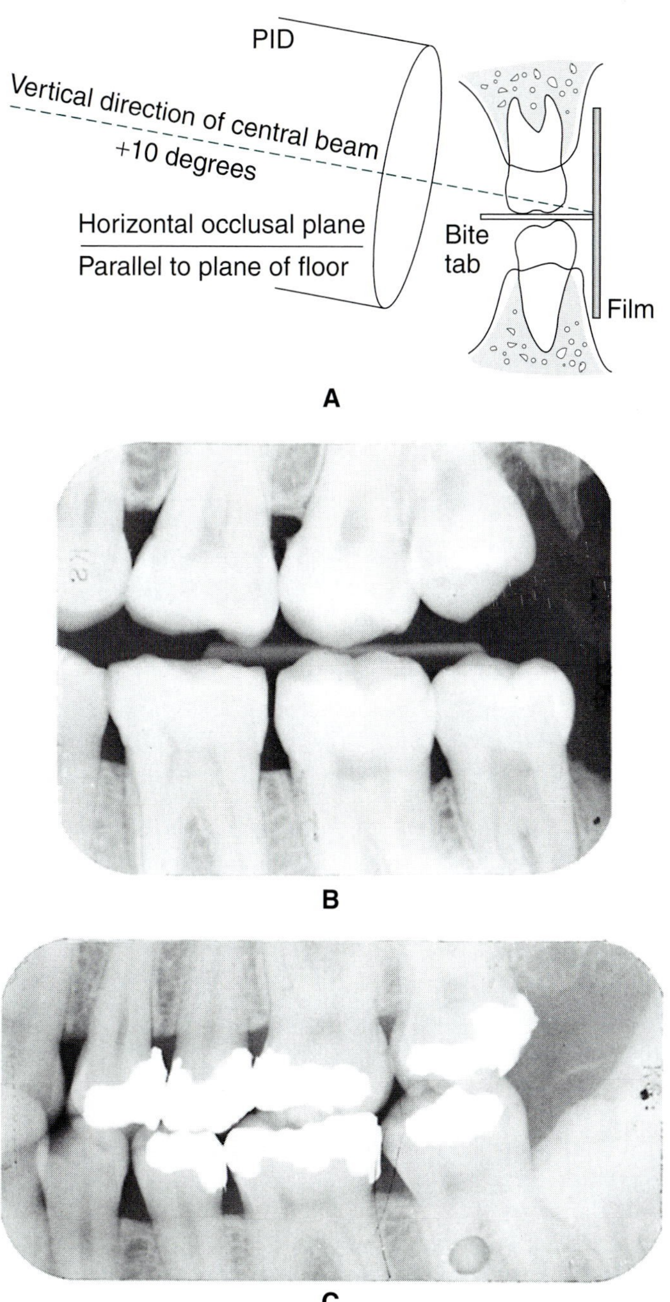

FIGURE 15-2. **Posterior interproximal area.** (**A**) Film slips into loop with widest dimension parallel to occlusal plane. Film packet is stabilized by bitetab that rests on the occlusal surfaces of the mandibular teeth. Patient closes on tab to immobilize the film. PID is projected vertically at +10 degrees toward center of film, and the central ray is directed horizontally through the interproximal spaces. Any size film packet form #0 through #3 may be used. (**B**) Radiograph of molar interproximal area made with standard #2 film. (**C**) Radiograph of premolar-molar interproximal area made with the long #3 film.

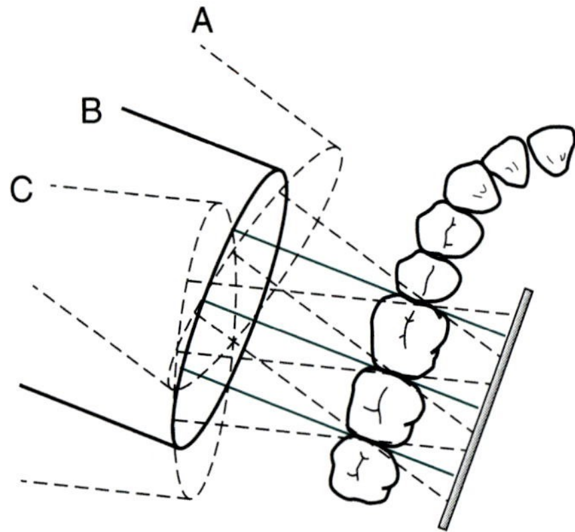

FIGURE 15-3. **Horizontal angulation.** (**A**) **Mesiodistal projection** shown here is deviated from a right angle by about 15 degrees, resulting in large overlapping of the contacts in the distal areas of the radiograph. (**B**) **Correct horizontal projection** of x-ray beam resulting in no overlapping. (**C**) **Distomesial projection** shown here is deviated from a right angle about 15 degrees, resulting in large overlapping in the mesial areas of the radiograph.

tal destruction. The bone loss can often be viewed by using more films placed vertically.

Care should be taken to ensure that the film is positioned in such a manner that it is evenly divided between the maxillary and mandibular teeth. The curvature of the palate or tongue interference has a tendency to disorient the film packet in its horizontal plane.

Once the film is satisfactorily positioned, the patient must close down on the tab or biteblock in an edge-to-edge relationship. Generally the bitetab or biteblock is visible after the film is placed. This serves as a guide for directing the central rays toward the center of the film.

It should be noted, posterior vertical bitewing radiographs have become more popular in periodontics.

Sequence for Film Placement

It is recommended to always follow a definite order for film placement when taking radiographs to prevent errors and to utilize time more efficiently. The following **sequence** is recommended.

- For patients requiring only bitewing radiographs:
  1. Premolar (bicuspid) bitewing films
  2. Molar bitewing films
- For patients requiring both periapical and bitewing radiographs:
  1. Anterior periapicals
  2. Posterior periapicals
  3. Bitewings

Patient Preparation

After completing the infection control procedures described in Chapter 22:

1. Seat the patient.
2. Explain the radiographic procedures to the patient.
3. Adjust chair to comfortable working level.
4. Adjust headrest to position patient's head so that the occlusal plane is parallel to the floor and the midsagittal plane (midline) is perpendicular to the floor.
5. Place the lead apron and thyroid collar on the patient.
6. Remove eyeglasses and objects from the mouth that can interfere with the procedure.

Following patient preparation, set the exposure factors (milliamperage, kilovoltage, and time).

Premolar (Bicuspid) Bitewing

To make the **premolar (bicuspid) bitewing exposure,** follow these steps.

1. Attach a bitetab or slip the film into a loop if special film is not available. The standard #2 film is generally most satisfactory. If necessary, slightly soften the film corners to conform to the curvature of the arch.
2. Insert the film into the patient's mouth and center the film over the second mandibular premolar (bicuspid). Cover the distal half of the mandibular canine (cuspid) with the anterior (front) edge of film.
3. Hold the tab firmly against the occlusal surface of the mandibular teeth. Ask the patient to close the mouth so that the teeth occlude normally. Biting down correctly on the tab is important to obtain the proper relationship of the teeth on the radiograph. Sometimes, practice without the film will help patients understand how to bite. Failure to hold the tab firmly permits the film to drift lingually and distally and increases the possibility that the tongue will move the film. This often results in a slanted occlusal plane. Caution the patient to bite firmly.
4. Center the PID over the point of entry, a spot on the occlusal plane between the maxillary and mandibular second premolars (bicuspids). Check to be sure the

PID is far enough anterior to cover the canines (cuspids) to avoid cone cutting.

5. Establish the vertical angulation, usually at +10 degrees.
6. Direct the horizontal angulation through the premolar (bicuspid) contacts toward the recording plane of the film.
7. Make the exposure.

NOTE: Patients with mandibular tori (bony growths) require special attention. Be gentle and place the film between the tori and the tongue. Do *not* rest the film *on* the tori.

Molar Bitewing

To make the **molar bitewing exposure,** follow these steps.

1. Attach a bitetab or slip the film into a loop if special film is not available. The standard #2 film is generally most satisfactory. If necessary, slightly soften the film corners to conform to the curvature of the arch.
2. Place the film in the patient's mouth. Grasp the tab and position the lower half of the film so that it is centered over the mandibular second molar. Cover the distal half of the second premolar (bicuspid) with the front edge of the film.
3. Hold the tab firmly against the occlusal surface of the mandibular teeth. Ask the patient to close so that the teeth occlude normally. Caution the patient to bite firmly.
4. Center the PID over the point of entry, a spot on the occlusal plane between the maxillary and mandibular first molars. Check to be sure the PID is far enough anterior to cover the second premolars (bicuspids) to avoid cone cutting.
5. Direct the vertical angulation at +10 degrees.
6. Direct the horizontal angulation through the molar contacts toward the recording plane of the film.
7. Make the exposure.

Premolar-Molar Bitewing Using the #3 Film

The **premolar-molar bitewing** exposure is identical to the exposures described, with these exceptions:

1. Unless the arch is extremely short use the **long #3 film** and center it over the embrasure between the mandibular second premolar and first molar. Cover the distal half of the mandibular canine with the front (anterior) edge of film.
2. Direct the central rays perpendicularly at the mean tangents of the interproximal spaces of both the premolars and molars. This is not always possible, particularly if the arch curves, and overlapping the proximal areas may result. That is why it is generally better to expose the premolar and molar areas separately.
3. Make the exposure.

Variations, Problems, and Corrections

Because the interproximal surfaces of the molars are in a mesiodistal relationship to the patient's sagittal plane, conventional film placement parallel to the buccal surfaces often results in overlapping of the contact areas and closure of the embrasure spaces. In such cases, position the film perpendicularly to the embrasures to avoid this distortion. Place the film slightly diagonally with the front edge of the film farther from the lingual of the teeth than the back part (Figure 15–4).

A sloping or slanting occlusal plane is a frequent reason for having to retake bitewing radiographs. **Probable causes** include:

1. The failure of the patient to maintain a steady pressure on the bitetab.
2. The patient swallowing while the exposure is being made.
3. Anatomical obstructions such as a torus or malpositioned tooth.
4. The top edge of the film contacting the lingual gingiva or curvature of the palate.
5. Poor placement of the bitetab or film holder.

Possible corrections include:

1. Cautioning the patient not to swallow or allow the teeth to separate.
2. Checking for anatomical obstructions before positioning the film packet.
3. If absolutely necessary, slightly bending a corner of the film.
4. Exercising care in selecting and positioning the correct size film.

Anterior Bitewing Examination

When making **anterior bitewing exposures,** position the patient and establish the horizontal angulation in the same manner as for the posterior exposures. Use a verti-

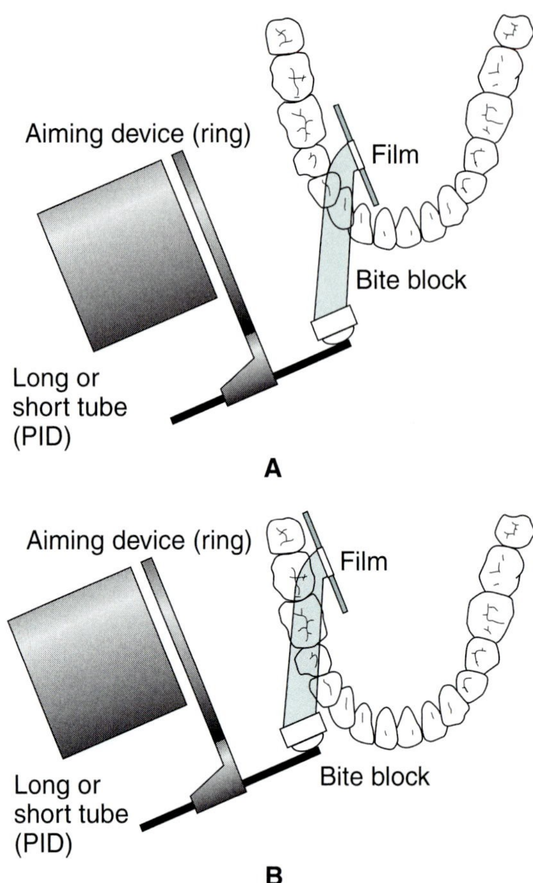

FIGURE 15-4. **Diagrams showing film and PID position with the Rinn bitewing instrument:** (**A**) Premolar position made in conventional manner. (**B**) Recommended molar position. Because the interproximal surfaces of the molar teeth are in a mesiodistal relationship to the sagittal plane, conventional positioning of the film parallel to the sagittal plane or to the buccal surfaces will result in overlapping of the contact areas and closure of the embrasure spaces. To avoid this distortion, it is recommended that the film be positioned perpendicularly to the embrasures, resulting in a diagonal placement of the film, with the anterior border at a slightly greater distance from the lingual surface of the teeth than the posterior border. (Courtesy of Dentsply/Rinn Corporation, Elgin,

cal angulation of +10 degrees. For ease of placement and least distortion, use the narrow #1 film. Use a longer bitetab, about 1 in. (25 mm) long, than used for the posterior exposures and attach it to the tube side in such a manner that the film can be placed in the mouth with its longest dimension vertically. This allows the film to be placed farther lingually in the mouth and prevents bending of the film in the middle as the tab is pulled forward when the patient is asked to bite with the teeth in edge-to-edge position on the tab.

Incisor Bitewing

To make an **incisor bitewing exposure** (Figure 15-5), follow these steps.

1. Slightly soften all four corners of the film for greater patient comfort. Grasp the bitetab and position the lower half of the film so that it is either centered at the midline, or if two films are to be used, between the central and lateral incisors. Direct the lower edge

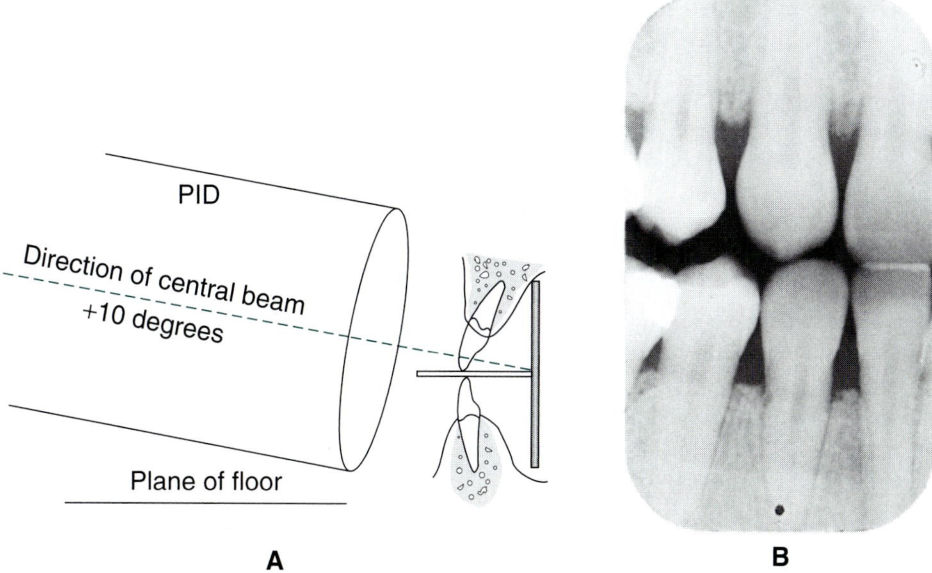

FIGURE 15–5. **Anterior interproximal area.** (**A**) Center film packet vertically at midline and stabilize by having the patient gently close on the tab at incisal edges of teeth. Teeth meet tab in end-to-end position. Suggested vertical angulation is +10 degrees toward the center of the film and horizontally the x-ray beam is directed through the interproximal spaces. (**B**) Bitewing film of the right canine area.

of the film into the space between the teeth and tongue.

2. Hold the bitetab so that it rests on the incisal edge of the mandibular incisor and ask the patient to close gently but firmly on it in an edge-to-edge position. Push the upper part of the film toward the lingual if it appears to prematurely come into contact with the palate. Exert only a gentle pull forward on the tab, just enough to take up any slack and prevent the film from turning.
3. Center the PID over the point of entry—a spot at the incisal line between the maxillary and mandibular incisors. Direct the vertical angulation at about +10 degrees. Establish the horizontal angulation by directing the central rays perpendicularly through the mean tangent of the embrasures between either the central incisors or between the central and lateral incisors toward the plane of the film.
4. Make the exposure.

Canine (Cuspid) Bitewing

To make the **canine (cuspid) bitewing exposure,** follow the same procedures as for the incisor area but center the film over the canine, with the front edge of the film including the distal of the mandibular lateral incisor. The point of entry is opposite the maxillary canine at the incisal edge.

Helpful Hints

- Explain the bitewing radiographic procedures to the patient.
- Set exposure factors before placing films in the mouth.
- Instruct the patient on how to close on the bitewing tab.
- Position the film between the torus and the tongue (not on top of the torus).
- Be gentle, but firm.
- Check the vertical angulation at +10 degrees.
- Direct the central ray through the contact areas of the teeth.
- Check for cone cuts before exposing the film.
- Use the word “uncomfortable” in place of “hurt.”
- Praise the patient for his or her cooperation.

CHAPTER SUMMARY

Bitewing films are exposed more often than any other type of dental film. The dentist considers them necessary to detect incipient caries in the tooth contact areas and early resorptive changes in the alveolar bony crest. Bitewing radiographs not only supplement and complete the full-mouth survey but are also exposed at most check-up examinations.

Any length PID may be used. Some form of film retention—bitetab, film loop, or biteblock—must be used. The patient prevents the film from moving by biting firmly on the tab or block in an edge-to-edge or centric relationship. Although many consider the bitewing exposure to be the easiest to make, it is the one most likely to fail.

Great care must be taken in placement of the film so that the radiograph will show the same amount of maxillary and mandibular structures. The vertical angulation is +10 degrees. An error in the horizontal angulation will cause an overlapping in the tooth contact areas and render the film useless for diagnostic purposes.

REVIEW QUESTIONS

1. How many standard-sized films are recommended to make the full bitewing survey of the posterior teeth?
   (a) 2
   (b) 4
   (c) 6
   (d) 8
2. Which of these conditions would not be visible on a bitewing radiograph?
   (a) Incipient caries
   (b) Recurrent caries
   (c) Apical abscess
   (d) Alveolar crest resorption
3. Which of these factors is most likely to reduce the usefulness of a bitewing radiography?
   (a) Error in horizontal angulation
   (b) Error in vertical angulation
   (c) Vertical instead of horizontal film placement
   (d) Horizontal instead of vertical film placement
4. Which size film is used and how is it positioned in the anterior area of a small and narrow adult arch?
   (a) Long-bitewing film placed vertically
   (b) Narrow film placed horizontally
   (c) Narrow film placed vertically
   (d) Standard film placed horizontally

5. Under what circumstances is the use of #3 film indicated?
   (a) When the patient is edentulous
   (b) When a child does not have permanent teeth
   (c) When it is desirable to show impacted third molars
   (d) When it is desirable to use a single film for the premolars and molars

6. What is the vertical angulation for most bitewing procedures?
   (a) −10 degrees
   (b) 0 degrees
   (c) +10 degrees
   (d) +20 degrees

7. The bitewing radiograph is used to examine:
   (a) The apical areas of teeth.
   (b) Odontogenic cysts.
   (c) Dental caries.
   (d) Root fractures.

BIBLIOGRAPHY

Eastman Kodak. *Successful Intraoral Radiography*. Rochester, NY: Eastman Kodak; 1998.

Rinn Corporation. *Intraoral Radiography with Rinn XCP/BAI Instruments*. Elgin, IL: Dentsply/Rinn Corporation, 1983.

White, S. C. & Pharoah, M. J. *Oral Radiology Principles and Interpretation*, 4th ed. St. Louis: Mosby,

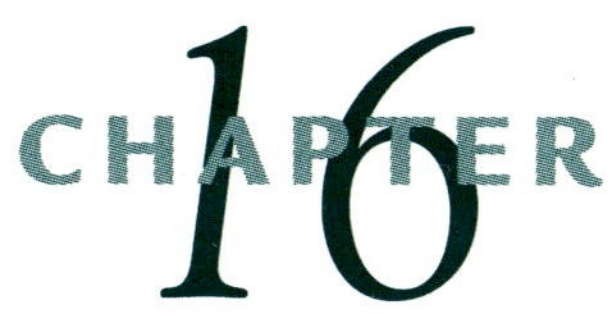

The Occlusal Examination

OBJECTIVES

By the end of this chapter the student should be able to:

- Define the key words.
- State the purpose of the occlusal examination.
- List the reasons for making occlusal radiographs.
- Discuss the technical considerations for the occlusal examination.
- Compare the topographical with the cross-sectional technique.
- State the sequence of steps for the maxillary and mandibular topographical surveys.
- State the sequence of steps for the maxillary and mandibular cross-sectional surveys.

KEY WORDS

Cross-sectional technique
Occlusal radiographs
Sialoliths
Topographical technique

Introduction

The purpose of the **occlusal examination** is to view large areas of the maxilla (upper jaw) or the mandible (lower jaw) on one radiograph. The film is placed in the mouth between the occlusal surfaces of the maxillary and mandibular teeth. The patient **occludes** (bites) lightly on the film to stabilize it.

The purpose of this chapter is to discuss the use and explain the procedures for the occlusal examination.

Reasons for Making the Occlusal Examination

The **occlusal examination** may be made alone or to supplement periapical or bitewing radiographs. The large #4 occlusal film is very useful for recording information that cannot be adequately recorded on the smaller periapical films. **Occlusal radiographs** are used to:

- Precisely locate supernumerary, unerupted, or impacted teeth (especially impacted canines [cuspids] and third molars).
- Locate retained roots of extracted teeth.
- Detect the presence, locate, and evaluate the extent of, disease and lesions (cysts, tumors, etc.).
- Locate foreign bodies in the jaws.
- Reveal the presence of salivary stones **(sialoliths)** in the ducts of the sublingual and submandibular glands.
- Aid in evaluating fractures of the maxilla or mandible.
- Show the size and shape of mandibular tori.
- Aid in examining patients with trismus who can open their mouths only a few millimeters.
- Evaluate the borders of the maxillary sinus.
- Examine cleft palate patients.

Although an occlusal film may not provide as complete and satisfactory information as a periapical film, the occlusal film can be used when it is desirable to view the area of interest in its entirety or when placement of periapical films is too difficult. For example, a patient with swollen cheeks may be unable to open the mouth wide enough for periapical film.

Children may misunderstand instructions for holding the film in place or may have tissues so sensitive that they cannot tolerate periapical film. Most children can cooperate by biting on a film. The smaller #1 or #2 films should be used for them.

Technical Considerations

The large 3 × 2 1/4 in. (7.7 × 5.8 cm) #4 occlusal film is used to make the occlusal survey. Smaller intraoral films may also be used, depending on the area to be examined. The standard #2 periapical film is frequently used with children, either to make a rapid survey of labiolingual or buccolingual unerupted tooth positions or in place of periapical positioning. The #2 film may also be used on adults when the mouth is too small for the large occlusal film.

A variety of film positions can be used to make the occlusal examination. The film may be placed horizontally or vertically. It may also be centered over one small sector, over the anterior portion of the arch, or over the entire right or left dental arch. Placement and size of film depend on how large the mouth opening is and the type of information that the radiograph is intended to reveal.

Most occlusal film packets contain two films. When they do, both films can be developed alike to give duplicate films. If duplicate films are not needed, one film can be developed fully for 5 min at 68°F (20°C), whereas the other film is developed for only 2 1/2 min. The fully developed film will show all details of the hard structures, whereas the underdeveloped film will show the soft structures.

The occlusal survey can be made with any length position indicating device (PID). The occlusal technique is based on the correlation of certain head positions with specific vertical angulations. Most occlusal exposures are made with the patient's midsagittal plane perpendicular to the plane of the floor. When maxillary exposures are made, the occlusal plane of the teeth is parallel to the plane of the floor; however, when the mandibular exposures are made, the patient is reclined in the chair, and the occlusal plane may be perpendicular to the plane of the floor.

Regardless of how the patient is positioned, the tube side of the film must always face toward the occlusal surfaces of the teeth in the arch being examined. The film is held in place during the exposure by slight pressure of the teeth of the opposite jaw. When the arches are edentulous, the patient holds the film with the thumbs.

Types of Occlusal Examinations

Occlusal radiographs are either **topographical** or **cross-sectional.**

Topographical Technique

When the **topographical technique** is used, the **film is placed** with the longest film dimension **anteroposteriorly (front-to-back)**. The rules of bisecting are followed, and the radiation is directed through the apices of the teeth perpendicularly toward the bisector. Because it is not always possible to use the most favorable vertical angle, the images of the teeth generally appear longer than they do on periapical radiographs (Figure 16–1).

Cross-Sectional Technique

In the **cross-sectional technique,** the **film is placed** with the widest film dimension (longest) **side-to-side.** The central ray is directed toward the area of interest and parallel with the long axes of the teeth and adjacent areas. This results in a circular or elliptical appearance of the teeth on the radiograph (Figure 16–2).

A topographical survey generally yields more detail in the alveolar crest and apical areas, whereas a cross-sectional survey yields more information about the location of tori and impacted or malpositioned teeth.

Preparation

Before exposing any films:

- Follow the infection control procedures described in Chapter 22.
- Seat the patient and explain the radiographic procedure.
- Set the exposure factors (kVp, mA, and time) on the control panel.

The Maxillary Occlusal Examination

Maxillary Topographical Survey

The following sequence of steps is suggested to make the **maxillary topographical survey** exposure (see Figure 16–1).

1. Adjust the headrest so that the midsagittal plane is perpendicular and the occlusal plane is parallel to the plane of the floor.
2. Insert the film packet (with the tube side toward the palate) into the patient's mouth with the **long edge anteroposteriorly (front-to-back)** between the occlusal surfaces of the teeth. Gently push it back as far as it will go.

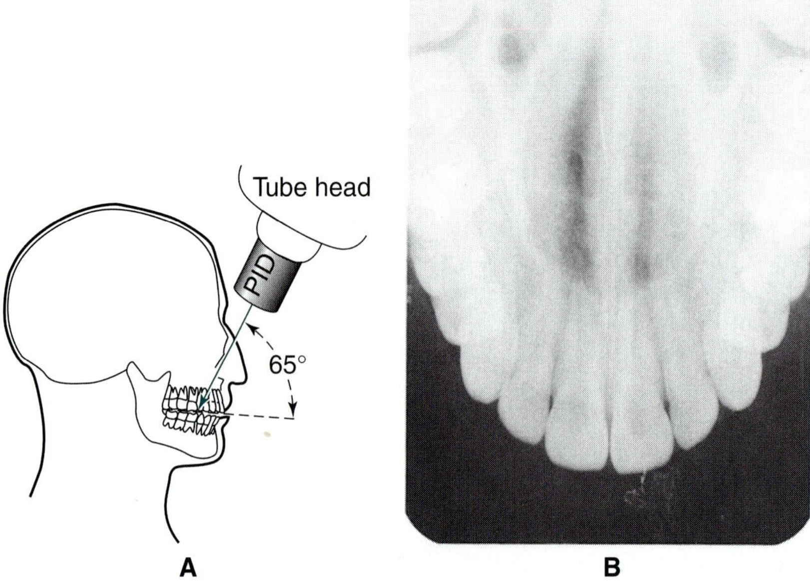

FIGURE 16–1. **Topographical technique.** (**A**) Diagram showing relationship of tube head and PID to occlusal film and patient for a topographical view of the maxillary incisor area. Exposure side of film faces maxillary arch with longest film dimension anteroposteriorly (front to back). The horizontal central ray is parallel with patient's midsagittal plane, and the vertical angulation is approximately +65 degrees through a point near the bridge of the nose. The x-ray beam is directed toward the center of the film. Slight modifications in film placement and angulation can be made when the center of interest is in the canine or molar area or when a cross-sectional view is desired. (**B**) Typical **radiograph of topographical maxillary incisor area.**

3. Instruct the patient to close gently but firmly with the teeth against the film to stabilize it.
4. **Establish the horizontal angulation.** Direct the central ray parallel with the patient's midsagittal plane and through the midline of the arch toward the center of the film.
5. **Establish the vertical angulation.** Direct the central rays at +65 degrees toward the center of the film through the point of entry above the bridge of the nose.
6. Make the exposure.

The Maxillary Cross-Sectional Survey

The following sequence of steps is suggested to make the **maxillary cross-sectional survey** (see Figure 16–2).

1. Adjust the headrest so that the midsagittal plane is perpendicular and the occlusal plane is parallel to the plane of the floor.
2. Insert the film packet (with the tube side toward the palate) into the patient's mouth with the widest dimension (longest) in a side-to-side direction between the occlusal surfaces of the teeth. Gently push it back as far as it will go.
3. Instruct the patient to close gently but firmly with the teeth against the film to stabilize it.
4. **Establish the horizontal angulation.** Direct the central ray parallel with the patient's midsagittal plane and through the midline of the arch toward the center of the film.
5. **Establish the vertical angulation.** Direct the central rays at +75 degrees toward the center of the film through the point of entry above the bridge of the nose.
6. Make the exposure.

If the maxillary arch is edentulous, position the film packet axis horizontally. The patient presses the film

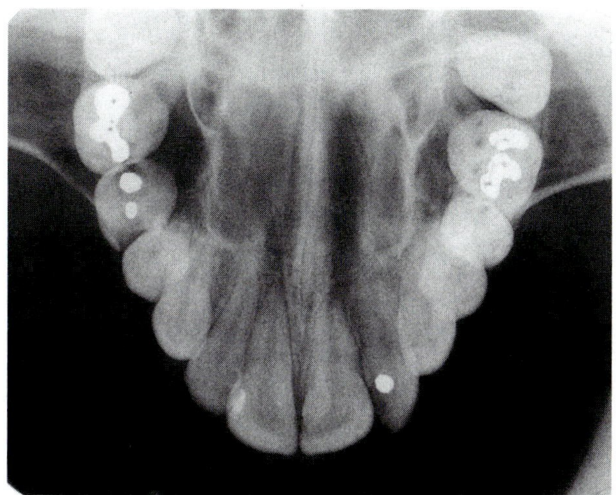

FIGURE 16–2. **Typical radiograph of a maxillary cross-sectional view.** Such a view can be made of a specific area or the entire dental arch. The film packet is placed between the occlusal surfaces horizontally (side to side). The central ray is directed toward the area of interest parallel to the long axis of the teeth. The teeth appear as round or elliptical areas on the film.

against the ridge with the thumbs and braces the other fingers against the side of the face to prevent the film from moving. If the patient has a lower denture, it may be left in the mouth to bite against the film.

Modified Techniques

The maxillary incisor technique can be **modified** for exposures of the canine, molar, or sinus areas by making slight changes in film placement and the central ray angulations.

Canine Survey

To make the **canine survey,** shift the film laterally to either the right or left side. Direct the central ray horizontally at about 45 degrees to the midsagittal plane and vertically at about +60 degrees. The point of entry is in the canine fossa, at a point near the infraorbital foramen.

Molar Survey

The film is shifted laterally in the same manner to make the **molar survey.** Use the same vertical angulation but change the horizontal angulation so it is at 90 degrees to the midsagittal plane. The point of entry is immediately below the outer canthus of the eye.

Sinus Survey

To make the **sinus survey,** establish the horizontal angulation at 0 degrees to the midsagittal plane, and set the vertical angulation at +80 degrees. Direct the central ray toward the center of the film through a point of entry in the canine fossa. In this procedure, the maxillary sinus is directly above the film. This exposure is occasionally made to locate root tips in the sinus.

The Mandibular Occlusal Examination

The Mandibular Topographical Survey

The following sequence of steps is suggested to make the **mandibular topographical exposure** (see Figure 16–3).

1. Adjust the headrest so that the midsagittal plane is perpendicular and the plane of occlusion is at a 45-degree angle to the plane of the floor. This can be done by either tilting the chair back or reclining the backrest.
2. **Insert the film packet** axis vertically between the occlusal surfaces of the teeth with the tube side toward the floor of the mouth, gently pushing it back as far as it will go.
3. Instruct the patient to close gently but firmly with the teeth against the film to immobilize it.
4. **Establish the horizontal angulation** so that the central ray is parallel with the patient's midsagittal plane and is directed through the arch toward the center of the film.
5. The problem in **establishing ideal vertical angulation** is in determining whether the patient has been reclined so that the plane of occlusion is at a 45-degree angle to the plane of the floor. A simple way to establish the vertical angulation is to first parallel the direction of the PID with that of the film and look at the angulation scale on the side of the tube head. Then subtract 60 degrees from whatever reading is shown. For example, if the reading shown is +40 degrees and 60 degrees are subtracted, the new reading is –20 degrees (PID is tilted upward). At that angle, direct the central rays toward the middle of the film through a point of entry at the tip of the chin.
6. Make the exposure.

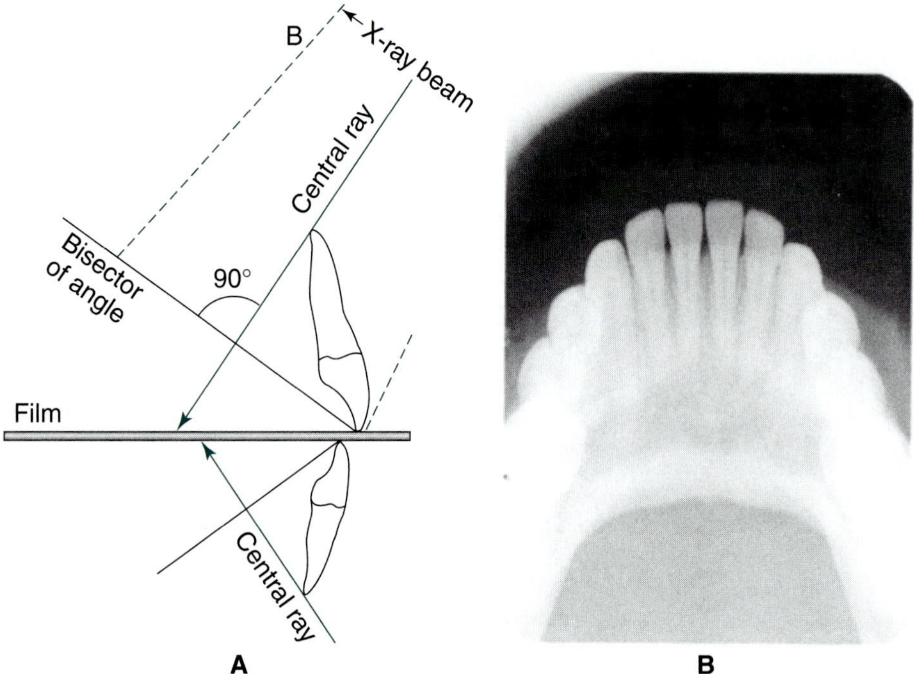

FIGURE 16–3. **Topographical projections.** (**A**) Diagram illustrating angulation theory of topographic projections. A topographic radiograph appears similar to ordinary periapical film except that it is larger. Angulation rules for topographical projections are identical to those for the bisecting technique. The central ray is directed through the apex of the teeth at right angles to the bisector. Vertical angulations are increased when examining areas in the distal part of the palate. (**B**) A **typical radiograph** of a mandibular anterior exposure.

The Mandibular Cross-Sectional Survey

The following sequence of steps is suggested to make the **mandibular cross-sectional survey** (see Figure 16–4).

1. Place the patient in a reclined position and insert the film packet axis horizontally in the mouth.
2. **Establish the horizontal angulation** at 0 degree to the midsagittal plane and set the vertical angulation at 0 degree and parallel to the plane of the floor.
3. Direct the PID toward the center of the film through the point of entry, approximately 1 in. (2.5 cm) below the point of the chin.
4. Make the exposure.

The technique for the mandibular incisor survey, with slight changes in film placement and in horizontal and vertical angulations, will give a canine, molar, or floor of the mouth survey.

If the patient is edentulous, position the film packet axis horizontally. The patient places the forefingers against the anterior border of the film to keep it from sliding forward and upward. If the patient has an upper denture, it may be left in the mouth to bite against the film.

For special results or in special situations, other head positions, film positions, or angulations may be used. Exposure procedures vary slightly according to the lesion or structure to be examined. The patient's size, age, and the density of the bone structures must be considered when determining the exposure factors.

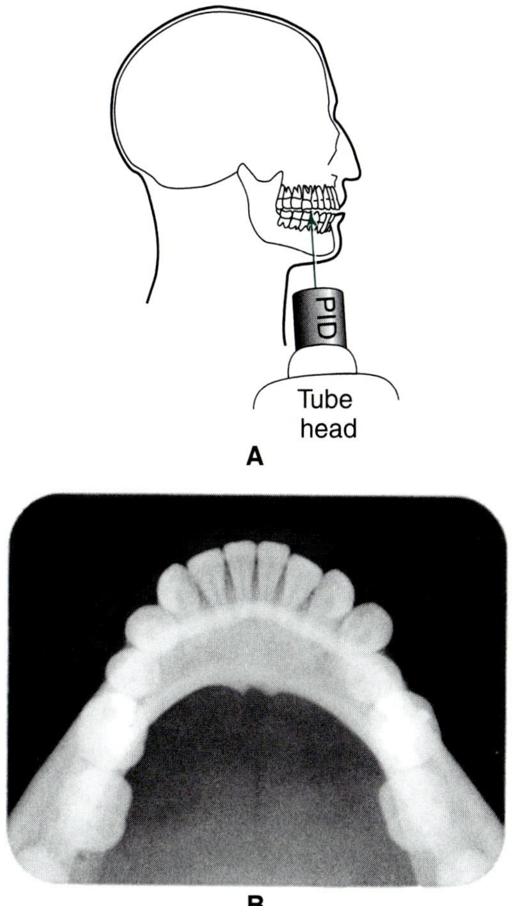

FIGURE 16–4. **Cross-sectional view.** (**A**) Diagram showing relationship of the tube head and PID to occlusal film and patient for a cross-sectional view of the entire mandibular arch. Exposure side of the film faces the mandibular arch with the widest dimension (longest) at right angles to the midsagittal plane. The central ray is directed perpendicularly to the occlusal plane through the inferior aspect of the mandible toward the center of the film. Slight modifications of this position must be made when the center of interest is in the canine or molar area of when a topographical view of the incisor area is desired. (**B**) Typical radiograph of cross-sectional view of the entire mandibular arch.

CHAPTER SUMMARY

The occlusal examination is made by inserting a film packet between the occlusal surfaces of the patient's teeth. Although the occlusal examination can be made alone, it is usually made to supplement the periapical survey. If the mouth opening is large enough, the #4 occlusal packet is preferred.

Advantages of the occlusal survey are the following:

1. A larger area than is possible on a periapical film can be visualized in its entirety.
2. A three-dimensional effect can be obtained by viewing an occlusal and periapical radiograph simultaneously.
3. The film packet is easy to position on a disturbed or uncooperative patient.

Two angulation techniques are employed.

1. The **topographical,** which is based on a modification of the bisecting principle. It is used to view fractures and large lesions.
2. The **cross-sectional,** which is based on directing the central rays toward the film at a right angle. It is used to establish buccolingual dimensions and to locate impactions or erupting teeth that are out of normal alignment.

REVIEW QUESTIONS

1. State the purpose of the occlusal radiographic examination.
2. Which of these film sizes is known as the occlusal?

   (a) #1
   (b) #2
   (c) #3
   (d) #4

3. How many films are generally inside the occlusal packet?

   (a) 1
   (b) 2
   (c) 3
   (d) 4

4. What term best describes the appearance of the image of the occlusal surfaces of the teeth when the cross-sectional technique is used for making the occlusal survey?

   (a) Overlapped
   (b) Elongated
   (c) Elliptical
   (d) Foreshortened

5. In which of these situations is an occlusal survey not indicated?

   (a) To determine the shape of the dental arch
   (b) To locate the position of an impacted canine
   (c) To reveal a fracture
   (d) To reveal the extent of periodontal lesions

6. When comparing the images of the teeth as shown on an occlusal topographical survey with the same images on a periapical survey, what will the images shown on the occlusal film appear to be?

   (a) Foreshortened
   (b) Elongated
   (c) Tilted mesially
   (d) Tilted distally

BIBLIOGRAPHY

Eastman Kodak. *Successful Intraoral Radiography*. Rochester, NY: Eastman Kodak, 1998.

White, S. C & Pharoah, M. J. *Oral Radiology Principles and Interpretation*. 4th ed. St. Louis: Mosby, 2000.

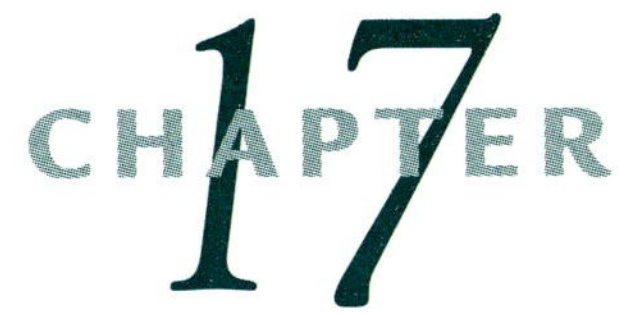

Radiographic Techniques for Children

OBJECTIVES

By the end of this chapter the student should be able to:

- Define the key words.
- Discuss the importance of making radiographic examinations on children.
- Identify the factors that determine when radiographs on children should be made.
- Discuss the suggested techniques for pediatric radiography.
- Discuss the film requirements for the pediatric survey.
- Explain the bitewing and periapical procedures for exposing radiographs on children.

KEY WORDS

Amelogenesis imperfecta
Anodontia
Aphthous ulcer
Deciduous teeth
Dentigerous cysts
Fistula
Herpes labialis
Parulis
Pediatric dentistry
Pulp polyp
Supernumerary teeth

Introduction

Pediatric dentistry (*pedia* is Greek for child) is the branch of dentistry dealing with the diagnosis and treatment of children's teeth. Children have the same basic needs for dental treatment, as do adults. In fact, the best time to prevent dental problems is in childhood. Although the teeth form and begin to calcify in the prenatal stage, much of the rapid growth of teeth and facial bones takes place between birth and 6 years. During these formative years the danger of permanent damage from dental neglect is greatest.

One frequent problem is infected teeth, which can seriously affect a child's health. The longer the source of infection remains hidden, the greater the effect on the patient. Because of infection, **deciduous teeth** may be lost too early and cause severe damage to the occlusion. Hidden lesions can only be detected by frequent periodic examinations including radiographs.

The purpose of this chapter is to discuss pediatric radiography and to present the techniques used for radiographing children.

Role of Radiography in Protecting Deciduous Teeth

Radiography is vital to both prevention and treatment. Through the use of radiographs, the dentist can locate dental caries in their beginning stages, detect lesions and infected teeth, and check how well treatment is progressing, The radiograph shows the roots of the deciduous teeth as well as the developing permanent teeth within the alveolar bone. Timely dental treatment can often avert the premature loss of the deciduous teeth and the subsequent malocclusion, which can turn the child into a dental cripple.

Disturbances in normal development, such as **anodontia** (absence of teeth), **supernumerary** (extra)

teeth, amelogenesis imperfecta (failure of the enamel to develop fully), the presence of **dentigerous cysts** (sacs containing fluid or producing teeth), and a host of other conditions can be discovered only through radiographs.

When to Expose Radiographs on Children

Several factors determine how often the child's teeth should be x-rayed and the size and number of films used. These include the:

- Dental needs of the child
- Cooperation and emotional stability of the child
- Size of the mouth opening
- Size and shape of the teeth and the dental arches
- Operator's ability to position the film
- Child's ability to retain the film and keep it still

The present position of the American Dental Association is that radiographs should only be made when, in the opinion of the dentist, there is a valid reason that they would benefit the patient (see Chapter 6). Unless an accident, toothache, or some other unusual circumstance causes a parent to bring a child to the dentist sooner, the **first radiographic survey** is often made soon after all the deciduous teeth have erupted **at 3 years.** A **second** complete radiographic survey may be made when the child is about **6 years;** the age when the first deciduous teeth are shed and the first of the permanent teeth erupt. A **third** survey may be made at **9 years,** when the child has a combination of deciduous and permanent teeth. The **fourth** survey is often made between **12 and 14 years,** when the last deciduous teeth are lost. After this, film placement, size, and number are the same as for adults.

Except in emergencies, bitewing surveys are made as needed between complete surveys to detect caries or other incipient lesions.

Suggested Techniques for Pediatric Radiography

Methods for exposing radiographs on children are basically the same as those for adults. Although either the bisecting or paralleling technique can be employed, many children are too small for periapical film positioning or often cannot manage film holders.

First Impressions

First impressions are always important and lasting. The young child's first visit to the dental office and the x-ray room should be pleasant and informative. Most children are extremely curious. Usually it is best to greet and take the child from the reception room to the x-ray room without the parents. Talking to and showing the child some of the equipment to be used and radiographs of other children will help in gaining the child's confidence. Since the child's first experience with radiography is such an important one, the visit should not be hurried and the operator must refrain from showing signs of impatience.

Only in emergencies should a child ever be forced to have any dental treatment. It is much better to delay until the second or third visit than to instill a lasting fear of dentistry. If the child remains uncooperative after the third visit, a telephone call to the child's physician may be advisable to arrange for sedation. The sedative should be administered shortly before the appointment.

Explain the Procedure

The radiographic survey should be explained to the child in simple terms. For example, the x-ray machine can be explained as a camera that takes pictures of the teeth.

Show and Tell

Conduct a **show and tell session** with the patient. The child should be given a film packet to feel and to handle. It may be unwrapped so that the child can see the film. If a film holder is to be used, the child should be allowed to examine and handle it, perhaps to put it in the mouth to become convinced that it is not an object to be feared. The entire procedure should be carefully explained and rehearsed. No exposure should be attempted before the child is emotionally prepared for the experience and understands what is to be done.

Sensitive Tissues

Special consideration must be given to the child whose oral tissues are still in the formative stage. The oral mucosa of the young child is extremely sensitive to the slightest pressure, especially when teeth are erupting or about to be shed.

Small mouths can make it hard to radiograph children. If film holders are used, they should not be too bulky or heavy. The plastic backing plate on some holders can be cut down to a smaller size.

The oral cavity should be examined thoroughly for loose or erupting teeth, any **parulis** (**fistula** or gum boil), **pulp polyps, herpes labialis** (cold sores), **aphthous ulcers** (canker sores), or swollen salivary glands.

Sequence

The easiest and most comfortable exposures, normally radiographs of the anterior teeth, should be exposed first to gain the child's confidence and to get the child accustomed to having a film in the mouth. A young child's span of attention is not very long, and one must repeat instructions with each exposure. Young children are often fidgety and restless, so when the child is finally ready, exposures should be made as rapidly as possible.

Be Confident

Most children react favorably to the authority of a confident, capable operator. Occasionally, a stubborn or frightened child proves difficult to manage. If such a child does not respond to firmness, a parent or older brother or sister may accompany the child into the x-ray room. In fact, if the child is too small to understand instructions or unable to hold the film, a parent or accompanying adult may have to hold the film while it is being exposed. The dentist, the dental hygienist, or the dental assistant should never hold the film in the mouth of a patient.

Problem Using Periapical Films

One problem in using periapical films is the distortion caused by the **flatness of the palate** and the **floor of the mouth** in children. Because of it, films lie flatter than they do in the mouths of most adults. This position results in an increase in the size of the angle between the teeth and the films, requiring an adjustment to compensate. When bisecting methods are used, the steepness of the vertical angulation is increased.

This problem can be solved by use of the **paralleling technique.** The biteblocks on the XCP instruments can be modified by reducing the size of the backing plate with shears or a knife to accommodate the #0 film. If the child objects to the film holder in the mouth or has difficulty biting hard enough to stabilize it, have the child hold the film with the thumb or index finger, guided by the radiographer.

When the child is too small to be seated in the dental chair, the child can sit on the parent's lap in the chair and the parent can hold the film. Under no circumstances should the radiographer hold the film packet.

Use of Lead Apron

A **lead apron** should always be placed over the patient. Special small lead aprons are available. As the bone structure on a child is smaller and less dense than that of an adult, average exposure time can be reduced by about one third.

Film Requirements for the Pediatric Radiographic Survey

Film requirements depend upon the age and size of the child.

Primary Dentition

Small size, tongue resistance, and gagging can be a problem in **small children** (3 to 6 years old). Ideally, it is advisable to expose **four films,** one anterior occlusal film in each jaw and one posterior bitewing on each side (see Figure 17–1).

Mixed Dentition

At **6 years,** the first permanent teeth have begun to erupt. Ideally, the **survey includes a minimum of 12 radiographs,** 10 periapical and two bitewing exposures. The periapical films are exposed in each of the four molar and canine (cuspid) areas and in the two incisor areas. As the child is now more mature, it may be possible to make the periapical exposures of all tooth areas. If using periapical films is still not feasible, the survey can be made with a minimum of six films, two occlusal, two extraoral, and two bitewings.

At **9 years,** the child has a mixed dentition. This examination may be made with **as few as 6 and as many as 18 exposures.** The larger #2 periapical films can often be used at this age; however, the smaller film sizes are most frequently used (see Figure 17–2).

Between **12 and 14 years of age,** the child may have all permanent teeth except the third molars. It is during this preadolescent period that growth is most rapid and metabolic changes occur that heighten the possibility of dental caries and increase the need for vigilance and preventive care. This survey may be made with **14 periapical and 4 bitewing films.** It is the same as that for the adult, and larger films can be used.

Panoramic Radiograph

A **panoramic radiograph** (see Chapter 21) of the entire dentition can be made to view the overall jaw develop-

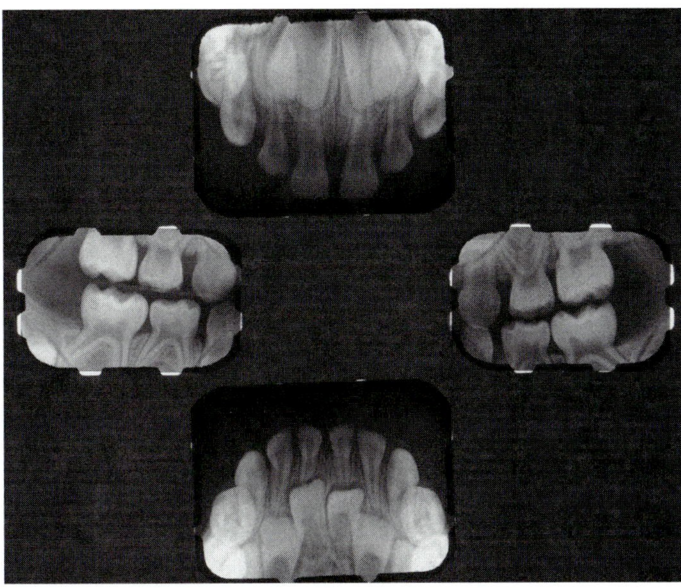

FIGURE 17–1. **Typical four film radiographic survey.** One anterior occlusal film in each jaw and one posterior bitewing film on each side. (Courtesy Dr. Dennis P. Gutz, University Nebraska Medical Center, College of Dentistry, Lincoln, NE)

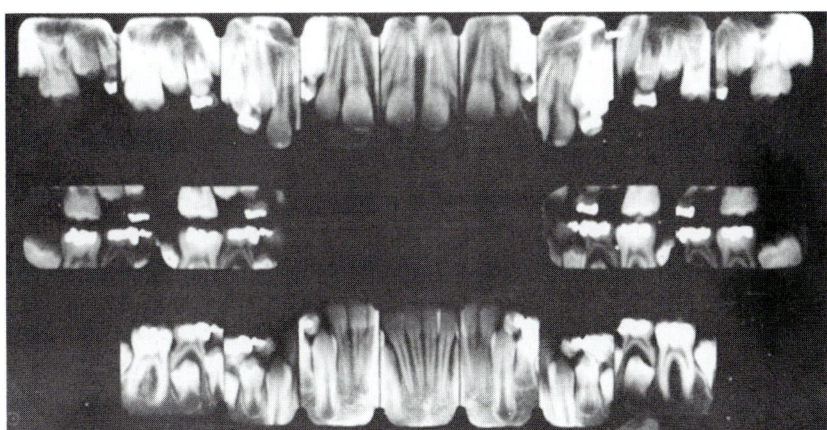

FIGURE 17–2. **Complete radiographic periapical and bitewing series on a 9-year-old child.** Depending on the size of the child, fewer films of several sizes may be used to make such a survey. (Courtesy of McCormack Dental X-ray Laboratory)

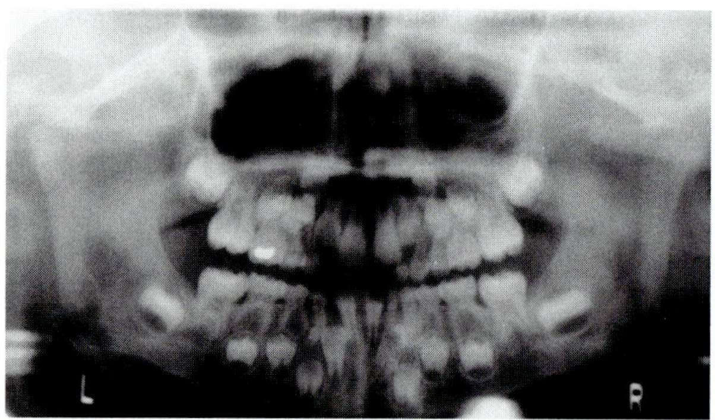

FIGURE 17-3. **Panoramic radiograph** of the entire dentition can be made to view the overall jaw development and growth of the teeth.

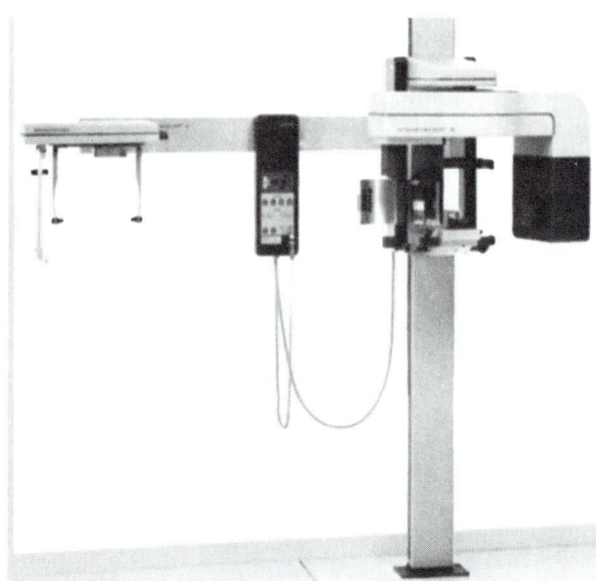

FIGURE 17-4. **Photograph of Orthoceph 10.** By having the child stand in position and adjusting the earplugs for size and height, it is possible to make cephalometric lateral skull and posteroanterior radiographs. The loaded cassette is inserted into the adjustable cassette holder and positioned parallel to the child's face. The head positioner can be rotated as needed. (Courtesy of Siemens Medical Systems, Inc., Dental Division, Iselin, NJ)

ment and growth of the teeth (see Figures 17–3 and 17–4). Such large radiographs may be supplemental to periapical exposures or may serve as the chief source of diagnostic information and be supplemented by periapical or bitewing films.

Bitewing and Periapical Exposures for Children

With few minor exceptions to compensate for the child's smaller mouth, the same technical procedures described in Chapters 14 and 15 are used when exposing radiographs on children. The main difference is in the use of smaller films and shorter exposure times. Depending on the age and size of the child, the exposure time is about one third less than used for making bitewing or periapical exposures on an adult. In addition, in some areas a slightly steeper vertical angulation than is customary in adults is used to compensate for the flatter palate and shallow floor of the mouth during bisecting. Other minor changes in technique are listed below for each of the exposures commonly made in a full-mouth series of radiographs for children.

Posterior Bitewing Survey

Only one **bitewing** film is required on each side unless the second permanent molars have already erupted (see Figure 17–5). Many dentists prefer two films on each side

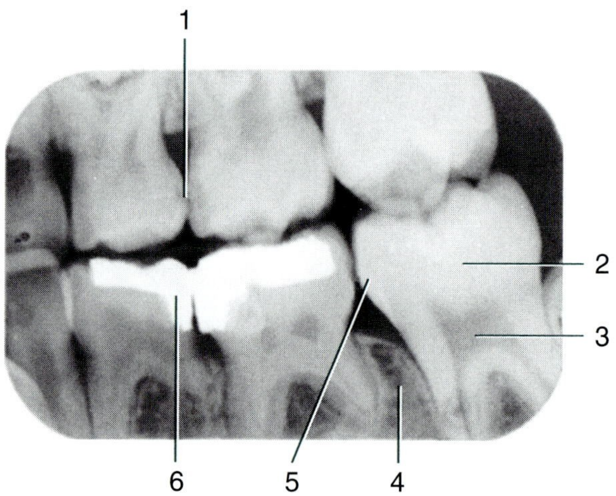

FIGURE 17-5. **Posterior bitewing radiograph of mixed dentition** exposed on #0 film shows (**1**) incipient caries in the interproximal areas between the maxillary first and second deciduous molars, (**2**) normal-appearing dentin in mandibular first permanent molar, (**3**) pulp chamber, (**4**) alveolar bone, (**5**) normal-appearing enamel covering of crown, and (**6**) metallic restorations on mandibular deciduous first and second molars.

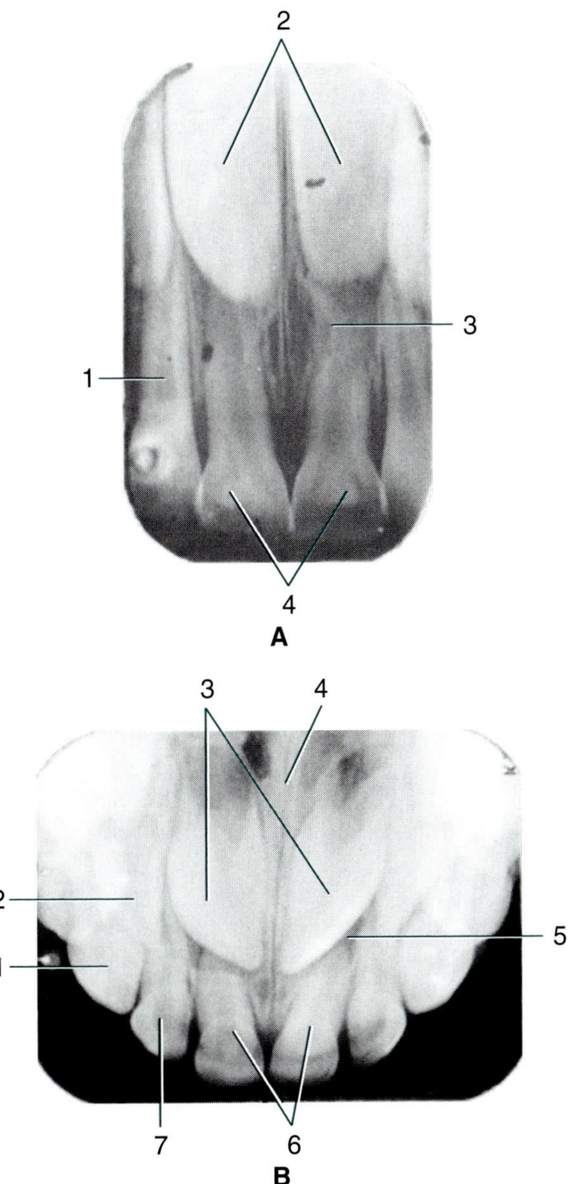

FIGURE 17-6. **Radiographs of maxillary incisor areas. A.** Exposure with #0 film shows (**1**) fully erupted deciduous lateral incisor, (**2**) crowns of unerupted permanent central incisors, (**3**) roots of deciduous central incisors showing signs of natural resorption, and (4) deciduous central incisors. **B.** An alternate method of exposing the maxillary anterior teeth is to use the occlusal technique with a standard #2 film. Observe the following: (**1**) deciduous canine, (**2**) crown of permanent lateral incisor, (**3**) unerupted permanent central incisors—note that root formation has not started yet, (**4**) thin radiolucent line indicating the location of the median palatine suture, (**5**) partially resorbed root of deciduous central incisor, (**6**) deciduous central incisors, and (**7**) deciduous lateral incisor.

if the child has permanent molars. The front edge of the film should cover the distal half of the mandibular canine (cuspid). Corners of the film packet may be softened so as not to bruise the delicate oral tissues. The vertical angulation is +10 degrees.

Maxillary Incisor Survey

Depending on the technique, the film is placed in the mouth vertically and held in place by the child's finger, or it is placed vertically in the biteblock on which the child closes (see Figure 17–6). The film is **centered at the midline.** The average vertical angulation is +45 to +50 degrees if using the bisecting method. Refer to Chapter 14 for procedures on the periapical exposures.

Maxillary Canine (Cuspid) Survey

Follow the same procedure as for the maxillary incisor survey but shift the film laterally so that it is **centered** over the long axis of the **maxillary canine (cuspid).** For the bisecting technique, the average vertical angulation ranges from +55 to +60 degrees (see Figure 17–7).

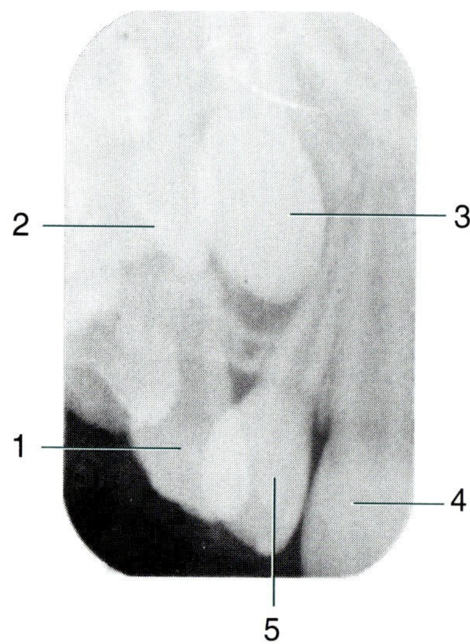

FIGURE 17–7. **Radiograph of maxillary canine area.** Exposure shows (**1**) deciduous canine, (**2**) crown of first premolar, (**3**) unerupted permanent canine with part of crown still in a follicle as indicated by radiolucent area around the tip of the crown, (**4**) permanent central incisor, and (**5**) permanent lateral incisor, which appears to be tipped distally and overlapping with deciduous canine.

Maxillary Molar Survey

Position the film horizontally over the molar area with the **front edge** covering the **distal half of the maxillary canine (cuspid).** For the bisecting technique, average vertical angulation ranges from +30 to +55 degrees (see Figure 17–8).

When making any of these exposures for the first time, review how to use the film holders (Chapter 14) and modify these procedures for the child patient. The paralleling technique is the method of choice.

Mandibular Incisor Survey

Depending on the technique, the film is placed in the mouth vertically and held in place by the child's finger, or it is placed vertically in the biteblock on which the child closes (see Figure 17–9). **Center the film** at the **midline** and allow about 1/8 in. (3 mm) of the film to protrude above the incisal edge to leave an incisal margin. The average vertical angulation for bisecting is –20 to –25 degrees.

Mandibular Canine (Cuspid) Survey

Except for minor positioning and angulation changes, follow the same procedures as for the mandibular incisors. **Center the film over** the long axis of the **mandibular canine (cuspid).** The average vertical angu-

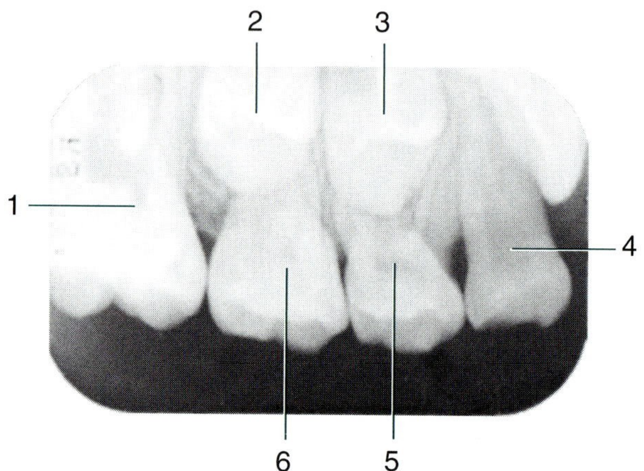

FIGURE 17–8. **Radiograph of maxillary molar area.** Exposure shows (**1**) permanent first molar, (**2**) crown of unerupted second premolar, (**3**) crown of unerupted first premolar, (**4**) deciduous canine, (**5**) deciduous first molar (note that the roots are almost completely resorbed), and (**6**) deciduous second molar. Note that the shadow of the still unresorbed lingual root is superimposed on the crown of the still unerupted second

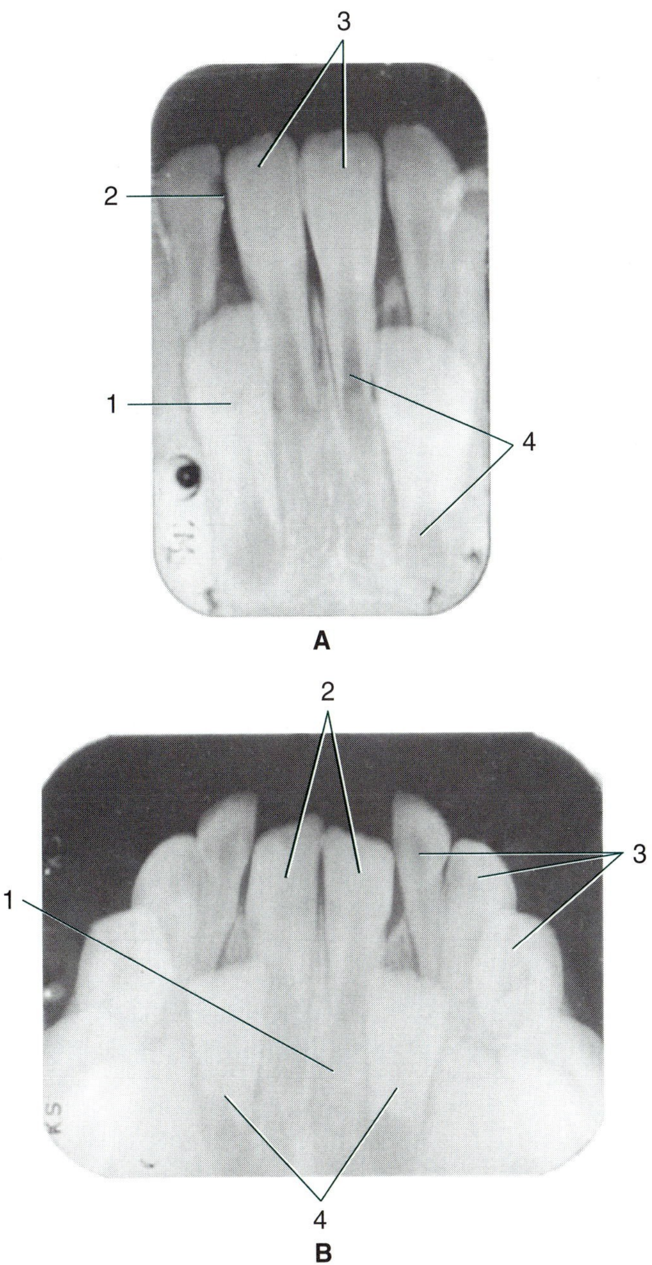

FIGURE 17-9. **Radiographs of the mandibular incisor areas**. **A.** (**1**) unerupted permanent lateral incisor, (**2**) incipient caries on mesial surface of deciduous lateral incisor, (**3**) fully erupted permanent central incisors, and (**4**) large open apex area on all permanent teeth indicating that root formation is still in progress. Root formation is generally not complete until about 2 or 3 years following tooth eruption. **B.** An alternate method of exposing the mandibular anterior teeth is to use the occlusal technique with a standard size #2 film. Observe the following: (**1**) alveolar bone, (**2**) partially erupted permanent central incisors, (**3**) deciduous teeth, soon to be exfoliated, and (**4**) unerupted permanent lateral incisors.

lation to −25 to −30 degrees if using the bisecting method (see Figure 17–10).

Mandibular Molar Survey

The film is positioned horizontally and held by the child's finger or is placed horizontally in the biteblock on which the child closes. The film is **centered** over the **mandibular molars.** If possible, the **front edge of the film** should **cover the distal half** of the **mandibular canine (cuspid).** The average vertical angulation is between −15 and −20 degrees if using the bisecting method (see Figure 17–11).

The Occlusal Survey for Children

The **occlusal technique** is the same for children as for adults, except that the exposure time is decreased. Although the film may be positioned several ways, the maxillary and mandibular topographical surveys described in Chapter 16 are the two variations used most often if the large occlusal film is used. When the child's mouth is too small to accommodate the occlusal film, a smaller film, usually the #2 posterior, is positioned in whatever direction will give the maximum coverage of the desired area.

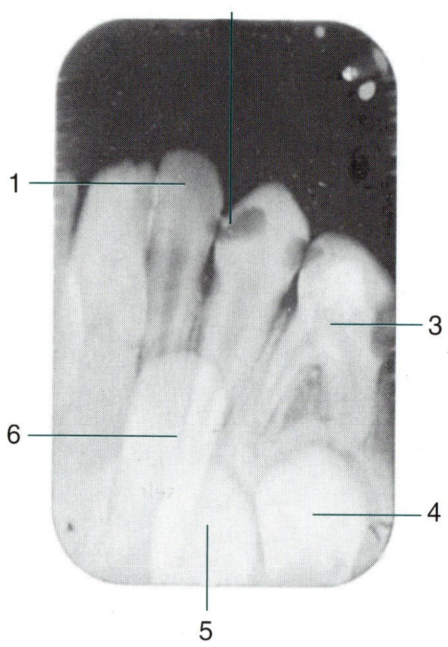

FIGURE 17–10. **Radiograph of mandibular canine (cuspid) area.** Exposure shows (**1**) deciduous lateral incisor, (**2**) radiolucent areas on mesial and distal of deciduous canine, which appear to be restored with silicate or acrylic resin; however, this must be confirmed by visual examination because the esthetic filling materials and dental caries often look similar on radiographs, (**3**) deciduous first molar, (**4**) unerupted first premolar, (**5**) unerupted canine, and (**6**) unerupted permanent lateral incisor.

The Lateral Jaw Survey for Children

The technique for making the **lateral jaw exposure** is fully described in Chapter 20. The exposure can be made with any size extraoral film or with an occlusal film placed against the cheek when the child is small.

If an occlusal film is used, line up the longest dimension of the film so that it is flush with the lower border of the mandible and line up the front edge of the film with the corner of the mouth. Place the tube side of the film against the cheek and ask the child to hold it with the fingers or palm of the hand. Use the ala-tragus line as a guide to parallel the child's occlusal plane with the plane of the floor, and press against the top of the child's head gently until the head is tipped about 20 degrees toward the side of the film. Then ask the child to close the mouth so that the upper and lower teeth touch each other. Direct the central ray through a point of entry toward the center of the film at a vertical angulation of about −10 degrees from a point slightly behind and below the angle of the opposite mandible.

When extraoral films are used, the film size depends on the size of the child's head and the structures that the dentist wishes to include. Place the tube side toward the cheek and center the film so that it covers ad structures of interest. Several head positions are used with extraoral films; the child may be upright or supine, or the cassette may be laid flat on a table and the child sits in front of it and bends the head until the face contacts the tube side. With some practice each operator develops a favorite technique.

Helpful Hints

- Be confident. Most children react favorably to the authority of a confident, capable operator.
- First impressions are always important and lasting. The young child's first visit to the dental office and the x-ray room should be pleasant.
- Explain the radiographic survey to the child in simple terms.
- Show and tell. Show the child the film and instruments that will be used and tell the child to handle them.
- Be gentle. The oral tissues of the young child are extremely sensitive to the slightest pressure.

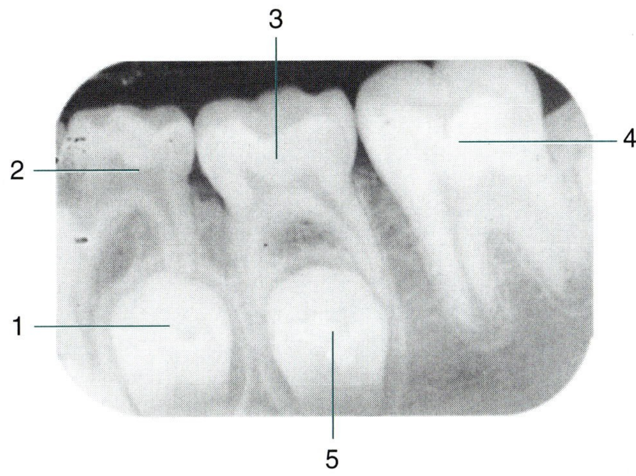

FIGURE 17–11. **Radiograph of mandibular molar area**. Mixed dentition shows (**1**) unerupted first premolar, (**2**) deciduous first molar with partial resorption of distal root, (**3**) deciduous second molar, (**4**) permanent first molar, and (**5**) unerupted second premolar.

CHAPTER SUMMARY

Good radiographs are essential if the dentist is to provide proper care for the child patient. Without radiographs incipient caries would be overlooked during a mirror and explorer examination, and studies of facial growth and development or tooth eruption could not be accurately made.

Any size film, in whatever number suits the purpose, may be used. The first exposures should be preplanned, rather than in frightening emergency situations, and at a preschool age, preferably when the child is about 3 years old.

The procedures may vary, intraoral or extraoral, with slight modifications because of the smaller size of the face, the dental arches, and the teeth, but they are similar to those performed on adults. A major difference is in the psychological approach. The child has a natural curiosity combined with a fear of the unknown. Securing the child's confidence and cooperation is absolutely essential because the radiograph is useless if the child moves suddenly or fails to hold the film in position.

Greater care must be exercised in positioning the film packet because some of the deciduous teeth may be loose. Because the bony structures are smaller, the exposure time required is about one third shorter.

REVIEW QUESTIONS

1. At what age is the first radiographic survey usually made on a child?
   (a) Age 3
   (b) Age 6
   (c) Age 9
   (d) Age 12

2. Which of these conditions would not interfere with film packet positioning in a child?
   (a) Herpes labialis
   (b) Loose teeth
   (c) Calculus deposits
   (d) Malpositioned teeth

3. Which of these factors does not need to be considered when deciding what size film to use on a child?
   (a) The size and shape of the dental arches
   (b) The degree of stain or calculus present
   (c) The size and shape of the mouth opening
   (d) The age and emotional stability of the child

4. What is the best time to give a nervous child sedation prior to radiographic procedures?
   (a) The evening before the appointment
   (b) Before breakfast on the day of the appointment
   (c) At least 2 hours before the appointment
   (d) About 20 minutes before the appointment

5. What change in angulation is usually required when using the bisecting technique on a child patient?
   (a) Direct the horizontal angulation mesiodistally.
   (b) Direct the horizontal angulation distomesially.
   (c) Increase the vertical angulation.
   (d) Decrease the vertical angulation.

6. Which of these is not a benefit derived from making radiographic surveys on children?
   (a) Incipient carious lesions can be detected.
   (b) Anodontia can be prevented.
   (c) Supernumerary teeth can be detected.
   (d) Abnormal tooth development can be detected.

7. Which film size is generally easiest to position on a 6-year-old child?
   (a) #1
   (b) #2
   (c) #3
   (d) #4

BIBLIOGRAPHY

Eastman Kodak. *Successful Intraoral Radiography*. Rochester, NY: Eastman Kodak, 1998.

Nowak, A. J., Creedon, R. L., & Musselman, R. J. et al. Summary of the conference on radiation exposure in pediatric dentistry. *J. Am. Dent. Assoc.* 103: 426–428, 1981.

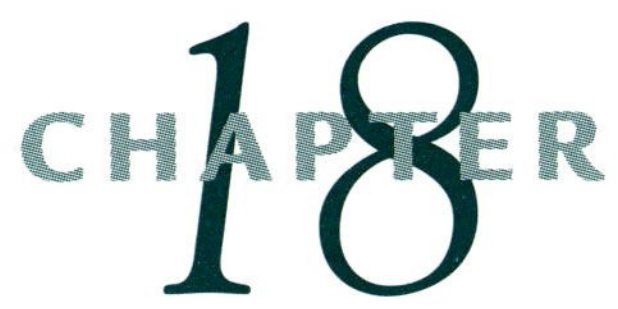

Radiographic Techniques for the Edentulous Patient

OBJECTIVES

By the end of this chapter the student should be able to:

- Define the key words.
- Explain the importance of making a radiographic survey of edentulous areas.
- Identify the film requirements for an edentulous survey.
- Name and describe the three techniques for radiographing edentulous patients.

KEY WORDS

Edentulous
Landmarks
Occlusal radiograph
Panoramic radiograph
Periapical radiographs
Preventive radiography
Ridges

Introduction

The term **edentulous** means "without teeth." Most edentulous patients (patients without teeth) have lost their teeth through neglect of decay, infection, or untreated periodontal conditions. A complete examination of the edentulous patient includes radiographs along with the visual and digital inspection.

The purpose of this chapter is to explain the importance and methods of radiographing the edentulous patient.

The Importance of Radiography for the Edentulous Patient

Preventive radiography is often of great benefit to the fully and partially edentulous patient because the normal appearance of the dental **ridges** may conceal problems underneath.

The dentist orders radiographs for the edentulous patient for the following reasons:

- To detect the presence of retained roots, impacted teeth, foreign bodies, cysts, and other pathological lesions.
- To establish the position of the mental foramen before constructing dentures.
- To establish the position of the mandibular canal before implant surgery.
- To determine the quantity of alveolar bone present.
- To observe the quality of the maxillary and mandibular bone.

Potential sources of difficulty may be present in a substantial number of edentulous ridges that interfere with the comfortable wearing of prosthetic appliances. The Dental Radiographic Patient Selection Criteria Panel, sponsored by the Food and Drug Administration, recommends a full-mouth intraoral radiographic or panoramic examination for newly edentulous patients (see Chapter 6).

Film Requirements

Several methods involving various combinations of intraoral, occlusal, or extraoral films are commonly used for a radiographic survey of the edentulous mouth using the conventional x-ray machine.

- Some dentists prefer to use **fourteen periapical films,** seven for the maxillary and seven for the mandibular ridge, placing the films over the same areas of the ridges as they would if the teeth were still present (see Figure 18–1).
- Others use only **ten periapical films,** five for the maxillary and five for the mandibular ridge (one in the incisor and four posterior films in each arch) (see Figure 18–2).

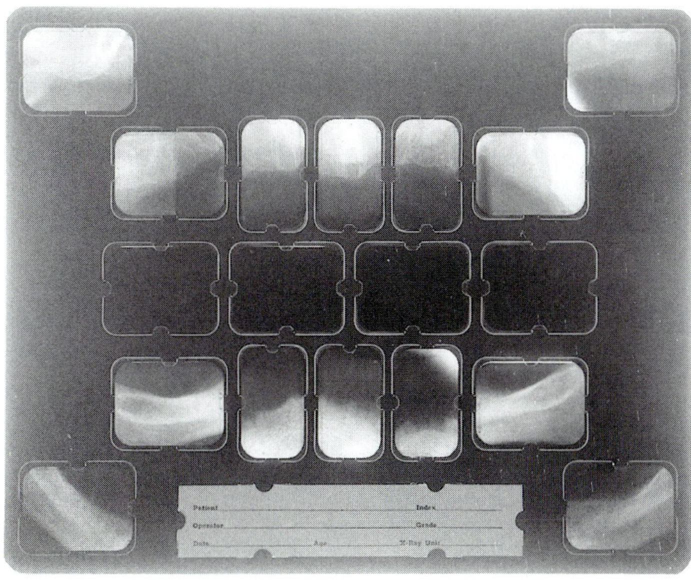

FIGURE 18–1. **Edentulous survey** made with 14 periapical films, seven for the maxillary and seven for the mandibular ridge. The films are placed over the same areas of the ridges as they would if the teeth were still present.

- Still others prefer a total of **seven films:** two occlusal films (one in each arch) and five periapical films (one in each of the four posterior regions and one in the mandibular incisor region).

Additional films can be used to supplement such a seven-film survey if the presence of some unsuspected object is detected and more information is required.

Edentulous Survey Techniques

The edentulous radiographic surveys can be made with **periapical radiographs, occlusal radiographs,** or a **panoramic radiograph.** Both the occlusal and panoramic radiographs do not show detail as well as periapical radiographs. Therefore, if suspicious areas are seen, periapical radiographs must be made as a supplement to the occlusal or panoramic radiograph to make a definitive diagnosis. As a rule, about 25 percent less exposure is required for an edentulous area than for one with teeth.

Periapical Technique

Periapical radiographs may be made using either the **paralleling technique** or the **bisecting technique.**

Fundamentally, the technique for exposing the 14 edentulous regions of the mandible or maxillae are very similar to the suggested procedures for exposing the periapical regions that were described in Chapter 14. The 6 anterior and 8 posterior exposures can be made with any size periapical film, but the standard #2 film is generally the film of choice.

Several minor modifications in technique are required for x-raying edentulous areas. Normally, the teeth serve as **landmarks** to guide film placement. Also, the center of interest is no longer the teeth but the ridge. Because the teeth are no longer present, visualizing the bisecting plane and establishing horizontal and vertical planes are more difficult, particularly when the bisecting technique is used. Fortunately, a fair amount of leeway in horizontal angulation is permissible, because the absence of teeth eliminates the problem of overlapping tooth images.

Paralleling Technique

The **paralleling technique** usually gives the best results. Radiographic detail is improved and dimensional distortion is minimized when film holders, properly supported by cotton rolls or styrofoam blocks, are used hold the film parallel to the long axis or the ridge.

When all the teeth are missing, cotton rolls, blocks of styrofoam, or a combination can be used, with ordinary biteblocks or film holders such as the XCP instruments.

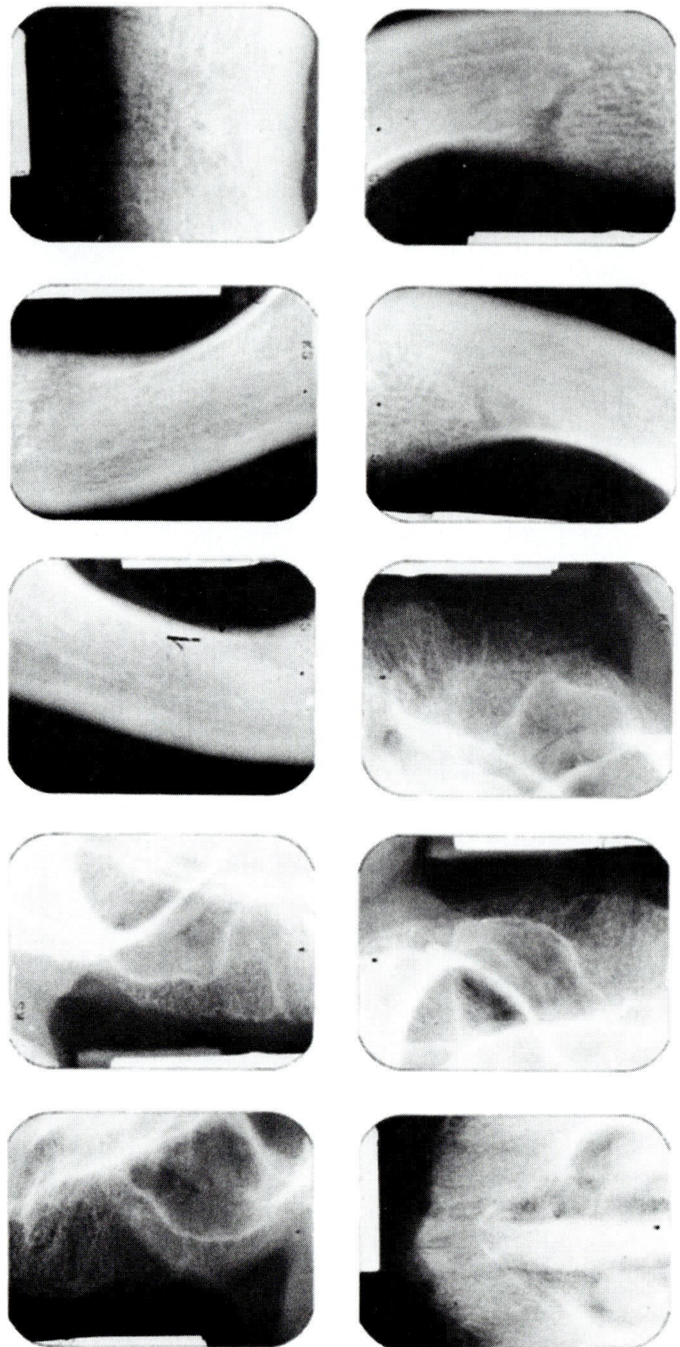

FIGURE 18-2. **Edentulous survey made with ten #2 periapical films.** All exposures were made with the paralleling technique, as evidenced by the radiopaque outline cast by the biteblocks. Can you mount these radiographs correctly? (Courtesy of UCLA School of Dentistry)

The thickness of the cotton rolls or styrofoam will determine the coverage of the edentulous ridge.

The film is placed vertically in the anterior biteblocks and horizontally in the posterior biteblocks. Because definite landmarks are seldom present, one must guess the best film position. Obviously, the incisor and molar regions are easiest to locate. Shifting the film distally or mesially is necessary to locate the canine and premolar regions. The biteblock or film holder is then placed in the mouth with the film parallel to the ridge being examined. The patient closes, holding the film in position. The final step is to direct the rays horizontally and vertically toward the center of the film perpendicularly to the mean tangent of the facial side of the ridge and to the plane of the film (Figure 18–3).

One can also modify this technique for use with the partially edentulous patient by substituting cotton rolls or a block of styrofoam for the space normally occupied by the crowns of the missing teeth and then following the standard procedures (Figure 18–4).

Bisecting Technique

In the **bisecting technique,** one determines vertical angulation by bisecting the angle formed between the recording plane of the film and an imaginary line through the ridge that substitutes for the long axes of the teeth (see Figure 18–5). Unfortunately, when the patient holds the film with the fingers, it lies much flatter than when teeth are present. This often results in a failure to show all the details of a small area, and in some, dimensional distortion of the visible structure occurs. However, acceptable radiographs can be produced.

Occlusal Technique

The **occlusal technique** is faster to take and subjects the patient to less radiation (see Figure 18–6). It has the advantage of pinpointing the location of root fragments, lesions, or other objects because two planes of reference are available instead of one. The occlusal film shows the buccolingual location of teeth or lesions in a horizontal

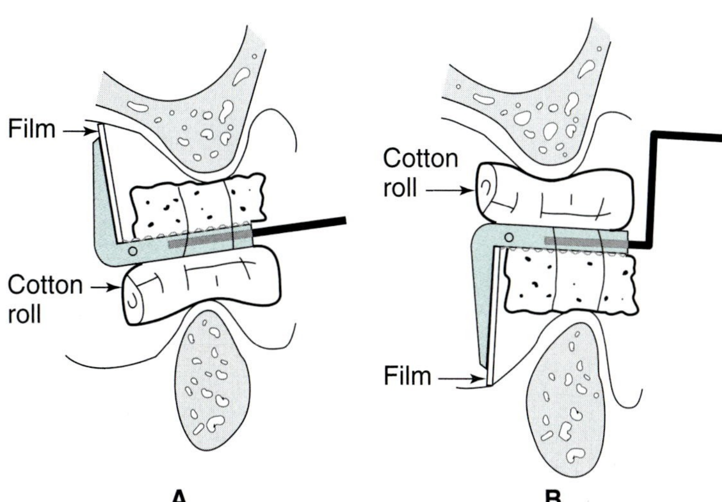

FIGURE 18–3. **Edentulous survey.** When all teeth are missing, cotton rolls, blocks of styrofoam, or a combination of both can be used with the XCP instruments. Their thickness will determine the amount of film coverage of the edentulous ridges. The instrument is positioned in the mouth with the film parallel to the ridge area being examined. The patient closes the mouth, stabilizing and holding the film in position, and the standard procedures are followed. (**A**) **Maxillary anterior region.** The film holder is rotated so the film is directed upward for the maxillary posterior areas. (**B**) **Mandibular posterior region.** The film holder is rotated so that the film is directed down for the mandibular areas. (Courtesy of Dentsply/Rinn Corporation)

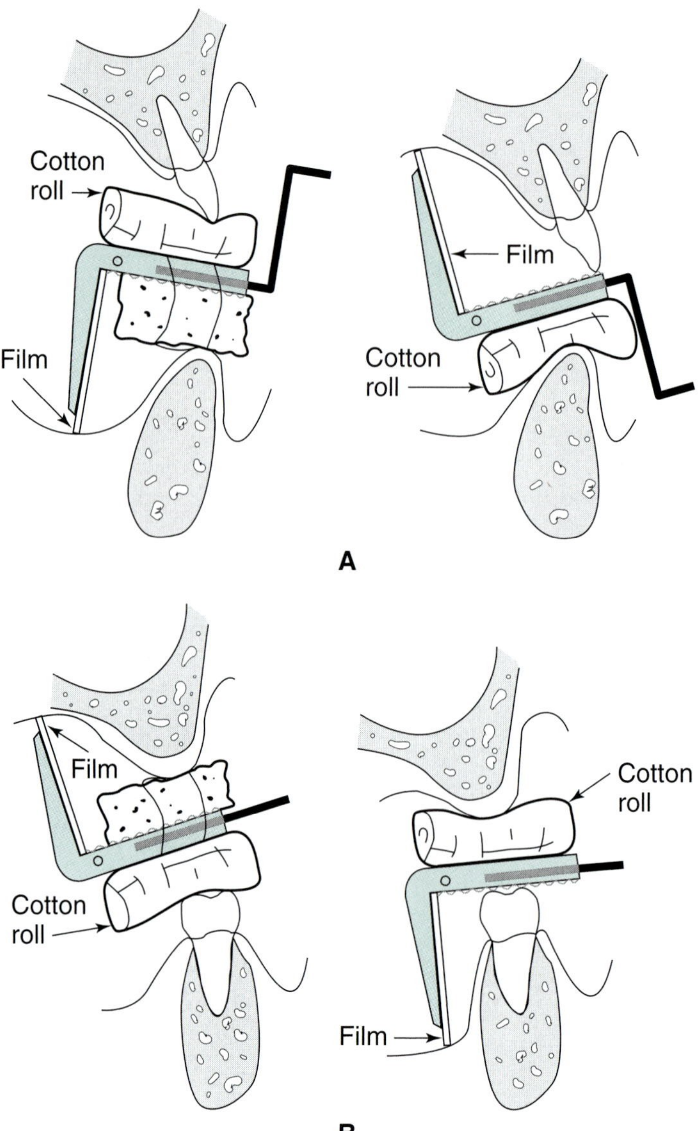

FIGURE 18–4. **Partially edentulous mouth.** The versatile XCP instruments can also be used in radiography of the partially edentulous mouth by substituting a cotton roll or block of styrofoam (or a similar radiolucent material) for the space normally occupied by the crowns of the missing teeth and then following standard procedures. (**A**) **Edentulous mandibular anterior region.** Opposite placement for the maxillary region. (**B**) **Edentulous maxillary posterior region.** Rotate the instrument the opposite way for the mandibular posterior areas. (Courtesy of Dentsply/Rinn Corporation)

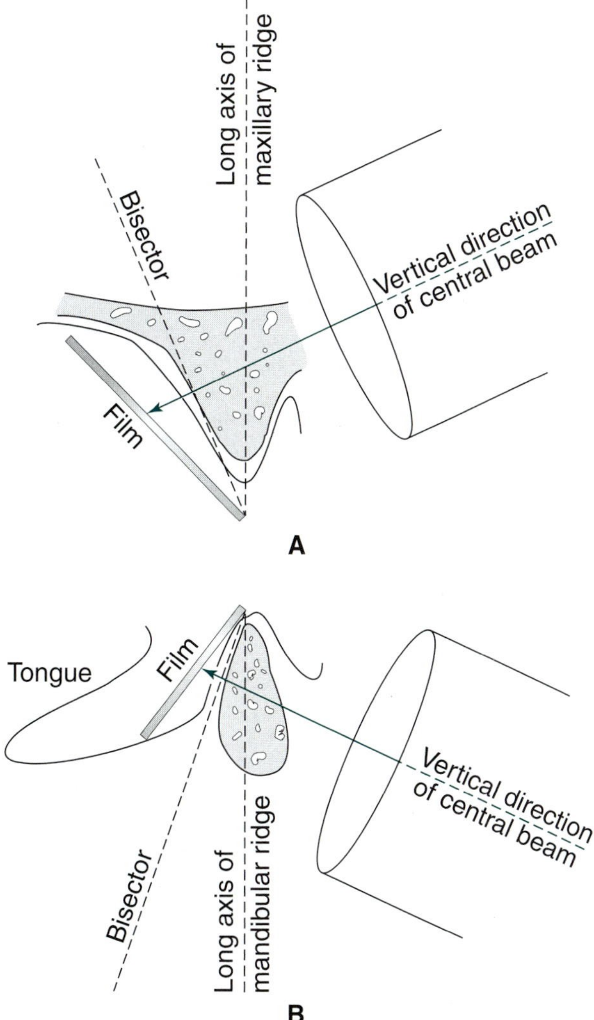

FIGURE 18–5. **Diagrams showing the relationship of the film to the ridge of an edentulous patient.** The film packet lies much flatter in the mouth when teeth are missing. Films are placed vertically for anterior and horizontally for posterior exposures. Unless film holders are used, the film is stabilized by the patient's thumb or index finger. When the rules of bisecting are followed, an imaginary line can be drawn vertically through the ridge to substitute for the long axis of the teeth formerly in the ridge. The central ray is directed perpendicularly to the bisector to determine the correct vertical angulation. The correct horizontal angulation is difficult to determine in the edentulous patient; however, it is not a major consideration since the absence of teeth eliminates overlapping. (**A**) Maxillary edentulous ridge, (**B**) Mandibular edentulous ridge.

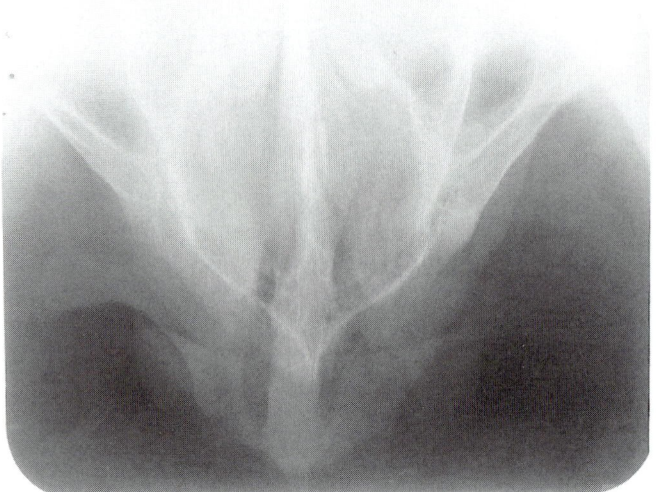

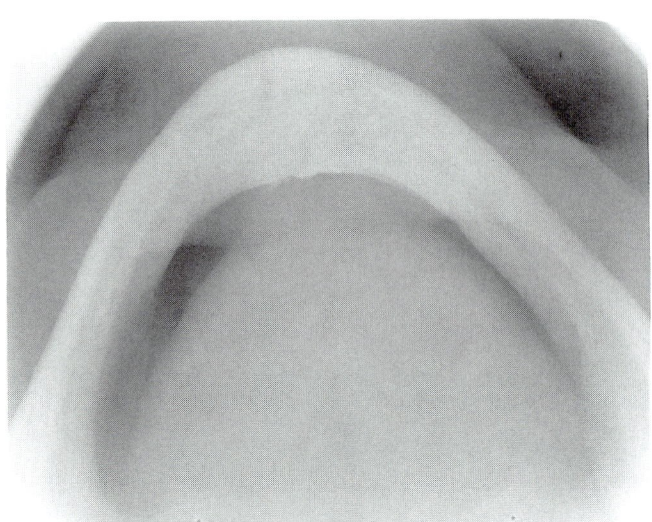

FIGURE 18–6. **Edentulous occlusal technique.** (**A**) Maxillary occlusal radiograph, (**B**) Mandibular occlusal radiograph.

plane, whereas the periapical films show them in a vertical plane.

The occlusal radiograph serves as an excellent guide in establishing the relative position of various structures or lesions to recognizable **landmarks.** However, it may not show some details that periapical radiographs do.

Periapical films are used in all four molar areas to supplement the occlusal film, because anatomical restrictions often keep the film from being inserted far enough back to include the third molar area. It is in this region that broken root fragments or unerupted teeth are most likely to be discovered.

The anterior region of the mandible is also radiographed, because the small size of the mandibular incisors and the deneseness of the bone near the front of the mandible often make the identification of small root fragments very difficult on occlusal radiographs.

Panoramic Technique

The easiest way of making the edentulous survey is with panoramic film (see Figure 18–7). Most edentulous surveys are made in this manner because it is convenient for the patient and requires only one film. All maxillary and

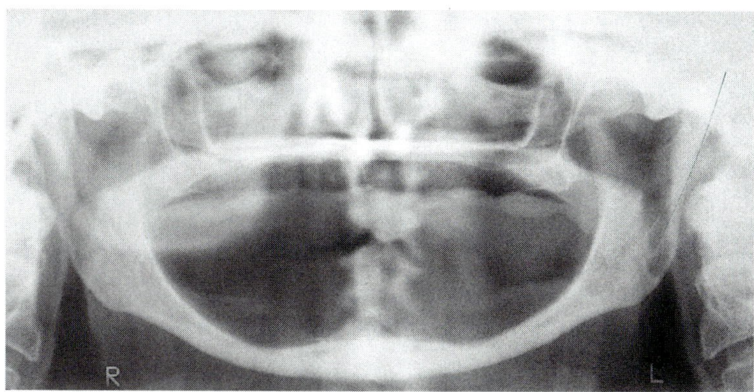

FIGURE 18–7. **Complete edentulous survey made on panoramic-type x-ray machine.** Relationship of the maxillary and mandibular structures is shown on a single radiograph.

mandibular structures can be visualized in proper relationship to each other. Panoramic techniques are explained in detail in Chapter 21.

If an examination of the panoramic radiograph reveals that unerupted teeth, root tips, or areas of suspected pathology are present, supplementary periapical films must be exposed. Periapical radiographs have greater definition and show more detail.

CHAPTER SUMMARY

It may be difficult to convince an edentulous person that radiographs are necessary, especially if there is no discomfort and the ridges appear healthy. However, the incidence of retained roots, impacted teeth, or other pathological conditions is high, and radiographs are a preventive measure.

The film requirements vary and are somewhat dependent on what equipment and film are available. A rapid survey of both ridges can be made on a panoramic film. By using a single film, all structures are shown in relation to each other. If necessary, supplemental films can be exposed.

Another procedure is to expose a series of 10 to 14 periapical films preferably by the paralleling method. The absence of teeth or landmarks makes positioning difficult. Horizontal angulation is less critical because there are no tooth structures to overlap.

It is irrelevant whether the exposures are intraoral or extraoral or a combination of both as long as all ridge areas are examined. Minor technique modifications are made when the patient is only partially edentulous.

REVIEW QUESTIONS

1. Which type of film is best suited to reveal the entire ridge?
   (a) Occlusal
   (b) Periapical
   (c) Bitewing
   (d) Panoramic

2. How much less exposure time is required when the patient is edentulous?
   (a) 10% less
   (b) 25% less
   (c) 45% less
   (d) 65% less

3. What type of film is never used when making edentulous exposures?
   (a) Occlusal
   (b) Periapical
   (c) Panoramic
   (d) Bitewing

4. What is the main cause of dimensional distortion on periapical films placed over edentulous areas?
   (a) Film movement
   (b) Flat position of film
   (c) Absence of normal landmarks
   (d) Shadow cast by styrofoam block

5. How is the location of the bisector determined in the edentulous patient?
   (a) By measuring the width of the ridge
   (b) By estimating the long axis of the ridge
   (c) By directing the central rays parallel to the ridge
   (d) By decreasing the vertical angulation.

BIBLIOGRAPHY

Matteson, S. R., Joseph, L. P., & Bottomley, W. et al. The report of the panel to develop radiographic selection criteria for dental patients. *Gen. Dent.* 39:264–270, 1991.

Rinn Corporation. *Intraoral Radiography with Rinn XCP/BAS Instruments*. Elgin, IL: Dentsply/Rinn Corporation, 1983.

Seals, R. R. Jr., Williams, E. O., & Jones J. D. Panoramic radiographs: Necessary for edentulous patients? *J. Am. Dent. Assoc.*123:74–78, 1992.

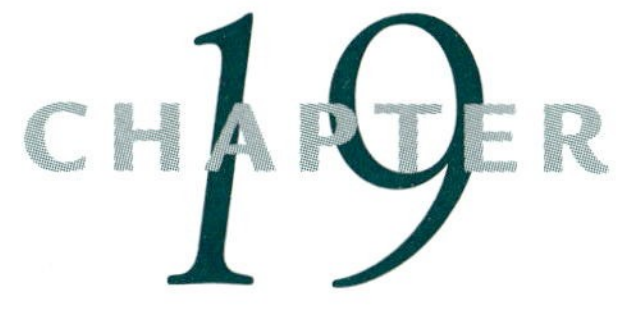

Digital Radiography

OBJECTIVES

By the end of this chapter the student should be able to:

- Define the key words.
- Differentiate a digital image from a radiograph.
- Discuss the fundamental concepts of digital radiography.
- Discuss the purpose and use of digital radiography.
- Describe the equipment used in digital radiography.
- State and describe the three types of digital imaging.
- List and discuss the advantages and disadvantages of digital radiography.

KEY WORDS

Analog
Charge-coupled device (CCD)
Digital imaging
Digital radiography
Digital subtraction
Digitize
Direct digital imaging
Gray scale
Indirect digital imaging
Pixel
Resolution
Sensor

Introduction

Digital radiography is the result of recent technological advances in the field of computer science. The introduction of a computed approach with instant images (both radiographic and photographic) has the potential to greatly improve the quality of dental care. This recent and exciting advance in computer technology has resulted in a unique "filmless" imaging system known as digital radiography (see Figure 19–1). This new age of imaging in dentistry began in 1987 when digital radiography was first introduced by Dr. Francois Mugnon with his RVG system (RadioVisioGraphy). Digital radiography will be an essential part of the modern dental office, along with digital cameras, surgical microscopes and electronic patient records. In order to use this very specialized technology, the dental radiographer must have an understanding of the basic concepts of digital radiography and a working knowledge of the equipment used in digital radiography.

The purpose of this chapter is to explain digital imaging, present the fundamental concepts of digital radiography, to introduce the types of digital imaging, and to discuss the advantages and disadvantages of digital radiography.

Terminology

First, the dental radiographer must become familiar with some of the basic terms used in digital radiography.

Analog: Relating to a mechanism in which data is represented by continuously variable physical quantities.

Charge-coupled device (CCD): A CCD is a solid-state detector used in many electronic devices such as the video camera, surgical microscope and fax machine. A CCD used in digital radiography is an image receptor found in the intraoral sensor, which converts x-rays to electrons.

Digital imaging: A filmless imaging system. The difference between digital images and radiographs is that digital images have no physical form. Digital images exist only as bits of information in a computer file which tells the computer how to construct an image to place upon a monitor or other viewing device.

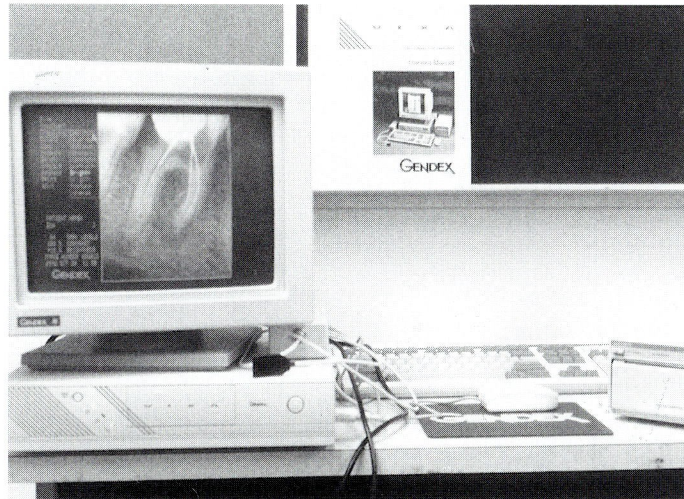

FIGURE 19–1. **Visualix digital intraoral radiographic system.** Instead of a film packet, a detector (sensor) is placed in the patient's mouth and exposed to x-rays. The picture is immediately available on the computer monitor. The image can be adjusted for brightness and contrast levels. (Courtesy Dr. Allan G. Farman and Dr. William C. Scharfe, School of Dentistry, University of Louisville, Louisville, KY)

Digital radiography: A method of producing a filmless radiographic image using a sensor (instead of film) and transmitting the electronic information directly into a computer, which serves to acquire, process, store, retrieve, and display the radiographic image.

Digital subtraction: A reversing of the gray-scale as an image is viewed. Radiolucent images appear radiopaque images and radiopaque images appear radiolucent.

Digitize: To convert an image into a digital form that can be processed by a computer.

Direct digital imaging: A method of directly obtaining a digital image by exposing an intraoral sensor to x-rays to produce an image that can be viewed on a computer monitor.

Gray scale: Refers to the total number of shades of gray visible in an image.

Indirect digital imaging: A method of obtaining a digital image in which an existing radiograph is scanned or photographed and then converted into a digital image.

Pixel (*pix*, plural of *pic*ture; *el*, *el*ement): Any of the small discrete elements that together constitute an image. Discrete units of information (also termed *picture element*). Any of the detecting elements of a charge-coupled device used as an optical sensor.

Resolution: The discernable separation of closely adjacent image details.

Sensor: An electronic or specially coated plate that is sensitive to x-rays. A small detector that is placed intraorally to capture a radiographic image when exposed to x-rays.

Digital Imaging

The term radiography is derived from the words, radiation and photography. That is to say, a radiograph is a photographic image created using radiation. Today, there are many different ways to create images of the patient. Images can be made within a computer using digital sensors, phosphor plates or ultra sound. Hence, we no longer need the photographic process. Therefore, the term *imaging* has come to replace the term *radiography* when referring to the different ways images of the patient are created. The term *image*, not *radiograph*, is used to describe the picture that is produced.

The difference between a digital image and a radiograph is that a digital image has no physical form. Digital images exist only as bits of information in a computer file which tells the computer how to construct an image to place upon a monitor or other viewing device.

Digital imaging systems used in dentistry replace film with an alternative sensor. In most instances this is a solid state electronic plate known as a charged-couple device (CCD). Signals from the CCD are transmitted directly into a computer, which serves to acquire, process, store, retrieve, and display the radiographic image

Fundamental Concepts

The term digital radiography refers to a filmless imaging system in which a radiographic image is created using a sensor, breaking it into electronic pieces, and storing the information into a computer (see Figure 19–2). In digital radiography, a **sensor,** or small detector, is placed inside the patient's mouth. The sensor is used instead of intraoral dental film that must be processed in a darkroom. As in conventional radiography, the x-ray beam is aimed to strike the sensor. The source of x-radiation is activated. An electronic charge is produced on the surface of the sensor; and the electronic signal is **digitized,** or converted into "digital" form. The digital sensor in turn transmits this information to a computer. After the image has been digitized by the sensor, it is processed by a computer. Software is used to store the image electronically. The image is displayed within seconds and may be readily manipulated to enhance the appearance for interpretation and diagnosis (see Figure 19–3).

Digital radiography systems are not limited to intraoral images; panoramic and cephalometric images may also be obtained. For example, the extraoral film traditionally used in panoramic radiography is replaced with an electronic sensor that delivers the image information to a computer for storage in digital format. As with intraoral radiography, the images are displayed on a computer monitor and may be stored for future use.

Characteristics of a Digital Image

The term **digital** image is used to distinguish it from an **analog** image. An analog image has been described as being like a painting with a continuous smooth blend from one color to another. A digital image is like a mosaic, made up of many small pieces put together to make a whole. The digital image is composed of structurally ordered areas called pixels. Each pixel is a single dot in a

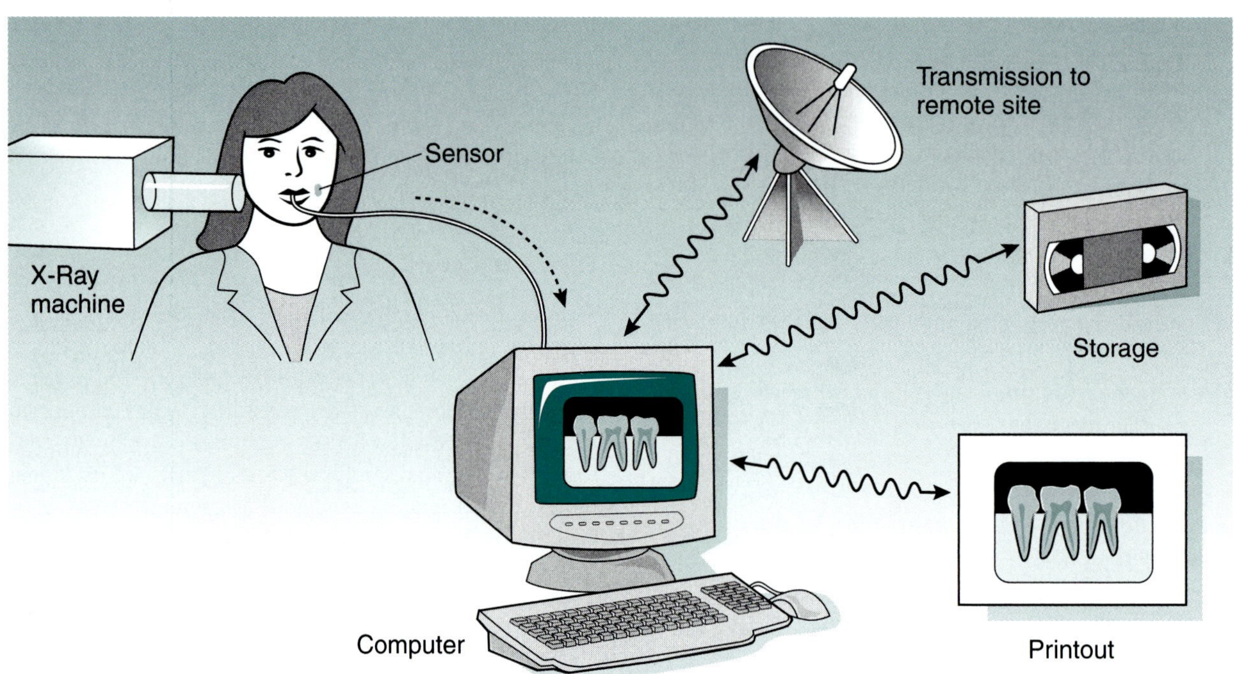

FIGURE 19–2. **Digital imaging system.** The image is made directly on a charge-coupled device (CCD) in the patient's mouth and sent to the computer. The image can then be displayed on the monitor, printed if required, transmitted to a remote site (such as a consultant, an insurance company, or a referring dentist), and stored for future use.

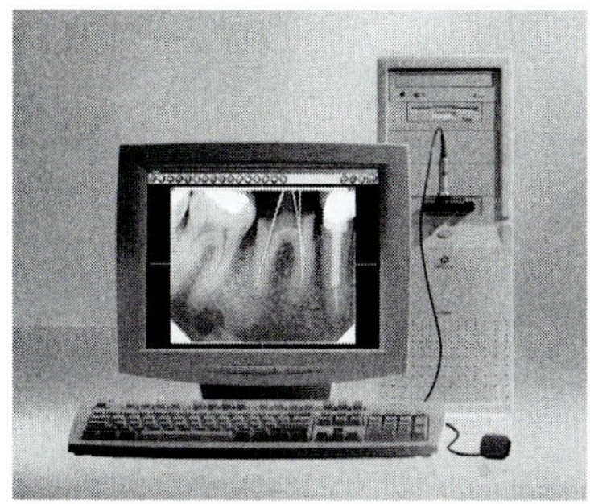

FIGURE 19–3. **Image displayed on computer screen.** Image may be readily manipulated to enhance the appearance for interpretation and diagnosis. (DEXIS x-ray images courtesy of ProVision Dental Systems, Inc., Redwood City, CA)

digital image. The more pixels that are present, the greater the resolution (detail) of the final image.

Spatial Resolution

The number and size of pixels determines the **spatial resolution** of an image. When the number of pixels is low, the image appears to have jagged edges and is difficult to see.

Spatial resolution is measured in terms of line pairs. A line pair refers to the greatest number of paired lines visible in 1 mm of an image. For example, a resolution of 10–line pairs/mm would mean that when 10 ruled lines are squeezed into 1 mm of an image, the individual lines can still be seen. The greater the resolution in an image, the sharper it looks.

Spatial resolution is also determined by pixel size. The smaller the pixel, the greater number of pixels can fit into the sensor. Manufacturers have been working to decrease pixel size.

Gray Scale Resolution

Gray scale resolution refers to the total number of shades of gray visible in an image. A number stored for each pixel determines the number of shades of gray visible. Each pixel has a number from 0 to 255, representing pure black at 0 to pure white at 255. Hence there are usually 256 gray levels in an image. However, the human eye can distinguish only about 32 shades of gray. In diagnosis, the dentist relies more on contrast discrimination (gray levels) than on spatial relations.

The combination of spatial resolution and gray scale resolution determines the quality of the final image. Therefore, these two characteristics should be maximized in an imaging system.

Purpose

The purpose of digital radiography is to produce images that can be used in the diagnosis and treatment of dental disease. The images produced are diagnostically equivalent to dental radiographs and enable the dental radiographer to identify conditions in underlying tissues that cannot be seen clinically. Like conventional radiographic procedures, digital radiography allows the radiographer to obtain important information about the teeth and supporting structures.

Use

Digital radiography is used to:

- Detect, confirm, and classify dental diseases and lesions
- Detect and evaluate trauma
- Evaluate growth and development
- Provide information during dental procedures such as root canal therapy and surgery
- Store images on a computer
- Educate patients about their dental health
- To reduce radiation

Digital Subtraction Radiography

Digital subtraction radiography is useful in the diagnosis of periodontal and carious lesions because of their relatively low rate of progression. Subtraction radiography requires two identical images. The subtracted image is a composite of the two images, representing their differing densities. Very small changes in density can be seen when the images are accurately matched.

Digital subtraction radiography is difficult to use clinically because each occasion requires reproducible alignment of the x-ray beam, the teeth, and the film.

Equipment

In digital radiography, the use of specialized equipment is necessary. The essential equipment needed for a digital imaging system include **x-ray machine, intraoral sensor,** and **computer** (see Figure 19–4).

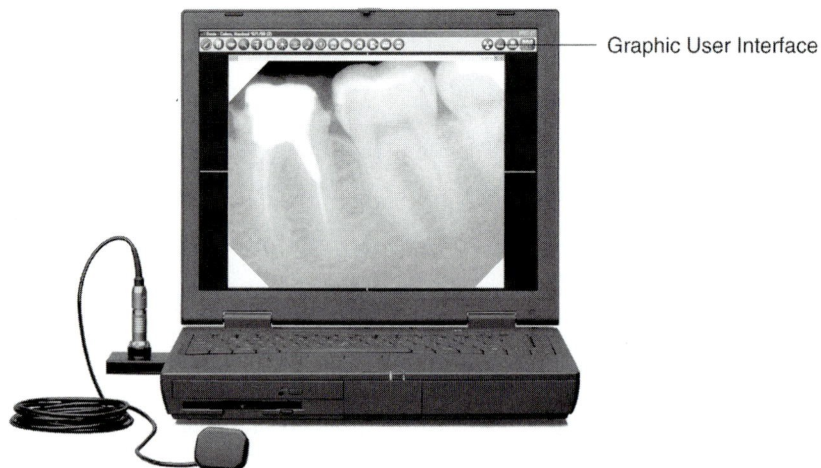

FIGURE 19–4. **Digital imaging system showing computer and sensor.** (DEXIS x-ray images courtesy of ProVision Dental Systems, Inc., Redwood City, CA)

X-ray Machine

In many dental offices, digital radiography can be used without replacing any existing radiographic equipment. However some systems require an x-ray machine capable of very short exposure times in the order of 1/100 of a second. Older x-ray machines using impulse timers may need replacement. New x-ray machines with electronic digital timers should be used. An x-ray machine adapted for digital radiography can still be used for conventional radiography.

Intraoral Sensor

In direct digital imaging, a sensor is used instead of intraoral dental film (see Figure 19–5). The sensor is an electronic or specially coated plate that is placed in the mouth of the patient. When exposed to x-rays the sensor converts the x-rays into an electronic form that can be read and used in a computer.

Intraoral sensors may be wired or wireless. Wired refers to the fact that the imaging sensor is connected by a fiber optic cable to a computer that records the generated signal. The cable may vary in length from 8 to 35 feet. The shorter the cable, the more limited the range of motion. Wireless means the imaging sensor is not connected by a cable to the computer.

Currently, there are three basic types of sensors:

1. Charge-coupled device (CCD)
2. Complementary metal oxide semiconductor/active pixel sensor (CMOS/APS)
3. Photo stimuable phophor (PSP)

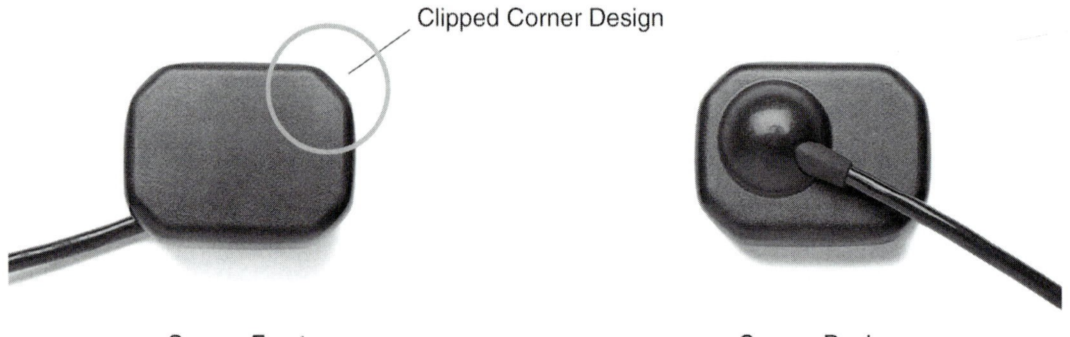

FIGURE 19–5. **Digital sensor showing front and back.** (DEXIS x-ray images courtesy of Pro Vision Dental Systems, Inc., Redwood City, CA)

1. **Charge-Coupled Device (CCD)**
The **charge-coupled device (CCD)** is the most common image receptor used in dental digital radiography. The CCD, first developed in the 1960s, is not a new technology. CCDs were first utilized in video cameras where they convert visible light images into a form that can be stored on tape. They were the first direct digital sensors to be used in dental radiology with the Trophy radiology system introduced in 1987 in France.

The CCD is a solid-state detector made up of a grid of small transistor elements that convert x-rays to electrons. When an x-ray strikes the transistor elements, electrons are trapped in proportion to the number of x-rays striking the element. The individual elements are arranged in a grid formation. Each element represents one **pixel** in the final image. A pixel is a small box or "well" into which the electrons produced by the x-ray exposure are deposited. Pixels, short for "picture elements," are tiny dots that make up a digital image. The more pixels in an image, the higher the resolution and the sharper the picture. A pixel is the digital equivalent of a silver crystal used in conventional radiography. As opposed to a film emulsion that contains a random arrangement of silver crystals, a pixel is structured in an ordered arrangement. The CCD is 640 by 480 individual pixels in size.

After exposure is complete, the elements are read and the electron charges are converted to brightness values and locations to form a digital image. This information is then passed through a wire to a circuit board inside the computer for processing and display on the monitor.

CCD sensors are designed with a scintillation screen that intercepts the x-rays and fluoresces with visible light to expose the CCD. In addition, CCD sensors utilize a fiber-optic plate between the scintillation screen and the active sensor. The fiber-optic plate provides additional blockage of x-radiation from destroying the active part of the sensor and also acts to focus the light from the screen onto the sensor and increase image sharpness. The addition of the scintillation screen and fiber-optic plate made early CCD sensors very thick and bulky. They were also very small so that often only one tooth could be imaged with each exposure. Patients had a difficult time tolerating the thick plastic, which was up to 15 mm thick as opposed to less than 1 mm thick for film. Today, CCD sensors have improved greatly with the use of thin leaded fiber optic plates and larger CCDs. Today, CCDs can be had in sizes similar to normal #2 periapical film and thickness as low as 3 to 5 mm.

Currently CCD technology is used in many devices; some examples include fax machines, home video cameras, microscopes, and telescopes.

The CCD technology used in digital radiography relies on a specialized fabrication process that is expensive to manufacture.

2. **Complementary Metal Oxide Semiconductor/Active Pixel Sensor (CMOS/APS)**
CMOS stands for **Complementary Metal Oxide Semiconductor,** a type of integrated circuit like CCDs. The advantages to CMOS technology are the individual pixels can be made smaller, power requirements are less, and the chip is more durable and less expensive to produce. However, until recently, the image quality has been poor. Recent technology has changed that. Manufacturers have been able to overcome the inherent noise and low signal output of the CMOS sensor by adding an active amplifying transistor to each pixel. This new sensor is known as a CNOS/APS where **APS** stands for **Active Pixel Sensor.** These sensors offer the capability of embedding microprocessors and other circuitry right on the sensor chip itself.

CMOS/APS sensors can be connected to the computer using low power external connections such as Universal Serial Bus (USB). They don't require an internal circuit card as with the CCD sensor. This makes laptop computer based systems very feasible. Other aspects of CMOS/APS sensor design are similar to the CCD sensor. CMOS/APS sensors use a wire connection and internal scintillation screen.

3. **Photo Stimuable Phosphor (PSP)**
The **photo stimuable phosphor (PSP) sensor** system utilizes a completely different technology than CCDs. They use rare earth phosphor (barium europium fluorohalide) coated plates that are exposed to x-rays. These storage phosphors do not fluoresce immediately, but "store" the x-ray energy until stimulated by a laser beam. This is done in a separate scanning device where the resulting fluorescent "signal" is read and converted into a digital image. This system is similar to film in that multiple images can be taken and the plates "developed" later. The plates are reusable and are erased by exposing them to bright light.

Computer

All digital images require a computer and a monitor in order to capture and view an image (see Figure 19–4). The computer digitizes, processes, and stores information received from the sensor. The monitor allows for immediate viewing. An image is recorded on a computer monitor in 0.5 to 120 sec; markedly less time than is required for conventional film processing. This speed of image recording is extremely useful during certain dental procedures, such as the placement of surgical implants or during root canal therapy instrumentation. The image may be stored permanently in the computer, printed on a hard copy for the patient record, or transmitted electronically to insurance companies or referring dental specialists.

The computer is responsible for converting the electronic signal from the sensor into a shade of gray that is viewed on the computer monitor. Each pixel is represented numerically in the computer by location and level of color of gray. The range of numbers for a pixel varies from 0 to 255, which creates 256 shades of gray. In comparison the human eye can only appreciate up to 32 shades of gray. This technology allows the dental professional to manipulate the image to enhance contrast and density without additional x-ray exposure of the patient.

Various computer-viewing features are available with digital radiography systems. Digital systems features split screen technology that allows the operator to view and compare multiple images on the same screen. This feature is helpful in the comparison and evaluation of disease progression involving caries or periodontal disease. For example, caries progression can be evaluated by comparing successive bitewing images.

Digital systems also provide a feature that allows specific images to be magnified up to four times their original size. This feature is helpful when evaluating the apical area of a tooth. Linear and angular measurements can also be obtained, a feature that is helpful in measuring the length of a root.

Radiation Exposure

The radiation exposure for digital imaging systems is up to 80% less than what is required for E-speed film used in conventional dental radiography. Digital imaging sensors are more sensitive to x-rays than conventional dental x-ray film. Exposure times for digital radiography are in the order of 0.05 sec (about 3 impulses), compared to 0.2 sec (about 12 impulses) required for E-speed intraoral film used in conventional dental radiography. Obviously, the lower the radiation exposure, the lower the absorbed dose to the patient.

Eastman Kodak F-speed film requires about 20% less exposure time than E-speed film.

Methods of Acquiring a Digital Image

In radiography, we "take a radiograph," whereas in digital imaging we "acquire an image." The two methods of acquiring a digital image are **direct digital imaging** and **indirect digital imaging.**

Direct Digital Imaging

In direct digital imaging, no film is used. The image is acquired directly by means of a sensor. A sensor is placed into the mouth of the patient and exposed to x-rays. The sensor captures in the radiographic image and then transmits the image to a computer monitor. Within seconds of exposing the sensor to x-rays, an image appears on the computer screen. Software is then used to enhance and store the image.

Indirect Digital Imaging

Indirect methods of making digital images were first to be used historically, dating back to the 1970s. In indirect imaging an actual film-based radiograph is still required (see Figure 19–6). An imaging device is used to either scan or photograph the radiograph.

Modern scanners offer a quick and convenient way to convert radiographs to digital images. Scanners pass a light beam through the radiograph to an imaging chip (charge-coupled device, or CCD). The CCD converts the light passed through into a digital image. This process is essentially the same as the CCD sensors. To scan radiographs requires a device called a transparency adapter that mounts in the lid of the scanner and passes light through the radiograph to be read by the scanner. Transparency adapters are available as options on most end flatbed scanners.

Video or digital cameras can be used to photograph existing radiographs placed on a viewbox. A digitizing board is needed with video cameras to transform the analog image into a digital image. With digital cameras, a digital image is created directly in the camera itself. The camera scans the image, digitizes or converts the image, and then displays it on the computer monitor. A copy stand or tripod should be used with this technique.

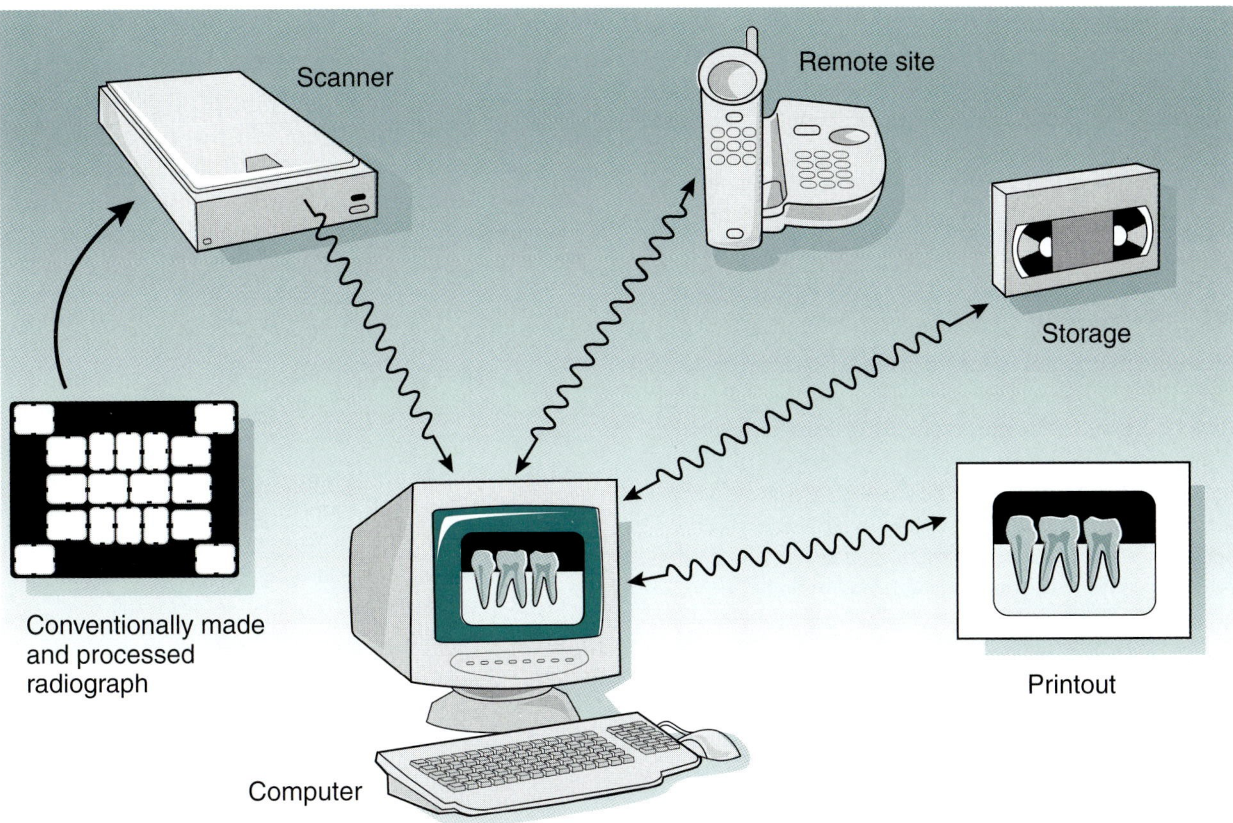

FIGURE 19-6. **Indirect digital imaging.** Conventional radiograph is converted into a digital image by scanning it into the computer. Changes may be made to the image before printout, storage, or transmitted to remote site (such as a consultant, an insurance company, or a referring dentist).

The quality of an indirect digital image is inferior to a direct digital image because the resultant image is similar to a "copy" of the image versus the "original."

Step-by-Step Procedures

The manufacturer's instructions must be followed concerning the equipment preparation, operation of the system, patient preparation, and exposure. Only general guidelines concerning patient preparation and sensor placement are included here.

Patient Preparation

After completing the infection control procedures described in Chapter 22, proceed by:

1. Seating the patient.
2. Adjust chair to comfortable working level.
3. Adjust headrest to position patient's head so that the occlusal plane is parallel to the floor and the midsagittal plane (midline) is perpendicular to the floor.
4. Place lead apron and thyroid collar on the patient.
5. Remove eyeglasses and objects from the mouth that may interfere with the procedure.
6. Explain the digital radiographic procedures to the patient.

Sensor Placement

Digital radiography involves placement of the intraoral sensor in the mouth of the patient; similar to the technique used in conventional film placement. Special care must be given to the intraoral sensor. Each sensor is sealed and waterproofed. For infection control purposes, the sensor must be protected with a disposable barrier because it cannot be sterilized.

The sensor is held in the mouth by biteblock attachments or instruments that aim the beam and sensor accurately (see Figure 19–7). As with conventional radiography, the paralleling technique is the preferred method. Paralleling technique film holders should be used to stabilize the sensor in the mouth. As with conventional intraoral film, the sensor is centered over the area of interest.

Legal Implications

Because the original digital image can be manipulated, there has been much concern about the legal implications of digital image processing. It is possible to modify an image to create caries where none exists. To address this concern, companies are producing software that will not permit an altered image to be saved (except as copy, clearly labeled as such). Eastman Kodak with its Digital Science Dental Scanning System, has included a warning feature that appears if the original image is not comparable with the image displayed on the monitor. Another technique, called digital watermarking, embeds an invisible ID into the image to make fraudulent modification of images too difficult to be practical. Most insurance companies are not concerned about accepting digital images because the cost savings greatly exceed the potential for fraud.

Advantages and Disadvantages

There are both advantages and disadvantages to using digital radiography.

Advantages

Advantages of digital radiography include instant viewing of the image, elimination of the photographic process and darkroom, improved gray-scale resolution, less radiation exposure to the patient, remote electronic consultation and transmission of images, the capability to enhance images, and serves as an effective method to educate patients.

- **Instant viewing of the image.** Images are created almost instantaneously, allowing immediate evaluation of the patient's condition. Speed of image viewing is one of the most important reasons for using this technology.
- **Elimination of the photographic process and darkroom.** Digital radiography eliminates the need for dental x-ray film, processing solutions and the darkroom. There are no darkroom processing errors and no disposal of processing chemicals, lead foil backings and film packets.
- **Improved gray scale resolution.** An important advantage to digital radiography is the improved gray scale resolution. Digital radiography uses up to 256 colors of gray compared to the 25 or less shades of gray seen on a conventional radiograph. The gray-scale resolution is important because diagnosis is often based on contrast discrimination. The density and contrast of the radiographic image can be manipulated to make the best possible diagnostic image.
- **Less radiation exposure to the patient.** The radiation exposure for digital imaging systems is up to 80% less than what is required for E-speed film used in conven-

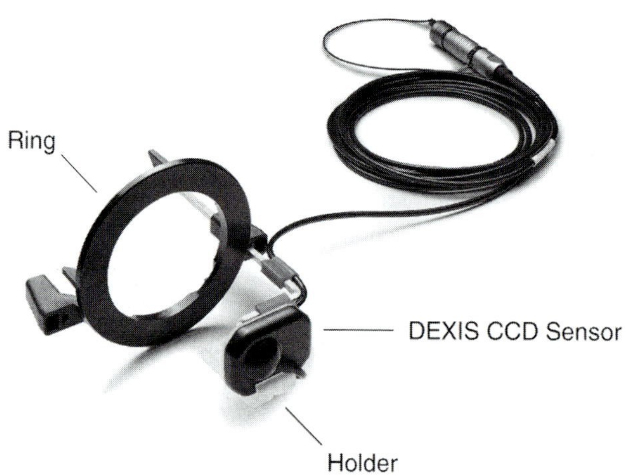

FIGURE 19–7. **Sensor-holding instruments used to align the primary beam.** (DEXIS x-ray images courtesy of Pro Vision Dental Systems, Inc., Redwood City, CA)

tional radiography. Digital imaging sensors are more sensitive to x-rays than conventional dental x-ray film.

- **Remote electronic consultation and sending of images.** The digital image can be placed into the electronic record of the patient and hard copies of the radiographic image can be printed when needed (see Figure 19–8). Digital radiographs can be electronically transmitted to consultants, insurance companies or referring dentists.
- **Improvement of the diagnostic image.** The diagnostic image can be improved by manipulating the controls. Features such as contrast modification, colorization and zoom allows the dental team to highlight conditions, such as bone resorption or small areas of decay. Another feature that can be used to enhance a diagnostic image is **digital subtraction.** With digital subtraction, the gray scale is reversed so that radiolucent images (normally black) appear white and radiopaque images (normally white) appear black. Digital subtraction eliminates distracting background information. For example, this feature permits the operator to remove all anatomic structures that have not changed between radiographic examinations for ease in identifying changes in diagnostic information.
- **Patient education.** Viewing digital images is an effective method of patient education (see Figure 19–9). Patients can view radiographic images with the dental radiographer or dentist. Such visualization can increase a patient's understanding of their dental condition. The size of the digitized image on a computer screen (compared with a 2-in. film) makes viewing easier for the patient.

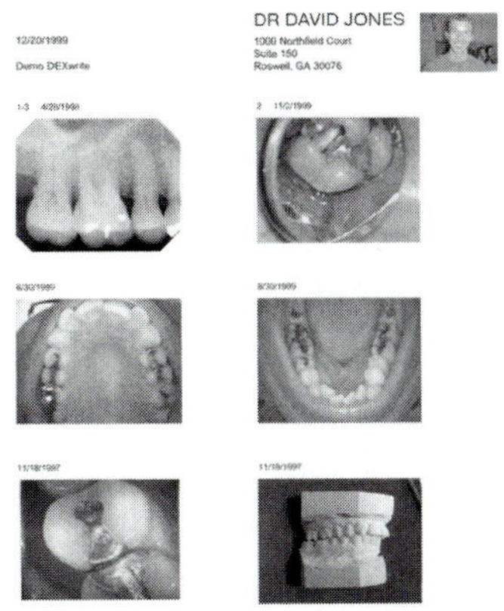

FIGURE 19–8. **Hard copies of radiographic images can be printed and sent to a referring dentist or insurance company.** (DEXIS x-ray images courtesy of Pro Vision Dental Systems, Inc., Redwood City, CA)

Disadvantages

Disadvantages of digital radiography include the following: high initial investment, image quality, sensor size, infection control issues, and legal issues.

- **High initial investment.** The initial cost of purchasing a digital imaging system is a significant disadvantage. The range of cost depends on the manufacturer, the level of computer equipment currently in the office, and auxiliary features, such as an intraoral camera. Service and maintenance for any repairs must also be considered. At the time of printing, typical start-up costs for one digital imaging system in the dental office is estimated at $6,000 to $16,000. This does not include the cost of the x-ray machine.
- **Image quality.** At this time, image quality continues to be a source of debate. The resolution of an image is defined as the number of line pairs per millimeter (lp/mm). Conventional dental x-ray film has a resolution of 12 to 20 lp/mm. A digital imaging system using a CCD has a resolution closer to 10 lp/mm. Given that the human eye can only resolve 8 to 10 lp/mm; a

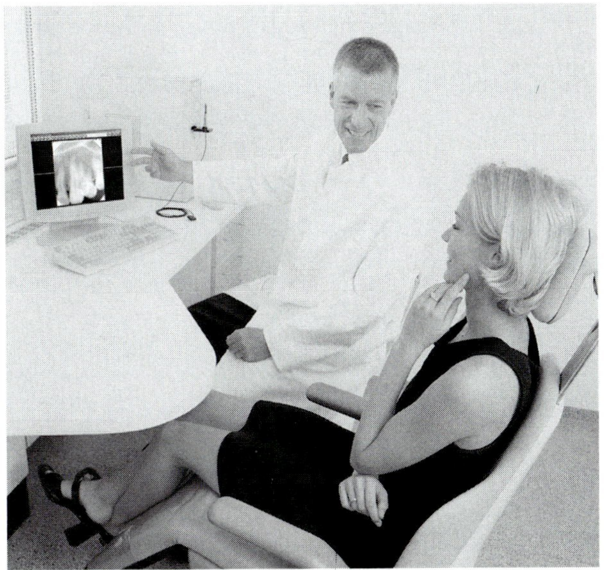

FIGURE 19–9. **Viewing digital images is an effective method of patient education.** (DEXIS x-ray images courtesy of Pro Vision Dental Systems, Inc., Redwood City, CA)

CCD system appears to be adequate for diagnosis of dental disease.

- **Sensor size.** Sensors are thicker than intraoral film. Patients may complain of the bulky nature of the sensor; the sensor may be uncomfortable or elicit the gag reflex.
- **Infection control.** The digital sensor cannot withstand heat sterilization. Therefore, the sensor requires complete coverage with disposable plastic sleeves that must be changed with each patient to prevent patient-to-patient cross-contamination.
- **Legal issues.** It is questionable whether digital radiographs can be used as evidence in court because the original image can be altered by manipulation. Manufacturers have addressed this problem and have developed a variety of solutions.

Despite the disadvantages, digital imaging represents a new age of imaging in dentistry. The modern dental office will have digital imaging equipment, digital cameras and electronic patient records.

CHAPTER SUMMARY

Digital radiography is a method of capturing a radiographic image and displaying it on a computer screen; no film is used and no film processing is required.

A conventional dental x-ray unit is used as the radiation source. A sensor or small detector is placed inside the mouth of the patient and the x-ray beam is aimed to strike the sensor. The electronic charge produced on the sensor is digitized (or converted into digital form) and can be viewed on a computer monitor.

Advantages of digital radiography include instant viewing of the image, elimination of the photographic process and darkroom, improved gray-scale resolution, less radiation exposure to the patient, remote electronic consultation and sending of images, the capability to enhance images, and serves as an effective method to educate patients.

Disadvantages of digital radiography include the following: high initial investment, image quality, sensor size, infection control issues, and legal issues.

REVIEW QUESTIONS

1. The term used to describe the picture produced using digital radiography is digital image.

   (a) True
   (b) False

2. Digital intraoral sensors should be heat sterilized after each use.

   (a) True
   (b) False

3. Digital radiography requires more x-radiation than conventional radiography.

   (a) True
   (b) False

4. The x-ray source used in most digital radiography systems is a conventional dental x-ray machine.
   (a) True
   (b) False
5. Digital radiography was introduced to dentistry in:
   (a) 1977.
   (b) 1978.
   (c) 1987.
   (d) 1988.
6. Digital radiography can be used for which of the following?
   (a) To detect caries
   (b) To evaluate growth and development
   (c) To detect dental disease
   (d) All of the above
7. Digital radiography requires less radiation than conventional radiography because the:
   (a) mA is increased.
   (b) Exposure time is increased.
   (c) Sensor is less sensitive to x-rays.
   (d) Sensor is more sensitive to x-rays.
8. The preferred exposure method for intraoral digital radiography is the:
   (a) Bisecting technique.
   (b) Paralleling technique.
9. The method of obtaining a digital image similar to scanning a photograph to a computer screen is termed:
   (a) Direct digital imaging.
   (b) Indirect digital imaging.
   (c) Composite digital imaging.
   (d) None of the above.
10. Digital radiography systems can be used for which of the following?
   (a) Bite-wing images
   (b) Periapical images
   (c) Panoramic images
   (d) Cephalometric images
   (e) All of the above
11. All of the following are advantages of digital radiography except:
   (a) Improved gray-scale resolution.
   (b) Size of the intraoral sensor.
   (c) Less radiation exposure to the patient.
   (d) Patient education.

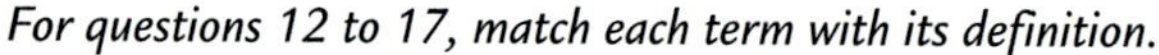

For questions 12 to 17, match each term with its definition.

a. analog
b. digital radiography
c. gray scale
d. pixel
e. resolution
f. sensor

_____ 12. A method of producing a filmless radiographic image using a sensor (instead of film) and transmitting the electronic information directly into a computer, which serves to acquire, process, store, retrieve, and display the radiographic image.

_____ 13. The discernable separation of closely adjacent image details.

_____ 14. Relating to a mechanism in which data is represented by continuously variable physical quantities.

_____ 15. Any of the small discrete elements that together constitute an image. Discrete units of information (also termed *picture element*). Any of the detecting elements of a charge-coupled device used as an optical sensor.

_____ 16. Refers to the total number of shades of gray visible in an image.

_____ 17. An electronic or specially coated plate that is sensitive to x-rays. A small detector that is placed intraorally to capture a radiographic image when exposed to x-rays.

BIBLIOGRAPHY

Dunn, S. M. & Kantor, M. L. Digital radiography: Facts and fictions. *J. Am. Dent. Assoc.* 124:28–47, 1993.

Jones, G. A., Behrents, R. C. & Baily, G. P. Legal considerations for digital images. *General Dentistry* 44:242–244, 1996.

Langland, O. E. & Langlais, R. P. Special radiographic techniques. In *Principles of Dental Imaging*. Baltimore: Williams & Wilkins, 1997, pp. 265–287.

Lusk, L. T. Comparison of film-based and digital radiography. *J Practical Hygiene* 7:45–50, 1998.

Razmus, T. F. & Williamson, G. F. An overview of oral and maxillofacial imaging. In *Current Oral and Maxillofacial Imaging*. Philadelphia: WB Saunders, 1996, pp. 1–22.

Tsang, A., Sweet, D., & Wood, R. Potential for fraudulent use of digital radiography. J. Am. Dent. Assoc. 130:1325–1329, 1999.

Tyndall, D. A., Ludlow, J. B., & Platin, E. et al. A comparison of Kodak Ektaspeed Plus film and the Siemens Sidexis digital imaging system for caries detection using receiver operating characteristic analysis. *Oral Surgery, Oral, Medicine, Oral Pathology, Oral Radiology and Endodontics* 85:113–118, 1998.

White, S. C. & Pharoah, M. J. *Oral Radiology Principles and Interpretation*, 4th ed. St. Louis: Mosby, 2000.

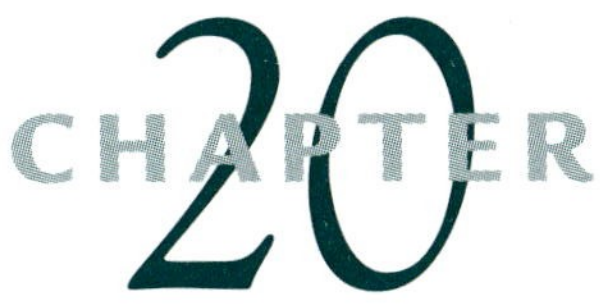

Extraoral Radiography

OBJECTIVES

By the end of this chapter the student should be able to:

- Define the key words.
- Describe the purpose and use of extraoral radiographs.
- Identify the types of film used in extraoral radiography.
- Give three reasons for making extraoral exposures.
- Identify the types of projections that can be performed extraorally.
- State the purpose and describe the procedure for each extraoral projection.

KEY WORDS

Acoustic meatus
Ankylosis
Cassette
Cephalometer
Cephalometric radiographs
Cephalostats
Condyle
Frankfort plane
Glenoid fossa
Head positioner
Intensifying screens
Lateral jaw projection
Lateral skull projection
Midsagittal plane
Occipital protuberance
Panoramic radiographs
Posteroanterior (PA) projection
Reverse-Towne projection
Screen film
Submentovertex projection
Temporomandibular joint (TMJ)
Tomograph
Tomography
Transcranial projection
Waters' (sinus) projection

Introduction

Extraoral radiographs are examinations made of the head and facial region using films located outside the mouth. They allow the dentist to view large areas of the jaws and skull on a single radiograph. The extraoral techniques described in this chapter can be performed by a trained operator using a conventional dental x-ray unit.

The purpose of this chapter is to present the purpose and use of extraoral radiographs, to describe the equipment needed, and to describe in detail the techniques for patient and film positioning.

Extraoral Radiographs

An **extraoral radiograph** is defined as a radiograph exposed outside the mouth. The dentist orders these views to examine areas not fully covered by intraoral films or to visualize the skull and facial structures.

Purpose and Use of Extraoral Radiographs

The purpose of extraoral radiographs is to examine structures of the skull, the maxilla and mandible, and the temporomandibular joint. Extraoral radiographs are used to:

- Examine large areas of the jaws and skull.
- Study growth and development of bone and teeth.
- Detect fractures and evaluate trauma.
- Detect pathological lesions and diseases of the jaws.
- Detect and evaluate impacted teeth.
- Evaluate temporomandibular joint (TMJ) disorders.

Extraoral radiographs are used when patients cannot or will not open their mouth. Handicapped patients or patients with trismus or temporomandibular joint disorders may not be able to tolerate the placement of intraoral film.

Extraoral radiographs can be used alone or in conjunction with intraoral radiographs. It is common to expose both a panoramic radiograph and intraoral radiographs on the same patient. Images on intraoral radiographs are sharper than the images seen on panoramic radiographs.

Except for the panoramic radiographs, extraoral radiographs are not frequently used by general practitioners. Major users are orthodontists, prosthodontists, and oral surgeons.

- **Orthodontists** use facial profile radiographs, cephalometric headplates ("cephalometric" meaning measuring the head), periodically to record, measure, and compare changes in growth and development of the bones and the teeth.
- **Prosthodontists** use facial profile radiographs to record the contour of the lips and face and the relationship of the teeth before removal (see Figure 20–1). This helps them construct prosthetic appliances that look natural.
- **Oral surgeons** use extraoral radiographs extensively to evaluate trauma, to determine the location and extent of fractures, to locate impacted teeth, abnormalities, and malignancies, and to evaluate injuries to the temporomandibular joint.

Many film positions and techniques require special equipment and a sound knowledge of the anatomical structures through which the radiation beam is directed. Most of these radiographs are made in hospitals, x-ray

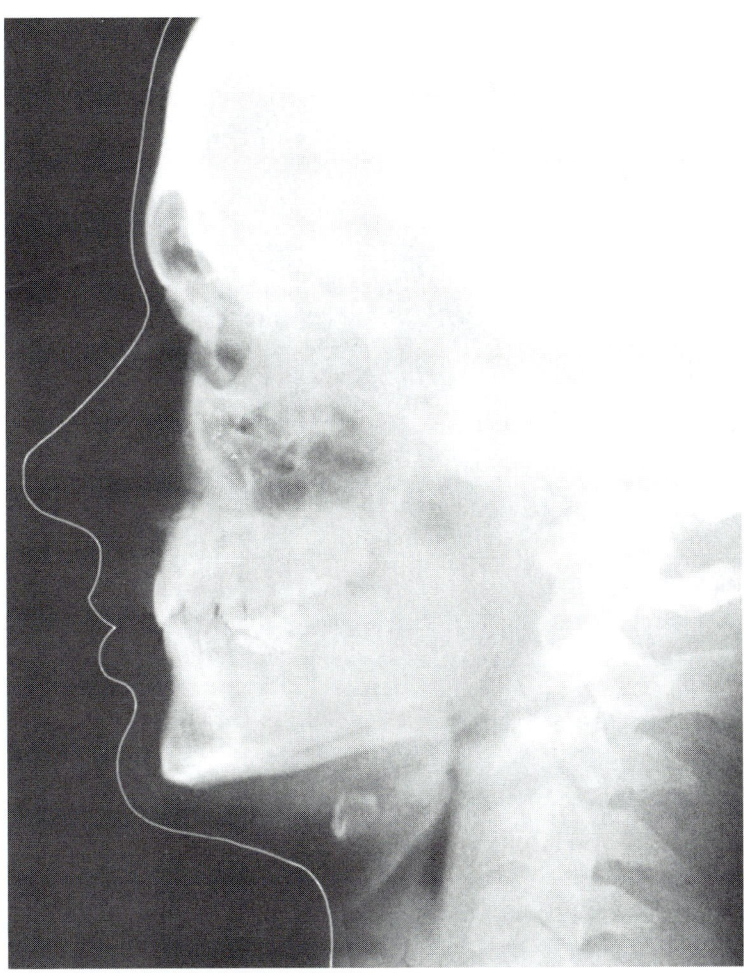

FIGURE 20–1. **Radiograph profile** exposed in extraoral cassette. Radiograph was underdeveloped to enhance the outlines of the soft tissues. Template can be made by cutting along the image of the facial outline, which then serves as a guide in maintaining the profile.

laboratories, or oral surgery offices by highly experienced operators. Only the more common techniques are described in this book.

Extraoral Film

No definite rule governs extraoral film size. Any film that will accomplish the intended purpose may be used. Other than panoramic film, the usual extraoral film sizes are 5 × 7 in. or 8 × 10 in. (13 × 18 cm or 21 × 26-cm).

As explained in Chapter 7, only the screen films are intended solely for extraoral use. Because they are extremely light-sensitive and not enclosed in a protective sealed wrapper like the periapical or occlusal films, they must be carefully loaded into a cassette under darkroom safelight illumination. The majority of extraoral projections are made with **screen film** placed in a **cassette** with **intensifying screens.**

As the larger extraoral films are packaged differently from intraoral films, they require special handling in the darkroom. Types of films and techniques for loading them are fully explained in Chapter 7.

Patient Preparation

After completing the infection control procedures described in Chapter 22:

1. Seat the patient.
2. Explain the radiographic procedures to the patient.
3. Adjust chair to comfortable working level.
4. Place lead apron on the patient.
5. Remove eyeglasses and objects from the mouth that may interfere with the procedure.

Extraoral Radiographic Techniques

Many methods can be used to make radiographs of the head and face. It is not within the scope of this book to describe all these techniques. The following projections are described: lateral jaw, lateral skull, posteroanterior, Waters, (sinus), reverse towne, submentovertex, and temporomandibular joint (TMJ).

Lateral Jaw Projection

The **lateral jaw projection** (see Figure 20–2), also known as the **lateral oblique projection,** is described first because it is the most frequent extraoral radiograph made with the conventional x-ray unit. Lateral jaw projections have been largely replaced by **panoramic radiographs,** but are still taken when greater image detail is needed or when panoramic equipment is not available.

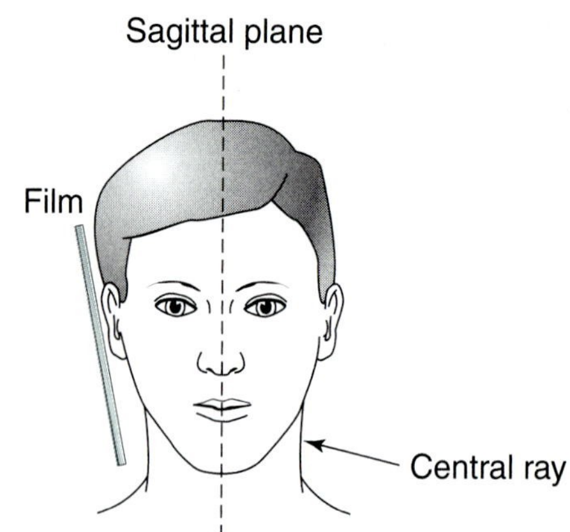

FIGURE 20–2. **Lateral jaw survey (lateral oblique survey).** Note that the central ray is directed at the cassette slightly underneath the opposite side of the mandible.

Purpose

The lateral jaw radiograph is used to examine the posterior region of the mandible. It is especially valuable to use with children (see Figure 20–3), with patients who have fractures or swelling, and with patients who are too young or senile to hold intraoral films. The lateral jaw radiograph is often made to evaluate the condition of the bone and to locate impacted teeth or large lesions.

Film Placement

The cassette is positioned flat against the cheek and centered over the mandibular first molar area. The front edge of the cassette should protrude slightly beyond the tip of the nose and the chin. The patient presses the tube side of the cassette firmly against the cheek with the palm of one hand and the thumb is placed under the lower edge of the cassette.

Head Position

The head is tilted (about 10 to 20 degrees) toward the side to be examined and the chin is protruded.

Central Ray Alignment

The central ray is directed toward the first molar region of the mandible from a point slightly underneath the opposite side of the mandible (see Figure 20–2). The cen-

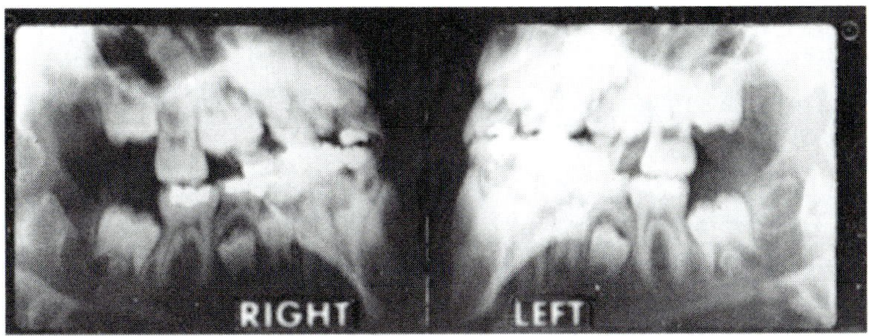

FIGURE 20–3. **Typical lateral jaw radiograph of a child with a mixed dentition**. This exposure is generally made with 5 x 7-in. (13 x 18-cm) film on adults.

tral ray should be directed as close to perpendicular to the horizontal plane of the film as possible.

Exposure Factors

The exposure factors vary considerably, depending upon the screen-film combination, target-film distance, and equipment used.

Figure 20–4 shows four possible centers of interest on the radiograph; the ramus area, the molars, the premolars, and the incisors. To change the center of interest, one varies the angle at which the film is held against the face and the direction of the central ray. The beam of radiation is directed perpendicularly to the desired area, usually at the level of the occlusal plane. Before making the exposure, ask the patient to thrust the mandible

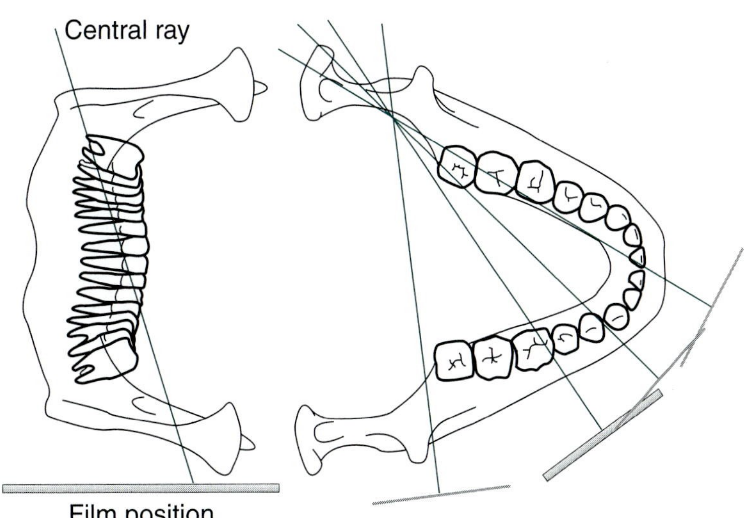

FIGURE 20–4. **X-ray beam direction for the lateral jaw projection**. Rays strike the film obliquely in the vertical plane but should be perpendicular in the horizontal plane. A true lateral projection of an entire side of the jaw is not possible because the image of the opposite side would be superimposed on it. The lateral jaw projection must be made with some oblique angulation. The beam of radiation can be directed toward the area of interest from two basic directions, underneath the mandible opposite the one being radiographed or behind the mandible opposite the one being radiographed. (Reproduced with permission from Wuehrmann, A.H. & Manson-Hing, L. R. *Dental radiology,* 5th ed. St. Louis: Mosby, 1981)

forward so that the vertebrae will not be superimposed on the mandibular structures.

Cephalometric Radiographs

Cephalometric radiographs may be either frontal (posteroanterior) or lateral skull projections (see Figure 20–5). The word "cephalometric" means measurement of the head. Cephalometric radiographs are made by placing the patient's head in a **cephalometer.** The cephalometer is a device used to standardize the placement of the head during exposure. Either conventional x-ray machines modified for cephalometric work or special units may be used. The patient's head must be completely stable. Devices called **cephalostats** have ear rods that stabilize the patient's head parallel to the film and at right angles to the direction of the beam of radiation. The cassette with intensifying screen is aligned in a definite relationship to the cephalostats so that the patient's head is between it and the source of radiation.

The cephalometer allows the head to be positioned identically at different times, for a series of identical exposures. Most orthodontists require cephalometric radiographs before treatment, at various stages of treatment, upon completion of treatment, and often as a follow-up procedure.

Lateral Skull (Cephalometric) Projection

The **lateral skull projection** shows the entire skull from the side. It is so named because the x-ray beam passes through the skull from side (lateral) to side (see Figure 20–6).

Purpose

The purpose of the lateral skull cephalometric projection is to evaluate growth and development, trauma, pathology, and developmental abnormalities. It also reveals the facial soft tissue profile when a filter is placed between the tube and the patient to remove some of the x-rays to enhance the image of the soft tissue profile of the face. It is the projection used by orthodontists for lateral cephalometric measurements. Prosthodontists and oral

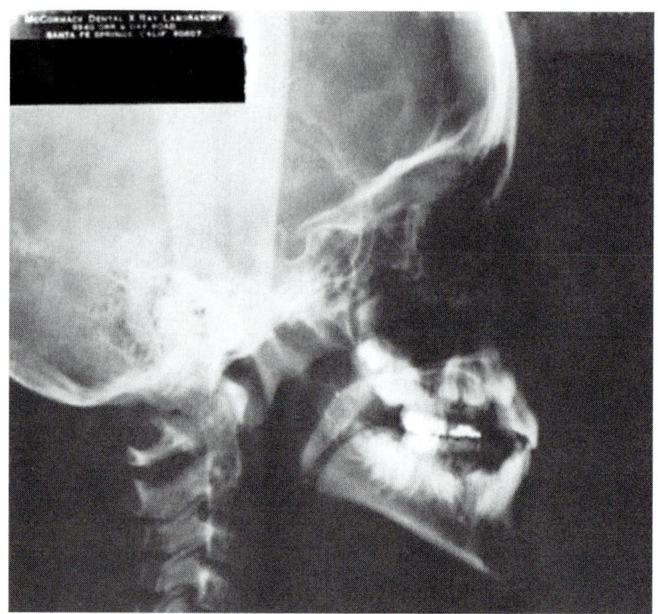

FIGURE 20–5. **Lateral skull cephalometric radiographs** are often required by orthodontists for making measurements of the head. A device is essential to position the head to achieve standardization and to establish a fixed relationship between the x-ray tube, the patient's head, and the film cassette. Ear rods are used to stabilize and maintain the head position. The film is positioned in a plane parallel to the midsagittal plane of the patient, and the central ray passes through both ear rods from the target-film distance of 60 in. (1.52 m) or more. Cephalometric tracings may be made from these radiographs. (Courtesy of McCormack Dental X-ray Laboratory)

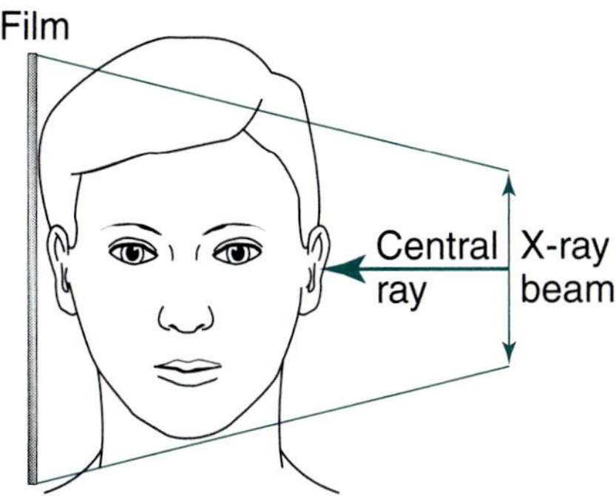

FIGURE 20–6. **Lateral skull survey**. The central ray is directed at 0-degree vertical angulation through the acoustic meatus of the ear and perpendicular to the cassette.

surgeons use the lateral skull cephalometric projection to establish pretreatment and post-treatment records.

Film Placement

An 8- × 10-in. (21- × 26-cm) cassette is positioned vertically in a holding device.

Head Position

The head is positioned with the left side of the face next to the cassette. The **midsagittal plane** is parallel to the cassette.

Facial Soft-tissue Profile

If a facial soft tissue profile is desired, a wedge filter is placed over the anterior side of the beam at the tube head. The filter absorbs some of the x-rays in the anterior region and results in the soft tissue outline of the patient's face on the radiograph.

Central Ray Alignment

The central ray is directed towards the **acoustic meatus** (opening of the ear) and perpendicularly toward the center of the film (see Figure 20–6).

Exposure Factors

The exposure factors vary considerably, depending upon the screen-film combination, target-film distance, and equipment used.

Posteroanterior (PA) Cephalometric Projection

The **posteroanterior projection** shows the entire skull in the posteroanterior plane. The PA radiograph is so named because the x-ray beam passes through the skull in a posterior-to-anterior direction.

Purpose

The purpose of the PA projection is to examine facial growth and development, disease, trauma, and developmental abnormalities. Because the right and left sides of the bony and facial structures are not superimposed on each other, this survey is often used to supplement the lateral skull survey.

Film Placement

An 8- × 10-in. (21- × 26-cm) cassette with intensifying screen is held in position vertically by a holding device.

Head Position

The patient faces the cassette. The patient's head is centered in front of the cassette so that the forehead and nose touch the face of the cassette (see Figure 20–7).

Central Ray Alignment

The central ray is then directed perpendicular to the film toward the external **occipital protuberance** (the large bump that can be felt by palpitating the occipital bone near the base of the skull) (see Figure 20–7).

Exposure Factors

The exposure factors vary considerably, depending upon the screen-film combination, target-film distance, and equipment used.

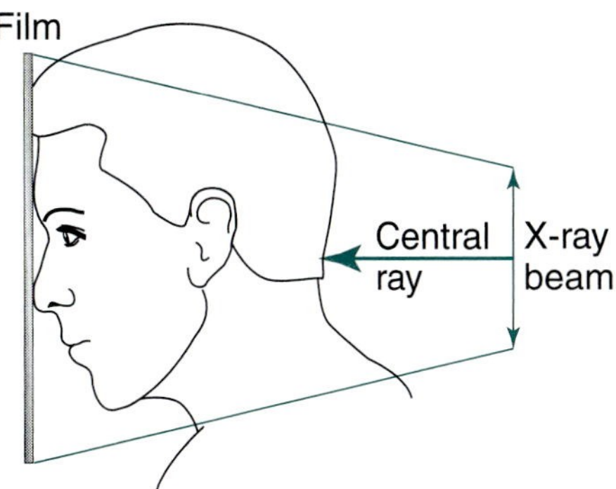

FIGURE 20–7. **Posteroanterior survey**. The nose and forehead touch the cassette. The central ray is directed at the occipital protuberance at a vertical angulation of 0-degree and perpendicular to the cassette.

Waters' (Sinus) Projection

The **Waters' projection** is also known as the **sinus projection.** It is similar to the posteroanterior projection except that the center of interest is focused on the middle third of the face (see Figure 20–8).

Purpose

The Waters' radiograph is particularly useful to evaluate the maxillary, frontal, and ethmoid sinuses.

Film Placement

The cassette is positioned vertically in a holding device.

Head Position

The patient faces the cassette. The patient's head is centered on the cassette with the midsagittal plane perpendicular to the floor. The chin touches the cassette and nose is positioned about 3/4 in. (18 mm) from the cassette.

Central Ray Alignment

As in the posteroanterior survey, the central ray is directed perpendicular to the center of the film through the occipital protuberance. The target-film distance is usually a minimum of 36 in. (0.9 m) (see Figure 20–8).

Exposure Factors

The exposure factors vary considerably, depending upon the screen-film combination, target-film distance, and equipment used.

Reverse-Towne Projection

Purpose

The **Reverse-Towne radiograph** is used to examine fractures of the condylar neck of the mandible (see Figure 20–9).

Film Placement

The cassette is positioned vertically in a holding device.

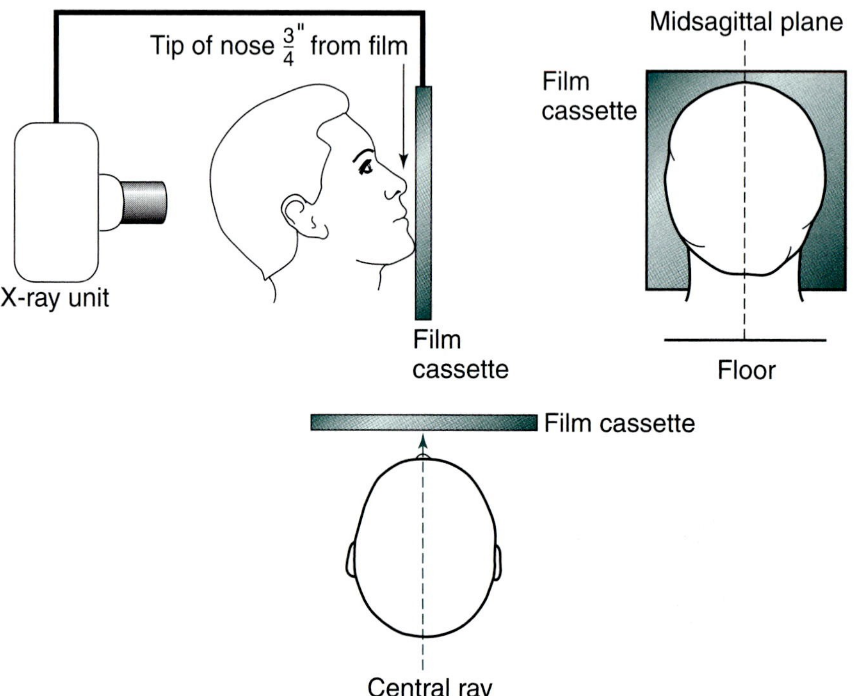

FIGURE 20–8. **Sinus survey (Waters' projection).** The chin touches the cassette and the nose is positioned about .75 in. (18 mm) from the cassette. The central ray is directed perpendicular to the center of the cassette through the occipital protuberance.

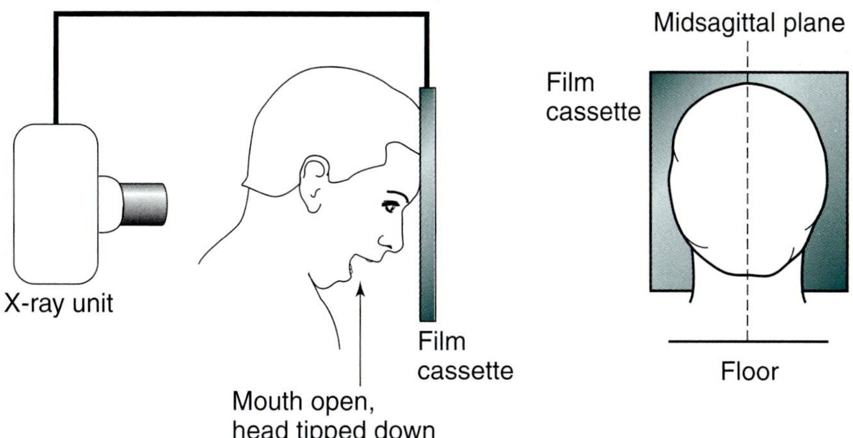

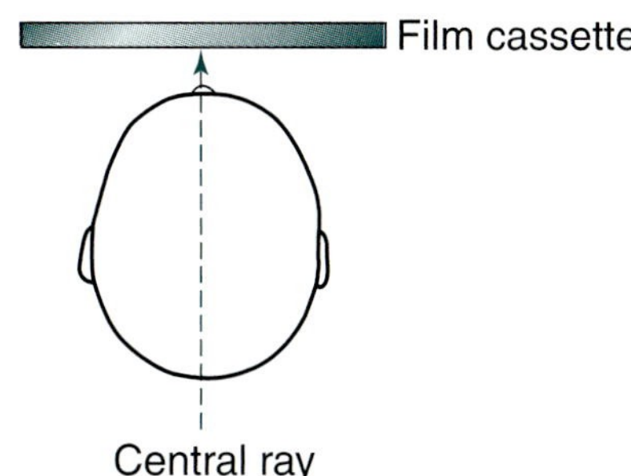

FIGURE 20–9. **Reverse-Towne projection.** The patient faces the cassette with the midsagittal plane perpendicular to the floor. With the mouth wide open, the patient's head is tipped down until the chin touches the chest. The top of the forehead rests against the cassette.

Head Position

The patient faces the cassette with the midsagittal plane perpendicular to the floor. With the mouth wide open, the patient's head is tipped down until the chin touches the chest. The top of the forehead rests against the cassette.

Central Ray Alignment

The central ray is directed perpendicular to the center of the film through the occipital protuberance. The target-film distance is usually a minimum of 36 in. (0.9 m).

Exposure Factors

The exposure factors vary considerably, depending upon the screen-film combination, target-film distance, and equipment used.

Submentovertex Projection

Purpose

The submentovertex radiograph is used to show the base of the skull, the position and orientation of the condyles, the sphenoid sinus, and fractures of the zygomatic arch (see Figure 20–10).

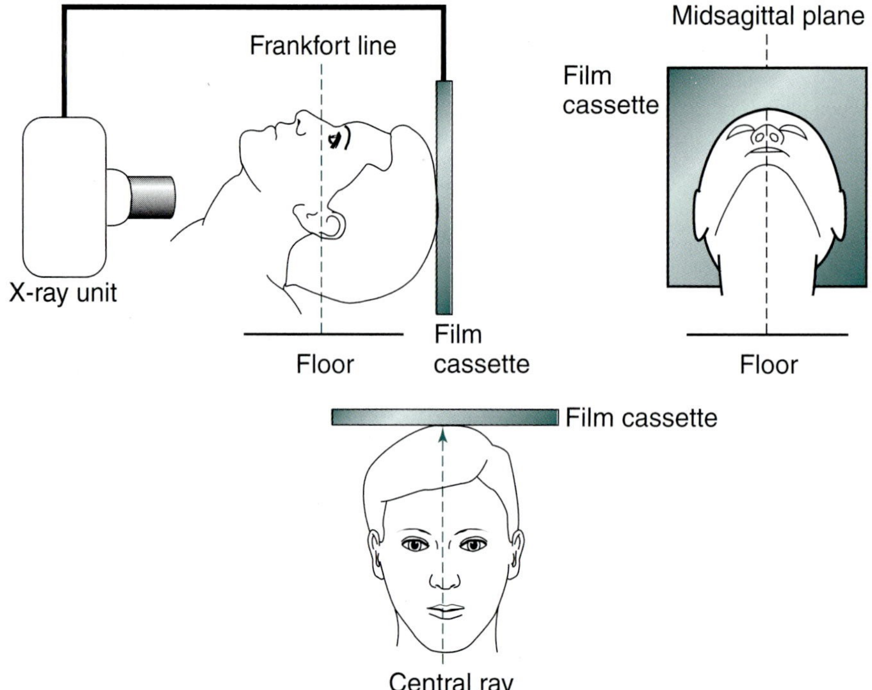

FIGURE 20–10. **Submentovertex projection.** The patient's head and neck are extended backward so the vertex (top) of the head touches the center of the cassette. The midsagittal plane is perpendicular to the floor. The Frankfort line is vertical and parallel with the film.

Film Placement

The cassette is positioned vertically in a holding device.

Head Position

The patient's head and neck are extended backward so the vertex (top) of the head touches the center of the cassette. The midsagittal plane is perpendicular to the floor. The **Frankfort plane** is vertical and parallel with the film.

Central Ray Alignment

The central ray is directed perpendicular to the film from below the mandible through the center of the head.

Exposure Factors

The exposure factors vary considerably, depending upon the screen-film combination, target-film distance, and equipment used.

Temporomandibular Joint Projection

The **temporomandibular joint (TMJ)** is very difficult to examine radiographically because the head of the mandibular **condyle** articulates with the **glenoid fossa** in an area where the structure of the temporal bone is extremely dense.

Purpose

The temporomandibular joint (TMJ) survey aids the dentist in diagnosing **ankylosis** (a stiffening of the joint caused by fibrous or bony union), malignancies, fractures, and tissue changes caused by arthritis. A radiograph, or series of radiographs, showing the head of the mandibular condyle in relation to the glenoid fossa of the temporal bone is essential for the dentist to make a diagnostic interpretation.

Some dentists make only one exposure, whereas others make several—with the mouth closed and the teeth in occlusion, at rest with the teeth slightly separated, and with the mouth fully open (see Figure 20–11). Because this exposure is made from the opposite side, the central ray has to pass first through a series of bones and soft structures. Therefore, the exposure requires extreme care and accuracy in adjusting the cassette to the head position and directing the PID so that the rays will strike the film at the best angle.

The two most common TMJ projection techniques are the transcranial projection and tomography.

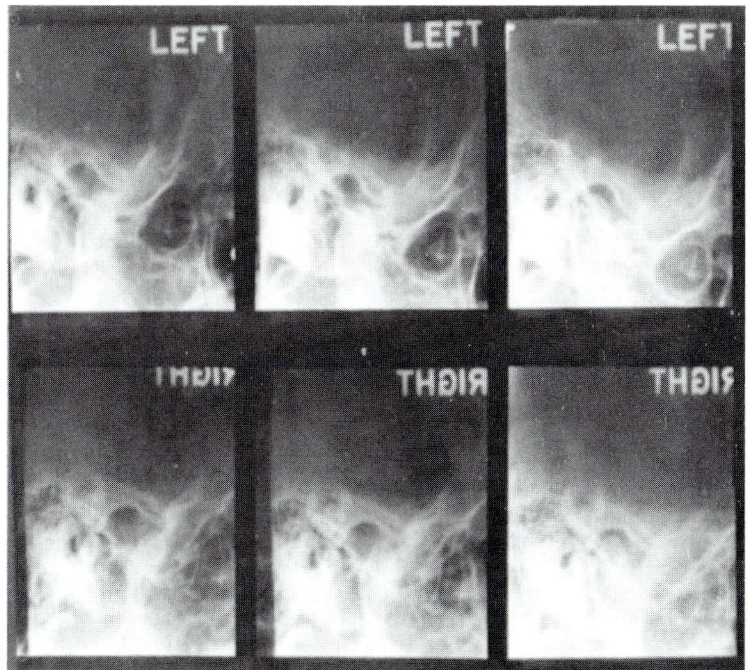

FIGURE 20–11. **Serial radiographs of the temporomandibular joint** showing the head of the condyle in the glenoid fossa with the mouth closed, in the at-rest position, and with the mouth open. A stabilizing device of some type is generally required to hold the patient's head in a firm position while the cassette is moved for each exposure on the same side. Such equipment for serial radiography is not available in most offices; single exposures can readily be made using techniques similar to those for the lateral jaw exposures. (Courtesy of McCormack Dental X-ray Laboratory)

Transcranial Projection

There are probably more ways to make a transcranial projection and more opinions about how to expose it than for any other extraoral radiograph. As the area to be examined is relatively small, a common practice is to use a single large film and make several exposures on it. Parts of the film are covered with lead so that only one part of the film is exposed each time. Thus three or four exposures, with the head of the condyle in a different position each time, can be made consecutively on the same film.

Purpose

The transcranial projection is used to view the TMJ in both an open and closed position.

Film Placement

The cassette is positioned against the ear and centered over the acoustic meatus (opening of the ear) (see Figure 20–12).

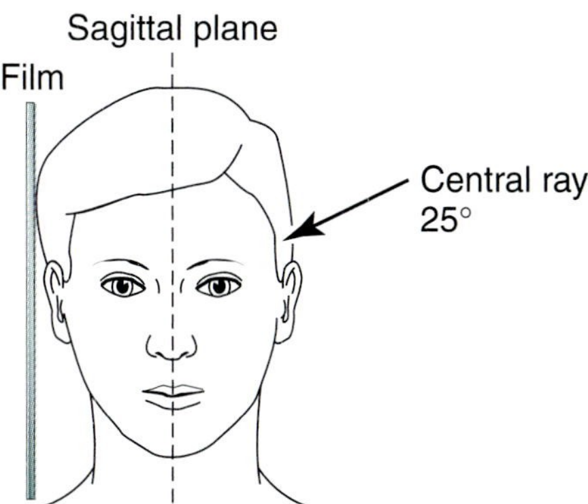

FIGURE 20–12. **Temporomandibular joint (TMJ) survey.** The central ray is directed at a vertical angulation of about + 25 degrees to the center of the film not covered by lead. The point of entry is located about 2.5 in. (6.4 cm) higher and slightly in front of the acoustic meatus of the ear.

Head Position

The midsagittal plane of the patient's head is positioned perpendicular to the floor and parallel to the cassette.

Central Ray Alignment

Direct the central ray at a vertical angulation of about +25 degrees to the center of the part of the film that is not covered with lead. The point of entry for the central ray is located about 2 1/2 in. (6.4 cm) higher and slightly in front of the acoustic meatus (opening of the ear). Caution the patient not to move or change position.

Exposure Factors

The exposure factors vary considerably, depending upon the screen-film combination, target-film distance, and equipment used.

The disadvantage of this technique is that it is difficult to stabilize the patient's head and prevent movement. Moreover, without special equipment, it is difficult to repeat the same exposure and get identical results. Manufacturers have produced new devices to assist the radiographer in positioning the patient and aligning the central ray. Such equipment is necessary to achieve reproducibility and permit comparison of radiographs.

Tomography

Tomography (see Chapter 21) is a special radiographic technique used to show images of structures located within a selected plane of tissue while blurring structures outside the selected plane.

Radiographs made using the tomography technique are called **tomographs.** Special tomographic x-ray equipment is required for TMJ tomography. Because of the high cost, few dentists own such equipment. Dentists usually refer patients requiring TMJ tomographs to hospitals or other radiographic imaging facilities.

CHAPTER SUMMARY

Extraoral radiography is the technique of producing radiographs by placing the film at the side of the face or head and positioning the source of radiation on the opposite side.

Three types of x-ray machines are used to produce radiographs: conventional x-ray machines, panoramic machines, and cephalometric machines.

Extraoral films should be the screen-type, so that the least amount of radiation is used. These films must be loaded into cassettes in the darkroom. Always check manufacturer's directions for safelight tolerance, exposure time, and processing.

Extraoral films are exposed for a variety of reasons including:

- Examination of large areas of the jaws and skull
- Study growth and development of bone and teeth
- Detection of fractures and evaluation of trauma
- Detection of pathological lesions and diseases of the jaws
- Detection and evaluation of impacted teeth
- Evaluate temporomandibular joint (TMJ) disorders

Initially films were exposed extraorally to supplement the intraoral survey. Several accessory or supplemental techniques that could be used with the conventional x-ray machine evolved. These include techniques for exposing impacted molar areas, the lateral jaw and skull, facial profiles, posteroanterior surveys, the temporomandibular joints, and the sinuses.

Cephalometric radiographs are generally exposed at the request of the orthodontist to assist in completing the diagnosis or treatment plan, to make tracings, and to record conditions before, during, and after treatment. Orthodontists, prosthodontists, and oral surgeons are major users of extraoral films.

REVIEW QUESTIONS

1. Which of these films is most often used in extraoral radiography?
   (a) Periapical film
   (b) Screen film
   (c) Occlusal film
   (d) Nonscreen film

2. What size film is generally used in cephalometric radiography?
   (a) 2 1/4 × 3 in. (57 × 76 mm)
   (b) 5 × 7 in. (13 × 18 cm)
   (c) 8 × 10 in. (20 × 25 cm)
   (d) 5 × 12 in. (13 × 30 cm)

3. For which of these purposes is extraoral film least suitable?
   (a) For detection of interproximal caries
   (b) For locating impacted teeth
   (c) For viewing the sinuses
   (d) For determining the extent of a fracture

4. Which of these surveys is most frequently ordered by the prosthodontist?
   (a) Sinus
   (b) Posteroanterior
   (c) Interproximal
   (d) Facial profile

5. Which of these radiographs would best show an impacted mandibular third molar?
   (a) Lateral jaw
   (b) Bitewing
   (c) Cephalometric
   (d) Temporomandibular joint

6. Which term describes a device used to stabilize the patient's head parallel to the film and at right angles to the direction of the x-ray beam?
   (a) Orbitale
   (b) Cephalostat
   (c) Exposure holder
   (d) Headplate

BIBLIOGRAPHY

Farman, A. G., Nortje, C. J., & Wood, R. E. *Oral and Maxillofacial Diagnostic Imaging*. St Louis: Mosby; 1993.

White, S. C. & Pharoah, M. J. *Oral Radiology Principles and Interpretation*, 4th ed. St. Louis: Mosby, 2000.

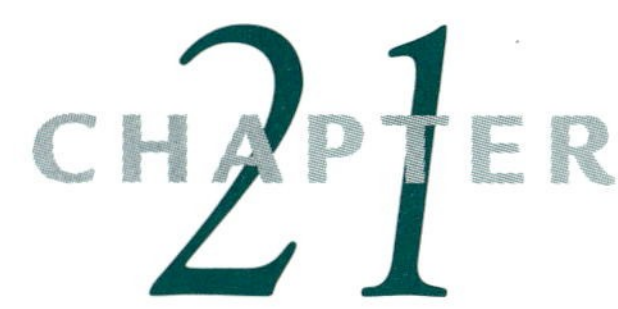

Panoramic Radiography

OBJECTIVES

By the end of this chapter the student should be able to:

- Define the key words.
- State the purpose and use of panoramic radiography.
- Differentiate between a conventional and a panoramic x-ray machine.
- Identify the main factor that determines the width of the focal trough.
- Identify the major factors that affect the geometry of the image.
- Identify the planes used to position the head correctly.
- Identify in sequence the basic steps in operating a panoramic x-ray unit.
- Compare the advantages and disadvantages of panoramic versus intraoral radiographic surveys.
- Identify five major head-positioning errors that result in faulty panoramic radiographs.
- List and identify the anatomic landmarks of the maxilla and surrounding tissues as viewed on a panoramic radiograph.
- List and identify the anatomic landmarks of the mandible and surrounding tissues as viewed on a panoramic radiograph.
- List and identify four soft tissue images as viewed on a panoramic radiograph.
- List and identify three air space images as viewed on a panoramic radiograph.

KEY WORDS

Cassette
Cassette holder
Drum
Flexible cassette
Focal trough
Frankfort plane
Head positioner
Laminography
Midsagittal plane
Orbitale
Orthopantomograph
Panelipse
Panoramic
Panoramic radiography
Panorex
Pantomography
Porion
Rotational center
Rotational panoramic radiography
Sagittal plane
Tomography

Introduction

Panoramic radiography refers to a technique for producing a radiograph that shows both the maxilla and mandible on a single radiograph. By placing an elongated screen film varying in width from 5 to 6 in. wide and 12 in. long (13 to 15 cm wide and 30 cm long) in a rigid or flexible cassette that is positioned extraorally, the dental professional is able to produce an image of the entire dentition, the surrounding alveolar bone, the sinuses, and the temporomandibular joints on a single film.

The purpose of this chapter is to explain the fundamental concepts of panoramic radiography and to describe the operational procedures of panoramic x-ray machines. Normal anatomy of the maxilla and mandible, soft tissue images, and air space images are also presented.

Terminology

The term **panoramic** means "wide view." The term **panoramic radiography** refers to an extraoral technique which produces a radiograph with a wide view of the maxilla and mandible. It is also known as **pantomography** (making graphic recordings of contours on radiographic film), **tomography** (making body sections on radiographic film), and **laminography** (from *lamina*, meaning "thin layer," and graphy, meaning "to record"), the recording of selected layers of body tissue on radiographic film. The term **panoramic radiography** is most common because the resulting radiograph shows a panoramic view of a large area of the face and lower portion of the head.

Purpose and Use

The **purpose** of panoramic radiography is to provide a radiograph with an image of the maxilla and mandible on a single film. The dentist uses a panoramic radiograph to:

- Examine large areas of the face and jaws
- Locate impacted teeth
- Evaluate trauma, lesions, and disease of the jaws
- Evaluate growth and development

Panoramic radiography **saves time.** Instead of exposing 16 or more intraoral radiographs, the entire panoramic exposure can be made in less than 3 min instead of the 15 min usually required for the full-mouth intraoral series. Time is also saved during processing by eliminating the sorting, arranging, and mounting of 16 separate films.

Not only is the exposure faster to make, but it is also more pleasant for the patient, as pressure against delicate tissues and gagging are eliminated.

The panoramic radiograph is **ideal for mass surveys,** as are common in the military services and public health clinics, for children, for invalids, and for any situation where a rapid survey is desired.

Diagnosis is simplified because all the teeth, whether erupted or not, and the sinuses are shown in a consecutive sequence, rather than in a series of separate and overlapping films. With the aid of a panoramic radiograph, the dentist is able to obtain a complete picture of the area of treatment.

Panoramic radiographs show poor image detail and should not be used to detect and evaluate caries or periodontal disease. For such evaluations, bitewing and periapical radiographs are required.

Fundamentals of Rotational Panoramic Radiography

During conventional intraoral radiography the x-ray source and the film remain stationary. The opposite happens in **rotational panoramic radiography,** which can be defined as a technique for making radiographic projections by utilizing a narrow beam of x-rays to image a curved layer.

Panoramic x-ray machines operate with the patient positioned between the tube head and the cassette that holds the film. The exposure is a continuous one, made as the tube head and cassette rotate slowly about the patient's head during the operational cycle (usually about 15 to 20 sec). These machines are said to operate on the principle of curved surface laminography.

The film in its cassette and the tube head move in opposite directions while the patient stands or is seated in a stationary position (see Figure 21–1). Through a series of rotational points or centers (differing according to the manufacturer), the x-ray beam is directed toward the moving cassette to reveal a select plane of dental anatomy. The **rotational center,** which is defined as the axis on which the tube head and the cassette rotate, is the functional focus of the projection. Unlike the concentric or rectangular beam of x-radiation common in intraoral radiography, the x-rays emerge from a narrow vertical slit opening in the tube head and are constricted to form a narrow band.

The radiation beam then passes vertically through the patient toward the cassette and through another vertical slit in the cassette holder to expose the film that is moving or rotating past (see Figure 21–2). By making use of this narrow opening in the tube head, the x-ray beam is collimated and much less tissue is irradiated as the x-rays pass through the patient to the slit in the cassette holder. This results in a panoramic radiograph showing a well-defined image of a curved layer of tissue including the teeth and tooth-bearing areas.

A variety of domestic and imported machines are available. The major differences between the machines are the number and location of rotational centers existing between the x-ray source and film. Following are descriptions of the three basic types, as shown in Figure 21–3.

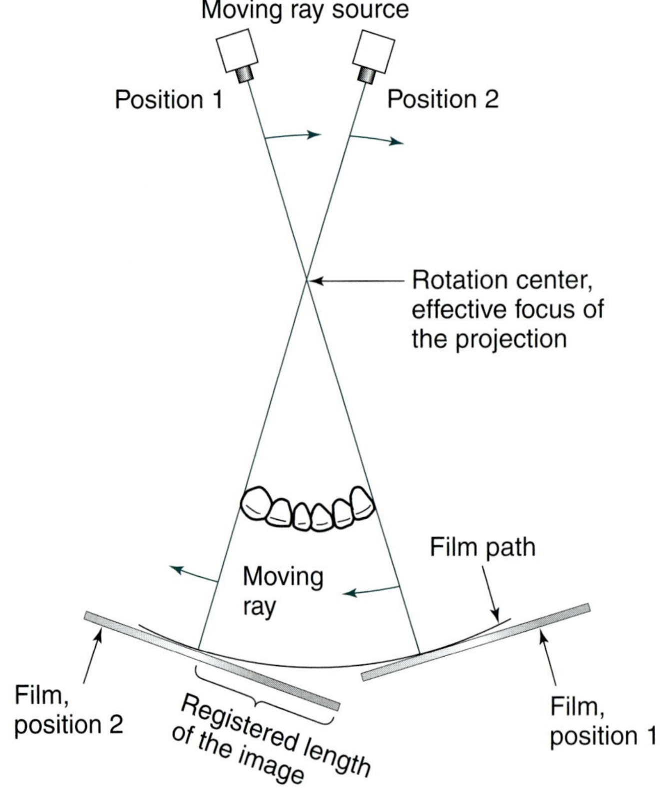

FIGURE 21–1. **Panoramic radiography.** Diagram showing the relationship of the moving x-ray beam as it passes through the center of rotation in a horizontal plane toward the path of the moving x-ray film. As the beam scans the object (usually the dental arches), a continuous image is registered on the moving film. (From a syllabus prepared for a symposium on Panoramic Radiography presented at Anaheim, California on October 3, 1983, by the American Dental Association (ADA) in cooperation with the University of Texas Health Science Center at San Antonio (UTHSCSA) Dental School. Particular thanks to the panelists Drs. Charles R. Morris, W. Doss McDavid, John W. Preece, Robert P. Langlais, Brigit J. Glass, and Olaf E. Langland)

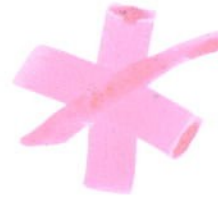

1. **Double-center rotation.** Here the left and right sides of the arc formed by the teeth and jaws coincide with arcs of two circles with centers at X and O as shown in Figure 21–3A. Two separate exposures are necessary, as the equipment shifts from one center to the other. This results in a "split" film image.
2. **Triple-center rotation.** With this method, three centers of rotation are used, as shown in Figure 21–3B. Although the examination contains three separate segments, the x-ray beam can be shifted from one center to the other with minor interruption, and a continuous image can be made.
3. **Moving-center rotation.** Good diagnostic results can be obtained with the beam rotating around a center that moves continuously in a path that is similar in shape to the anatomy being examined. The elliptical pattern made by the machine shown in Figure 21–3C very closely matches the arc of the teeth and jaws. A continuous image is provided. Both horizontal and vertical magnification of the image are relatively constant, and this system allows adjustment of the size of the elliptical path to match the varying size dental arches.

It is important to be aware that the projections in the horizontal (see Figure 21–1) and the vertical (see Figure 21–2) directions do not have the same **focus of projection.** In the horizontal plane, it is at the center of

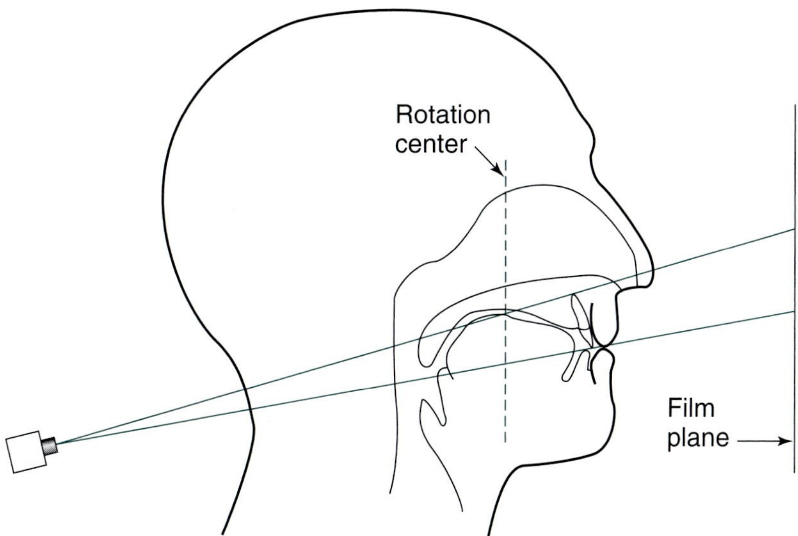

FIGURE 21–2. **Rotational center.** Diagram showing the relationship in a vertical plane of the tube head to the center of rotation and the film as the moving x-ray beam passes through the patient's head toward the moving film. (From a symposium syllabus on Panoramic Radiography by the ADA in cooperation with the UTHSCSA Dental School)

rotation, whereas in the vertical plane it is located at the target in the tube head. This difference in the location of the foci of projection accounts for the fact that a degree of image distortion is characteristic of rotational panoramic radiographs.

Concept of the Focal Trough

The **focal trough** is not an anatomical structure; rather, it is a theoretical concept used in rotational panoramic radiography to determine where the dental arches, the sinuses, or other areas that are to be examined should be positioned in order to achieve the clearest image. The focal trough (see Figure 21–4) is that area of the dental anatomy that is reproduced distinctly on the panoramic radiograph. Theoretically, a plane extends through this trough, and objects in that plane are recorded with diagnostic sharpness. Objects located at various distances from the plane become less sharp as they get farther from the plane.

Size and Shape of the Focal Trough

The **focal trough** is three-dimensional, and its actual shape varies depending on the equipment used. The size and shape of the focal trough are controlled by the manufacturer.

The main factor that determines the **width** of the focal tough is the distance from the functional center of rotation to the object (the structures to be radiographed). As a general rule the width of the focal trough increases whenever the distance from the rotational center to the object is increased. The width of the focal trough and distance from the rotation center is controlled by the speed of the moving cassette. This means that the manufacturer can program the width and the shape of the focal trough to conform to the shape of an average dental arch by varying the speed of the moving cassette.

The drawings in Figure 21–5 show **variations** in the **shape** of the **focal trough** produced by panoramic x-ray machines having:

1. Double-center rotation
2. Triple-center rotation
3. Moving-center rotation

The double-center system (see Figure 21–5A) trough is wide both anteriorly and posteriorly, with the distal ends of the trough curving medially. The inward curving is unfavorable to obtaining the best sharpness in the temporomandibular joint areas.

The other focal troughs show wide posterior and narrow anterior thickness. The clinical implication is that the

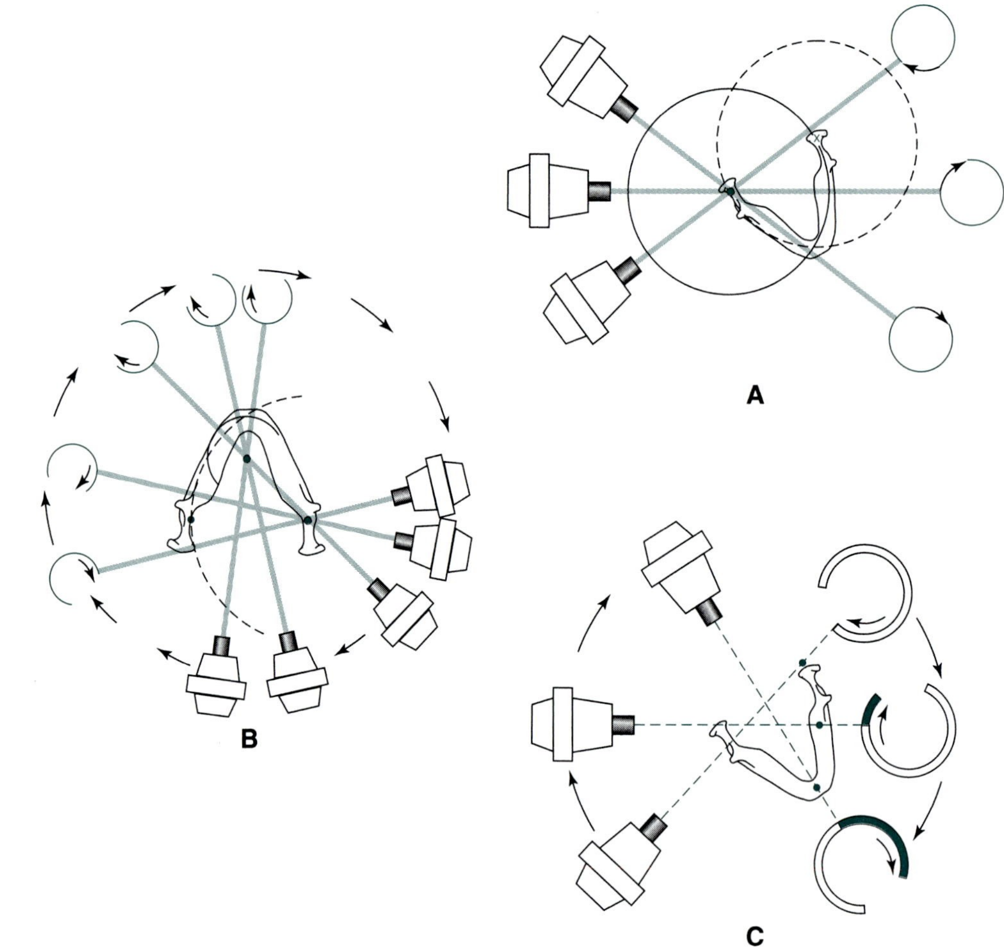

FIGURE 21–3. **Rotational panoramic radiography machines.** (**A**) Double-center rotation system used by Panorex (made by Keystone X-ray, Inc.). (**B**) Triple-center rotation system used by Orthopantomograph (made by Siemens Corporation, West Germany). (**C**) Moving-center rotating system used by Panelipse (made by Gendex Corporation). (Panoramic illustrations reproduced with permission from Manson-Hing LR. *Principles of panoramic radiography.* Springfield, IL: Thomas, 1976)

anterior teeth must be positioned very accurately. The distal ends shown in Figure 21–5B flair laterally, whereas in Figure 21–5C, they extend straight posteriorly. The moving-center system has the widest trough in the posterior areas, facilitating temporomandibular joint studies.

Geometry and Sharpness of the Panoramic Image

Consideration must also be given to those factors that affect the **geometric shape** (distortion) and **sharpness** of the image. **Distortion** can be defined as unequal vertical and horizontal magnification. In conventional radiography, the x-ray images may be magnified equally in a horizontal and vertical direction by using the paralleling technique. The amount of magnification is proportional to the target-object distance and the object-film distance.

In rotational panoramic radiography, vertical and horizontal magnification are controlled by two different factors. The focal spot in the vertical direction is the actual focal spot in the anode of the x-ray tube, whereas the apparent focal spot in the horizontal direction is the center of rotation (effective rotation center). The magnification in the vertical dimension is proportional to the target-

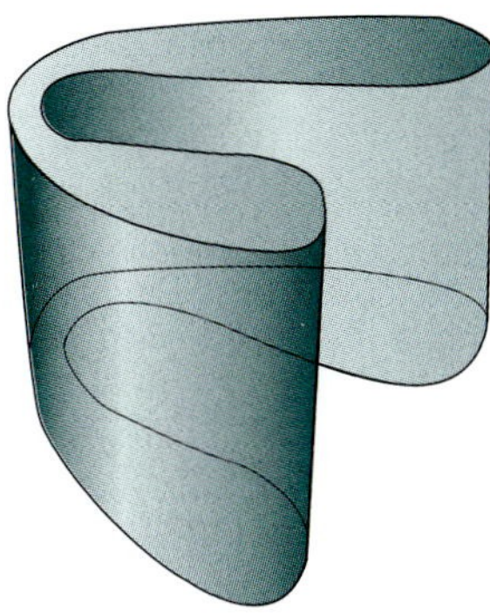

FIGURE 21–4. **Diagrammatic sketch of focal trough.** (Panoramic illustrations reproduced with permission form Manson-Hing LR. *Principles of panoramic radiography.* Springfield, IL: Thomas, 1976)

object distance and the object-film distance (same as conventional radiography). The magnification in the horizontal dimension is controlled by the effective rotation center-object distance and the object-film distance.

If there were no film movement, the amount of magnification would be much greater in the horizontal dimension than in the vertical dimension. But the slow movement of the film compensates for this so that the horizontal and vertical magnification are equal for objects in the focal trough. Therefore, movement of the film not only controls the width of the focal trough, and the shape of the focal trough, movement of the film also compensates to make the horizontal and vertical magnification equal for objects in the focal trough.

It is easier to visualize image geometry if one imagines the focal trough to be that layer of tissues or area of space within the head that is occupied by the teeth and the alveolar bone. The factors of image magnification or diminution are equal if the structures or objects to be viewed are positioned in the center of the focal trough. These same structures or objects, if displaced backward (toward the center of rotation) will appear wider, and if displaced forward (toward the film) will appear narrower (see Figure 21–6).

For the machines that have fixed centers of rotation, the magnification varies within a certain range. The range exists because the object's position relative to the film and x-ray tube is constantly changing. This happens because the curve of the jaw does not identically follow the curve of a circle.

However, in machines with moving centers of rotation, the object, tube, and film positions are more constant, making the magnification virtually constant. When considering factors that influence the geometry or sharpness of the image, it is helpful to realize that the path of the sliding center of rotation (see Figure 21–7) is predetermined by the manufacturer and cannot be changed by the operator. What can, and unfortunately does, occur is that the operator malpositions the patient's head in relation to the focal trough. When that happens, some of the images may be magnified, diminished, or blurred.

Although undesirable in a panoramic film, a minor degree of magnification of the image is generally acceptable. Blurring or lack of sharpness of the image often reduces the amount of diagnostic information that can be obtained from the radiograph.

The manufacturer gives the film a speed that matches the projected speed of points lying within a selected curved plane. Consequently, these points are sharply depicted on the radiograph. The projection of object points outside the focal trough, either toward the center of rotation or toward the film, has a different projected speed at the film plane from the film itself. Thus, the projection of these points moves in relation to the film and appears blurred. Because the difference between the speed of the film and the speed of the projection of the points in the

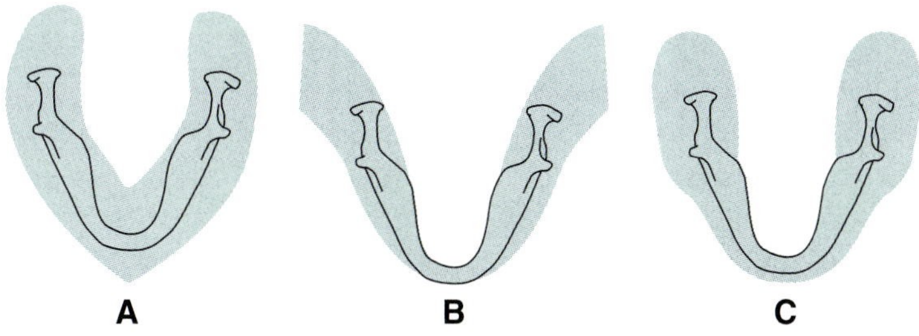

FIGURE 21–5. **Variations in shape of focal trough** produced by panoramic x-ray machines having (**A**) double-center rotation, (**B**) triple-center rotation, (**C**) moving-center rotation. (Panoramic illustrations reproduced with permission form Manson-Hing LR. *Principles of panoramic radiography.* Springfield, IL: Thomas, 1976)

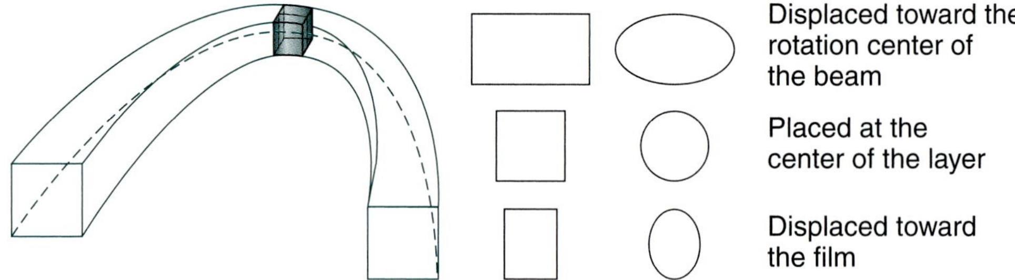

FIGURE 21-6. **Image geometry.** At the center of the layer the magnification, factors in the horizontal and vertical directions are equal. This implies that a small flat object positioned at the center of the layer will be portrayed in proper proportion. Outside the center of the layer, the magnification factors in these two dimensions are unequal. This results in distortion effects. If three planes are cut out from the layer at different object depths, the images of objects in these planes will exhibit different proportions. The plane at the center is correctly depicted. The positioned toward the rotational center of the beam will be magnified more in the horizontal than in the vertical dimension and will appear too narrow. (From a symposium syllabus on Panoramic Radiography by the ADA in cooperation with the UTHSCSA Dental School)

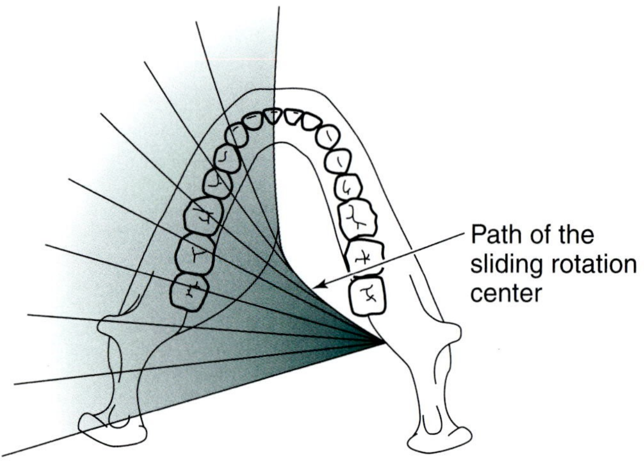

FIGURE 21-7. **Path of sliding center of rotation.** In systems creating continuous images, several different movement patterns of the beam are utilized to achieve the desired projection of the jaws. The objective is to project each part of the jaws as close to perpendicular as possible. The beam may be given a sliding movement throughout the total excursion, so that the effective projection center (the functional focus) is constantly shifted along a defined path. The central ray of the beam is always at a tangent to this path at some point. The form of the path defines the direction of the beam and hence the projection of each successive part of the jaws. (From a symposium syllabus on Panoramic Radiography by the ADA in cooperation with the UTHSCSA Dental School)

object (usually the teeth) increases with the distance from the sharply depicted object plane, the lack of clarity increases in both directions from this plane. At some distance, this lack of clarity reaches a level where an object point is no longer visible on the radiograph. This can be avoided by proper head positioning.

Importance of Correct Head Positioning

The most important **factor** that can be **controlled by the operator** is the correct **positioning** of the **patient's head.** Failure to do so will result in a radiograph with reduced or no diagnostic value. The head positioning will vary, depending on whether the major area of interest is in the region of the temporomandibular joints, the sinuses, or the teeth. The manufacturers supply detailed instructions on how each of these areas should be positioned within the focal trough.

Because the area of interest in the majority of panoramic radiographs is centered on the teeth and the surrounding alveolar structures, methods of correctly positioning the dental arches are of prime importance.

Most rotational panoramic x-ray machines have some type of **head positioner** (see Figure 21–8) that assists the operator in determining the optimum position. Each machine is different, and the operator must follow the manufacturer's instructions. Easier-to-adjust head positioners are being introduced.

The **Orthopantomograph 10** casts three separate beams of light on the patients face to indicate the location of important planes. The first beam indicates the position of the **Frankfort plane,** a horizontal line between the **porion** and the **orbitale.** When properly adjusted, this line should be parallel with the floor to give the correct skull inclination. The second beam helps to locate the **sagittal plane,** which must be positioned at midline to locate the vertical center of the focal trough. The third beam indicates to the operator the location of the layer of maximum sharpness in the central incisor region.

Since most panoramic machines have relatively wide focal troughs in the posterior area, the posterior teeth can usually be positioned in the trough. In the anterior region, many of the machines have narrow focal troughs and must be positioned with extreme precision. If maxillary incisors are to be placed in the trough, the apices must be brought slightly forward. Since mandibular incisors also tend to have their apices placed posteriorly, the operator will have the patient bring the incisors into an edge-to-edge position for better visualization.

The operator may have difficulty checking these head positions when using equipment requiring the patient to face the wall. Extra care must be taken to visualize the midline of the patient's face and the sagittal plane. To maintain image quality and uniform x-ray absorption, the operator should keep the patient's spine as erect as possible. If the patient is seated, rather than standing, the system should have a movable backrest for proper positioning.

When correctly positioned, the anterior teeth are in the focal trough, and there is an equal magnification and sharpness over all parts of the radiographic image (see Figure 21–9). If the patient has been positioned too far forward (toward the film), the anterior teeth are in front of the focal trough and appear blurred and diminished, particularly in width (see Figure 21–10). If the patient has been positioned too far backward (toward the x-ray tube head), the anterior teeth are behind the focal trough and the anterior teeth appear magnified and blurred (see Figure 21–11). If the patient's head has been rotated, the anterior teeth are correctly positioned in the focal trough, but the teeth on the side closer to the film are diminished, whereas those on the side closer to the center of rotation are enlarged (see Figure 21–12).

Numerous other position errors, such as tilting the chin up or down (see Figures 21–13 and 21–14), can be made. An exposure should never be made until the operator is satisfied that all planes are correctly aligned.

Types of Panoramic X-ray Machines

New types of machines with varying capabilities are being introduced, and changes are being made by the manufacturers so rapidly that it is not feasible to give a detailed description here.

The various manufacturers use trade names such as **Orthopantomograph, Orthoceph,** and **Status X** (Siemens); **Panorex** (Keystone); **Panelipse** (Gendex); **Versaview** (Morita); and others. Many panoramic machines now have cephalometric capabilities.

Rotational Machines

All of the x-ray machines mentioned except the Status X (Siemens) are of the **rotational** type. As stated previously, rotational panoramic x-ray machines have a mechanism that moves the tube and film in opposite directions simultaneously while the specific tissue layer remains in a fixed relationship to the tube. The film produces a clear image of the layer that is being examined while at the same time blurring and eliminating the

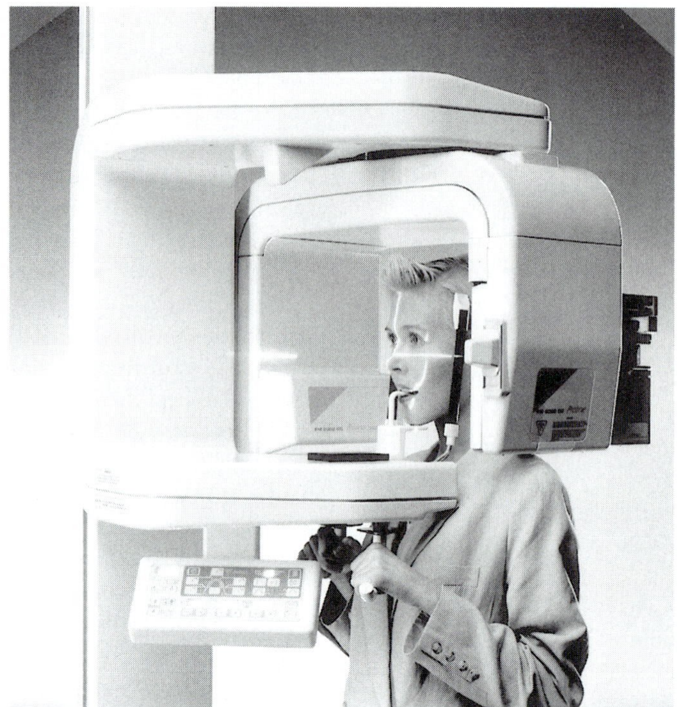

FIGURE 21-8. **Head positioner.** Photo of patient with head properly positioned in head positioner of Planmeca 2002 CC Proline Pan. The beams of light on the patient's face indicate the location of important planes. (Courtesy of Planmeca)

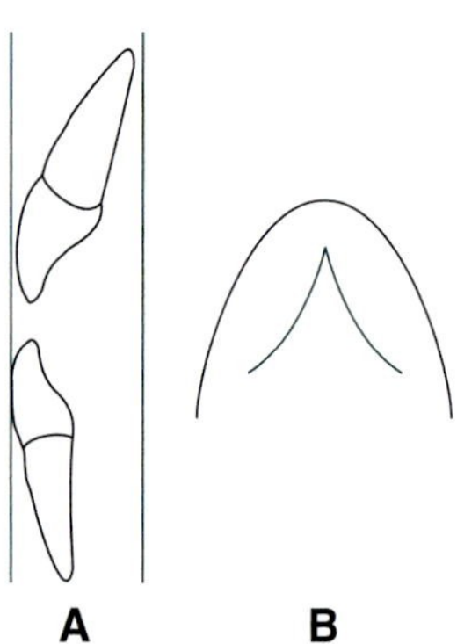

FIGURE 21-9. **Correct positioning** with equal magnification and sharpness all over the image. (**A**) Anterior teeth on focal trough. (**B**) Relationship of center of rotation to dental arches. (From a symposium syllabus on Panoramic Radiography by the ADA in cooperation with the UTHSCSA Dental School)

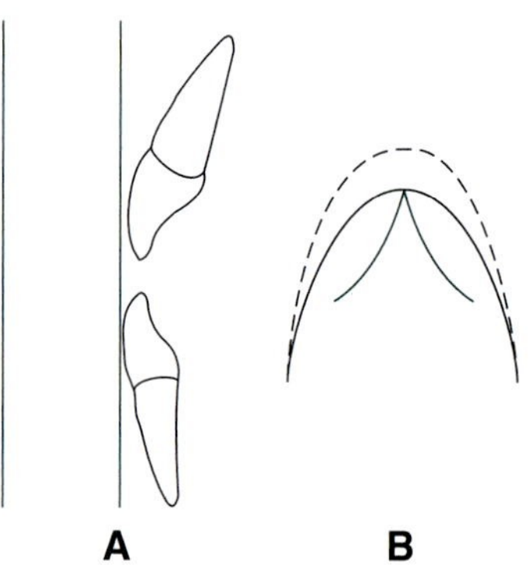

FIGURE 21-10. **Incorrect positioning. The patient has been positioned too far forward (toward the film),** and the anterior teeth appear blurred and diminished. (**A**) Anterior teeth outside focal trough. (**B**) The dental arches (unbroken line) are positioned forward in relation to focal trough (dotted line). (From a symposium syllabus on Panoramic Radiography by the ADA in cooperation with the UTHSCSA Dental School)

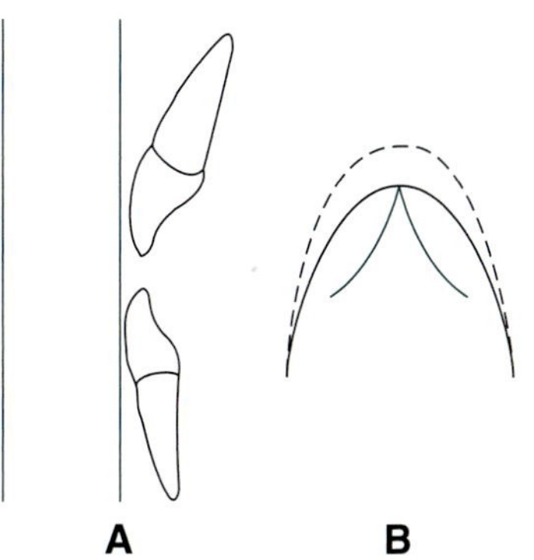

FIGURE 21-11. **Incorrect positioning. The patient has been positioned too far backward (toward the x-ray tube head),** and the anterior teeth appear magnified and blurred. (**A**) Anterior teeth outside focal trough. (**B**) The dental arches (unbroken line) positioned backward in relation to the focal trough (dotted line). (From a symposium syllabus on Panoramic Radiography by the ADA in cooperation with the UTHSCSA Dental School)

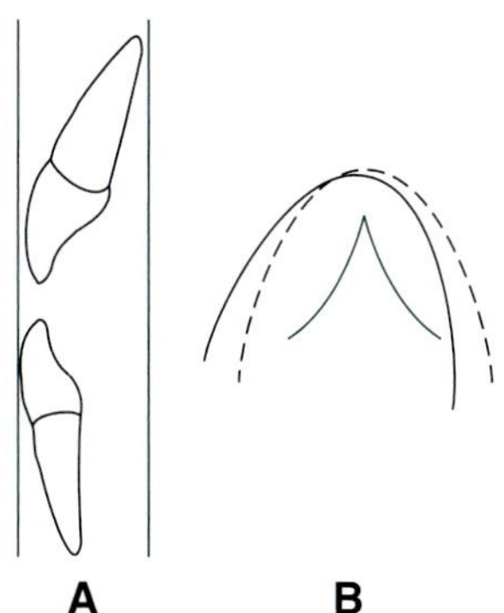

FIGURE 21-12. **Incorrect positioning. The patient's head has been rotated.** Diminution will be apparent on the side malpositioned toward the film and magnification will be apparent on the side malpositioned toward the rotation center of the beam. On both sides the distortion will be most marked in the horizontal dimension; the width of the teeth and jaw structures is affected more than their height dimension. (**A**) Anterior teeth correctly positioned in focal trough. (**B**) Dental arches (unbroken line) rotated around the anterior teeth. One side will be malpositioned outside the focal trough (dotted line). The other side will be malpositioned inside the focal trough. (From a symposium syllabus on Panoramic Radiography by the ADA in cooperation with the UTHSCSA Dental School)

images in the adjacent tissues. Hence, when the tissues of the right side are in the path of the x-ray beam, the tissues of the left side are out of focus and do not superimpose on those of the right side and vice versa. This blurring of the other layer is necessary to prevent interference from the structures of the other layers that were not selected for viewing.

Intraoral Source

A second method of exposure employed in panoramic radiography is to use an **intraoral source** of x-rays. This method has been tested in Europe and used there but has little following in the United States. It is included here for comparison of exposure techniques. The Status X operates on the principle of using an intraoral source of radiation. The anode is located at the tip of the unit containing the tube and is placed inside the patient's mouth. A complete survey is made with two exposures, one of the mandible and one of the maxillae. An alternative procedure is to make an exposure of the right or left side. The film is placed in a **flexible cassette** on the surface of the face.

Operational Procedures for Panoramic X-ray Machines

Although considerable differences exist in the size and configuration of modern rotational panoramic x-ray units, the operational procedures are similar and relatively simple. Obviously, all manufacturers claim that their unit is the best, and each has features that may have special appeal to one dentist or another. Each manufacturer provides an instruction manual that must be carefully read and followed. Most errors can be avoided, and high-quality panoramic radiographs can be produced, with any modern unit if the operator understands the instructions and follows them correctly.

Although a detailed description of all panoramic x-ray units cannot be given, some major differences are visible at a glance. The unit may be constructed in such a manner that the patient must be seated or remain standing during the exposure, or the chair may be positioned so that the patient faces toward or away from the operator.

For example, the patient remains standing and faces toward the back of the unit on the Orthopantomograph 10 (see Figure 21–15) and the Versaview; however, it is possible to lower the assembly that controls the height of the tube head, cassette, and head positioner so that a patient seated on a movable stool or wheelchair can be ac-

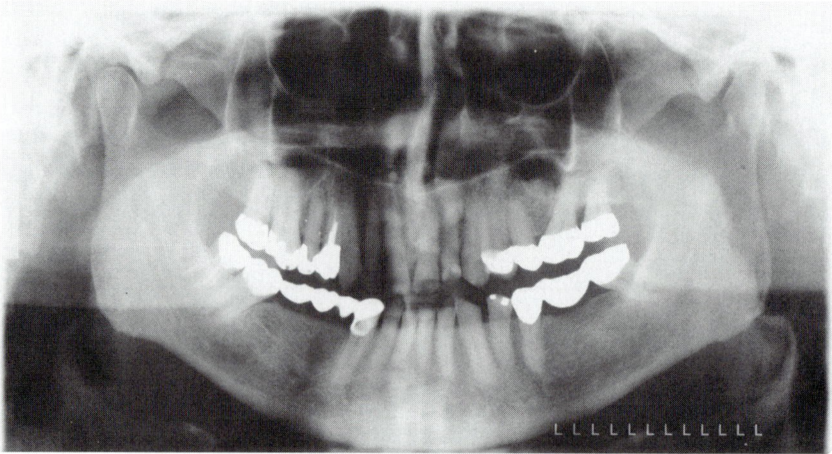

FIGURE 21–13. **Incorrect positioning. Radiograph showing chin tipped too low.** Radiograph appears to be "smiling."

commodated. By comparison, the patient must be seated and facing the operator during the exposure when the Panelipse II (see Figure 21–16) is used.

Less obvious differences are found in the size and shape of the cassette, the manner in which the positioning system is adjusted, and the method used to stabilize the head (see Figure 21–8) and to determine the zone desired to be in focus. The cassette may be in the shape of a circular drum that rotates, or the chair in which the patient is seated may have an automatic lateral shifting device, such as in the older Panorex models. Midway through the exposure cycle, as the tube passes behind the spinal column, the machine automatically shuts down the radiation, producing a **split image** (see the clear area in the middle of Figure 21–17). The Panorex 2 is equipped with a mode selector control, and the operator has the option of producing a radiograph of either a split image or one with a continuous image as shown in Figure 21–18. Most current panoramic x-ray machines produce only continuous image radiographs.

Operational Procedures

With minor variations, the following **operational sequence** is required with most panoramic x-ray machines:

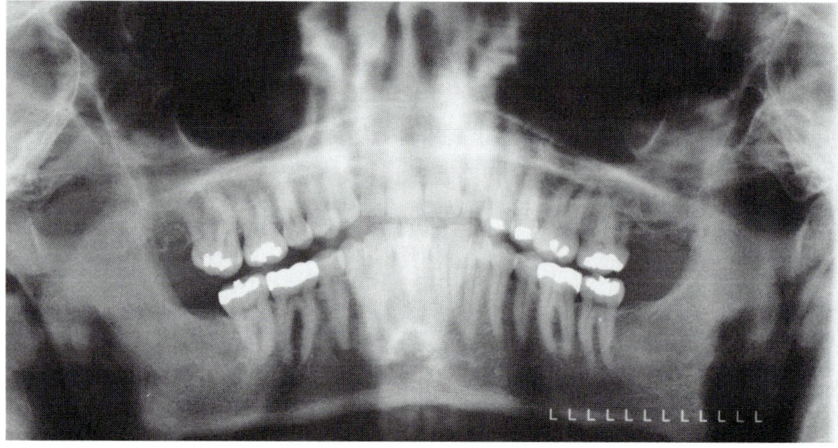

FIGURE 21–14. **Incorrect positioning. Radiograph showing chin raised too high.** Radiograph appears to be "frowning."

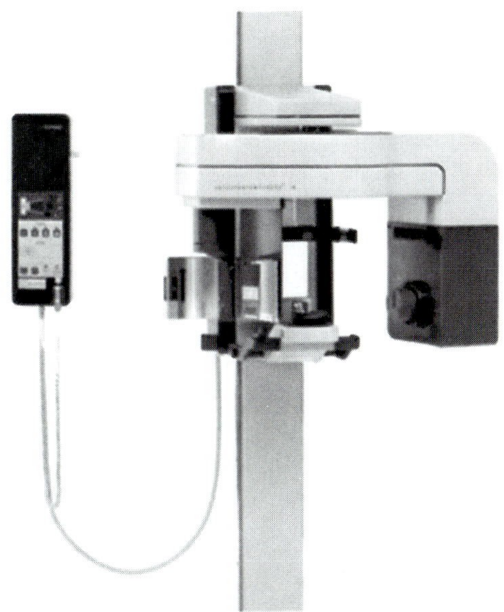

FIGURE 21–15. **Photograph of Orthopantomograph 10.** The patient can be examined standing or seated. This unit has a motorized head positioner with digital readout and is height adjustable. Correct patient head positioning can be controlled in three planes by light beam indicators that show the correct location of the Frankfort horizontal plane, the sagittal plane, and the layer of optimum sharpness in the central incisor region. (Courtesy of Siemens Medical Systems, Inc., Dental Division, Islelin, NJ)

1. Load the film into the **cassette** in the darkroom and identify the film. Use the safelight recommended by the film manufacturer.
2. Handle the film carefully. Be sure that it is inserted between the screens of the cassette. Close the cassette completely before leaving the darkroom.
3. Depending on the type of cassette, either place it into the **cassette holder** or securely fasten it to the **drum.** Check that the drum can turn.
4. Turn the machine on to check that it is operational. Raise or lower the overhead assembly, and swing the head positioner out of the way so that the patient can be positioned.
5. Ask the patient to remove glasses, earrings, body piercing jewelry, or other appliances that might become superimposed on the image. This includes necklaces, napkin chains, or any other metal objects on the back of the neck.
6. Depending on the machine used, ask the patient to stand or sit up straight. Drape the patient with a lead apron. Make sure the lead apron is out of the primary beam and does not interfere with the rotation of the machine.
7. Swing the head positioner assembly into place. According to the unit used, follow the manufacturer's directions in positioning the patient's head and chin. Make sure that the **midsagittal plane** of the patient's face is perpendicular to the floor.
8. Confirm that the manufacturer's recommendations on mA, kVp, and duration of exposure time are followed. Alert the patient to the fact that certain parts of the machine will revolve around the head. Stress the importance of remaining still during the time required to make the exposure.
9. Make a final check to determine that the anterior teeth are in the proper (edge-to-edge) position and ask the patient to place the tongue against the roof of the mouth.
10. Stand behind protective covering or an adequate distance away while making the exposure. Watch the patient during this time to make sure that there has been no undesired movement.
11. Swing the head positioning assembly out of the way. Remove the protective apron and release the patient. Return glasses, earrings, or appliances.
12. Deactivate the x-ray machine, and swing the head positioner back into place. Remove the cassette from the cassette holder or drum.
13. Unload the cassette under proper safelight conditions, and process the film according to the manufacturer's instructions.

The procedures for making the exposures are similar on most panoramic machines. As the complexity of the controls and head holder adjustments varies from unit to unit, read the manufacturer's instructions carefully before attempting to operate an unfamiliar machine. If possible, have someone who is familiar with the machine give a demonstration.

Advantages and Disadvantages of Panoramic Radiography

A panoramic radiograph is less confusing to the patient than a series of small separate intraoral radiographs, making it easier for the dentist to explain the diagnosis and the proposed treatment plan in a manner that is clear

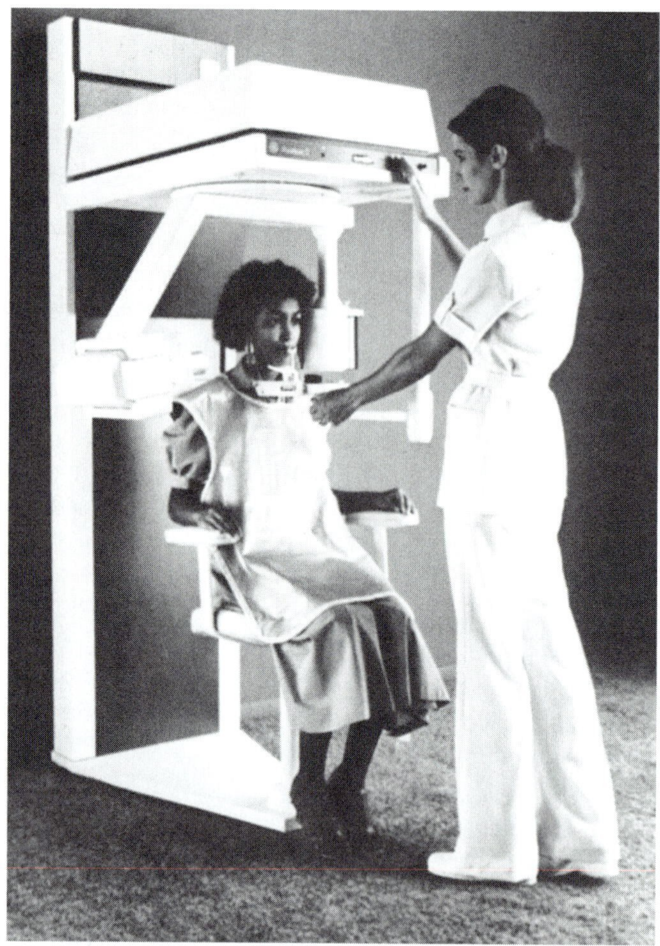

FIGURE 21–16. **Panelipse II.** The Panelipse II produces an elliptical path of the plane in focus that is adjustable to any size dental arch. All teeth, sinuses, and maxillary and mandibular structures can be displayed in a uniform continuous image. The exposure is made in approximately 20 sec. (Courtesy of Gendex Corporation)

and understandable to the patient. Because a greater area can be examined than is possible by the conventional full-mouth survey, the patient benefits if conditions are revealed that otherwise would not have been detected.

However, panoramic radiography has limitations because such factors as magnification, distortion, and poor definition are inherent with panoramic techniques. For example, most dentists agree that incipient caries can be visualized better on periapical or bitewing radiographs. Therefore, it should be emphasized that panoramic radiography is an adjunct or additional diagnostic aid but does not replace conventional radiography.

To summarize, the major advantages and disadvantages of panoramic radiographycompared with conventional full-mouth radiography are as follows.

Advantages

1. The procedure for exposing panoramic films is relatively simple to perform and requires considerably less time.
2. Panoramic exposures are better tolerated by the patient, especially when gagging problems exist.
3. Visualization is greater because all parts of the maxillae and the mandible that lie within the zone of the focal trough of any given panoramic machine can be seen on a single film.
4. The area covered exceeds that of the full-mouth survey and may reveal conditions that otherwise might remain undetected.
5. The radiation dose is relatively low.

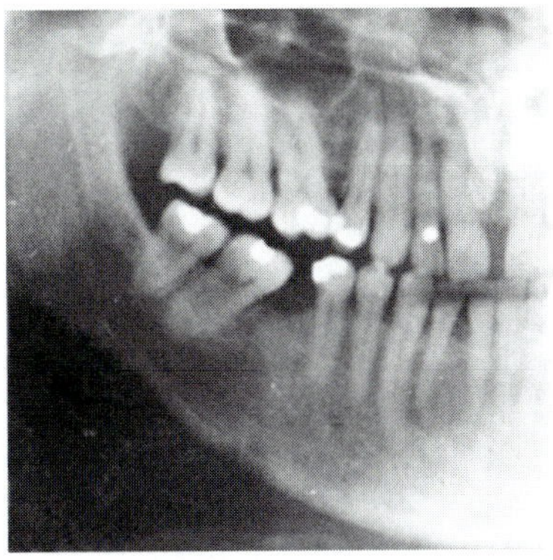
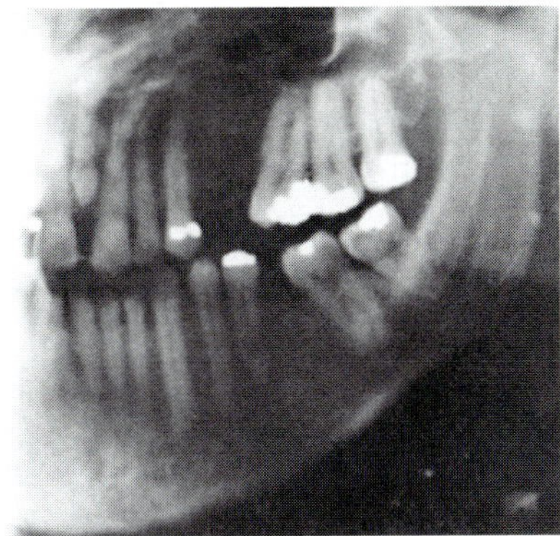

FIGURE 21-17. **A panoramic radiograph exposed with a Panorex machine.** The blurring in the center of the film and the duplication of tooth structures in the incisor regions are caused by the shift in position of the moving parts of the machine during the middle of the exposure. This does not materially detract from the diagnostic quality of the radiograph.

6. Less operator time is required in processing, as only one film instead of a series must be handled.
7. Mounting time is eliminated. Panoramic film is easier to file and store. The danger of losing or damaging a film of the series is removed.
8. Panoramic film is useful in patient education and as a visual aid. The absence of a series of overlapping films makes it easier for the patient to follow the dentist's explanations.

Disadvantages

1. Areas of diagnostic interest out of the focal trough may be visualized poorly or not at all.
2. A varying degree of magnification, geometric distortion, and poor definition is inherent in panoramic radiographs.
3. It is common to overlap teeth, particularly in the premolar (bicuspid) area.
4. It is difficult to obtain good images of the anterior teeth when they have a sharp inclination toward either the labial or lingual.
5. The spinal column often becomes superimposed on structures of interest.
6. The amount of vertical and horizontal distortion is not constant—it varies from one part of the radiograph to another.

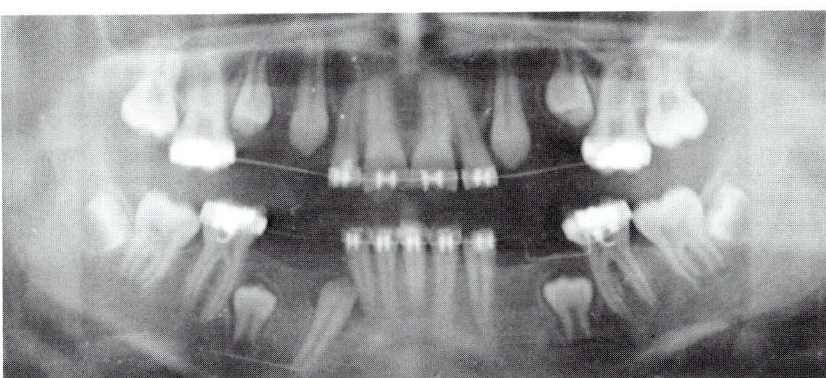

FIGURE 21-18. **Panoramic radiograph produced by Panelipse.** Note the presence of orthodontic bands and wires. Radiograph also shows erupting teeth, impacted teeth, and anodontia. Teeth are shown in an uninterrupted sequence.

7. Incipient caries are difficult to detect and are frequently missed. Supplementary films are required for this purpose.
8. Artifacts are common and may easily be misinterpreted.

Technique Errors Resulting in Faulty Panoramic Radiographs

Panoramic imagery differs vastly from conventional imagery, and some **technique errors** are unique to it. Because a narrow x-ray beam is used to image a curved layer and only the plane at the center of the layer is reproduced correctly, all errors in positioning the patient or the movable parts of the panoramic unit result in:

1. Distortion of the image.
2. Superimposition of the vertebrae over the anterior region.
3. The inclusion of artifacts.
4. The formation of "ghost" images.

When the head is positioned correctly, all parts of the image have the same degree of magnification and sharpness. Conversely, unequal magnification (or diminution) and unsharpness (blurring) are clear indications of malpositioning.

Positioning Errors

The following are **common positioning errors** in rotational panoramic radiography.

1. **Patient is too far forward, too close to the film** (see Figure 21–10). This results in all of the anterior teeth appearing blurred and diminished, particularly in width.
2. **Patient is too far back toward the tube head** (see Figure 21–11). This results in all the anterior teeth appearing blurred and magnified.
3. **Patient's head is rotated** (see Figure 21–12). The teeth on the side closer to the film are diminished, whereas those on the side closer to the center of rotation are enlarged.
4. **Patient's chin is tipped too low** (see Figure 21–13). Frankfort plane angled downward giving the appearance of an exaggerated smile. When this happens the maxillary anterior teeth or the mandibular anterior teeth are placed outside the focal trough and are blurred. When the maxillary teeth are positioned within the focal trough, the mandibular teeth will be blurred and magnified. Conversely, when the mandible teeth are positioned within the focal trough, the maxillary teeth are blurred and diminished, most prominently in width.
5. **Patient's chin is raised too high** (see Figure 21–14). Frankfort plane angled upward giving the appearance of a reversed smile (frown). When this happens, the bottom of the nasal cavity and the palatial plate form a line of low density that partially overlaps the apices of the maxillary teeth. The maxillary anterior teeth or the mandibular anterior teeth are positioned outside the focal trough and are blurred. When the mandibular teeth are positioned within the focal trough, the maxillary teeth appear blurred and magnified. When the maxillary anterior teeth are positioned within the focal trough, the mandibular teeth appear blurred and diminished, most prominently in width.

Additional, **less common patient positioning errors** include the following:

1. Failure to position the chin on the chin rest
2. Failure to use the bite guide or failure to use it correctly
3. Setting the machine too high or too low
4. Failure to remove earrings or prostheses
5. Failure of the patient to keep lips closed
6. Failure to keep the tongue on the palate
7. Patient movement

Other **errors** are **caused by improper exposure and film handling.**

1. Improper manipulation and loading of the film
2. The presence of paper or lint on the **intensifying screens**
3. Failure to start the film at the proper line
4. Interference of the thyroid collar with the rotation of the cassette
5. Artifacts caused by fingernail pressure or static electricity
6. Chemical stains
7. The use of "unsafe" safelights
8. Overexposure
9. Underexposure
10. Double exposure

Normal Panoramic Anatomical Landmarks

The way that a panoramic radiograph is formed results in a unique projection of many anatomical structures. This produces several unusual anatomical relationships in the panoramic image which is not seen in any other type of radiograph. In the panoramic radiograph, the mandible and maxilla as well as the spine are imaged as if they were split vertically in half down the midsagittal plane with each half folded outward. This leaves the nose in the middle of the radiograph and the right and left sides of the jaws on each side. The split cervical spine appears beyond the mandibular rami at the extreme right and left edges of the radiograph.

The dental professional must be able to recognize normal anatomic structures viewed on the panoramic radiograph. The radiographer should review Chapter 11 and the anatomy of the human skull to assist them in identifying the normal anatomy seen on the panoramic radiograph. Then locate the anatomic landmarks of the maxilla and surrounding tissues, the anatomic landmarks of the mandible and surrounding tissues, the soft tissue images, and the air space images as viewed on the panoramic radiograph.

Anatomic Landmarks of the Maxilla and Surrounding Tissues

Find each of the following anatomic landmarks of the maxilla and surrounding tissues on Figures 21–19 and 21–20.

Mastoid Process

The **mastoid process** of the temporal bone is located posterior and inferior to the temporomandibular joint (TMJ). On a panoramic radiograph, it appears as a rounded radiopacity located posterior and inferior to the TMJ.

Styloid Process

The **styloid process** is a long, pointed spine that extends downward from the inferior surface of the temporal bone, just anterior to the mastoid process. On a pamoramic radiograph, it appears as a long, narrow radiopaque spine that extends downward, just anterior to the mastoid process.

External Auditory Meatus

The **external auditory meatus** (external acustic meatus) is a round opening in the temporal bone located anterior and superior to the mastoid process. On a panoramic radiograph, it appears as a round radiolucency anterior and superior to the mastoid process.

Glenoid Fossa

The **glenoid fossa** (mandibular fossa) is a concave, depressed area of the temporal bone located anterior to the external auditory meatus. The head of the mandibular condyle rests in the glenoid fossa. On a panoramic radiograph, it appears as a concave radiopacity superior to the mandibular condyle.

Articular Tubercle

The **articular tubercle** (articular eminence) is a rounded projection of the temporal bone located anterior to the glenoid fossa. On a panaramic radiograph, it appears as a rounded radiopaque bony projection located anterior to the glenoid fossa.

Lateral Pterygoid Plate

The **lateral pterygoid plate** is a wing-like bony projection of the sphenoid bone located posterior to the maxillary tuberosity. On a panoramic radiograph, it appears as a radiopaque plate of bone posterior to the maxillary tuberosity.

Maxillary Tuberosity

The **maxillary tuberosity** is a rounded prominence of bone on the distal portion of the maxillary alveolar ridge. On a panoramic radiograph, it appears as a radiopaque rounded prominence distal to the third molar region.

Infraorbital Foramen

The **infraorbital foramen** is a small round opening in the maxilla, inferior to the border of the orbit. On a panoramic radiograph, it appears as a round radiolucency inferior to the orbit.

Orbit of the Eye

The **orbit** is the bony cavity that contains the eyeball. On a panoramic radiograph, it appears as a large round radiolucency with radiopaque borders superior to the maxillary sinuses. Often, only the inferior border of the orbit is visible as a radiopaque line.

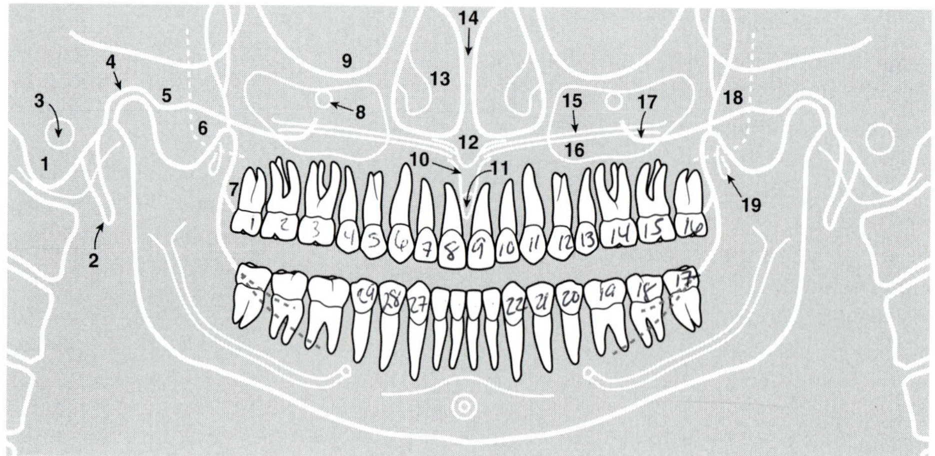

FIGURE 21-19. **Panoramic drawing of the maxilla and surrounding tissues showing normal anatomic landmarks.** The drawing shows the (**1**) mastoid process, (**2**) styloid process, (**3**) external auditory meatus, (**4**) glenoid fossa, (**5**) articular tubercle, (**6**) lateral pterygoid plate, (**7**) maxillary tuberosity, (**8**) infraorbital foramen, (**9**) orbit of the eye, (**10**) incisive canal, (**11**) incisive foramen, (**12**) anterior nasal spine, (**13**) nasal cavity, (**14**) nasal septum, (**15**) hard palate, (**16**) maxillary sinus, (**17**) zygomatic process of the zygoma, (**18**) zygoma, and (**19**) hamulus.

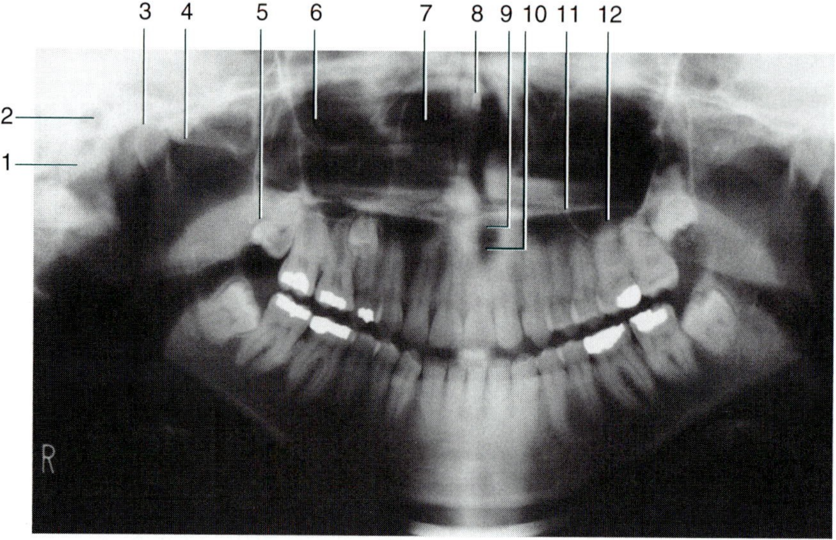

FIGURE 21-20. **Panoramic radiograph of the maxilla and surrounding tissues showing normal anatomic landmarks.** The radiograph shows the (**1**) mastoid process, (**2**) external auditory meatus, (**3**) glenoid fossa, (**4**) articular tubercle, (**5**) maxillary tuberosity, (**6**) orbit of the eye, (**7**) nasal cavity, (**8**) nasal septum, (**9**) incisive canal, (**10**) incisive foramen, (**11**) hard palate, and (**12**) maxillary sinus.

Incisive Canal

The **incisive canal** (nasopalatine canal) is a Y-shaped passageway that extends from the floor of the nose to the hard palate lingual to the central incisors. The upper arms of the Y open on the floor of the nose and the base of the Y opens on the anterior of the hard palate. On a panoramic radiograph, it appears as a tunnel-like radiolucency with radiopaque borders located between the maxillary central incisors.

Incisive Foramen

The **incisive foramen** (nasopalatine foramen) is an opening in bone located in the anterior midline of the hard palate directly posterior to the maxillary central incisors. On a panoramic radiograph, it appears as a round pea-shaped radiolucent area located between the roots of the maxillary central incisors.

Anterior Nasal Spine

The **anterior nasal spine** is a pointed bony projection of the maxilla located at the most anterior point of the floor of the nasal cavity. On a panoramic radiograph, it appears as a V-shaped radiopacity located at the intersection of the floor of the nasal cavity and the nasal septum.

Nasal Cavity

The **nasal cavity** (nasal fossa) is a pear-shaped compartment of bone located superior to the maxilla. On a panoramic radiograph, it appears as a large radiolucency above the maxillary incisors.

Nasal Septum

The **nasal septum** is a vertical bony wall that separates the right and left nasal fossae. On a panoramic radiograph, it appears as vertical radiopacity that divides the nasal cavity into two parts.

Hard Palate

The **hard palate** is a bony wall that separates the oral cavity from the nasal cavity. On a panoramic radiograph, it appears as a horizontal thick radiopaque band superior to the maxillary teeth.

Maxillary Sinus

The **maxillary sinuses** consist of two paired cavities located within the maxilla apical to the maxillary posterior teeth. On a panoramic radiograph, they appear as paired radiolucent cavities apical to the maxillary posterior teeth.

Zygomatic Process of the Maxilla

The **zygomatic process of the maxilla** is a J- or U-shaped bony process of the maxilla that extends laterally to articulate with the zygoma. On a panoramic radiograph, it appears as a J- or U-shaped radiopacity located apically to the maxillary first molar.

Zygoma

The **zygoma** (malar bone) is the cheekbone that articulates with the zygomatic process of the maxilla. On a panoramic radiograph, it appears as a thick radiopaque band that extends posteriorly from the zygomatic process of the maxilla.

Hamulus

The **hamulus** (hamular process) is a very small hook-like process of bone that extends downward and slightly backward from the medial pterygoid plate of the sphenoid bone. On a panoramic radiograph, it appears radiopaque and can be seen posterior to the maxillary tuberosity.

Anatomic Landmarks of the Mandible and Surrounding Tissues

Find each of the following anatomic landmarks of the mandible and surrounding tissues on Figures 21–21 and 21–22.

Mandibular Condyle

The **mandibular condyle** is a rounded bony process extending from the posterior superior border of the ramus of the mandible. It articulates with the glenoid fossa of the temporal bone. On a panoramic radiograph, the mandibular condyle appears as a rounded radiopaque process extending from the posterior superior border of the ramus of the mandible.

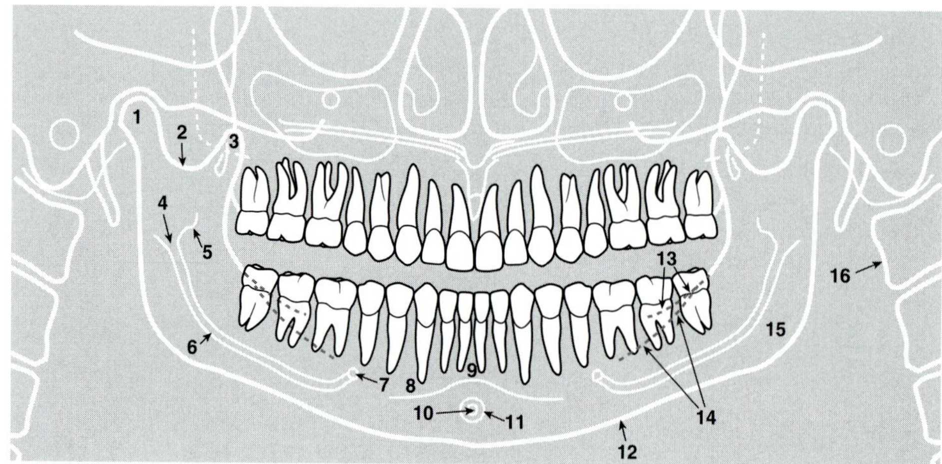

FIGURE 21–21. **Panoramic drawing of the mandible and surrounding tissues showing normal anatomic landmarks.** The drawing shows the (**1**) mandibular condyle, (**2**) signoid notch, (**3**) coronoid process, (**4**) mandibular foramen, (**5**) lingula, (**6**) mandibular canal, (**7**) mental foramen, (**8**) mental ridge, (**9**) mental fossa, (**10**) lingual foramen, (**11**) genial tubercles, (**12**) inferior border of the mandible, (**13**) mylohyoid ridge, (**14**) oblique ridge, (**15**) angle of the mandible, (**16**) cervial spine.

Sigmoid Notch

The **sigmoid notch** (coronoid notch or mandibular notch) is a concavity of bone located posterior to the coronoid process on the superior border of the ramus of the mandible. On a panoramic radiograph, it appears as a radiopaque concavity located posterior to the coronoid process on the superior border of the ramus of the mandible.

Coronoid Process

The **coronoid process** is a large triangular prominence of bone located on the anterior superior ramus of the mandible. On a panoramic radiograph, it appears as a large triangular radiopaque area anterior to the coronoid notch.

Mandibular Foramen

The **mandibular foramen** is an ovoid opening in bone on the lingual aspect of the ramus of the mandible. On a panoramic radiograph, it appears as a round radiolucency located in the center of the ramus of the mandible.

Lingula

The **lingula** (means "little tongue") is a small tongue-shaped projection of bone located anterior and adjacent to the mandibular foramen. On a panoramic radiograph, it appears as a small radiopacity anterior to the mandibular foramen.

Mandibular Canal

The **mandibular canal** is a long tunnel-like passageway extending from the mandibular foramen on the medial aspect of the ramus of the mandible to the mental foramen on the lateral aspect of the body of the mandible. The canal carries nerves and blood vessels that supply most of the teeth in the mandible. On a panoramic radiograph, the canal appears as a radiolucent tube outlined by two thin radiopaque lines representing the walls of the canal.

Mental Foramen

The **mental foramen** is an opening through which the mental nerve and related blood vessels emerge on the lateral aspect of the body of the mandible in the region of the premolars. On a panoramic radiograph, it appears as a small round radiolucent area near the roots of the mandibular premolars.

Mental Ridge

The **mental ridge** is a thick prominence of bone located on the external surface of the mandible and extends anteriorly from the premolar area to the midline. On a

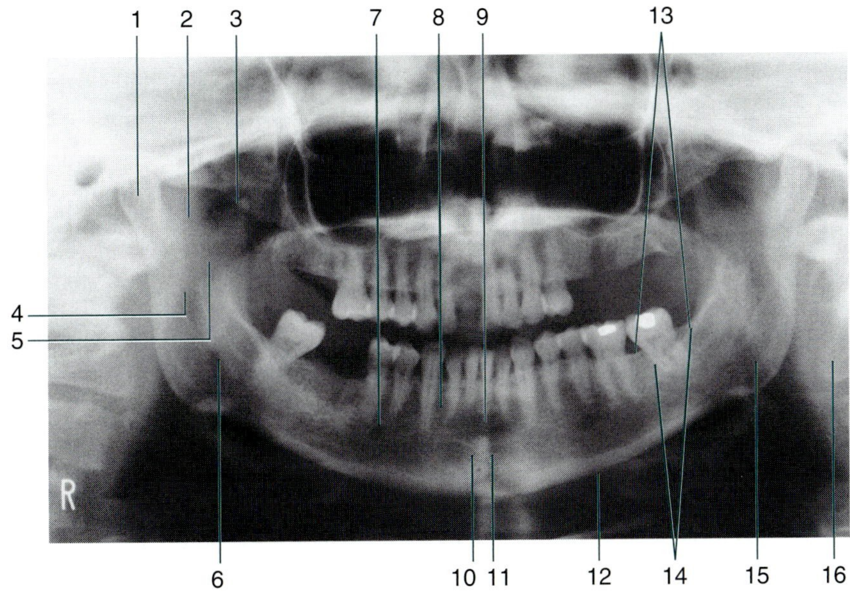

FIGURE 21–22. **Panoramic radiograph of the mandible and surrounding tissues showing normal anatomic landmarks.** The radiograph shows the (**1**) mandibular condyle, (**2**) signoid notch, (**3**) coronoid process, (**4**) mandibular foramen, (**5**) lingula, (**6**) mandibular canal, (**7**) mental foramen, (**8**) mental ridge, (**9**) mental fossa, (**10**) lingual foramen, (**11**) genial tubercles, (**12**) inferior border of the mandible, (**13**) mylohyoid ridge, (**14**) oblique ridge, (**15**) angle of the mandible, (**16**) cervial spine.

panoramic radiograph, it appears as a thick radiopaque band that extends from the premolar area to the midline.

Mental Fossa

The **mental fossa** is a depressed area of bone located on the external surface of the anterior mandible in the mandibular incisor region. On a panoramic radiograph, it appears as a radiolucent area in the region of the roots of the mandibular incisor teeth.

Lingual Foramen

The **lingual foramen** is a very small round opening located in the center of the genial tubercles on the lingual side of midline of the mandible. On a panoramic radiograph, it appears as a small round radiolucency located inferior to the apices of the mandibular incisor teeth.

Genial Tubercles

The **genial tubercles** are four small projections of bone located on the lingual surface of the midline of the mandible. On a panoramic radiograph, they appear as a radiopaque donut-shaped circle surrounding the lingual foramen.

Inferior Border of the Mandible

The **inferior border of the mandible** is the corticle bone that outlines the lower border of the mandible. On a panoramic radiograph, it appears as a dense radiopaque band that outlines the lower border of the mandible.

Mylohyoid Ridge

The **mylohyoid ridge** is a ridge of bone running diagonally downward and forward on the lingual aspect of the ramus of the mandible to near the apices of the molar roots. On a panoramic radiograph, it appears as a dense radiopaque band that extends downward and forward from the ramus of the mandible to near the apicies of the molar teeth.

Oblique Ridge

The **oblique ridge** is a ridge diagonal ridge of bone on the lateral aspect of the mandible. The ridge runs downward and forward from the anterior border of the ramus to the level of the cervical portion of the molar and premolar roots. On a panoramic radiograph, it appears as a dense radiopaque band that extends downward and forward from the anterior border of the ramus of the mandible.

Angle of the Mandible

The **angle of the mandible** is the area at the posterior and inferior corners of the mandible, where the body of the mandible meets and joins the ascending ramus of the mandible. On a panoramic radiograph, it appears as a radiopaque structure where the body of the mandible meets and joins the ascending ramus of the mandible.

Cervical Spine

On a panoramic radiograph, the **cervical spine** appears as a radiopaque area beyond the rami of the mandible at the extreme right and left edges of the radiograph.

Soft Tissue Images Viewed on the Panoramic Radiograph

The panoramic radiograph is unique in that some soft tissue structures attenuate the beam of radiation enough to become visible in the radiograph. Various soft tissues may be visualized such as the tongue, soft palate, lipline, and ear. Find each of the following soft tissue images on Figures 21–23 and 21–24.

Tongue

The **tongue** is a movable muscular organ located on the floor of the mouth. On a panoramic radiograph, it appears as a large radiopaque area superimposed over the maxillary posterior teeth.

Soft Palate

The **soft palate** is located posterior to the hard palate and separates the oral cavity from the nasal cavity. On a panoramic radiograph, it appears as a diagonal radiopaque area above and posterior to the maxillary tuberosity.

Lipline

The **lipline** is the outline of the patient's lips. On a panoramic radiograph, it appears as a radiopacity superimposed over the anterior teeth.

Ear

On a panoramic radiograph, the **ear** appears as a radiopaque area that is superimposed over the styloid process, anterior and inferior to the mastoid process.

Air Space Images Viewed on the Panoramic Radiograph

Air does not attenuate the beam of radiation as much as hard or soft tissue. For this reason air spaces appear radiolucent (black) on a panoramic radiograph. Air spaces that may be seen include the palatoglossal, nasopharyngeal, and glossopharyngeal. Due to the uniqueness of the

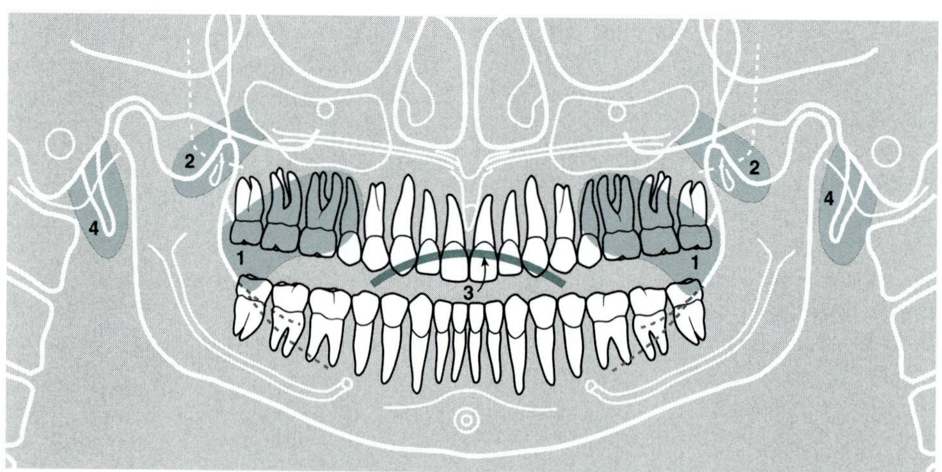

FIGURE 21–23. **Drawing of soft tissue images as viewed on the panoramic radiograph.** The drawing shows the (**1**) tongue, (**2**) soft palate, (**3**) lipline, and (**4**) ear.

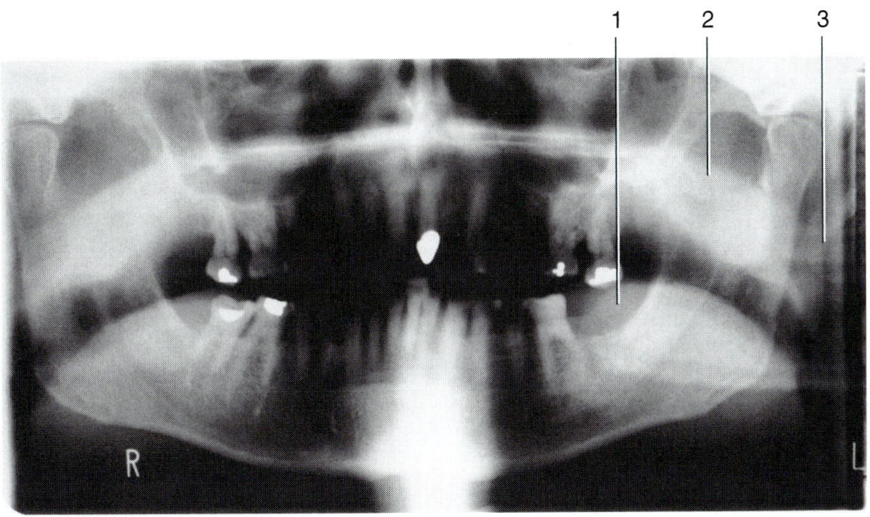

FIGURE 21–24. **Radiograph showing soft tissue images as viewed on the panoramic radiograph.** The radiograph shows the (**1**) tongue, (**2**) soft palate, and (**3**) ear.

machine it should be remembered that air obscures hard tissues (bone), soft tissues obscures air spaces, and hard tissues obscure soft tissues. Find each of the following air space images on Figures 21–25 and 21–26.

Palatoglossal Air Space

The **palatoglossal air space (glossopalatine air space)** is the air space between the palate and the tongue. On a panoramic radiograph, it appears as a radiolucent horizontal band located above the apices of the maxillary teeth.

Nasopharyngeal Air Space

The **nasopharyngeal air space** is the air space located posterior to the nasal cavity. On a panoramic radiograph, it appears as diagonal radiolucent area located superior to the radiopaque soft palate.

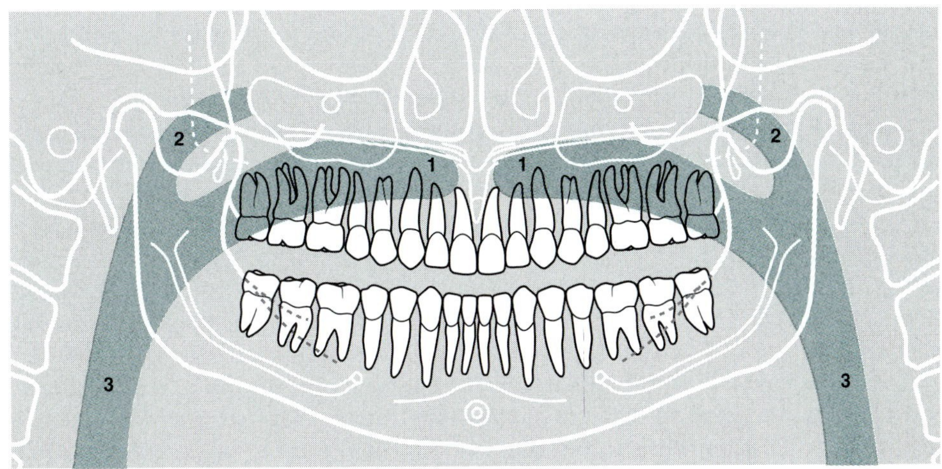

FIGURE 21–25. **Drawing of air space images as viewed on the panoramic radiograph.** The drawing shows the (**1**) palatoglossal air space, (**2**) nasopharyngeal air space, and (**3**) glossopharyngeal air space.

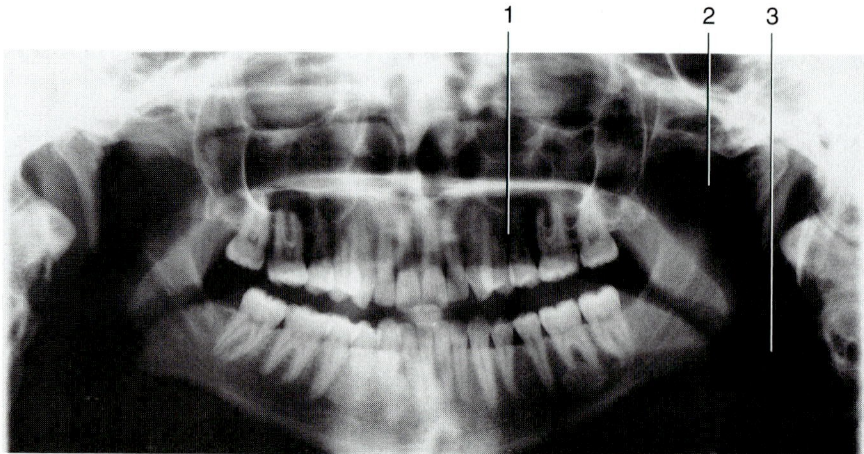

FIGURE 21-26. **Radiograph showing air space images as viewed on the panoramic radiograph.** The radiograph shows the (**1**) palatoglossal air space, (**2**) nasopharyngeal air space, and (**3**) glossopharyngeal air space.

Glossopharyngeal Air Space

The **glossopharyngeal air space (oropharyngeal air space)** is the portion of the pharynx located posterior to the tongue and oral cavity. On a panoramic radiograph, it appears as vertical radiolucent band superimposed over the ramus of the mandible.

CHAPTER SUMMARY

Panoramic radiography is an important new technique that has been refined in the last two decades. Almost all panoramic x-ray machines used in the United States work on a system by which the patient's head is carefully positioned between the tube head and the film. The tube head and film rotate at a predetermined speed around the patient's head. A narrow beam of x-rays is used to project the image on the film.

Several different continuous movement patterns of the x-ray beam (centers of rotation) are built into the machines by the manufacturers to achieve the desired projection of the jaws. The form of the path determines the direction of the beam and hence the projection of each successive part of the jaws. The target in the tube serves as the focus of the projection in the vertical dimension, whereas the center of rotation serves as the functional focus in the horizontal direction. Distortion effects are characteristic of panoramic radiographs because the focus of projection is different in the horizontal and vertical planes.

The panoramic radiograph, often called the tomograph, is produced by a special technique used to show in detail the images of structures located within a predetermined plane of tissues, while at the same time eliminating or blurring those structures located in the planes that were not selected. The plane in focus or depth of field, also known as the focal trough, is the sharply defined area that in most tomographs corresponds to the size and shape of the dental arches. Correct patient positioning and head and jaw alignment are the decisive determining factors for the quality of the radiograph produced.

The best image is obtained when the teeth and jaws are positioned in the center of the focal trough. Displacement toward rotation center of the beam (backward) causes the anterior teeth to appear magnified horizontally and blurred. Conversely, if displaced toward the film (forward), the anterior teeth will appear narrower and blurred.

The procedure for exposing panoramic radiographs varies from unit to unit but generally involves the following steps.

1. Identify and load the film into the cassette.
2. Activate the unit and attach the cassette to the holder or drum.
3. Prepare the patient, making required head measurements and positioning the patient's head so that the teeth will be in the focal trough.
4. Select the proper mA and kVp and holding the button on the hand switch, pressed down firmly until the exposure is completed.
5. Deactivate the machine, releasing the patient, and removing the cassette from the holder or drum.

There are advantages and disadvantages to using panoramic radiographs. Among the **advantages** are the following:

1. Simplicity and rapidity of procedure
2. Minimal patient resistance to film positioning
3. Large areas, even sinuses and temporomandibular joints, can be viewed on a single film
4. Useful for making mass surveys
5. Easier for the patient to visualize and understand the dentist's plan of treatment

Among the **disadvantages** are the following:

1. Loss of radiographic detail
2. Inherent magnification and image distortion
3. The difficulty experienced by many operators in correctly positioning the patient's head so that the dentition is centered on the focal trough when using panoramic machines

Many of the technique errors that result in producing substandard panoramic radiographs are the result of mistakes in film handling and exposure. However, most errors are caused by malpositioning the head. Excellent radiographs can be produced when the operator follows the technique procedures carefully and adheres to the manufacturer's instructions.

Panoramic anatomy should be studied by the dental radiographer to become familiar with all normal panoramic landmarks.

REVIEW QUESTIONS

1. A panoramic film shows an unexposed area in the center that was caused by the shifting of the chair. Which make of panoramic machine was used to make the exposure?
   (a) Orthopantomograph
   (b) Panelipse
   (c) Orthoceph
   (d) Panorex

2. In what position should the incisors be during a panoramic exposure?
   (a) Mandibular incisors should protrude.
   (b) There should be an edge-to-edge relationship.
   (c) Maxillary incisors should protrude.
   (d) Mouth should be open with incisors at least 1/2 in. (13 mm) apart.

3. Which term describes the area of the dental anatomy that is reproduced distinctly on the panoramic radiograph?
   (a) Focal trough
   (b) Rotation center
   (c) Sagittal plane
   (d) Laminograph

4. Which of these factors is a disadvantage of extraoral radiography that is often observed when a panoramic and an intraoral film are compared?
   (a) More teeth are shown on a panoramic film.
   (b) The sinuses may be shown on a panoramic film.
   (c) The images are magnified on a panoramic film.
   (d) The temporomandibular joints may be shown on a panoramic film.

5. In panoramic radiography, the focal trough is the:
   (a) Slit in the cassette holder.
   (b) Collimated radiation beam.
   (c) Zone of sharpness.
   (d) Path that the cassette holder follows while rotating.

6. A panoramic radiograph is of little value when diagnosing:
   (a) An impacted molar.
   (b) Recurrent caries.
   (c) A cyst.
   (d) A supernumerary tooth.

7. Which of these is an advantage of using panoramic instead of periapical film?
   (a) Mounting time is eliminated.
   (b) The image is magnified.
   (c) Distortion is eliminated.
   (d) Definition is improved.

8. What is the effect on the shape of the focal trough when the distance from the center of rotation to the dental arches is increased?
   (a) There is no effect.
   (b) The width increases.
   (c) It is eliminated.
   (d) The width decreases.

9. Which type of film is best for detecting incipient caries?
   (a) Extraoral film
   (b) Bitewing film
   (c) Occlusal film
   (d) Panoramic film

10. Where is the center of rotation located?
    (a) Between the teeth and the film
    (b) Between the tube head and the film
    (c) Between the Frankfort plane and the cassette
    (d) Between the focal trough and the cassette

11. What is the effect on the image geometry of the central incisors when the patient's head is positioned too far forward?
    (a) The incisors are diminished and blurred.
    (b) There is no effect.
    (c) The incisors are magnified vertically.
    (d) The incisors are magnified and blurred.

12. In a panoramic radiograph, the teeth on the right side are magnified and the teeth on the left side are very small. This error was caused by positioning the patient's head:
    (a) Too far forward.
    (b) Too far backward.
    (c) To the left of the midline.
    (d) To the right of the midline.

13. Air spaces on a panoramic radiograph:
    (a) Appear radiolucent.
    (b) Block out soft tissue shadows.
    (c) Are more radiopaque then bone.
    (d) Do not show up on any type of radiograph.

14. The spine is seen:
    (a) In the middle of a panoramic film if the patient is positioned correctly.
    (b) At the left edge of a panoramic film if the patient is positioned correctly.
    (c) At the right edge of a panoramic film if the patient is positioned correctly.
    (d) At both the left and right edges of a panoramic film if the patient is positioned correctly.

15. Anatomical objects which may form a double image include:
    (a) Hard palate.
    (b) Soft palate.
    (c) Hyoid bone.
    (d) All of the above.

16. Which of the following appears radiolucent on the panoramic radiograph?
    (a) Nasal cavity
    (b) Nasal septum
    (c) Nasal spine
    (d) Hard palate

17. Which of the following appears radiopaque on the panoramic radiograph?
    (a) External auditory meatus.
    (b) Zygomatic process of the maxilla.
    (c) Mental fossa.
    (d) Mandibular foramen.

BIBLIOGRAPHY

Eastman Kodak. *Successful Panoramic Radiography*. Rochester, NY: Eastman Kodak, 2000.

Farman, A. G., Nortje, C. J. & Wood, R. E. *Oral and Maxillofacial Diagnostic Imaging*. St Louis: Mosby, 1993.

Langland, O. E., Langlais, R. P., & McDavid W. D. et al. *Panoramic Radiology*, 2nd ed. Philadelphia: Lea & Febiger, 1989.

White, S. C. & Pharoah, M. J. *Oral Radiology Principles and Interpretation*, 4th ed. St. Louis, Mosby, 2000.

PART VII: Dental Radiographer Fundamentals

CHAPTER 22

Infection Control

OBJECTIVES

By the end of this chapter the student should be able to:

- Define the key words.
- State the purpose of infection control.
- Describe the possible routes of disease transmission.
- Discuss the "chain of infection."
- State the infection control guidelines that directly relate to dentistry.
- Identify the benefits of infection control.
- Discuss protective barriers and give four examples.
- Discuss protective attire and state which ones are optional for dental radiology.
- Differentiate between disinfection and sterilization.
- Discuss in detail the infection control procedures used before film exposure.
- Discuss in detail the infection control procedures used during film exposure.
- Discuss in detail the infection control procedures used after film exposure.
- State step-by-step film handling procedures with barrier envelopes.
- Discuss daylight loaders and state the step-by-step film handling procedures used without barrier envelopes.

KEY WORDS

AIDS (acquired immunodeficiency syndrome)
Antiseptic
Asepsis
Barrier
Bloodborne pathogens
Contamination
Cross-contamination
Disinfect
Disinfection
Exposure incident
Hepatitis B
HIV (human immunodeficiency virus)
Immunization
Infection control
Infectious waste
Occupational exposure
Parenteral exposure
Pathogen
Protective barrier
Sanitation
Sepsis
Sharp
Sterilization
Universal precautions

Introduction

Infection control is a major concern of patients, health agencies, and dental personnel in the practice of dentistry. Infection control procedures are used in dentistry to minimize the transmission of disease. Dental personnel must understand and use infection control procedures to protect their patients and themselves.

One major problem is that most infections cannot be seen and become visible only when viewed through a microscope. This makes the task of infection control more difficult because there is a natural tendency to assume that there is nothing wrong because nothing unusual can be seen.

The purpose of this chapter is to present the need for infection control, infection control terminology, infection control guidelines, and to describe step-by-step infection control procedures used in dental radiology.

Purpose of Infection Control

The **primary purpose of infection control** is to prevent the transmission of infectious diseases. People have always lived with the possibility of infection occurring through invasion of the body by pathogens such as bacteria or viruses. (A **pathogen** is a microorganism capable of causing disease.) But now with the advent of **acquired immunodeficiency syndrome (AIDS),** the **human immunodeficiency virus (HIV),** the highly infectious **hepatitis B** virus (HBV), and the resurgence of tuberculosis (TB), concern over infection control in the dental office has heightened dramatically.

Infectious diseases may be transmitted from patient to dental personnel, from dental personnel to patient, and from patient to patient.

Routes of infection transmission are:

- Direct contact with pathogens in open lesions, blood, saliva, or respiratory secretions
- Direct contact with airborne contaminants present in aerosols of oral and respiratory fluids
- Indirect contact with contaminated objects or instruments

Chain of Infection

For infection to occur, **four conditions** must be present (see Figure 22–1).

1. A **susceptible host** (i.e., not immune)
2. A **disease-causing microorganism** present (**pathogen**)
3. **Sufficient numbers of the pathogen** present to initiate infection
4. An **appropriate route (portal of entry) for the pathogen to enter the host**

The **purpose of infection control** is to alter one of these four conditions to prevent the transmission of disease.

Breaking the Chain of Infection

The **chain of infection** can be broken by:

1. **Immunization of the susceptible host.** The Centers for Disease Control and Prevention (CDC) recommends dental personnel working with blood or blood-contaminated substances be vaccinated for hepatitis B virus (HBV). All dental healthcare workers should be vaccinated against influenza, measles, mumps, rubella, and tetanus.
2. **Removing the pathogen.** Use sterilization techniques and/or protective barriers.
3. **Reducing the sufficient numbers of pathogens.** Use disinfection and sterilization techniques and/or protective barriers.
4. **Blocking the portal of entry.** Use protective attire (barriers) such as protective clothes, gloves, masks, and eyewear.

Infection Control Terminology

The following terms are frequently used in infection control. They should be studied and understood.

Antiseptic: An agent used on living tissues to destroy or stop the growth of bacteria. An example would be antiseptic soaps used by dental personnel for washing hands.

Asepsis: Describes the absence of septic matter or freedom from infection (*a* means without, *sepsis* means infection). The term is used to describe procedures that prevent infection of tissues by microorganisms.

Barrier: Used to describe any material that is used to prevent the transmission of infective microorganisms to the patient. Barriers include gloves, masks, protective eyewear, surface covers and operating gowns.

Bloodborne pathogens: Pathogens present in blood that causes disease in humans.

Contamination: Soiling by contact or mixing.

Cross-contamination: To contaminate from one place or person to another place or person.

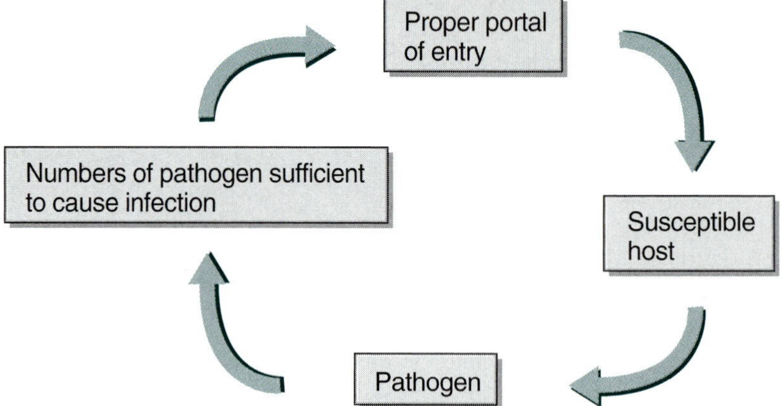

FIGURE 22-1. **Chain of infection.**

Disinfect: The use of a chemical or physical procedure to reduce the disease-producing microorganisms to an acceptable level on inanimate objects. This is done by wiping off those portions of the equipment that come into contact with the patient or operator with gauze saturated with a chemical disinfectant such as an EPA-registered surface disinfectant. Spores are not necessarily destroyed. Disinfecting agents are usually only used on surfaces and instruments because they are too toxic for living tissues.

Disinfection: The act of disinfecting.

Exposure incident: An incident that involves contact with blood or other potentially infectious materials and that results from procedures performed by dental personnel.

Immunization: The process of making someone immune to a disease. All dental personnel should have the recommended immunizations, including that for the hepatitis B virus.

Infection control: The prevention and reduction of disease-causing (pathogenic) microorganisms.

Infectious waste: Waste (such as blood, blood products, and contaminated sharps) that may contain pathogens.

Occupational exposure: A worker (dental personnel) coming in contact with blood, saliva, or other infectious material that involves the skin, eye, or mucus membrane.

Pathogen: A microorganism that can cause disease (*pathos* means disease). Infection control procedures are used to prevent the cross-contamination of pathogens between patients and dental personnel.

Parenteral exposure: Exposure to blood that results from puncturing the skin barrier.

Sanitation: A term used when microorganisms are reduced to a level of concentration considered to be safe. Food-handling facilities are usually concerned about adequate sanitation.

Sepsis: Infection, or the presence of septic matter.

Sharp: Any object that can penetrate the skin, such as needles or scalpels.

Sterilize: The total destruction of spores and disease-producing microorganisms. This is accomplished by autoclaving or dry heat processes. Ideally, all equipment or instruments used should be sterilized. Unfortunately this is not feasible with most radiographic equipment because of their large size.

Sterilization: The act of sterilizing.

Universal precautions: A method of infection control in which blood and certain body fluids are treated as if known to be infectious for HIV, HBV, and other bloodborne pathogens.

"Cold sterilization" is a term that has been commonly misused in medicine and dentistry for many years. It has usually been applied to procedures resulting in disinfection, not sterilization.

Benefit of Infection Control

Everyone in the dental office—the patient, the dental staff, and the dentist—benefits when measures are implemented that decrease the likelihood of transmitting bacterial, fungal or viral infections. A lawsuit can be defended easier if it can be proved that the office adheres to an approved infection control plan. Infection control, properly carried out, gives the entire professional staff a feeling of security or peace of mind.

It is a well-known fact that some patients who are infected are reluctant to admit their condition. In situations where a double standard was used, and protective measures were only used when the patient was known to be infectious, everyone was at risk. The failure to use a single standard for all patients provided inadequate protection. Taking a thorough medical history and making a dental examination will not always identify potential infected patients.

Any risk, no matter how small must be evaluated. It is far better to be safe than to be sorry. Therefore, practice **universal precautions,** where all patients, whether known to be infected or not, are assumed to be infected and the necessary precautions are applied.

Guidelines for Infection Control

Present research activity involves ways of keeping the risk of infection as low as it can be reasonably achieved—the **ALARA** principle. The goal of these and future guidelines will be to set standards for controls that are simple enough to be practical. Since we cannot be certain, it must be assumed that each patient is potentially infected and that the development of a single standard of patient care is essential.

Each dental installation, whether a teaching institution, clinic, single or multiple practice should have a written infection control policy which should be practical and compatible with local or state regulations. The dentist (or designated personnel) has the authority and the responsibility see to it that the infection control policy is correctly carried out.

Currently there are publications available from the American Dental Association that provide detailed information about infection control and treatment of patients with infectious diseases. These include *Proceedings of the National Symposium on Hepatitis B and the Dental Profession*, and *Facts About AIDS for the Dental Team.*

The Centers for Disease Control and Prevention (CDC) has published infection control guidelines entitled *Recommended Infection-Control Practices for Dentistry (1993)*(see Table 22–1). CDC has contributed its **universal precaution** approach to infection control procedures. Their recommendation is to **"treat everyone as if known to be infectious."** The **CDC's infection control guidelines** that directly relate to dental radiology are:

- Use protective barriers
- Wear protective attire
- Handwashing
- Sterilize and disinfect instruments
- Clean and disinfect the dental unit and environmental surfaces

TABLE 22–1. **Recommended Infection-Control Practices for Dentistry by Centers for Disease Control and Prevention (CDC)**

- Vaccination of all dental personnel.
- Use protective barriers.
- Wear protective attire.
- Hand washing and use of gloves.
- Proper care and use of sharp instruments and needles.
- Sterilization or disinfection of instruments.
- Cleaning and disinfection of the dental unit and environmental surfaces.
- Disinfection of the dental laboratory.
- Use and care of handpieces and other intraoral dental devices attached to air and water lines of dental units.
- Single use of disposable instruments.
- Proper handling of biopsy specimens.
- Proper use of extracted teeth in dental educational settings.
- Proper disposal of waste materials.
- Implementation of recommendations.

Protective Barriers

The term **barrier** is used to describe any material that is used to prevent the transmission of infective microorganisms to the patient. The use of barrier techniques is the foundation of any successful infection control program. **Protective barriers** should be used whenever practical. Gloves, masks, gowns, and protective eyewear are worn by dental personnel and plastic wrap, plastic bags, paper towels, paper cups, aluminum foil and etc. are used on appropriate surfaces, equipment and supplies.

Surfaces not covered must be disinfected after the radiographic procedures are completed. Disinfectants have several drawbacks. They, like all liquids, have the potential to affect electrical connections. Also, disinfecting solutions may not reach all irregular surfaces.

Protective Attire

Protective attire (clothing, gloves, masks, and protective eyewear) worn by dental personnel act as protective barriers (see Figure 22–2). They prevent the transmission of

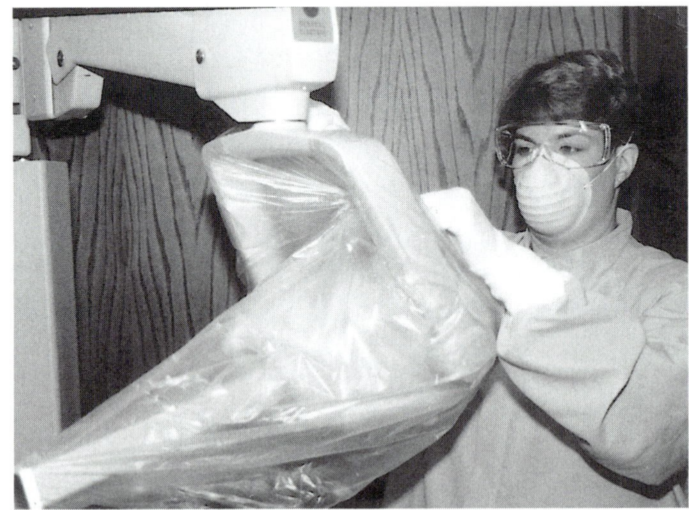

FIGURE 22–2. **Picture of a dental operatory.** Operator wearing gloves, mask, and protective eyewear is placing barrier bag to cover PID, tube housing, and yoke.

infective microorganisms to the dental staff and to the patient.

Protective Clothing

Protective clothing, such as gowns, uniforms, and lab coats, provides protection from exposure to blood and saliva when large quantities are expected. Change protective clothing daily, or more frequently if soiled with blood or saliva. Remove protective clothing before leaving the dental office. Choose clothes made of fabrics that can be effectively washed in normal laundry cycles. Follow manufacturer's laundering instructions.

Gloves

Gloves should be worn at all times when taking intraoral x-rays (just as with any other dental procedure) to prevent skin contact with blood, saliva, or mucous membranes. Gloves should always be changed and discarded between patients. Punctured, torn, or cut gloves should be changed immediately.

A variety of gloves are available for specialized uses. Sterile gloves for surgical procedures, non-sterile gloves for non-surgical procedures, and utility gloves for cleaning and disinfection. Gloves are made of latex or vinyl material. Gloves should never be washed or disinfected for reuse. Washing may damage gloves and increase the flow of liquid through undetected holes in the gloves.

All personnel must be instructed to avoid touching areas such as doorknobs, unexposed film packets, or records with contaminated gloves. Care should be taken to avoid touching anything that is not essential to the procedure being carried out.

Do not wear powdered gloves, as the powder can cause radiographic artifacts.

Hands should always be washed before gloving. And hands should always be washed after removing a pair of gloves. Potentially infectious pathogens can grow rapidly inside a warm, moist glove.

Masks

Snug fitting **masks** may be worn as an additional precaution. The mask offers protection against pathogens transmitted by airborne particles and from spatter containing blood and saliva. Change masks when wet or soiled and between patients. The mask should be removed before removing gloves.

Protective Eyewear

A variety of **eyewear** is available to protect against saliva and/or blood spatter. Traditional protective glasses, goggles, side shields, and full-face shields are popular. Protective eyewear must be washed with appropriate cleaning agents following treatment and as needed.

Because aerosol contaminants are not created during radiographic procedures, the use of masks and protective eyewear are optional.

Handwashing

Hands should be washed thoroughly with an antiseptic skin cleanser before and after treating each patient (before gloving and after removing gloves). Don't wear rings, fingernail polish, or false fingernails at work. Handwashing is most effective when nails are cut short and well manicured. Lather hands well with soap and rub them vigorously together for at least 10 sec.

Care should be taken to avoid hand injuries during dental treatment.

Disinfection and Sterilization of Instruments

Disinfection and **sterilization** of instruments breaks the "chain of infection" to prevent the transmission of infective microorganisms.

Disinfection

Disinfection is the use of a chemical or physical procedure to reduce the disease-producing microorganisms (pathogens) to an acceptable level on inanimate objects. Spores are not necessarily destroyed. Disinfecting agents are usually only used on surfaces and instruments because they are too toxic for living tissues.

One mandate of the U. S. Environmental Protection Agency (EPA) is the regulation and registration of surface disinfectants. EPA-registered sterilants-disinfectants are classified as:

- **High-level disinfectant.** Chemical germicides that can be used to disinfect heat-sensitive semicritical dental instruments.
- **Intermediate-level disinfectant.** Chemical germicides labeled as both hospital grade disinfectants and tuberculocidals. Examples are iodophors, phenolics, and chlorine-containing compounds.
- **Low-level disinfectant.** Chemical germicides labeled as hospital grade disinfectants.

Sterilization

Sterilization is the total destruction of spores and disease-producing microorganisms. Sterilization is usually accomplished by autoclaving or dry heat processes. Ideally, all equipment or instruments used should be sterilized. Unfortunately, this is not feasible with most radiographic equipment because of their large size.

Acceptable methods of sterilization in the dental office are:

- Steam under pressure (steam autoclave)
- Dry heat
- Heat/chemical vapor (chemical autoclave)
- "Sterilant/disinfectant" that has been registered by the EPA

A variety of sterilizers are available. Manufacturer's operating instructions should be followed.

Classification of Dental Instruments

Dental **instruments are classified** according to their risk of transmitting infection and to the need to sterilize them between uses.

- **Critical instruments** are those used to penetrate soft tissue or bone. Examples are scalpels, forceps, and scalers. Critical instruments must be sterilized after each use. No critical instruments are used in dental radiology.
- **Semicritical instruments** are those that contact but do not penetrate soft tissue or bone. Examples are x-ray film-holding instruments, mirrors, and burrs. Semicritical instruments must be sterilized after use. Heat sensitive semicritical instruments may be sterilized with EPA-registered chemicals classified as high-level disinfectant.
- **Noncritical instruments** are those that do not come into contact with the mucus membrane. Examples are the lead apron, the position-indicating device PID, and the exposure button. Noncritical instruments can be disinfected using EPA-registered chemicals classified as intermediate-level and low-level disinfectants.

Certain biteblocks and intraoral film holders, panoramic biteblocks, and beam aligning devices can be sterilized by autoclave. Head positioners, chin rests, and ear rods that are not practical for sterilization may be disinfected with EPA-registered chemicals classified as intermediate-level and low-level disinfectants.

Mirror, explorer or necessary biteblocks should be kept covered when not in use. Obviously standard sanitation procedures are followed in any correctly maintained dental installation.

Cleaning and Disinfection of the Dental Unit and Environmental Surfaces

Cleaning is the first step in sterilization and in high-, intermediate-, and low-level **disinfection**. The dental unit, counter tops, and environmental surfaces must be thoroughly cleaned after each patient. Scrub any area contaminated with blood and/or saliva with cleaning agents and disposable towels.

All surfaces must be disinfected with EPA-registered hospital grade disinfectants. Be sure to use the correct immersion time when using a chemical disinfectant. Intermediate-level disinfectants are recommended for all contaminated surfaces. Low-level disinfectants are recommended for general housekeeping duties such as cleaning walls and floors.

Disinfect the headrest, the arm rests, the bracket table, and the handles of the operating light. When x-ray equipment is involved, the tube head, PID, cassettes, and any other items handled by the operator or contacted by the patient should be disinfected.

Protective barriers should be used whenever practical. Plastic wrap, plastic bags, paper towels, paper cups, aluminum foil and etc. are used on appropriate surfaces, equipment and supplies. Barrier material is commonly placed over surfaces likely to be contaminated (chair headrest and controls, PID, tube head yoke, control panel, exposure switch, counter surfaces, etc.) (see Figures 22–3 to 22–5). Areas covered do not need to be disinfected.

REMEMBER: Surfaces not covered must be disinfected after the radiographic procedures are completed. **Disinfectants** have several drawbacks. They, like all liquids, have the potential to affect electrical connections. Also, disinfecting solutions may not reach all irregular surfaces.

Infection Control Procedures

Infection control procedures are to be used on all patients. This is the **universal precaution** approach where we **treat everyone as if known to be infectious.** The infection control procedures have been divided into before, during, and after film exposure.

Procedures before Film Exposure

The following are infection control procedures that are carried out before film exposure (see Table 22–2).

Prepare the Treatment Area

All **treatment area surfaces** likely to be contaminated should be covered with a protective barrier material or

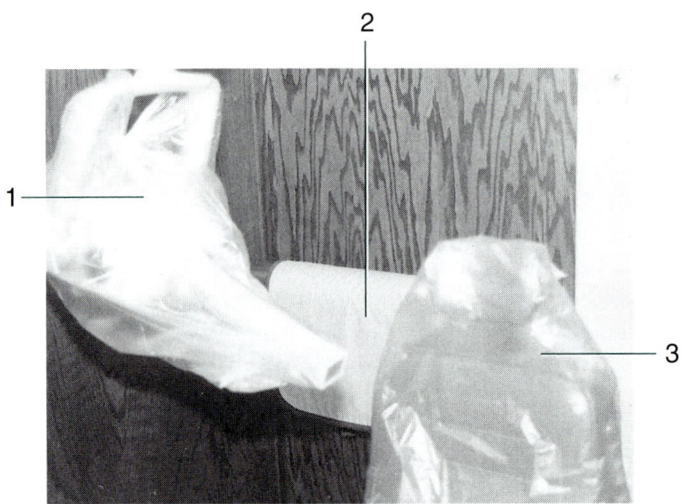

FIGURE 22-3. **Picture of dental operatory.** This figure shows: (**1**) plastic barrier bag covering PID, tube housing and yoke, (**2**) lead apron draped over storage rack, and (**3**) plastic barrier bag covering chair, headrest and chair controls.

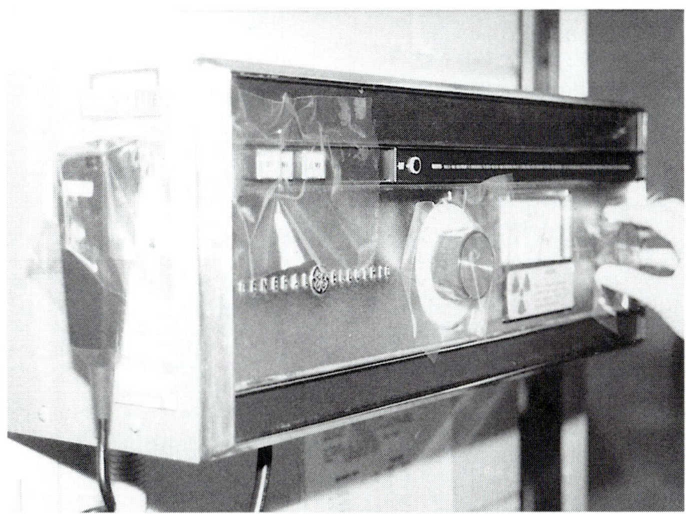

FIGURE 22-4. **Plastic barrier wrap covering exposure switch and controls on control panel.**

disinfected. Protective barriers are impervious (can not be penetrated) materials (such as plastic wrap, plastic backed paper, and aluminum foil) that are used to cover exposed surfaces. Protective barriers save time by eliminating the need for surface cleaning and disinfection between patients.

REMEMBER: Those surfaces not covered shall be cleaned and disinfected with an EPA-registered disinfectant after the radiographic procedures are completed. Disinfectants have several drawbacks. They, like all liquids, have the potential to affect electrical connections. Also, disinfecting solutions may not reach all irregular surfaces.

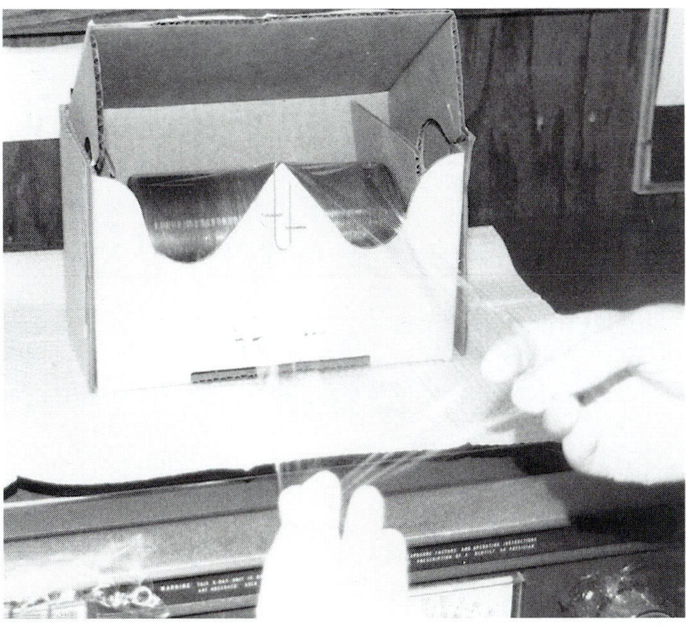

FIGURE 22-5. **Operator dispensing plastic barrier wrap.**

TABLE 22-2. **Infection Control Checklist: Before Film Exposure**

Prepare Treatment Area
Cover or disinfect:
- Dental chair
- X-ray machine
- Lead apron
- Thyroid collar
- Work area

Prepare Supplies and Film-holding Devices
Prepare:
- X-ray film
- Supplies
- Film-holding devices

Seat Patient
Adjust chair
Adjust headrest
Place lead apron and thyroid collar
Remove objects

Radiographer
Wash hands
Put on gloves
Prepare film-holding devices

1. **Dental chair.** Cover or disinfect the headrest, headrest adjustment, arm, backrest, seat, and chair adjustment controls.
2. **X-ray machine.** Cover or disinfect the tubehead, yoke, PID, control panel, and exposure button. Large plastic bags do an excellent job of covering the PID, tubehead, and yoke (see Figures 22–3 and 22–4).
3. **Lead apron and thyroid collar.** Wipe the lead apron and thyroid collar with an EPA-registered disinfectant between patients.
4. **Environmental work area.** Cover or disinfect all work area surfaces.

Prepare Supplies and Film-Holding Devices

All supplies and film-holding devices should be dispensed from the central supply area.

1. **Dental x-ray film.** Film packets should be dispensed in disposable containers such as a paper cup or small envelope. The film packet must be handled carefully to prevent cross-contamination. The film packet with its heat-sensitive emulsion cannot be disinfected or sterilized in the dental office. Therefore the operator should protect the packet by keeping it in the factory-sealed package or dispenser until ready to use.

   There are two methods used to prevent the transmission of microorganisms by the film packet, **barrier protection** and proper infection control **handling technique.**

   Barrier protection: Barrier envelopes are commercially available for film sizes #0, 1, and 2. Film packets from the factory-sealed package are placed and sealed in the plastic envelopes (see Figure 22–6). Film packets sealed in barrier plastic envelopes at the factory are also available commercially (see Figure 22–7). The film packet in the barrier envelope is then exposed. The barrier envelope is opened, allowing the film packet to drop on a clean surface (see Fig. 22–8). Then with clean hands (or new gloves), the film packets are opened and the film is processed.

   Handling technique: Exposed film packets should be placed in a container (usually a paper cup or towel) that is outside the radiographic operatory. When all the exposures have been made, the container is carried to the darkroom. In the darkroom, under safelight conditions, the film packets are opened. Take care not to touch the films as they drop onto a paper towel or clean disinfected surface. Throw away packets. Remove and discard the contaminated gloves and wash hands. The films are then processed.
2. **Supplies.** Cotton rolls, paper towels, rubber bands, and disposable containers should be dispensed from the central supply area.
3. **Film-holding devices.** Film-holding devices should be packaged in sterilized bags.

Seat the Patient

After the treatment area is prepared and supplies and film-holding devices dispensed, it is time to seat the patient.

1. **Adjust the chair.** The patient is seated in an upright position and the chair adjusted to the working height of the radiographer.
2. **Adjust the headrest.** Adjust the headrest to support the patient's head. The occlusal plane should be parallel to the floor.

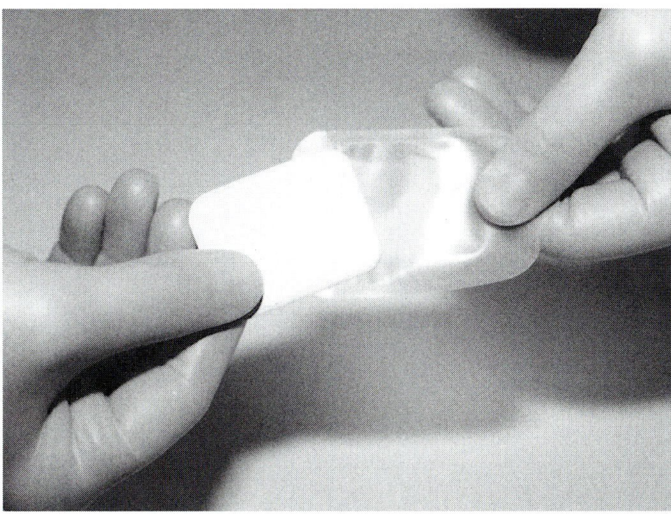

FIGURE 22-6. **Film handling.** Film packet is placed (and then sealed) in a plastic barrier envelope.

3. **Place the lead apron and thyroid collar.** Drape patient with the lead apron and thyroid collar.
4. **Remove patient's eyeglasses, dentures, etc.** Any object that may interfere with film exposure should be removed.

Radiographer Preparation

Final radiographer preparation procedures are:

1. **Wash hands.** Wash and dry hands thoroughly.
2. **Put on gloves.** Mask and eyewear are optional.
3. **Remove film-holding devices from sterilized package with gloved hands.**

Procedures during Film Exposure

Once film exposures begin, care must be taken to touch only covered surfaces. The best way to minimize contamination is to touch as few surfaces as possible.

The following are infection control procedures that are carried out during film exposure (see Table 22–3).

Dry Exposed Film Packets

Exposed film packets should be dried thoroughly with a paper towel and placed in a disposable container (usually a paper cup or towel). The container should be located inside a barrier-lined lead box or outside the radiographic operatory to prevent scattered radiation from fogging the

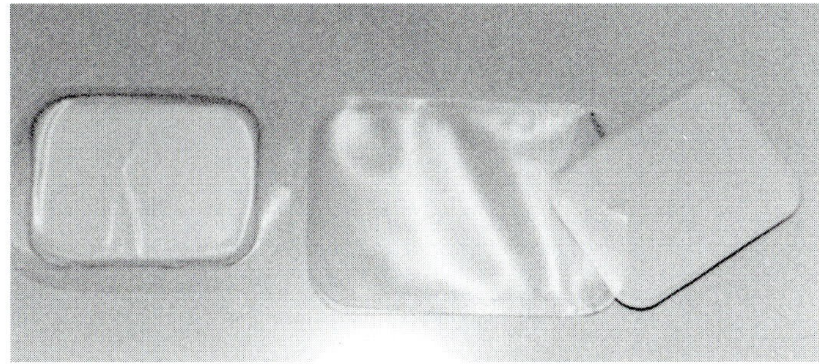

FIGURE 22-7. **Barrier envelope.** Left, film sealed in barrier packet ready to use from the manufacturer. Right, barrier envelope with film packet partially inserted.

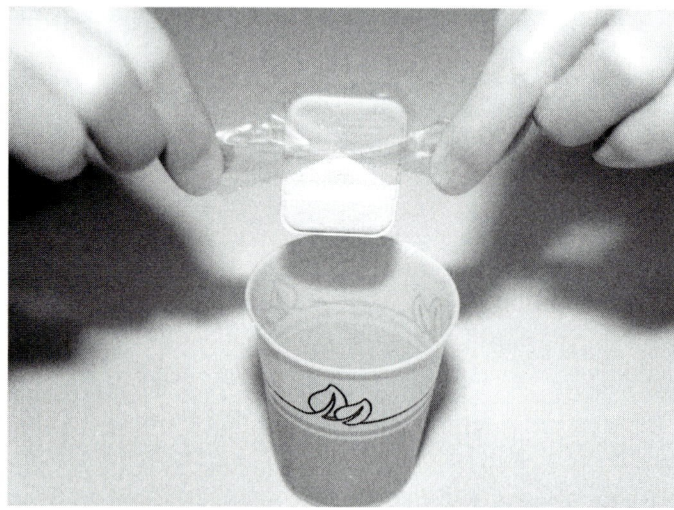

FIGURE 22–8. **Opening the envelope of the barrier packet.** A steady pull is used, allowing the film packet to drop in a clean cup.

film. Label the container with the patient's name to prevent possible errors. **Never put exposed films in your pocket!**

Care of Film-Holding Devices

Always **transfer film-holding devices** from a covered surface to the patient's mouth and then back to the same covered surface. Never place contaminated instruments on an uncovered surface.

> **NOTE:** If work is interrupted for any reason and you have to leave the room, remove and dispose of your gloves. Wash hands and put on a new pair of gloves before resuming work.

TABLE 22–3. **Infection Control Checklist: During Film Exposure**

Dry Exposed Film Packet
Place film in disposable container
Care of film-holding devices
Transfer film-holding device from work area to patient and back to work area.
Never place film-holding device on uncovered surface.

Procedures after Film Exposure

The following are infection control procedures that are carried out after film exposure (see Table 22–4).

Remove Film-Holding Devices

Film-holding devices are removed from the treatment area and placed with contaminated instruments while still wearing gloves.

Remove and Discard All Disposable Contaminated Items

Contaminated items (cotton rolls, paper towels, protective barrier coverings) are disposed of while the radiogra-

TABLE 22–4. **Infection Control Checklist: After Film Exposure**

Place film-holding devices with contaminated instruments
Remove and discard all contaminated items
Remove and discard gloves
Wash hands
Remove lead apron and thyroid collar
Dismiss patient from x-ray area
Disinfect all uncovered surfaces

pher is still wearing gloves. Carefully unwrap all covered areas making sure not to touch the surfaces with gloved hands. Dispose all contaminated items following local and state regulations.

- **Remove and discard gloves**
- **Wash hands**
- **Remove lead apron and thyroid collar** from patient
- **Dismiss patient from x-ray area**
- **Disinfect all uncovered surfaces** that were contaminated using an EPA-registered hospital-grade disinfectant.

> **NOTE: After the gloves have been removed, hands washed, patient dismissed, and the area cleaned, the exposed films must be processed. Carry the disposable film container holding the contaminated films to the darkroom.**

It has been suggested that exposed film packets be sprayed with disinfectant prior to processing. This may result in artifacts if moisture reaches the film. Paper film packets would be especially vulnerable.

Infection Control Procedures Used for Processing

Film handling procedures depend upon whether or not barrier envelopes are used to protect the film packets.

Film Handling without the Use of Barrier Envelopes

The following is the recommended step-by-step procedure for handling film **without** the use of barrier envelopes.

1. Cover darkroom work surface with disposable towel.
2. Place container holding contaminated films next to towel (see Figure 22–9).
3. Wash hands.
4. Put on clean gloves.
5. Work under darkroom conditions.
6. Remove one film and open film packet tab (see Figure 22–10A).
7. Slide out black paper and lead foil backing.
8. Discard film packet wrapping.
9. Discard lead foil backing (see Figure 22–10B).
10. Open black paper wrapping, being careful not to touch the film (see Figure 22–10C).
11. Drop film onto clean paper towel (see Figure 22–10D). Be careful not to touch film with gloved hands.
12. Discard black paper wrapping.
13. After opening all film packets, discard container.
14. Remove and dispose of gloves.
15. Wash hands.
16. Process uncontaminated film manually or by automatic processor.
17. Mount films or store in labeled envelope.

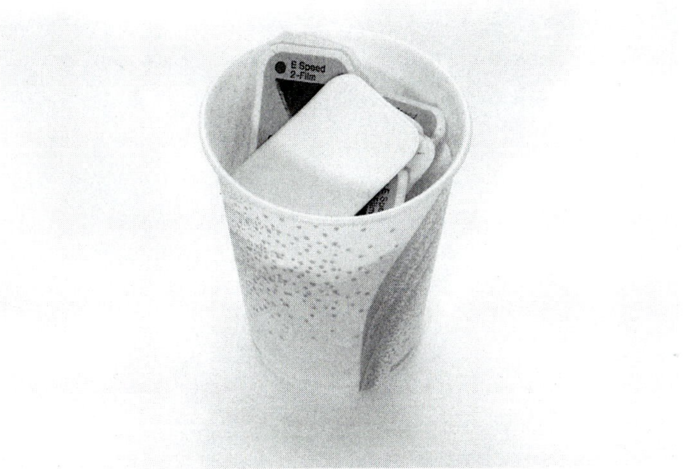

FIGURE 22–9. **Cup holding contaminated films.**

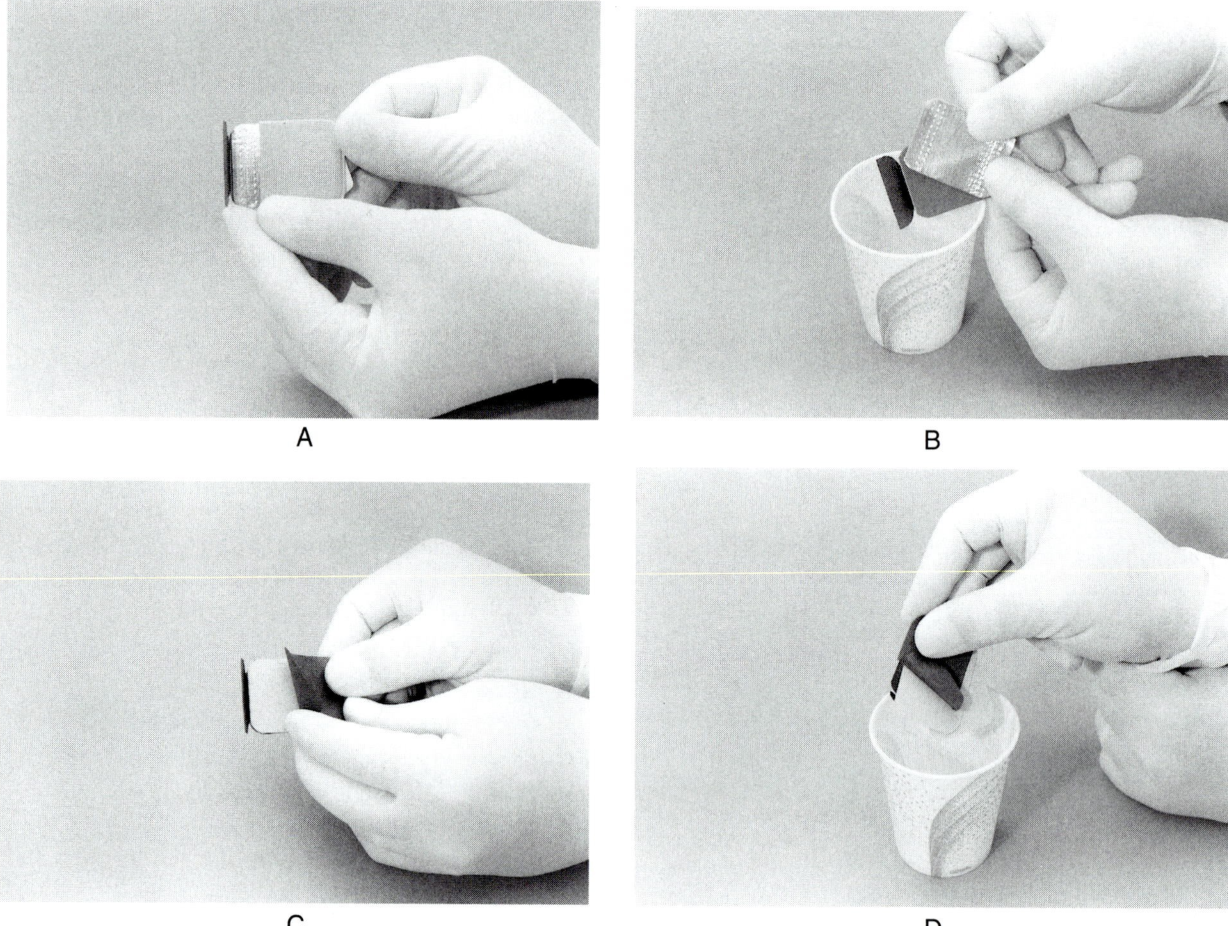

FIGURE 22–10. **Steps for removing film from packet without touching film with contaminated gloves.** (**A**) Open packet and slide black paper and lead foil from wrapping. (**B**) Remove and discard lead foil. (**C**) Bend black paper away from film. (**D**) Drop film into a clean cup.

NOTE: All contaminated supplies that cannot be disinfected or sterilized for reuse must be disposed of as required by local regulations to minimize health hazards to patients and employees.

Film Handling Procedures with the Use of Barrier Envelopes

The following is the recommended step-by-step procedure for handling film **with** the use of barrier envelopes.

1. Cover darkroom work surface with disposable towel.
2. Place container holding contaminated films next to towel.
3. Wash hands.
4. Put on clean gloves.
5. Remove one contaminated film from container.
6. Tear open barrier envelope.
7. Allow film to drop onto paper towel (or into a clean paper cup).
8. Be careful not to touch the film with gloved hands.
9. Discard barrier envelope.
10. After opening all barrier envelopes, discard container.
11. Remove and dispose of gloves.

12. Wash hands.
13. Work under darkroom conditions.
14. Unwrap and process film manually or by automatic processor.
15. Mount films or store in labeled envelope.

Daylight Loaders

Daylight loaders require special consideration. Some organizations discourage the use of daylight loaders because contamination is difficult to avoid. However, many offices use them, therefore strict infection control procedures must be followed.

Daylight loaders may be used without barrier envelopes and with barrier envelopes. The following is the recommended step-by-step procedure for handling film without barrier envelopes.

Film Handling Procedures without the Use of Barrier Envelopes

1. Wash hands before using the loader.
2. Open cover from daylight loader.
3. Place gloves inside the loader.
4. Place container of contaminated film packets inside the loader.
5. Close daylight loader cover.
6. Put hands into the loader.
7. Put on gloves.
8. Take one contaminated film out of the container.
9. Unwrap film packets as described in *Film Handling Procedures without the Use of Barrier Envelopes*.
10. Drop the film onto paper towel. Be careful not to touch films with gloved hands.
11. Place contaminated film packet wrappings in paper cup.
12. After all film packets have been unwrapped, remove gloves.
13. Place gloves in paper cup with packet wrappings.
14. Feed all unwrapped films into processor.
15. Remove hands from daylight loader.
16. Wash hands.
17. Open cover from daylight loader.
18. Remove and discard cup containing film wrappings and gloves.
19. Remove and discard container that held contaminated films.
20. Close daylight loader cover.
21. Collect processed films.
22. Mount films or store in labeled envelopes.

Film Handling with the Use of Barrier Envelopes

Follow recommendations as described in *Film Handling Procedures with the Use of Barrier Envelopes*.

Darkroom Disinfection

Remove and discard all materials used as protective barriers. **Clean and disinfect darkroom** counter surfaces and/or areas touched by gloved hands. Use EPA-registered hospital-grade disinfectants.

CHAPTER SUMMARY

Dental personnel must understand and practice infection control procedures to prevent the transmission of infectious diseases. Universal precautions must be taken to treat every patient as if known to be infectious.

The "chain of infection" involves a susceptible host, pathogens in sufficient numbers to initiate infection and an appropriate route for the pathogen to enter the host.

Protective barriers are used to prevent the transmission of infective microorganisms to the patient by breaking the chain of infection. Protective clothing, gloves, masks, and eyewear worn by dental personnel act as barriers to prevent the transmission of infective microorganisms.

Disinfection and sterilization of instruments breaks the "chain of infection" to prevent the transmission of infective microorganisms. Specific step-by-step infection control procedures are carried out before, during and after film exposure.

Recommended step-by-step procedure for handling film with and without barrier envelopes is presented. Strict infection control procedures must be followed when using daylight loaders.

REVIEW QUESTIONS

1. What is the purpose of infection control?

2. Define pathogen.

3. List the four conditions that must be present for disease transmission to occur.

4. EPA-registered chemical germicides labeled as both hospital disinfectants and tuberculocidal are classified as:

   (a) High-level disinfectants.
   (b) Intermediate-level disinfectants.
   (c) Low-level disinfectants.
   (d) None of the above.

5. Gloves should be worn when exposing dental radiographs to prevent skin contact with:

   (a) Blood.
   (b) Saliva.
   (c) Mucous membranes.
   (d) All of the above.

6. Which of these terms describes efforts made to reduce disease-producing microorganisms to an acceptable level?

   (a) Sterilization
   (b) Asepsis
   (c) Disinfection
   (d) Sepsis

7. Which of these items is not suitable for sterilization?

   (a) Film packet
   (b) Explorer
   (c) Forceps
   (d) Cutting instruments

8. The best method for sterilizing instruments that come into contact with saliva or blood is by:

   (a) Autoclaving.
   (b) Wiping with alcohol.
   (c) Washing with soap and water.
   (d) Immersing in an ADA-approved surface disinfectant.

9. The responsibility for carrying out infection control measures is the responsibility of the:
   (a) Patient.
   (b) Dental assistant.
   (c) Entire office staff.
   (d) Person that makes the exposure.

10. List the infection control procedures that are carried out before film exposure.

11. List the infection control procedures that are carried out during film exposure.

12. List the infection control procedures that are carried out after film exposure.

13. What is the recommended step-by-step procedure for handling film without the use of barrier envelopes?

BIBLIOGRAPHY

American Dental Association. Infection control recommendations for the dental office and the dental laboratory. *J. Am. Dent. Assoc.* 127:672, 1996.

Brand, J., Benson, B., & Ciola, B. American Academy of Oral and Maxillofacial Radiology infection control guidelines for dental radiographic procedures. *Oral Surg. Oral Med. Oral Pathol.* 3:48–249, 1992.

Centers for Disease Control and Prevention. Recommended infection-control practices for dentistry, 1993. *MMWR* 41:1–12, 1993.

Centers for Disease Control and Prevention. Recommendations for preventing transmission of human immunodeficiency virus and hepatitis B virus to patients during exposure-prone invasive procedures. *MMWR* 40:1–9, 1991.

Cottone, J. A., Terezhalmy, G. T., & Molinari, J. A. *Practical Infection Control in Dentistry*. Philadelphia; Williams and Wilkins, 1996.

Karpay, R. I., Plamondon, T. J., & Dove, S. B. Infection control in dental radiology. *Operatory Infection Control Update* 5:1–6, 1997.

Proceedings of the National Symposium on Hepatitis B and the Dental Profession. *J. Am. Dent. Assoc.* 110:613–650, 1995.

Puttaiah, R., Langlais, R. P., Katz, J. O., & Langland, O. E. Infection control in dental radiology. *J. Calif. Dent. Assoc.* 23:21–28, 1995.

CHAPTER 23

Patient Relations and Education

OBJECTIVES

By the end of this chapter the student should be able to:

- Define key words.
- Discuss the importance of appearance and first impression.
- Explain how the patient should be greeted.
- Discuss five personality traits.
- Discuss communication and listening skills.
- Explain the necessity for patient education in radiography.
- Identify the benefits that the patient derives from preventive radiation procedures.
- Describe three methods by which the patient can be educated to appreciate the value of dental radiography.
- Identify the goals of the dental radiographer.

KEY WORDS

Attitude
Chairside manner
Cheerfulness
Communication
Empathy
Enthusiasm
Honesty
Trait
Patient education
Patient relations
Preventive radiation

Introduction

The dental radiographer must not only be capable of technically making radiographs, but must also have a professional attitude, be able to communicate with patients, and be capable of educating patients. The purpose of this chapter is to discuss patient relations, present communicating skills, and review patient education.

Patient Relations

Patient relations refers to the relationship between the patient and the dental office personnel. Patient relations are important to the dental radiographer. Pleasing **appearance,** good **personality traits,** and **communication** help build solid patient relations.

Appearance

The patient's first impression of the dental radiographer is important. And the first impression is often made by the radiographer's **appearance.** The dental radiographer should always maintain a professional appearance in the presence of a patient. Careful attention should be given to personal hygiene and grooming. Wear a clean uniform and appear well groomed. Personal hygiene such as trimmed nails, clean hands, and fresh breath are important. Never eat or chew gum while working with patients. A clean, neat appearance makes people feel good about themselves and helps self-confidence.

Greeting the Patient

The patient should be greeted in the reception room and then escorted to the treatment area. Always greet the patient by name. Address the patient using their proper title (Miss, Mrs., Ms., Mr., Dr., etc.) and last name. If you are uncertain of the correct pronunciation of the patient's name, ask the patient to pronounce it for you. Always introduce yourself to the patient, using both your name and title.

You might say: "Good morning, Mrs. Smith. My name is Linda Johnson. I'm the dental assistant who will be taking your radiographs today. Please follow me to the x-ray room and we will get started."

Chairside Manner

Chairside manner refers to the conduct of the radiographer while working at the patient's chairside. Always make the patient feel comfortable. Work in a confident manner and the patient will feel at ease. Avoid comments such as "Oops!" which indicates lack of control. Whenever possible, praise the patient for any assistance they may give you and tell them what a good patient they are.

Personality Traits

A **trait** is defined as a distinguishing quality or characteristic. Positive **personality traits** include **attitude, enthusiasm, cheerfulness, honesty,** and **empathy** (see Figure 23–1).

Attitude

Attitude is the most important trait. Attitude is defined as the position assumed by the body in connection with a feeling or mood. Your attitude towards your employer, coworkers, and patients will determine the degree of your success or failure.

Approach each task with a positive attitude. Radiographers with a good attitude who believe they can do a task (like make radiographs) will produce good results. The person with a poor attitude will produce poor results (such as poor radiographs). Learn from your mistakes and strive for excellence. The radiographer should always exhibit a friendly attitude in both speaking and facial expression. People can sense your attitude by the way you walk, talk, and behave. Maintain a pleasant, positive attitude, and you will have a successful future.

Enthusiasm

Enthusiasm is from the Greek work *enthousiasmos*, which means to be inspired by God. Enthusiastic people are expressing this inspiration with excess energy to do anything they wish to do. Be enthusiastic about your work and soon it will not seem like work at all. Challenge yourself to be come an expert dental radiographer. Show your coworkers overabundance of energy, and some will rub off on them.

Cheerfulness

Everyone likes to be around a **cheerful** person. Cheerfulness is contagious. When you are cheerful, people around you will be cheerful.

Honesty

Be **honest** with your patients and they will have confidence in your procedures. Radiography can cause the patient some discomfort but rarely causes great pain.

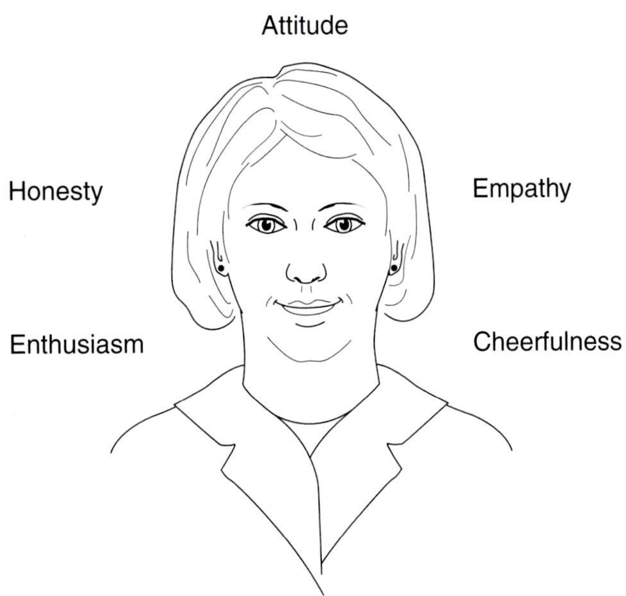

FIGURE 23–1. **Personality traits.**

Explain to the patient possible discomfort and request cooperation and assistance.

Honesty develops trust. When a patient trusts the dental radiographer, the patient is more likely to cooperate with the radiographic procedure. Also the patient is more likely to return for future dental care.

Empathy

Empathy is defined as the ability to share in another's emotions or feelings. The radiographer must have empathy for all patients, but especially for children and handicapped patients. Be courteous and polite at all times even in difficult situations.

Follow the golden rule, do unto others as you would have them do unto you. Treat your patient as you want to be treated. Threat your coworkers as you want your coworkers to treat you. And treat your dentist as you want your dentist to treat you.

Communication

Communication is defined as the process by which information is exchanged between two or more persons. It may be accomplished by words or signs. The radiographer and the patient must communicate during radiographic procedures. Effective communication is the basis for developing a successful relationship between the radiographer and the patient.

The radiographer's choice of words is very important. Choose words at a level the patient can understand. For instance, young children may understand "pictures of the teeth made with a camera" rather than "radiographs made with an x-ray machine." Highly technical words may confuse the patient and result in a misunderstanding. Certain words are more professional than others. For example, say, "extract the tooth" rather than "pull the tooth" and "restore the molar" rather than "fix the molar." Words that imply negative images such as drill, shot, or cut should not be used.

Nonverbal communications, such as facial expressions and body movement, are important when delivering dental care. A nod of the head indicates yes or agreement, while a shake of the head indicates no or disagreement. Facial expression conveys the attitude of the radiographer. A smile by the radiographer relaxes the patient and reduces apprehension.

The use of **show and tell** method of communication is useful in dental radiography. Show a radiograph to help explain it. Show a film holder and demonstrate PID placement. Showing while telling provides the patient with more information in a shorter period of time.

Listening

A good **listener** communicates attention and interest. Whenever possible use eye contact when listening. Careful attention to listening results in fewer misunderstandings. Never interrupt the patient or finish the patient's sentences. If the radiographer must perform a task while the patient is talking, an occasional comment will indicate the radiographer is still listening to the patient.

Patient Education in Radiography

One of the greatest services that the dental radiographer can render the patient is **dental health education**. This includes not only education in oral health and restorative dentistry but also education in the value of dental radiography (see Figure 23–2). It is surprising how many patients, even today, do not comprehend the enormous value of a radiographic examination of their teeth.

Value of Patient Education

The value of **patient education** is twofold. First, the understanding that dental radiographs disclose cavities and lesions that can become a source of danger if not treated in time. Second, the educated patient is more inclined to

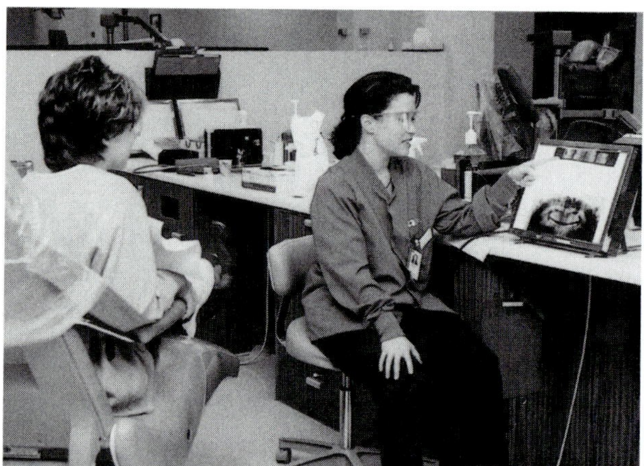

FIGURE 23–2. **Patient education.** The dental radiographer should educate the patient concerning dental health and radiography. (Courtesy Michelle L. Sensat, RDH, MS, University Nebraska Medical Center, College of Dentistry, Lincoln, NE)

understand and accept the dentist's treatment plan and prevention program. Such patient acceptance helps to develop a spirit of confidence and mutual trust in the dentist and the staff.

Necessity for Patient Education

Most dental patients have heard about the bad effects of overexposure to radiation. Rightfully, they are concerned. It is only natural that they may on occasion question the necessity of having more radiographs exposed. It is the responsibility of the dentist or a member of the staff to provide the patient with a clear, concise, and satisfactory explanation.

The dental radiographer must take the time to educate the patient. The patient may be shown collimated position indicating devices (PIDs), thyroid collars, and protective lead aprons. Tell the patient that the films now used require only a fraction of the radiation previously necessary to expose them and that modern equipment is better constructed to prevent unnecessary radiation.

Further, the radiographer should stress all standard safety practices as suggested by the National Council on Radiation Protection and Measurements are adhered to in the office. The patient must be made aware that the use of radiographs entails many benefits and few risks.

The patient should be assured that everyone in the office who works with radiography is trained in its use and the safety aspects of radiation. If the state issues a license or a certificate of compliance to show that a radiation safety examination has been passed, that can be offered in evidence. Many radiographers display their certificates near the x-ray machine.

Methods of Patient Education

Several methods can be used to educate the patient on the value of **preventive radiation.** An **oral presentation, printed literature,** or a **combination** of both may be used to educate the patient. What is successful in one office may not be in another. Everyone concerned in the performance of radiation duties shares the responsibility for teaching patients. Be sure to use terms that the patients can understand.

Oral Presentation

An effective method of educating the patient is to give an **oral presentation** using a series of radiographs showing typical dental conditions, both normal and abnormal. Placed in convenient mounts, the radiographs are shown to the patient on a screen or an illuminated viewer.

The viewer-enlarger shown in Figure 12–7 is extremely well suited for enlarging radiographs. Patients are generally able to identify the areas that are pointed out to them on the radiographs better if the images are magnified and the brightness of the light is controlled. Although many trained radiographers can interpret radiographs correctly, they should limit their presentations by showing slides or radiographs of someone other than the patient. This avoids the appearance that the radiographer is making the diagnosis. In the event that the patient's own radiographs are to be shown, the dentist should make the presentation.

There are many persons who seldom or never visit the dental office unless an emergency forces them to do so. Such nonpatients are occasionally reached when they attend meetings or lectures devoted to dental health at schools, health centers, or PTA meetings. The entire dental staff is encouraged to make presentations at such meetings.

Printed Literature

An effective education method is to place **printed literature** in the reception room or to hand it to the patients before their x-ray appointment. The literature may be obtained from the American Dental Association or produced in the dental office. Two such pamphlets, *Answers to Common Questions about Dental X-Ray Examinations (w209)* and *The Benefits of Dental X-Ray Examinations (w138)* can be obtained from the American Dental Association. These pamphlets explain in simple terms what x-rays can do and how x-rays work for you.

Producing your own brochure may require some time, thought, imagination, and a degree of artistic ability. The preparation of such a brochure can be fun, helpful to the patient, and very satisfying. For example, such a brochure could be titled "Why Dental X-Rays?" or something similar. The narration should be simple and in language that is professional, yet not overly technical. Depending on the amount of available space, pictures of a few radiographs illustrating conditions that can be identified easily may be shown. Such a brochure might be constructed by formulating a series of questions and then presenting a very short answer.

Giving pamphlets to the patient opens the door for two-way communication between the patient and the dentist or staff member on the advisability and necessity of regular radiographic examinations. Most dental offices do not have a specific method or program by which the benefits of periodic x-ray examinations are taught. All too often the patient is simply told that the doctor requires them and will not treat the patient unless they are taken, or else the explanation is limited to a few short and often unsatisfactory answers.

Combination

Whether the patient receives the information at chair-side, in a specially equipped room, or at a talk given at some meeting is irrelevant. A mixture of information presented at chair-side **combined** with a pamphlet and some form of x-ray slide presentation is probably the most effective method of educating the patient.

Goals of the Dental Radiographer

The dental radiographer should develop pride in his or her work and strive for professional improvement. One achieves this by setting **goals.** Such goals are closely related, and all are equally important.

- One goal is to **achieve perfection** with each radiograph. It is accomplished by careful attention to all details. Each step in the process, whether in film placement, exposure technique, or processing and identification, though small, can be significant.
- A closely related goal is to **work rapidly** but without undue haste. Haste often makes waste and results in having to retake radiographs.
- Another goal is to **take pride in work** and professional advancement. This is accomplished by reviewing techniques, reading professional journals and books, and attending lectures and seminars.
- Still another goal is to **keep radiation levels as low as possible.** This includes using protective devices that minimize radiation to the patient and remaining in a distant area during the exposure.
- An additional goal is to always **keep in mind the needs of the patient.** Avoid making two exposures when one can produce the required result.
- A final goal of every radiographer is to **develop integrity, dedication, and competence** to such a degree that the patient can be motivated and educated.

By constantly keeping these goals in mind, the radiographer benefits both the patient and dentistry by rendering the finest professional service.

Helpful Hints

- **Attitude** is the most important trait. Maintain a pleasant, positive attitude and you will have a successful future.
- Be **enthusiastic** about your work.
- **Cheerfulness** is contagious.
- **Be confident.** Most patients react favorably to the authority of a confident, capable operator.
- **First impressions** are always important and lasting.
- **Treat others as you want to be treated.**

Questions and Answers

Many patients have questions concerning radiographic procedures. The dental radiographer can answer some questions and some must be answered only by the dentist. For example, the dentist must answer questions about diagnosis. Questions to be answered only by the dentist should be established by the dentist and understood by all staff members. The dental radiographer must be prepared to answer questions in terms the patient understands.

Some of the following questions and answers are taken from the American Dental Association brochure "Dental X-ray Examinations: Your Dentist's Advice."

Question: Are dental radiographs really necessary?

Answer: Many diseases of the teeth and surrounding tissues are not always visible when your dentist simply looks into your mouth. Small carious lesions (cavities) between the teeth, infections in the bone, cysts, developmental abnormalities, and some types of tumors may go unnoticed for a long period of time. Dental radiographs are taken for the patient's benefit. Finding and treating dental problems at an early stage can save time, money and unnecessary discomfort. If you have a hidden tumor, early diagnostic x-rays may even help save your life.

Question: How often should I have dental x-ray examinations?

Answer: The frequency of dental radiographic examinations depends on the patient's individual health needs. It is important to recognize that just as each patient is different from the next, so should x-ray exams be individualized for each patient. Your dentist will review your history, examine your mouth and then decide whether you need radiographs and what type. If you are a new patient, the dentist may recommend radiographs to determine the present status of the hidden areas of your mouth.

The schedule for needing radiographs at recall visits varies according to age, risk for disease, and signs and symptoms. Patients with cavities and gum disease need radiographs more often than patients without disease.

Question: How often should children have dental radiographs?

Answer: Radiographic examinations should be based on the individual needs of the child. Children with tooth decay need more frequent radiographic examinations than children without tooth decay.

Children may need x-ray exams more often than adults. This is because their teeth and jaws are still developing and because their teeth are more likely to be affected by dental caries (tooth decay) than those of adults.

Question: Can I refuse dental x-rays and still be treated?

Answer: No. Treatment without necessary radiographs is considered negligent care. Even if you signed a paper stating that you refused radiographs and released the dentist from all liability, you would be consenting to negligent care. You cannot, legally, consent to negligent care.

Question: What is a bitewing radiograph?

Answer: A bitewing radiograph shows the crowns of several upper and lower teeth on one small film. Films of this type are especially useful for showing cavities between the teeth and changes in bone caused by gum disease.

Question: What is a panoramic radiograph?

Answer: A panoramic radiograph shows all the upper and lower teeth, large portions of the jaws and other structures on one relatively large film. It is often used to find unerupted or impacted teeth, cysts, retained root fragments, fractures and other conditions of the jaws.

Question: How are x-rays measured?

Answer: Special units are used to measure x-rays. When human tissue or other materials are exposed to x-rays, some of the energy is absorbed and some passes through without effect. The amount of energy absorbed by the tissue is the dose. The dose is often measured in rads. Another unit of measurement, the rem, is used to compare the biological effects of different kinds of radiation.

In modern diagnostic dental x-ray procedures, the exposure and dose are usually so small that they are expressed in "milli" units—that is, units that are equal to one-thousandth of a rad, or rem.

Question: How much radiation is involved in a dental x-ray exam?

Answer: A full mouth x-ray examination of 21 films will deliver an effective dose equivalent of approximately 13 millirem (mrem). This is equivalent to approximately 16 days of exposure to naturally occurring environmental radiation.

For purposes of comparison it is useful to know that, according to federal and mostÏ state regulations, persons whose occupations involve some exposure to radiation are permitted to receive up to 5,000 mrem of whole body radiation per year.

Question: Do people receive radiation from sources other than medical and dental x-ray exams?

Answer: Yes, people are exposed to natural background radiation all their lives. This radiation comes mainly from naturally radioactive substances (mostly radon) but also from outer space in the form of cosmic radiation.

Natural background radiation varies greatly in different geographic areas. It has been estimated that the average person receives about 100 to 300 millirem (mrem) of radiation every year from the natural environment.

Question: What effects can x-rays have on the body?

Answer: Scientists have known for some time that exposure to very large amounts of x-radiation is harmful. Changes can occur in the reproductive system, altering the genetic material that determines the health of future generations. Large amounts can cause changes in the tissues of the body, including the possibility of cancer.

On the other hand, diagnostic procedures involve very low doses. With modern techniques and equipment, the amount of radiation received in a dental exam is minuscule. Also only a small part of the body is exposed (approximately the region corresponding to the size of the film). Therefore, the risk of harmful effects from dental x-ray exams is extremely small.

Question: Why do you use a lead apron?

Answer: Because a lead apron and thyroid collar absorbs the x-rays and protects you from unnecessary radiation.

Question: Why do the dentist and other members of the dental staff leave the room when x-ray exposures are made?

Answer: If a dentist and other members of a dental staff did not leave the room or stand behind a barrier, they would be exposed many times a day to radiation. Although the amount of radiation they would receive each time is quite small, over a long period of time they would receive a needless dose that provides no benefit to them.

Question: If I am pregnant or think I may be pregnant, should dental x-ray exams be postponed?

Answer: No. Only x-ray exams in which a fetus or embryo would be in, or near, the primary x-ray beam should be avoided. Since dental x-ray exams are limited to the head and neck region, it is unlikely that the developing baby receives any detectable radiation. There is no dose to the developing baby when a lead apron is used.

Question: If I have had radiation therapy for cancer of the head or neck, should I avoid a x-ray exam?

Answer: No. The dose of radiation required for dental x-ray exams is extremely small compared to that used for radiation therapy. The effects of very high doses involved in therapeutic radiation may increase your susceptibility to diseases, such as tooth decay. This can occur as a result of a decrease in secretions of the salivary glands. It is especially important for you to have x-ray exams as needed, to detect problems at an early stage.

Question: Can dental x-rays cause skin cancer?

Answer: There is not a single recorded case of a patient developing cancer from diagnostic dental x-rays. Dentists have developed cancer on their fingers after receiving repeated exposures for many years from holding the film in the patient's mouth.

Question: Does my dentist take special precautions to minimize the amount of radiation I receive?

Answer: Yes. There are several ways your dentist minimizes the amount of radiation that you receive. Your dentist should take only necessary radiographs, use the fastest type of x-ray film, use equipment that restricts the beam to the area that needs to be examined, use the lead apron and thyroid shield when appropriate, and finally, develop films according to the manufacturer's recommendations.

Question: Who owns my dental radiographs?

Answer: The dentist owns all your dental records including the radiographs. You have the right of reasonable access to your dental records but they remain the property of the dentist.

Question: Should I have my previous radiographs sent to my new dentist?

Answer: Yes, if possible. These radiographs can reveal your previous disease activity and may assist in determining the need for a new x-ray exam. Although the dentist who treated you in the past is considered the owner of you records, including your x-rays, arrangements can usually be made to have x-rays duplicated and sent to your new dentist. You should contact your former dentist and request that this is done.

CHAPTER SUMMARY

Dental health education is not limited to demonstrations on toothbrushing and flossing techniques or to slogans such as "visit your dentist twice a year." It does and must include education in how x-rays can benefit the patient. The emphasis of this education must be on the preventive aspect of radiography. The exposing of bitewing radiographs during the checkup appointment to disclose incipient caries is a perfect example of preventive radiation.

Patient education is necessary not only to secure the patient's cooperation and motivation to return to the office for regular examination but also to allay any fear about the safety of the procedures involved.

The patient must be told or shown why a complete diagnosis is not possible without x-rays, as hidden lesions may remain undetected until it is too late to repair the damage. Dental neglect results in pain, discomfort, loss of function and esthetics, and a needless expenditure of time and money.

The methods of patient education include oral presentations at chair-side, the distribution of pamphlets, and showing the patient enlarged pictures or slides of radiographs projected on a screen. Lectures may be given to children or adults at schools or at meetings. Often a combination of these measures is most effective.

As the dental radiographer develops expertise, a set of standards and goals must be developed. This is essential if the finest service is to be rendered to the patient. These goals include producing radiographs of good diagnostic quality, avoiding careless actions that result in retakes, keeping radiation levels low, and always keeping the patient's interests supreme.

REVIEW QUESTIONS

1. Dental radiographers with a positive attitude produce high-quality radiographs.
   (a) True
   (b) False
2. The use of highly technical words may confuse the patient and result in miscommunication.
   (a) True
   (b) False
3. When a patient trusts the radiographer, the patient is more likely to cooperate with the radiographic procedures.
   (a) True
   (b) False
4. What is the value of patient education?
   (a) The dentist can schedule the patients better.
   (b) More patients will call for appointments.
   (c) An informed patient is inclined to accept the dentist's treatment plan.
   (d) The patient will demand more radiographs at each appointment.
5. Why is patient education in radiography necessary?
   (a) To increase the demand for radiographic services
   (b) Because it is legally required
   (c) To assure the patient that all radiographers are licensed
   (d) Because patients must be reassured that dental radiation procedures are safe

6. Why does the patient benefit from preventive radiation?
   (a) Because incipient decay may be disclosed
   (b) Because radiation inhibits dental decay
   (c) Because fewer cavities will have to be restored
   (d) Because radicular cysts can be eliminated by radiation treatment

7. Which of these is not a method of patient education in radiography?
   (a) Information given orally at chair-side
   (b) Follow-up letters from the dentist
   (c) Visual presentation of enlarged radiographs
   (d) Pamphlets on radiation protection

8. Which of the following is not a goal of the radiographer?
   (a) Professional improvement and advancement
   (b) Reducing the levels of radiation used during an exposure
   (c) Increasing the demand for dental x-ray services
   (d) Taking only such radiographs as are needed for diagnosis of the patient's needs

BIBLIOGRAPHY

American Dental Association. *Facts about AIDS and Infection Control*. Chicago: ADA, 1993.

American Dental Association. *The Benefits of Dental X-ray Examinations*. Chicago: ADA, 2000.

American Dental Association. *Answers to Common Questions about Dental X-rays*. Chicago: ADA; 2000.

Thunthy, K. H. X-rays: Detailed answers to frequently asked questions. *Compendium of Continuing Education in Dentistry*. 14:394–398, 1993.

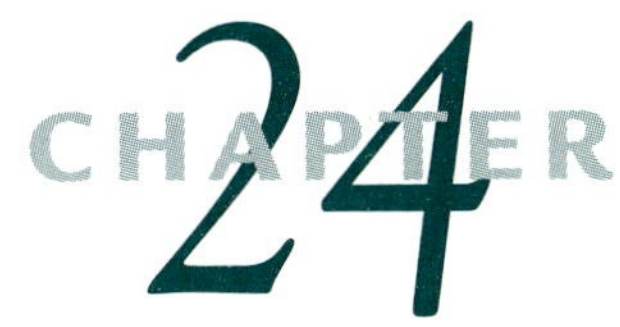

Managing Patients with Special Needs

OBJECTIVES

By the end of this chapter the student should be able to:

- Define key words.
- List the areas of the oral cavity that are most likely to initiate the gag reflex.
- List the two stimuli that commonly initiate the gag reflex.
- Describe seven methods to reduce psychogenic stimuli to control the gag reflex.
- Describe four methods to reduce tactile stimuli to control the gag reflex.
- Discuss the procedures for managing the wheelchair-bound patient.
- Discuss the procedures for managing visually and hearing impaired patients.
- Discuss the procedures for managing the apprehensive patient.
- Discuss the procedures for film placement in patients with maxillary or mandibular tori.
- Discuss the procedures for film placement in patients with low palatal vaults.

KEY WORDS

Apprehensive
Disability
Gagging
Gag reflex
Tori

Introduction

Dental radiographic techniques cannot be standardized for all patients. The dental radiographer must be competent in altering procedures to meet the needs of individual patients.

The purpose of this chapter is to provide specific information on how to manage patients with the gag reflex, patients with physical disabilities, the apprehensive patient, and patients with anatomical variations.

The Gagging Patient

The term **gagging** means to make an involuntary effort to vomit. Gagging is caused by the **gag reflex,** which is a protective mechanism that serves to clear the airway of obstruction. The receptors for the gag reflex are located in the soft palate and lateral posterior third of the tongue.

Two reactions occur prior to the gag reflex.

- First, a cessation of respiration.
- Second, a contraction of the muscles of the abdomen and the throat. (Sometimes food is regurgitated.)

All patients have gag reflexes, but some are more sensitive than others. A hypersensitive gag reflex is probably the most troublesome problem the radiographer encounters. Two stimuli that commonly initiate the gag reflex are:

- **Psychogenic stimuli** (stimuli originating in the mind)
- **Tactile stimuli** (stimuli originating from touch)

These stimuli must be diminished or eliminated to reduce gagging.

Reducing Psychogenic Stimuli

Patients with a hypersensitive gag reflex are usually nervous and high-strung individuals with very sensitive oral tissues. The dental radiographer can **reduce psychogenic stimuli** by use of the following techniques.

1. **Convey a confident attitude to reduce anxiety.** Every effort should be made to give the patient confidence in the radiographer's ability to perform radiographic procedures.
2. **Have patience and be understanding.** Make every effort to relax and reassure the patient. Explain the procedure to be performed and then compliment the

patient as each exposure is completed. Thank the patient for their "help." As patients become more comfortable with radiographic procedures, they become more confident and are less likely to gag.

3. **Radiograph anterior regions first.** Anterior films are less likely to initiate the gag reflex. Always expose the premolar (bicuspid) film before the molar film. The maxillary molar film is the most likely film placement to initiate the gag reflex. Hopefully, the patient's fears from psychic stimuli will have been forgotten by the time the maxillary molar exposure is made.
4. **Give the patient a task to perform.** For instance, bite hard on the bite block, raise an arm or clench a fist. Anything that helps to divert the patient's attention may lessen the likelihood of initiating the gag reflex.
5. The dental radiographer should **never suggest gagging** or ask the question "are you a gagger?" The power of suggestion is a strong psychogenic stimulus and can initiate the gag reflex. If the patient brings up the subject of gagging, do not use the terms gag, gagger, or gagging. Instead, refer to the gag reflex as "a tickle in the throat."
6. The radiographer should try to **divert the patient's attention** away from the procedure. This can be done by maintaining a running dialogue or telling the patient to think of something pleasant such as their favorite vacation.
7. **Give the patient breathing instructions.** Instruct the patient to breathe deeply through the nose during film placement and exposure. For the gag reflex to take place breathing must stop; therefore, if the patient is breathing, the gag reflex cannot occur.

Reducing Tactile Stimuli

Some patients have an accentuated gag reflex because of hypersensitive pharyngeal tissues. The worst gaggers are patients suffering from chronic sinus problems (postnasal drip). Mucus and saliva accumulate into the nasopharynx area and initiate the gag reflex. The dental radiographer can **reduce tactile stimuli** by use of the following techniques.

1. **Place film positively** and retain in position without movement. For maxillary molar projections, carry the film into the mouth parallel with the plane of occlusion. When in proper position, rotate the film to touch the palate.
2. **Expose the film as quickly as possible.** Plan ahead, have everything organized. Immediately after the exposure tell the patient how well he or she did. Reassure the patient that gagging is not unusual.
3. **Use a desensitizing agent** to confuse the sensory nerve endings and lessen the likelihood of stimulating the gag reflex.
   - **Ice water.** Hold ice water in the mouth for several seconds.
   - **Salt.** Place some salt on the tip of the patient's tongue.
4. **Use a topical anesthetic.** A topical anesthetic spray can be used to numb the areas that initiate the gag reflex. Spray the soft palate and posterior third of the tongue. **Be sure to instruct the patient to exhale while the anesthetic is sprayed.** Caution must be taken to make sure the patient does not inhale the anesthetic or an inflammation of the lungs may occur. The anesthetic takes effect in 1 minute and lasts for about 20 minutes. Do not use topical anesthetic sprays in patients who are allergic to benzocaine.

Extreme Cases of the Gag Feflex

Occasionally, the radiographer will encounter a patient with an accentuated gag reflex that will not allow intraoral radiographs to be made. Thankfully, these patients are few and far between. The radiographer should take as many intraoral radiographs as possible and then supplement them with extraoral radiographs.

Suggested alternatives are:

- Panoramic radiograph
- Lateral jaw radiographs
- Maxillary and mandibular occlusal radiographs
- Bitewings using the smaller #1 or #0 size

The Disabled Patient

A **disability** is defined as a physical or mental impairment that substantially limits one or more of an individual's major life activities. The dental radiographer must be prepared to accommodate patients with disabilities. When treating a patient with a disability:

- **Talk directly to the patient.** Do not ask the patient's caretaker questions that should be directed to the patient. For example, do not say to the caretaker, "Can he (or she) stand up?" Instead, speak directly to the patient and say, "Can you stand up?"

- **Offer assistance to disability patients.** Ask the patient if he or she would like you to push the wheelchair.
- **Do not ask personal questions about the patient's disability.**

The Wheelchair-bound Patient

Usually, the patient in a wheelchair is accompanied to the dental office by a family member or a caretaker.

Wheelchair patients can be **transferred to the dental chair** by use of the following techniques.

- **Wheelchair patients who can temporarily support their weight** are transferred to the dental chair by placing the wheelchair alongside the dental chair. Set the brakes of the wheelchair and elevate the dental chair to the height of the wheelchair. Move the dental chair arm from between the chairs. Have the patient move or slide sideways into the dental chair with the caretaker and radiographer assisting.
- **If the patient is totally unable to walk,** the immobile patient may be transferred to the dental chair. The radiographer and caretaker may lift the patient from the wheelchair into the dental chair.

If the chair transfer is not possible, radiographs may be made with the patient seated in the wheelchair. Some panoramic machines permit a wheelchair to be substituted for the machine chair.

Patients that do not have the use of their arms or hands may need the assistance of a relative or caretaker to hold the film. In such cases the relative or caretaker should wear a lead apron and thyroid collar during the exposures. The radiographer must never hold the film in the patient's mouth during the x-ray exposure. In most cases the radiographer can use a biteblock type of film holder to keep the film in position. Most film holders only require the patient to close the jaws.

The Visually Impaired Patient

If a patient is **visually impaired** or blind, the radiographer must communicate verbally. Explain each procedure before performing it. Keep the patient informed of each step as it is being done. The visually impaired or blind patient requires special consideration. The radiographer must communicate using clear verbal explanations of each procedure before performing it. Keep the patient informed of each step as it is being performed.

Never gesture to another person in the presence of a patient who is blind. Blind persons are sensitive to gesture communication and may feel you are "talking behind their back."

The Hearing Impaired Patient

The **hearing impaired** or deaf patient requires special consideration for communication. Several options are:

- Use of written instructions.
- Ask a relative or caretaker to act as an interpreter.
- Use of gestures.

If the patient can read lips, face the patient and speak slowly and clearly. When a hearing aid must be removed for extraoral radiographs, be sure to explain the procedures before removing it.

The Apprehensive Patient

Apprehensive means to be anxious or fearful about the future. Apprehensive patients are usually nervous individuals with sensitive oral tissues and a low pain threshold. These patients tend to avoid dental care and do not have regular dental check-ups. It is important that the apprehensive patient's contact with the dental radiographer be pleasant and reassuring.

Apprehensive patients should be assessed regarding their degree of apprehension, which can range from mild concern to extreme fear. A program should be set up to systematically desensitize and control their fear. Apprehensive patients can become cooperative dental patients when cured of their fears. To **reduce the patient's apprehension,** the dental radiographer should:

- **Be organized** so that the procedure can be rapid and accurate.
- **Expose the easier maxillary anterior projections first**, and then progress to the more difficult posterior areas.
- **Reassure the patient** that all is going well.
- **Compliment apprehensive patients on their cooperation.** Thank them for their "help."

Anatomical Variations

The dental radiographer should be familiar with some of the more common anatomical variations.

Maxillary and Mandibular Tori

Tori (torus, singular) are commonly seen in the oral cavity. Tori are outgrowths of bone. A **maxillary torus** (called torus palatinus) is an outgrowth of bone along the midline of the hard palate. A **mandibular torus** (called torus mandibularis or lingual torus) is an outgrowth of bone along the lingual aspect of the mandible in the canine premolar area.

Torus Palatinus

A patient with a large **torus palatinus** presents a problem when radiographing the maxillary posterior area. Place the film on the far side of the torus before exposing the film. Do not place the film on the torus itself (see Figure 24–1).

Torus Mandibularis

Mandibular tori are usually bilateral on the lingual aspect of the mandible in the canine-premolar area.

- **Periapical film placement.** Place the film between the torus and the tongue (see Figure 24–2). Do not place the film on top of the mandibular tori, as it would result in only a partial image of the roots of the teeth. Be gentle and careful when placing the film, as the mucosa covering the torus is thin and sensitive.
- **Bitewing film placement.** Place the film between the torus and the tongue. Mandibular tori may cause problems when exposing bitewing radiographs. When bitewing tabs are used, and the patient has large tori, the film must be pushed away from the teeth making the patient bite on the very end of the bitewing tab. In such cases, proper film placement is difficult and may require a bitewing film holder to be used.

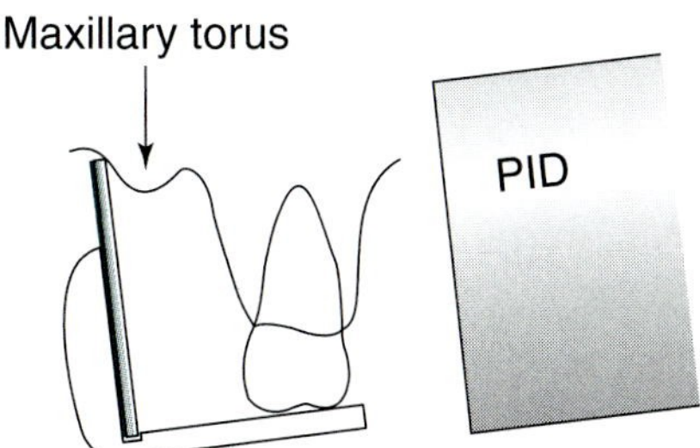

FIGURE 24–1. **Maxillary torus.** Film is shown placed on the far side of the torus away from the teeth.

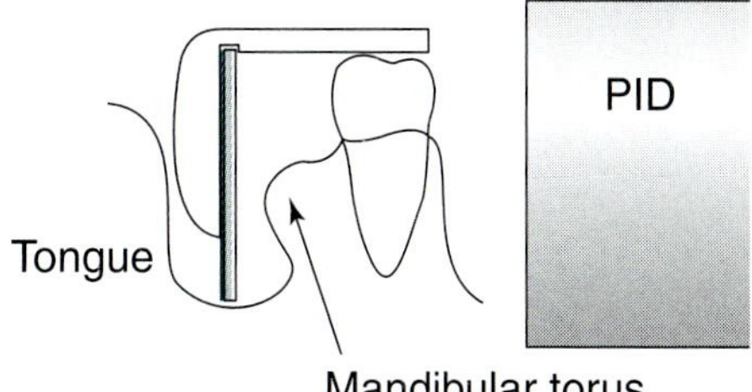

FIGURE 24–2. **Mandibular torus.** Film is shown placed between the torus and the tongue.

Shallow Palate

Some patients have **shallow maxillary palates** (also called low palatal vault) making it difficult to place the film parallel to the long axis of the teeth. If the film and teeth are parallel, the apices of the teeth may be cut off. In such cases, one of three methods may be used.

1. **Tip the tissue edge of the film away from the teeth** (see Figure 24–3). If the discrepancy of parallelism between the film and teeth does not exceed 15 degrees, the resultant radiograph is usually acceptable.
2. **Increase the vertical angulation 15 degrees greater than the XCP instrument indicates.** The resultant radiograph will be acceptable, however, there will be some foreshortening of the teeth and a portion of the cusp tips may be cut off.

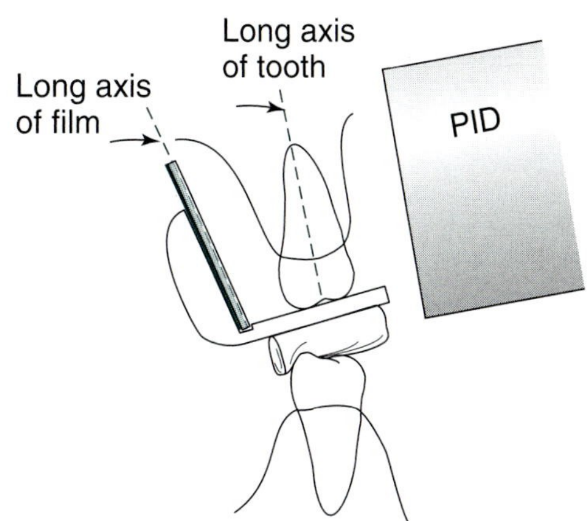

FIGURE 24–3. **Shallow palate.** The tissue edge of the film is shown tipped away from the teeth. When the lack of parallelism is less than 15 degrees, the resultant radiograph will generally be acceptable.

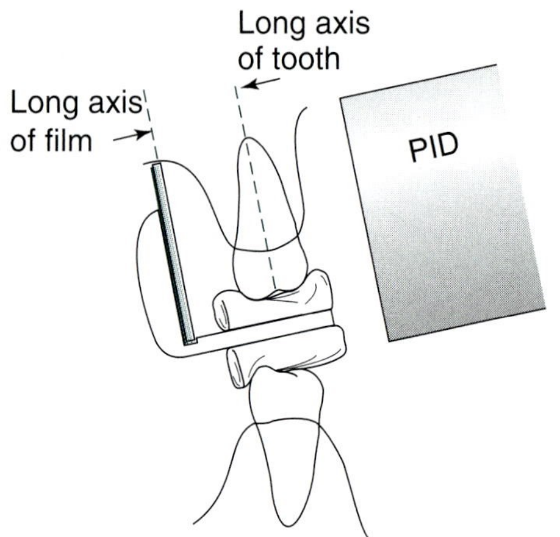

FIGURE 24-4. **Parallelism.** Use of two cotton rolls to achieve parallelism of the film and teeth. One cotton roll is placed on each side of the biteblock.

3. **Two cotton rolls are used, one on each side of the biteblock** (see Figure 24-4). However, care must be taken because periapical coverage is reduced and the apices of the teeth may be cut off.

Helpful Hints

- Be confident.
- Work rapidly, but accurately.
- Never suggest gagging.
- If a patient gags, remove the film as quickly as possible and reassure the patient.
- Do not ask questions about a disability.
- Be gentle when placing film near tori.

CHAPTER SUMMARY

Dental radiographic techniques cannot be standardized for all patients. The dental radiographer must be competent in altering procedures to meet the needs of individual patients.

Gagging is caused by the gag reflex, which is a protective mechanism that serves to clear the airway of obstruction. A hypersensitive gag reflex is probably the most troublesome problem the radiographer encounters. Psychogenic and tactile stimuli must be diminished or eliminated to reduce gagging.

A disability is a physical or mental impairment that substantially limits one or more of an individual's major life activities. The dental radiographer must be prepared to accommodate patients with disabilities.

The dental radiographer should be familiar with some of the more common anatomical variations.

REVIEW QUESTIONS

1. The film most likely to initiate the gag reflex is:
   (a) Maxillary premolar (bicuspid).
   (b) Maxillary molar.
   (c) Mandibular premolar (bicuspid).
   d) Mandibular molar.
2. Breathing and the gag reflex cannot take place at the same time.
   (a) True
   (b) False

3. The longer the film stays in the mouth, the less likely the patient is to gag.
   (a) True
   (b) False

4. Confident dental radiographers have fewer gagging problems with their patients.
   (a) True
   (b) False

5. Diverting the patient's attention often helps to suppress the gag reflex.
   (a) True
   (b) False

6. The dental radiographer should talk to the caretaker of a patient with a disability instead of talking directly to the patient.
   (a) True
   (b) False

7. Film placement for a patient with a torus palatinus is:
   (a) Between the torus and the tongue.
   (b) On the top of the torus.
   (c) On the near side of the torus, close to the teeth.
   (d) On the far side of the torus, away from the teeth.

8. Film placement for a patient with a mandibular torus is:
   (a) On top of the torus.
   (b) On top of the tongue.
   (c) Between the torus and the tongue.
   (d) None of the above.

BIBLIOGRAPHY

Langland, O. E. & Langlais, R. P. *Principles of Dental Imaging*. Baltimore: Williams & Wilkins; 1997.

White, S. C. & Pharoah, M. J. *Oral Radiology Principles and Interpretation*, 4th ed. St. Louis: Mosby, 2000.

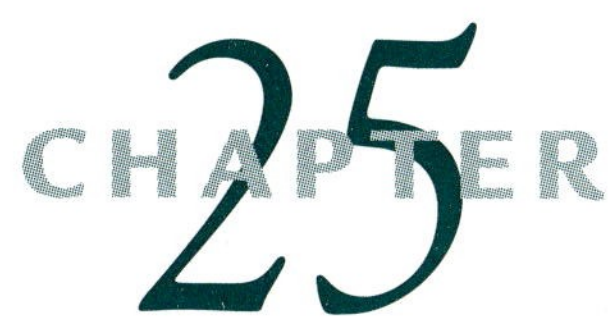

Regulations and Legal Aspects

OBJECTIVES

By the end of this chapter the student should be able to:

- Define the key words.
- Discuss the federal and state regulations concerning the use of dental x-ray equipment.
- Describe licensure requirements for exposing dental radiographs.
- Discuss risk management.
- Discuss the relationship of the patient and the radiographer.
- Discuss informed consent.
- List the items that must be documented in the patient's record.
- Explain what should be said to patients who refuse radiographs.

KEY WORDS

Disclosure
Informed consent
Liable
Malpractice
Negligence
Risk management
Self-determination
Statute of limitations

Introduction

The dental radiographer must understand the legal considerations involved in taking dental radiographs. Local and federal laws exist that regulate the use of dental x-rays. Every radiographer must be aware of and comply with these laws.

The purpose of this chapter is to discuss regulations that apply to dental radiology and to present the legal aspects of dental radiography.

Regulations and Licensure

The dental radiographer should be aware of the laws and regulations pertaining to dental radiology.

Federal and State Regulations

There are both **federal and state regulations** that control the manufacture and use of x-ray equipment. The Federal Performance Act of 1974 requires that all x-ray equipment manufactured or sold in the United States meet federal performance standards. These standards include safety requirements for filtration, collimation, and other x-ray machine characteristics.

In addition to federal regulations, there are city, county, and state laws that affect the use of dental x-ray equipment. Most state laws require registration and inspection of x-ray machines. Inspections are conducted every 2 to 4 years and usually fees are collected.

NOTE: State regulations vary. Be familiar with your state and local regulations!

Licensure Requirements

State laws require that **operators** of x-ray equipment be trained and certified or licensed to take dental radiographs. The **dental hygienist** is a licensed professional in all states. However, some states may require the hygienist to take an additional examination to be certified to make radiographs.

State laws vary considerably for dental assistants exposing radiographs. **Dental assistants** may only need the national certifying examination to be authorized to take dental radiographs, or they may need to take special training and/or pass an examination. Some states allow the uncertified dental assistant to take radiographs under the direct supervision of a dentist. Direct supervision means the dentist is present in the office when the radiographs are taken.

State laws and regulations change constantly. This text cannot list the requirements of every state. Be sure to become familiar with your state's regulations.

Legal Aspects

The dental radiographer should be familiar with the legal aspects of dental radiography.

Risk Management

The most important legal aspect of dental radiology is **risk management.** Risk management can be defined as the policies and procedures to be followed by the radiographer to reduce the chances that a patient will file legal action against the dentist and staff. Malpractice actions have increased in number and amount of awards in recent years. All members of the dental staff must participate to make an effective risk management program

Patient Relations

Patient relations refers to the relationship between the patient and the dental radiographer. It is important to make the patient feel comfortable by establishing a relaxing and confident chairside manner (see Chapter 23).

Avoid negative remarks about procedures, equipment, and the dental staff. Statements like, "The films were left in the developer too long" or "The timer switch always sticks" should never be said. If equipment is not working properly, one should discuss it with the dentist in private.

To avoid misunderstandings, the office staff should explain in advance financial payments, filing of insurance claims, and other office policies. Always explain to the patient what and how procedures are to be performed. Answer all questions the patient may have concerning the procedures. Good patient relations reduces the risk of possible legal actions.

Informed Consent

Informed consent is the consent the patient gives for treatment after being informed of the nature and purpose of all treatment procedures.

All patients have the legal right to make choices about the health care they receive. This is called **self-determination**. Self-determination includes the right to refuse treatment. The patient must be informed of the following:

- The purpose of the procedure
- The benefits of receiving the procedure
- The possible risks of receiving the procedure
- The possible risks of not receiving the procedure
- The person who will perform the procedure

It is the responsibility of the dentist to explain the nature and purpose of all treatment procedures. When taking radiographs, the risks and benefits must be explained in lay terms. The informing process is called **disclosure.** The patient should be given the opportunity to ask questions prior to radiography. Answer all questions completely in terms the patient understands. State laws vary concerning informed consent. Be sure to become familiar with your state laws.

Liability

Liable means to be legally obligated to make good any loss or damage that may occur. State law requires dentists to supervise the performance of dental radiographers. Both dentists and dental radiographers are **liable** for procedures performed by the dental radiographer. Therefore, it is important to understand that even though radiographers work under the supervision of the dentist, they are legally liable for their own actions. In malpractice cases, both the supervising dentist and the dental auxiliary may be sued for the actions of the auxiliary.

Patient Records

A **record** of all aspects of dental care must be kept for every patient. Dental radiographs are considered a part of the patients record and are therefore legal documents.

Documentation

The exposure of dental radiographs should be documented in the patient's record. Entries in the patient's record should be made by the dentist or under the dentist's supervision. Be sure the following items are documented in the patient's record.

- The patient's informed consent
- The number and type of radiographs, including retakes
- The date and radiographer
- The reason for taking the radiographs
- The interpretive results

Confidentiality

State laws govern **confidentiality** to protect the patient's privacy. The patient's records, including the radiographs, are confidential and should never be shown or discussed with anyone outside the dental office without first obtaining a current, signed release form from the patient.

Ownership

The courts have ruled that **radiographs are the property of the dentist.** The patient pays for the dentist's ability to interpret the radiographs and to arrive at a diagnosis. However, patients may have reasonable access to their radiographs. They may request a copy of their radiographs if they decide to change dentists or request a consultation with a dental specialist (see Table 25–1). The original radiographs, however, belong to the dentist. Because of statute of limitation laws, it is recommended that all records (including radiographs) be retained indefinitely.

Retention

Dental radiographs must be **retained for 7 years** after the patient ceases to be a patient. Legal actions that can be brought against the dentist depend on the malpractice and limitation statues that vary from state to state.

For adult patients, the statute of limitations generally begins to run at the time of the injury, or when the injury should have reasonably been discovered. For children, the statute of limitations does not begin to run until the child reaches the age of majority (18 to 21 years old, depending on the state). If you work for a governmental entity, the statute of limitations may be affected by certain notice statutes, which may greatly reduce the time in which a suit may be brought. Because the time period is so indefinite, it is recommended that radiographs be retained forever.

TABLE 25–1. **Steps to Follow when Patient Transfers to Another Dentist**

1. Request for radiographs should be in writing.
2. Keep the letter requesting radiographs in the patient's record.
3. Duplicate the original radiographs.
4. Send the duplicate radiographs by registered or certified mail.
5. Keep the postal receipt in the patient's record.

Insurance Claims

Insurance companies have the right to request pretreatment radiographs to evaluate the dental treatment plan. Only duplicate radiographs should be sent out of the dental office.

Malpractice Issues

Malpractice results when one is negligent. **Negligence** occurs when the dental diagnosis or treatment is below the standard of care provided by dentists in a similar locality and under similar conditions.

Negligence

Negligence is defined as the failure to use a reasonable amount of care when failure results in injury or damage to another. Negligence may result from the care (or lack of care) of either the dentist or the dental radiographer.

Statute of Limitations

Statute of limitations is the time period during which a patient may bring a malpractice action against a dentist or radiographer. State laws govern this time period which begins when the patient discovers, or should have discovered, an injury due to negligent dental treatment.

Sometimes negligence is not discovered until years later when a patient changes dentists and discovers an injury has occurred. In such cases, the statute of limitations begins years after the negligent dental treatment occurred. An example would be where appropriate radiographs were not taken on a patient with periodontal disease. Years later, the patient is examined by another dentist and is informed of the irreversible periodontal condition that might have been prevented if detected earlier.

Besides the statute of limitations, many states have separate malpractice laws that may limit damages or, in the case of governmental entities, may provide limited or complete immunity from suit, under certain circumstances. Because the laws vary greatly from state to state, it is desirable to bring in a lawyer experienced in this area to provide training and answer questions for the staff, as part of the risk management program.

Patients who Refuse Radiographs

Occasionally, for a variety of reasons, patients express opposition to the dentist's proposal that x-rays be taken. Typically those patients believe that such radiographs are unnecessary and just add to the cost, or that they are fearful that additional x-ray exposure will be hazardous to their health. When this happens, the dentist or radiographer must carefully explain in clear terms why the suggested radiographs are needed to complete the diagnosis, prognosis, or treatment plan and therefore are of benefit to the patient.

Frequently a patient may say, "I will sign a paper to assume the responsibility for not taking x-ray pictures if something later goes wrong because of this." At this juncture the patient must be informed in a diplomatic manner that legally, such documents to release the dentist from liability are not valid because the patient cannot legally consent to negligent care. If the patient still refuses to be radiographed, the dentist must carefully decide whether treatment can be provided. Usually, in such cases, the dentist cannot treat the patient.

CHAPTER SUMMARY

The dental radiographer should be aware of the laws and regulations pertaining to dental radiology. There are both federal and state regulations that control the manufacture and use of x-ray equipment.

State laws require that operators of x-ray equipment be trained and certified or licensed to take dental radiographs. Some states may require the dental hygienist to take an additional examination to be certified to make radiographs.

State laws vary considerably for dental assistants exposing radiographs. The dental assistant may only need the national certifying examination to be authorized to take dental radiographs, or they may need to take special training and/or pass an examination.

The dental radiographer should be familiar with the legal aspects of dental radiography. Always explain to the patient what and how procedures are to be performed. Answer all questions the patient may have concerning the procedures. Both the dentist and the dental radiographer are liable for procedures performed by the dental radiographer.

The patient's records, including the radiographs, are confidential and should never be shown or discussed with anyone outside the dental office. The courts have ruled that radiographs are the property of the dentist; the patient pays only for the diagnosis. However, patients may have access to their films.

REVIEW QUESTIONS

1. Most state laws require registration and inspection of x-ray machines.
   (a) True
   (b) False
2. State laws require that operators of x-ray equipment be trained and certified or licensed to take dental radiographs.
   (a) True
   (b) False
3. It is all right to make negative remarks such as, "The timer switch always sticks" to the patient.
   (a) True
   (b) False

4. Dental radiographs should be retained for:
   (a) 3 years.
   (b) 5 years.
   (c) 7 years.
   (d) 9 years.

5. Every patient has the legal right to make choices about the health care they receive. This is called:
   (a) Disclosure.
   (b) Informed consent.
   (c) Self-determination.
   (d) Liability.

6. Both the dentist and the dental radiographer are liable for procedures performed by the dental radiographer.
   (a) True
   (b) False

7. When patients express opposition to having dental radiographs taken, the auxiliary should:
   (a) Ask the patient to sign a document to release the dentist of all liability.
   (b) Explain in clear terms why the radiographs are needed.
   (c) Ask the patient to return at a later date.
   (d) Take the radiographs immediately.

8. The courts have ruled that radiographs are the property of the dentist.

BIBLIOGRAPHY

Bundy, A. L. *Radiology and the Law.* Rockville, MD: Aspen, 1988.

Morris, W. O. *The Dentist's Legal Advisor.* St Louis: Mosby; 1995.

PART VIII: Radiographic Interpretation

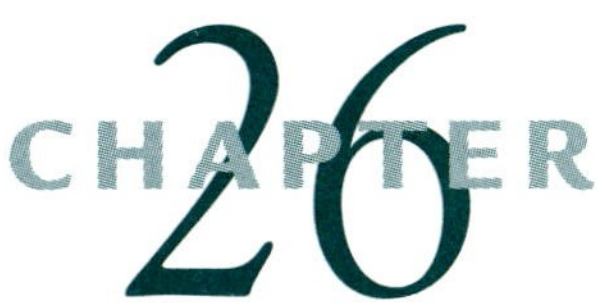

Introduction to Radiographic Interpretation

OBJECTIVES

By the end of this chapter the student should be able to:

- Define the key words.
- Differentiate between interpretation and diagnosis of the radiograph.
- Identify all radiopaque- and radiolucent-appearing restorative materials.
- Identity at least four types of cysts.
- Describe the appearance of at least eight anomalies.
- Differentiate between normal and pathological resorption of bone structures and teeth.
- Differentiate between calcifications and ossifications.
- Describe the radiographic appearance of odontogenic tumors.
- Describe the radiographic appearance of dental injuries.
- Identify two methods used to localize objects in the jaws by applying the buccal-object rule.

KEY WORDS

Abscess
Amalgam tattoo
Ameloblastoma
Amelogenesis imperfecta
Ankylosis
Anodontia
Anomalies
Benign
Buccal-object rule
Calcification
Cementoma
Clark's rule
Concrescence
Condensing osteitis
Cyst
Dens in dente
Dentinogenesis imperfecta
Diagnosis
Dilaceration
Exostosis
Follicular (eruptive) cyst
Foreign body
Fracture line
Fusion
Gemination
Giant cell tumor
Globulomaxillary cyst
Granuloma
Hypercementosis
Impacted tooth
Incisive canal cyst
Interpretation
Macrodontia
Malignant
Malposed tooth
Mesiodens
Microdontia
Nonodontogenic cyst
Odontogenic cyst
Odontoma
Ossification
Osteoma
Osteomyelitis
Phlebolith
Pulp stone
Radicular cyst
Radiolucent
Radio-osteosclerosis
Radiopaque
Rarefying osteitis
Residual cyst
Resorption
Retained root
Rhinolith
Sarcoma
Sclerosis
Sialolith
Supernumerary tooth
Taurodontia
Torus
Tumor

Introduction

Dental hygienists and dental assistants play an important role in radiographic interpretation. It is the dentist's responsibility for the final diagnosis and treatment of dental disease, however, all members of the dental team should be able to recognize radiographic deviations from the normal. Patient care is enhanced when radiographs are interpreted and findings discussed by the entire dental health care team.

The dental hygienist must be able to utilize radiographic findings when preparing the dental hygiene diagnosis. The ability to identify periodontally involved teeth and to locate irritating factors such as calculus and overhanging restorations is vital to treatment planning.

Developing interpretation skills fosters an appreciation for producing quality radiographs. Understanding what information is being sought from the radiographic image motivates the dental radiographer to obtain precise images.

Interpretation is a skill that requires a great deal of practice. The beginning student is often frustrated by not being able to "see" what the expert easily identifies. Students should first identify normal radiographic anatomy and then systematically progress through a sequence of evaluation, naming each radiopaque and radiolucent structure observed.

Chapter 11 dealt with the radiographic appearance of normal anatomical structures and landmarks. In this chapter the emphasis is on the recognition of the radiographic appearance of restorative dental materials, periodontal disease, cysts, anomalies, bone pathology, and dental injuries. Chapter 27 is devoted exclusively to interpreting periodontal disease and Chapter 28 to interpreting dental caries.

The purpose of this chapter is to present the basic concepts of radiographic interpretation and to present an overview of common radiographic features of dental anomalies, periapical pathology, trauma and restorative materials. Also, methods of localizing objects in the jaws are presented.

Interpretation by the Dental Radiographer

Just a few years ago, all that was expected of a competent dental radiographer was to recognize sufficient anatomical landmarks or structures to be able to mount the radiographs correctly. Today, dentists expect their radiographers to have a sound knowledge of the normal and abnormal (pathological) conditions that may occasionally be visible on dental radiographs. The final diagnosis of dental radiographs is the task of dentists, whose years of training and study have prepared them to render a diagnosis. However, a preliminary interpretation can be made by the trained dental radiographer.

The terms **interpretation** and **diagnosis** are often used interchangeably. This book, however, defines interpretation as the ability to read the radiographs. Diagnosis means correlating the patient's case history, clinical findings, test results, and radiographs. The dentist makes the diagnosis only after considering all the evidence pertaining to the patient's condition.

To produce consistently good radiographs, the radiographer must not only be familiar with dental anatomy and exposure techniques but must know how to tell whether or not all the desired information appears on the radiograph.

Viewing Radiographs

As explained in Chapter 12, proper radiographic viewing is essential for the interpretation of dental radiographs. A **viewbox** and a **magnifying glass** are required for optimal viewing.

- **Viewbox.** The viewbox must have lighting of uniform intensity and evenly diffused. A variable light intensity viewbox is best. The viewing surface should be large enough to accommodate a full set of intraoral radiographs as well as uncounted extraoral radiographs. A cardboard template should be used to mask out distracting light round the mount.
- **Magnifying glass.** A handheld magnifying glass should be used to aid the viewer. Some viewers are equipped with a magnifying device (Figure 12–7).

Always use subdued room lighting to allow the eyes to adapt to the light level of the radiographs.

Radiographic Appearance of Dental Restorative Material

The radiographic appearance of normal tooth structures was discussed in Chapter 11. These are readily identified by most students. The differentiation between the various restorative materials is a little more difficult and requires additional experience.

Some restorative materials are easy to identity. Others can be differentiated only by the size and contour of the restoration, its probable location on the tooth, and the relative degree of radiopacity or radiolucency.

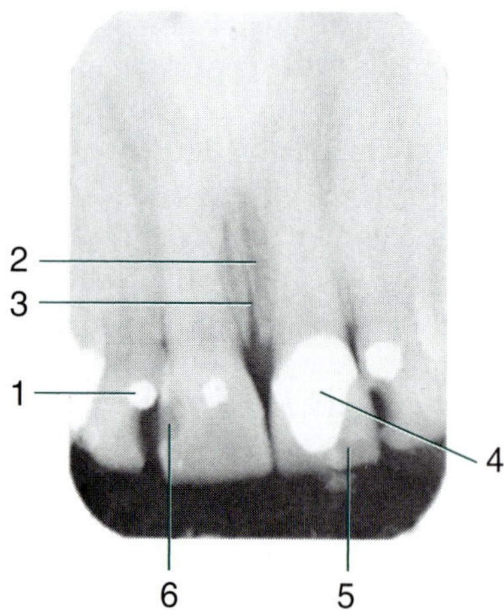

FIGURE 26–1. **Radiograph of maxillary incisor region.** This radiograph shows a (**1**) small radiopaque metallic restoration, which could be a gold foil or amalgam. These materials cannot be differentiated on a radiograph and must be determined by a visual inspection. Also seen is the (**2**) incisive (anterior palatine) foramen, (**3**) thin dark line as median palatine suture, and (**4**) metal core of porcelain jacket crown. (**5**) A fused porcelain crown. Porcelain is the most dense of the aesthetic (natural appearing) dental restorative materials and described as being slightly radiolucent. (**6**) A silicate restoration (radiolucent). Observe that the silicate in the adjacent tooth has partially disintegrated. A visual inspection is required to verify any preliminary interpretation of the radiographs.

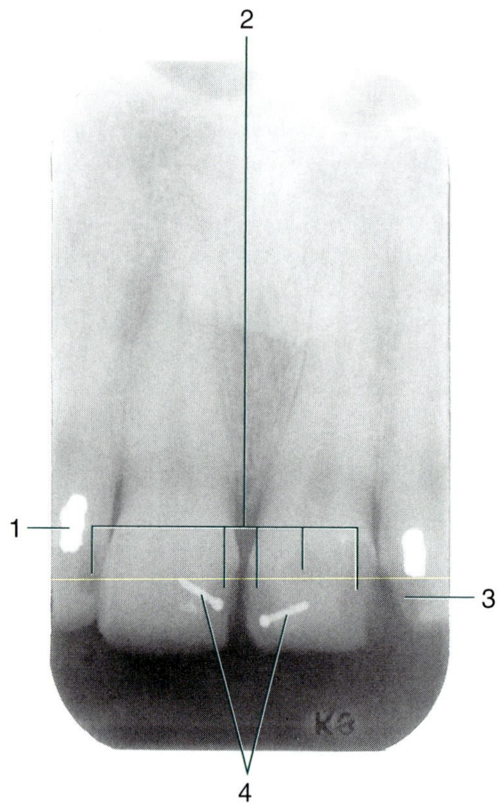

FIGURE 26–2. **Radiograph of maxillary incisor region.** This radiograph shows a (**1**) small radiopaque metallic restoration, probably amalgam on the lingual surface. (**2**) Radiolucent areas, possibly restorative materials (composites, acrylic resins or silicates) or caries. A visual inspection is required to verify any preliminary interpretation of the radiographs. (**3**) A fractured mesial incisal angle. (**4**) Radiopaque metallic pins holding the radiolucent composite restorations.

The image of a restoration on one surface may be superimposed on the image of another large restoration on the same tooth, thus giving the appearance of only one restoration instead of two, or even more. Some materials, such as the cements used in dentistry, can be differentiated only by the location on the tooth and the degree of radiopacity. Dental restorative materials are identified on the radiographs in Figures 26–1 through 26–3.

Metallic Restorations

The image outlines of all **metallic restorations** of approximately equal density appear extremely radiopaque. Thus it is impossible to determine whether the material used was gold, silver, or a base metal alloy. Only by looking at the size and contour of the restoration is it possible to make an educated guess based on what materials are generally used in such circumstances.

Further, it is not always possible to determine on which tooth surface the restoration is located. A filling looks the same whether it is on the facial (buccal) or lingual side of the tooth because radiographs are merely shadow pictures. Methods of localization are presented at the end of this chapter.

All metals used in dentistry, whether in the form of fillings, crowns, bridges, or orthodontic wires, are **radiopaque** (white). Gutta percha points used in root canals, the zinc phosphate cements used in bases and for

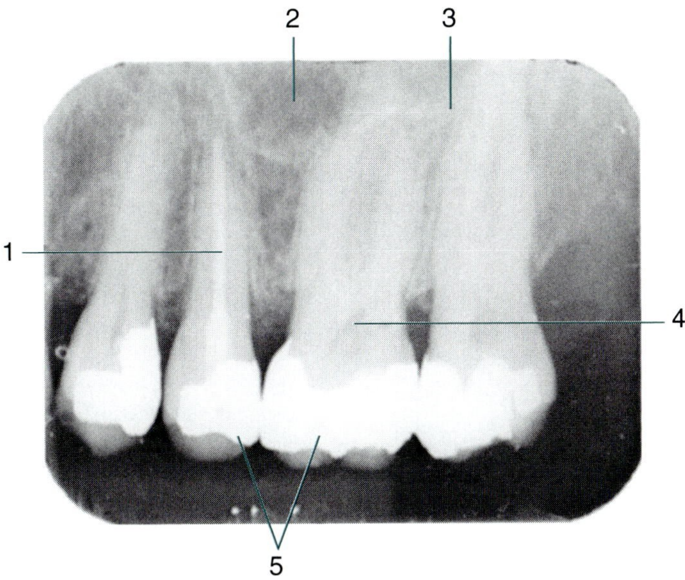

FIGURE 26–3. **Radiograph of maxillary premolar (bicuspid) region.** Shown in this radiograph are: (**1**) Gutta-percha root canal (radiopaque), (**2**) maxillary sinus, (**3**) dense bone lining the inferior border of the maxillary sinus, (**4**) small radiopaque pulp stone in the center of the pulp chamber, and (**5**) metallic restorations.

cementation, and the zinc oxide-eugenol pastes used as protective bases are also radiopaque. The composite filling materials and calcium hydroxide pastes used in pulp capping have opaque materials added to them to exhibit some degree of radiopacity.

Aesthetic Materials

Aesthetic materials, such as fused porcelain, silicate, acrylic resins (plastics), composites, and the sealants may be barely visible and exhibit only slight differences in radiolucency. Of these, fused porcelain is the most dense and least radiolucent, whereas the acrylic resins are least dense and most radiolucent.

The identification of composite resin restorations is difficult because some manufacturers add radiopaque particles to their product so that the viewer will not mistake it for dental caries. Thus, it should be obvious that a visual and digital examination is required to verify the conditions shown on a radiograph.

The fused porcelains used for crowns and as facings for bridgework appear radiolucent (dark). Silicates used for filling anterior teeth, acrylic resins used for fillings and crowns, composite fillings, and most calcium hydroxide pastes exhibit some degree of radiolucency. Several of these materials are identified on the radiographs in Figures 26–1 through 26–3.

Radiographic Appearance of Apical Disease

Radiolucencies surrounding the **apices** of the teeth indicate pathological changes in the hard (bony) tissues. Their radiographic appearance may be misleading unless carefully correlated with other diagostic information.

Periapical Lesions

The three common periapical lesions are **abscesses, granulomas,** and **cysts.**

Periapical Abscesses

Periapical infections usually result from pulpal inflammation. Bacteria from caries infect the pulp and gain access to the periapical bone by way of the root canals. As a rule, **acute abscesses** (early stages of pulpal or periapical infections) are barely discernible, becoming more radiolucent as they become chronic. In fact, in the very early acute stages there may be no radiographic evidence at all. The earliest sign may be a break in the **lamina dura.** Clinically such teeth are often tender to percussion.

Chronic abscesses may appear as circular dark areas around the apices and eventual turn into **granulomas.**

Periapical Granulomas

Granulomas are masses of granulation tissues usually surrounded by a fibrous sac continuous with the periodontal ligament and attached to the root apices. Under certain conditions epithelial elements may proliferate to form a **radicular cyst** (also known as apical cyst, periapical cyst, apical periodontal cyst, or root end cyst)—a cyst around the end of the root. Radiographically all the described lesions assume various configurations and it is not possible to accurately differentiate between a periapical abscess, a granuloma, or a cyst (see Figure 26–4).

Periapical Cysts

Cysts are epithelium-lined sacs filled with fluid or semisolid material. Because of osmotic imbalance, pressure is exerted in all directions; therefore, cysts tend to be spherical unless unequal resistance is encountered. Cysts follow the path of least resistance. Cysts tend to be slow-growing and push aside adjacent structures. Although usually unilocular (made up of one compartment), cysts may also be multilocular (made up of several compartments). Radiographically cysts may appear as fairly uniform radiolucent cavities within the bone and surrounded by a well-defined radiopaque border that resembles the lamina dura.

Cysts

There are many types of **cysts.** The most common are **odontogenic cysts** (of tooth origin); a few of the rarer ones are **nonodontogenic.** A cyst frequently observed on radiographs of young patients is the **dentigerous cyst** (see Figure 26–5). When found, this type of cyst occurs frequently with imbedded teeth—third molars and supernumerary teeth—and is always associated with the crown of a tooth. If the tooth causing the cyst continues to develop and is able to erupt, the cyst is often destroyed by natural means. Hence it is also known as a **follicular cyst** or **eruptive cyst** (see Figure 26–6).

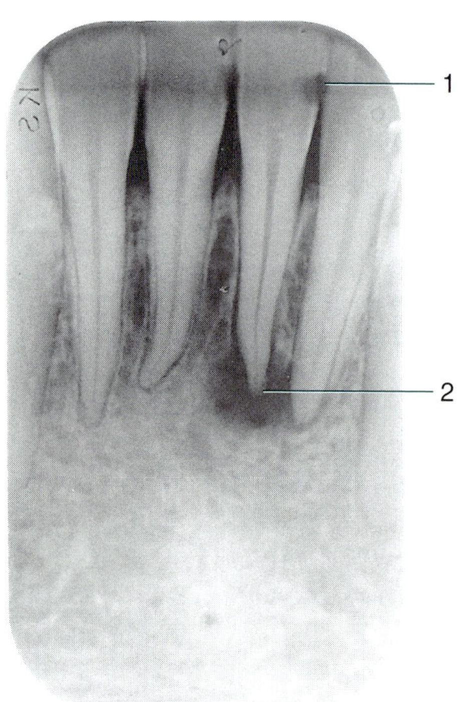

FIGURE 26–4. **Radiograph of mandibular incisor region.** This radiograph shows (**1**) caries on the distal surface of the left central incisor, and (**2**) a round radiolucent lesion that may be a periapical abscess, a granuloma, or a cyst.

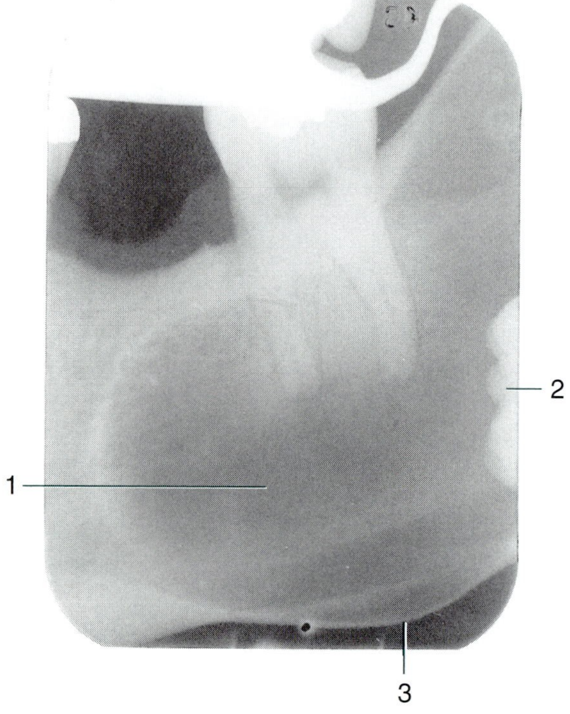

FIGURE 26–5. **Radiograph of mandibular molar region.** This film was placed in a vertical position instead of the usual horizontal position and shows (**1**) dentigerous cyst involving (**2**) imbedded third molar, and (**3**) expansion and thinning of the cortical bone.

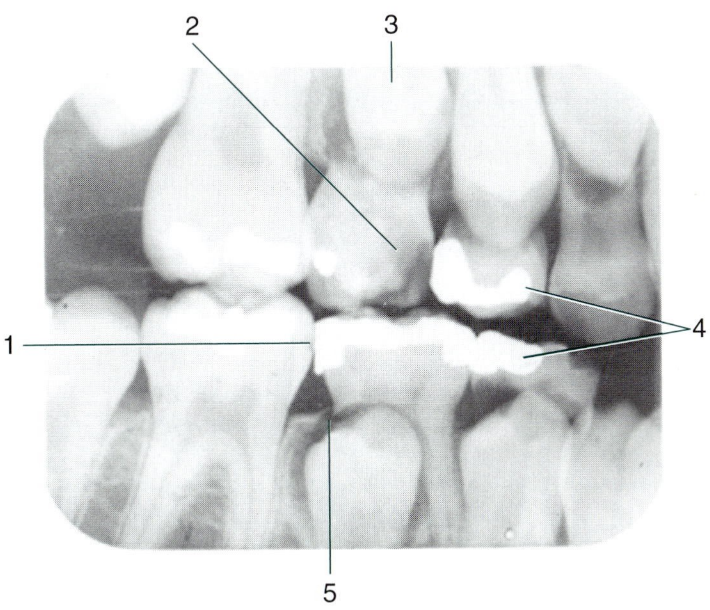

FIGURE 26-6. **Bitewing radiograph of mixed dentition.** This radiograph shows (**1**) incipient caries on permanent molar, (**2**) deep caries on deciduous second molar, (**3**) an erupting second maxillary premolar, (**4**) deciduous first molars about to be exfoliated, and (**5**) a follicular (eruptive) cyst around the crown of second mandibular premolar.

Unless radicular cysts are completely removed at the time of the extraction or surgery, they will remain and are then called **residual cysts.**

Nonodontogenic cysts arise from epithelium other than that associated with tooth formation. Two types are the **incisive canal** (nasopalatine) **cyst** (see Figure 26–7), located within the incisive canal, and the rare **globulomaxillary cyst** (see Figure 26–8), which arises between the maxillary lateral incisor and the canine (cuspid).

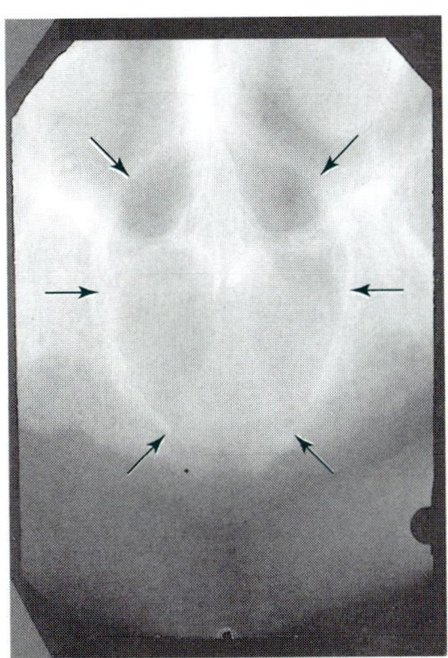

FIGURE 26-7. **Incisive canal cyst.** Arrows outline an incisive canal (nasopalatine) cyst in an edentulous maxilla.

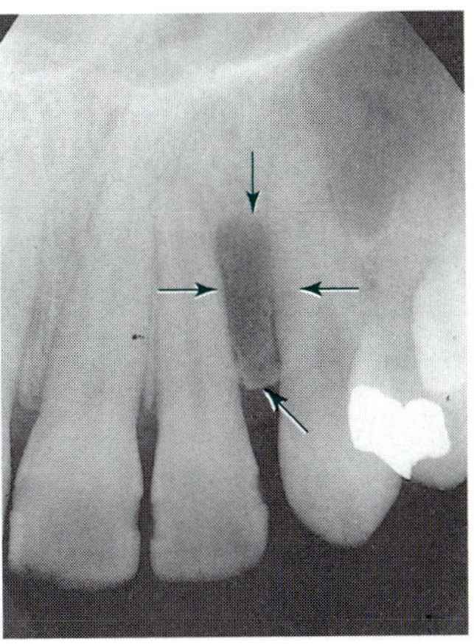

FIGURE 26-8. **Globulomaxillary cyst.** Arrows outline a globulomaxillary cyst that arises between the maxillary lateral incisor and the canine (cuspid).

Radiographic Appearance of Anomalies

An **anomaly** is defined as any deviation from normal. Dental anomalies are numerous. Such anomalies include:

- **Anodontia,** Absence of the teeth (may be complete or partial). Congenitally missing teeth often include the third molars, the premolars (bicuspids) (see Figure 26–9), and the maxillary lateral incisors.
- **Supernumerary teeth** (extra teeth), radiopacities that may or may not resemble normal tooth form (see Figure 26–10). Complications caused by supernumerary teeth include the possibility of cyst formation and the malposition, noneruption, or both of the normal teeth. Radiographic examination at an early age will reveal the presence of supernumerary teeth so that they may be removed.
- **Mesiodens,** so named because they are located in the maxillary mid-line, are small extra teeth that are almost always conical in shape (see Figure 26–10).

Additional anomalies include the following:

- **Malposed teeth** are teeth that are often unerupted and not in normal location.
- **Dens in dente** (dens invaginatus) is, literally, a tooth within a tooth, an invagination of the enamel within the body of the tooth. This anomaly occurs most frequently in the maxillary lateral incisor (see Figure 26–11).
- **Hypercementosis** usually appears radiopaque and is caused by excessive cementum formation. The excessive cementum on the roots often causes a bulbous enlargement along the root surface with the area near the apex appearing most bulbous (see Figure 26–12).
- **Ankylosis** is a radiopacity produced by the fusion or union of part or all of a tooth to the alveolus. It is caused by mineralization and hardening of the periodontal ligament fibers that normally surrounds the roots and separates them from the alveolus.
- **Dilaceration** is a tooth with a sharp bend in the root (see Figure 26–13). It usually develops as a result of trauma during root formation.

Other less frequently encountered **anomalies** include the following:

- **Dentinogenesis imperfecta** (hereditary opalescent dentin) is characterized by imperfectly formed dentin that has an opalescent or amber color. Radiographs reveal small underdeveloped roots and obliterated pulp chambers.
- **Amelogenesis imperfecta** is characterized by scant or totally missing enamel.

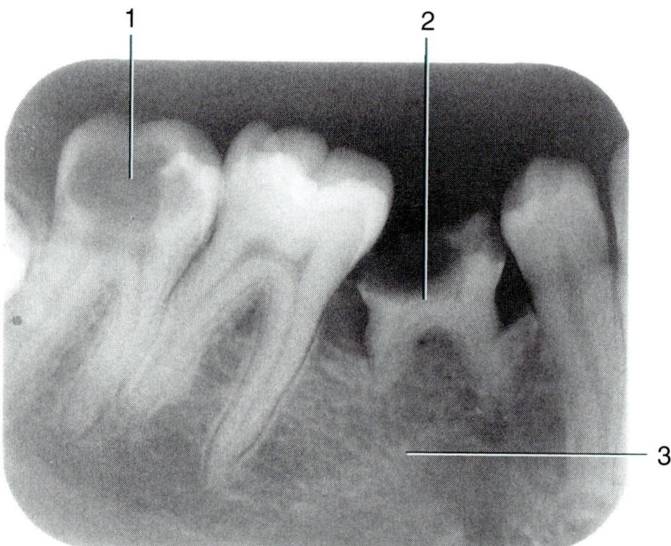

FIGURE 26–9. **Radiograph of mandibular premolar (bicuspid) region.** This radiograph shows (**1**) extensive caries in second molar, (**2**) second primary molar, and (**3**) congenitally missing second premolar (bicuspid).

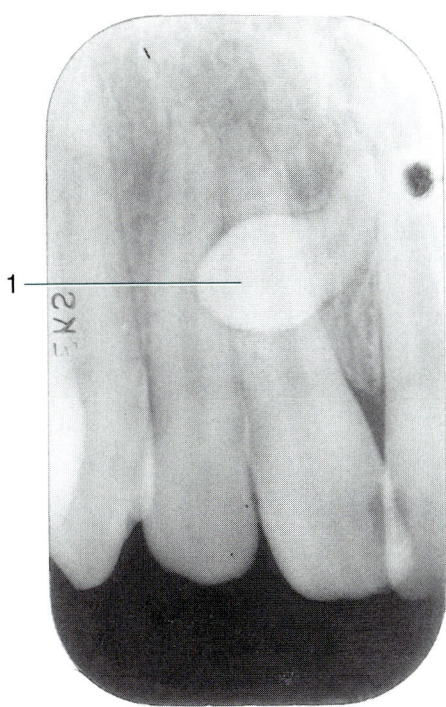

FIGURE 26–10. **Radiograph of maxillary incisor region.** (**1**) A mesioden, or small supernumerary tooth, located in the midline between the central incisors is seen.

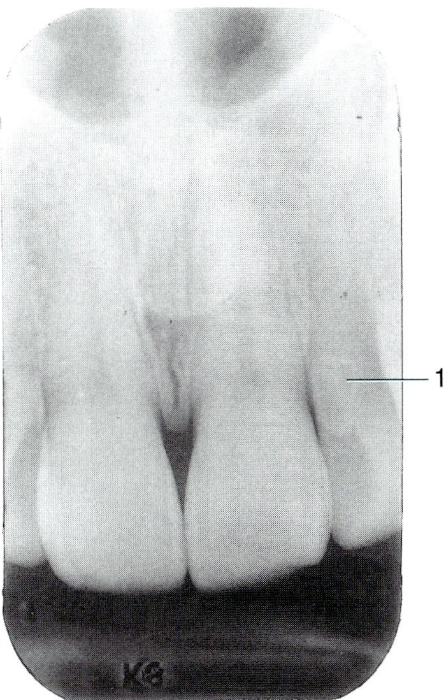

FIGURE 26–11. **Radiograph of maxillary incisor region.** This radiograph shows (**1**) dens in dente, an invagination of the enamel within the body of the lateral incisor.

- **Taurodontia** is characterized by very large pulp chambers and very short roots.
- **Macrodontia** is characterized by teeth that appear too large for the individual
- **Microdontia** is characterized by teeth that appear too small for the individual.
- **Gemination** (twinning) is a single tooth bud that divides and forms two teeth.
- **Fusion** is a condition where the dentin and one other dental tissue of adjacent teeth are united (see Figure 26–14).
- **Concrescence** is a condition where the cementum of adjacent teeth is united.

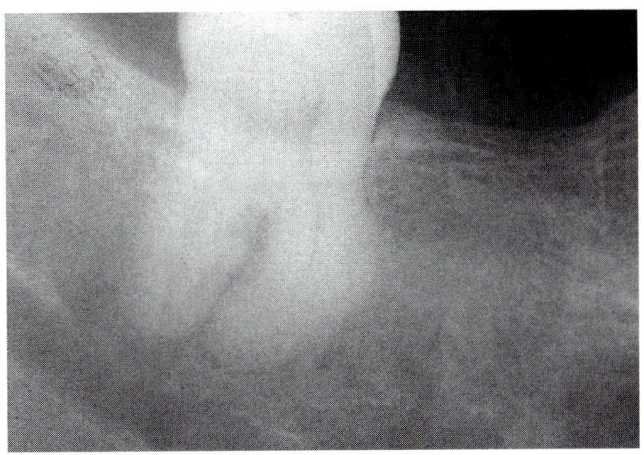

FIGURE 26–12. **Radiograph of mandibular molar region.** This radiograph shows (**1**) hypercementosis on the roots of the molar.

Radiographic Appearance of Bone or Tooth Resorption

Evidence of **resorption** is a common finding in dental radiographs. Resorption, such as the roots of deciduous teeth or the gradual diminution of the alveolar process in the elderly, can be considered normal. Most resorptive

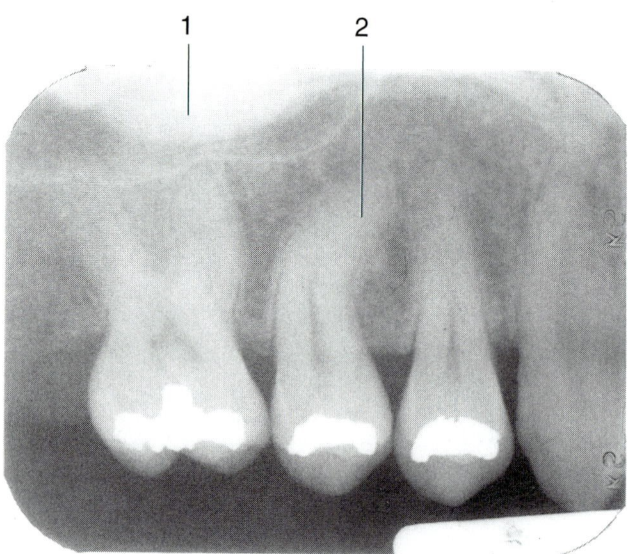

FIGURE 26–13. **Radiograph of maxillary premolar (bicuspid) region.** This radiograph shows (**1**) torus palatinus, a radiopaque overgrowth of bone on the midline of the palate, and (**2**) dilaceration, a sharp bend in the root of the tooth.

processes, however, are the result of infection, trauma, or some unusual condition. An example of such resorption is the gradual destruction of the vertical and horizontal bone loss that is typical of **periodontal disease** as seen in Figure 26–15.

Other examples include the resorption of the adjacent tooth by pressure from an impacted or erupting tooth, resorption caused by slowly growing tumors, or trauma that causes root-end resorption when teeth are moved too rapidly during orthodontic treatment (see Fig. 26–16).

Less common is **idiopathic resorption,** where the cause is unknown (see Fig. 26–17).

Radiographic Appearance of Calcifications and Ossifications

Calcifications, the deposition of calcium salts from the saliva into the tissues surrounding the teeth, and **ossifications,** the pathological or abnormal conversion of soft tissues into bone, appear radiopaque.

Calculus is the most frequently observed form of calcification. Calculus, although not classified as a lesion because its formation is a normal process for many persons, is a gradual deposition of calcium and other inorganic salts and organic matter around the gingival areas of the teeth. The accumulation and growth of these calculus deposits contributes to periodontal disturbances. Although there are several forms of supragingival and subgingival calculus, all forms appear radiopaque on the radiographs (see Figure 26–15).

Calcifications in the dental pulp occur in the form of small nodules called **pulp stones** (see Figure 26–3). They appear in the radiograph as radiopaque structures of varied size and may appear singly, but more often are multiple. Pulp stones are very common but of little significance because they never cause inflammation of the pulp. They do present a problem in root canal therapy if they are large and adhere to the pulpal wall.

Other less frequently encountered calcifications are **sialoliths,** depositions of calcium salts in the salivary glands and ducts (see Figure 26–18); **rhinoliths,** stones within the maxillary sinuses; and **phleboliths** or calcified thrombi, calcified masses that are observed as round or oval bodies in the soft tissues of the cheeks.

Two forms of **ossification** are often radiographically visible. **Condensing osteitis** occurs when **sclerotic** (hardened) bone is formed as a result of infection (see Figure 28–9). This condition may develop in periapical areas prior to complete pulp degeneration and appear as a widening of the periodontal ligament and surrounded by dense bone. **Osteosclerosis** occurs when regions of abnormally dense bone form that are not a direct result of

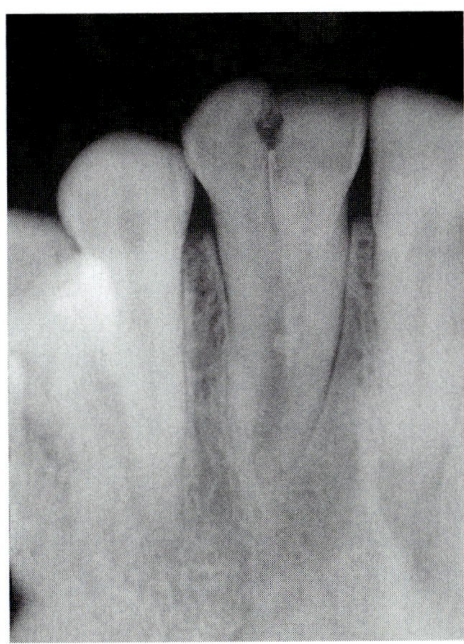

FIGURE 26-14. **Radiograph of mandibular incisor region.** This radiograph shows (**1**) fusion of two adjacent incisors.

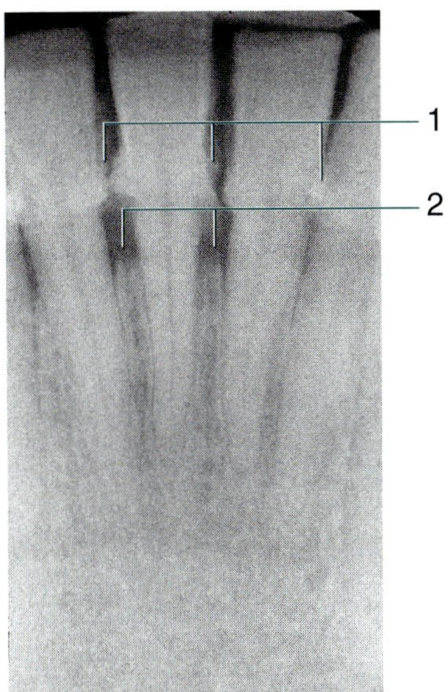

FIGURE 26-15. **Radiograph of mandibular incisor region.** This radiograph shows (**1**) large deposits of calculus around the necks of teeth and (**2**) radiolucent areas indicating bone loss that is typical of periodontal disease.

infection (see Figures 26–19 and 26–20). Although the cause is unknown, it commonly occurs in the interseptal premolar area and may be associated with fragments of retained deciduous roots. This condition tends to remain following extraction of the teeth.

Radiographic Appearance of Odontogenic Tumors

Odontogenic tumors result from abnormal proliferation of cells and tissues involved in odontogenesis (the formation of the teeth). The three types occasionally seen on radiographs are ameloblastomas, odontomas, and cementomas. **Ameloblastomas** have the greatest potential for serious implications for the patient. These appear as large radiolucencies of enamel origin. Radiographically, ameloblastomas may be monolocular (one compartment) or multilocular (many compartments). The monolocular form closely resembles a dentigerous cyst (see Figure 26–21). The multilocular form has a characteristic "soap bubble" appearance.

Odontomas are the most common ondontogenic tumors (see Figure 26–22). These are tumors of small misshaped teeth whose number in each odontoma varies widely. These toothlike structures appear radiopaque and are located within a radiolucent fibrous capsule that often resembles a cyst.

Cementomas, also called cementifying fibromas, are derived from the periodontal ligaments of fully developed and erupted teeth. Early cementomas are radiolucent and appear identical to radicular cysts. In the later stages of development cementomas appear as radiopaque masses surrounded by a radiolucent line (see Figure 26–23). Cementomas occur most frequently in the mandibular incisor region of women. The teeth are vital and the cementomas need no treatment.

Radiographic Appearance of Nonodontogenic Tumors

The tumors described here include a few pathologically insignificant ones as well as some that are life threatening. The majority of these lesions do not have a characteristic radiographic appearance that enables us to determine the diagnosis from the radiograph alone. In fact, a diagnosis of a malignant tumor cannot be made until the pathologist, the clinician, and the radiologist have com-

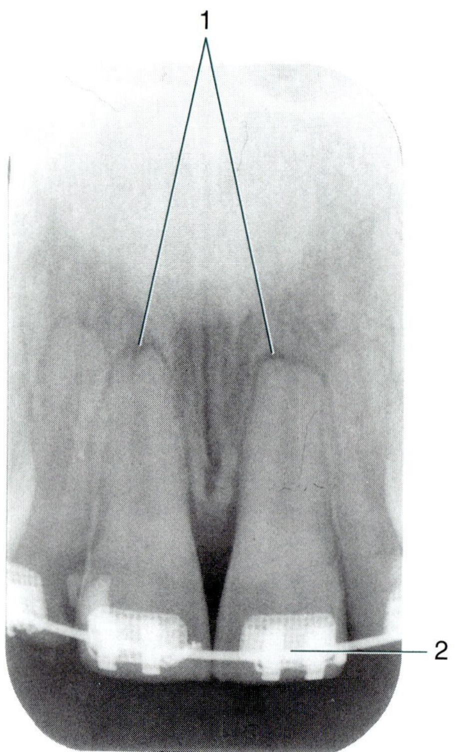

FIGURE 26–16. **Radiograph of maxillary incisor region**. This radiograph shows (**1**) root-end resorption, caused by trauma of orthodontic treatment, and (**2**) orthodontic appliance.

bined their findings. However, radiologists can detect the presence of lesions in bone and frequently can determine the nature of the lesion. As dental personnel we may on occasion be the first to detect malignancies and alert the patient.

Tumors are classed as **benign** (doing little or no harm) and **malignant** (very dangerous or life threatening). Fortunately most tumors that we see in the dental office are benign. Careful examination of the radiograph can often help to differentiate benign from malignant lesions.

Benign tumors may be either radiolucent or radiopaque. The cortex (outer layer) tends to remain intact, even though it may be thinned or expanded. The margins are usually well defined. Benign tumors do not metastasize (spreading of disease from one part of the body to another).

Malignant tumors tend to produce destruction of the cortex or elevation of the periosteum. They tend to have irregular margins and are less distinct, blending into the adjacent bone. Malignant tumors frequently metastasize.

Exostoses and tori are the most frequently encountered forms of benign tumors. An **exostosis** (plural exostoses) is a localized overgrowth of bone. The term **torus** (plural tori) is often used to describe an exostosis that occurs near the midline of the palate (**torus palatinus**) (see Figure 26–13) and on the lingual surface of the mandible (**torus mandibularis**) (see Figures 11–23 and 11–26). Ra-

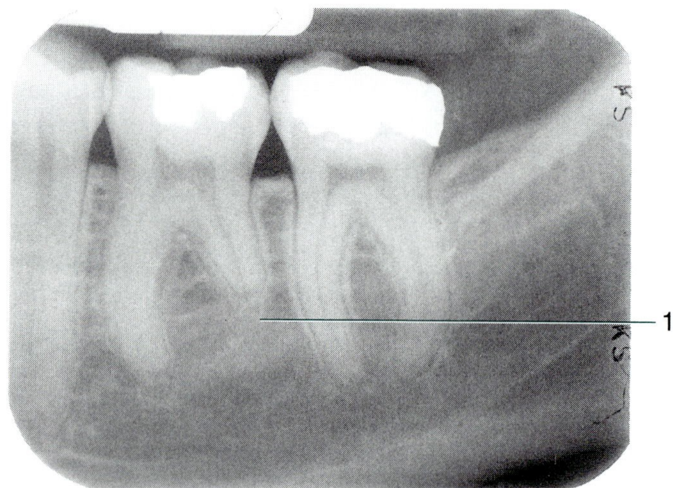

FIGURE 26–17. **Radiograph of mandibular molar region.** This radiograph shows (**1**) idiopathic resorption of the distal root of the first molar.

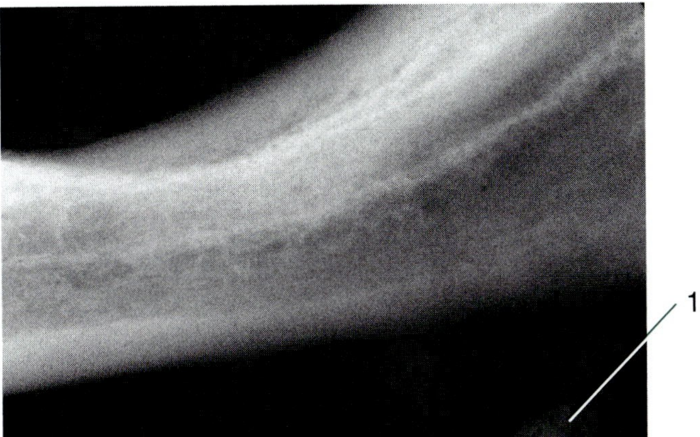

FIGURE 26-18. **Radiograph of edentulous mandibular posterior region.** This radiograph shows (**1**) sialolith in a salivary gland.

diographically both appear as an area of increased radiographic density (radiopaque).

Another common benign tumor is the **osteoma,** a noninflammatory type of bone tumor that varies greatly in size and shape and is radiopaque.

Still another variety of benign tumor is a **giant cell tumor** or **granuloma,** a radiolucent area of varying size that frequently can be observed anterior to the molars in children and young adults.

The two main types of oral malignancies are carcinomas and sarcomas. Both grow rapidly and spread into adjacent tissues. **Carcinomas** are malignant tumors of epithelial origin. These are of many types and may arise from any organ in which there is epithelial tissue. The

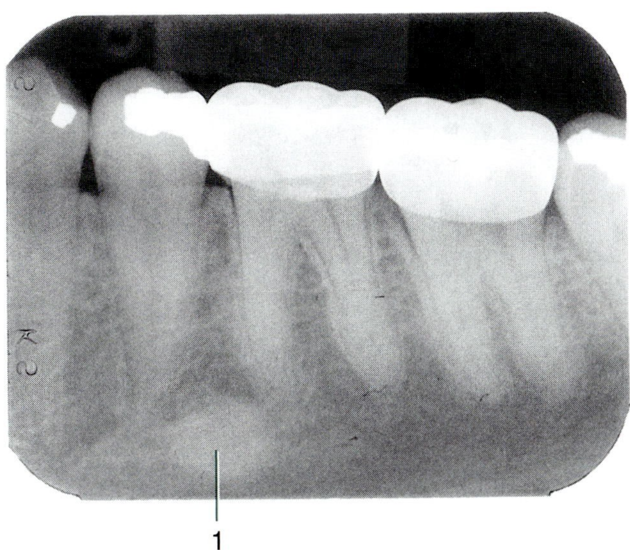

FIGURE 26-19. **Radiograph of mandibular posterior region.** Shown is the radiographic appearance of (**1**) radiopaque osteosclerosis, a hardening of the bone. The cause is unknown.

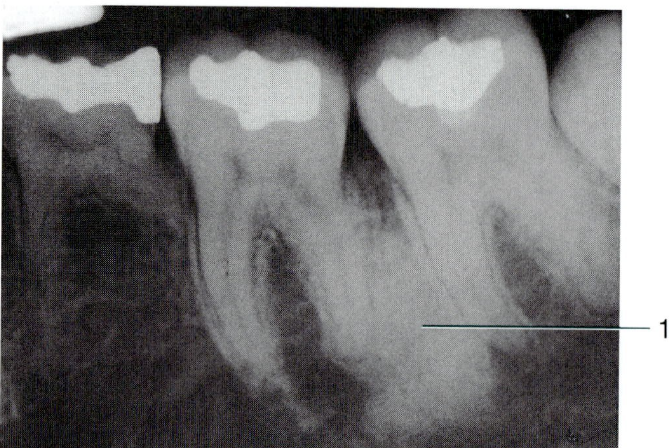

FIGURE 26–20. **Radiograph of mandibular molar region.** This radiograph shows (**1**) diffuse idiopathic osteosclerosis.

radiographic appearance is radiolucent with irregular and poorly defined borders.

Sarcomas are malignant tumors of connective tissue origin. Radiographically many of these appear as radiolucent, irregularly shaped and diffuse destructions of bone having a "patchy" appearance with no demarcation from normal surrounding bone. Some types may appear radiopaque because of excessive cartilage or bone formation in or on the bone. Such radiographs are vitally important in early detection because sarcomas produce changes in bone early in their development.

Radiographic Appearance of Injuries

The two most common injuries are fractures of facial bones and teeth. **Fracture lines** are thin radiolucent lines that demarcate the region of bone or tooth separation. Radiographic evidence of healing may later show as a radiopaque line in the fracture area (see Figure 26–24),

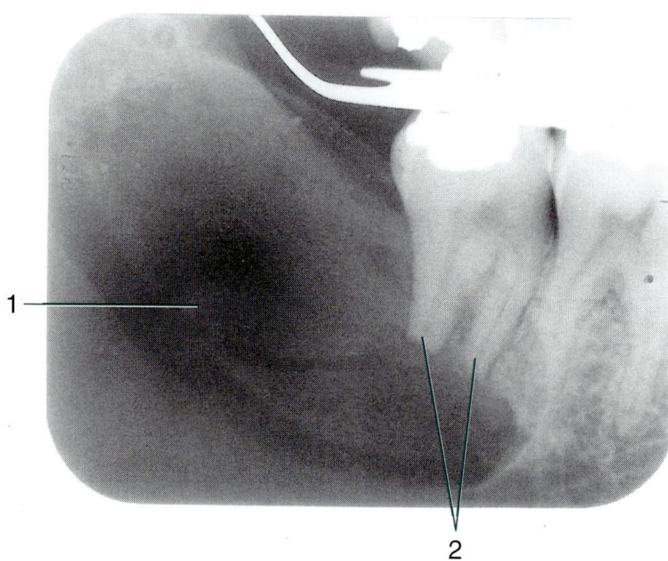

FIGURE 26–21. **Radiograph of mandibular molar region.** This radiograph shows (**1**) a large radiolucent ameloblastoma, and (**2**) resorption of the molar roots caused by pressure of the tumor.

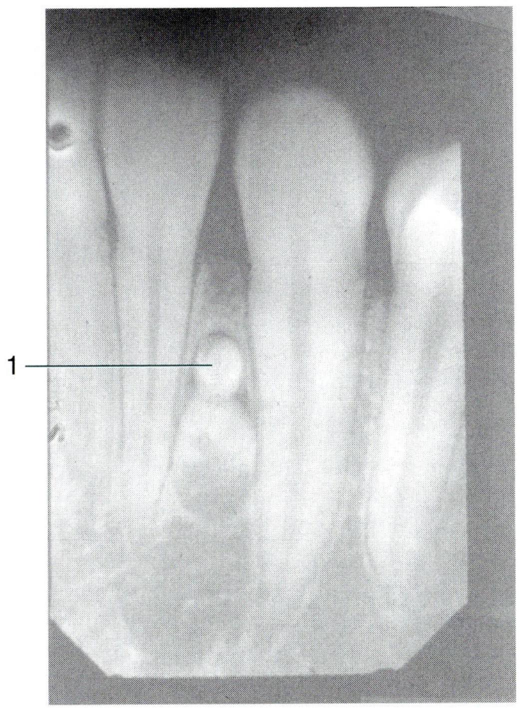

FIGURE 26–22. **Radiograph of mandibular canine (cuspid) region.** Radiograph shows (**1**) an odontoma consisting of small-misshaped teeth located within a radiolucent fibrous capsule.

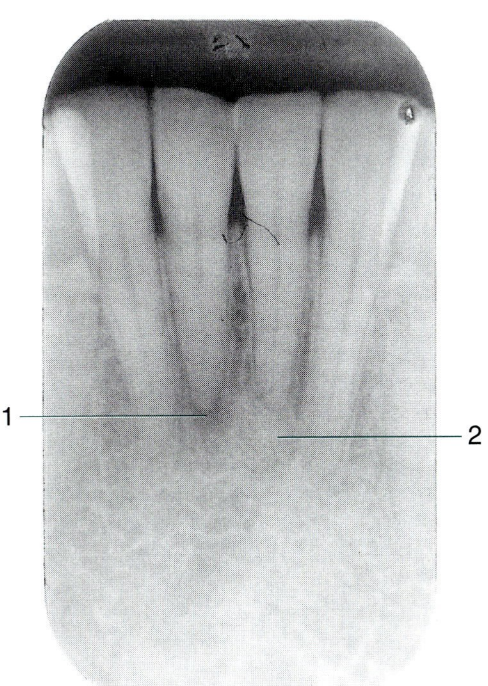

FIGURE 26–23. **Radiograph of mandibular incisor region**. This radiograph shows (**1**) early cementoma (radiolucent), and (**2**) cementoma in late stage of development (radiopaque). The teeth are vital.

however, such evidence of union may take a long time and is generally not visible radiographically until long after the healing has taken place. Fractures may on occasion have a similar appearance to the nutrient canals described in Chapter 11.

The radiographic examination sometimes reveals **foreign bodies** in the jaws and soft tissues. The most common foreign body seen in the jaw is amalgam (see Figure 26–25). Most particles of amalgam are found in the edentutous areas of the mandible. Often amalgam is fractured during extractions and fragments fall into the root socket or under the gingival tissue. Amalgam situated under the gingival tissue may impart a bluish-purple color to the tissue called an **amalgam tattoo.**

Other foreign bodies of the jaws include cements, gutta-percha, and dental instruments such as files, broaches, and burrs (see Figure 26–26). Foreign bodies of the soft tissues are apt to be hypodermic needles, pins, birdshot, glass, sand, and metal objects from automobile and other accidents.

Frequently encountered on radiographs are **retained roots,** which appear radiopaque (see Figure 26–27).

One other form of injury that is not often seen is **radio-osteosclerosis.** Generally limited to cancer patients, osteosclerosis is a devitalization of bone subjected to large doses of ionizing radiation.

A radiolucency that may involve large areas of bone is **osteomyelitis,** an inflamation of the bone marrow. Although not common, osteomyelitis may be either chronic or acute.

NOTE: What has been described in this chapter (and Chapters 27 and 28) is only a partial list of structures or lesions that may be visible on radiographs; any attempt to describe them fully belongs in a text devoted entirely to radiographic interpretation. Furthermore, anyone who attempts to make a preliminary interpretation must constantly be aware that many of the lesions described look very similar and that a biopsy report may be required before a final diagnosis can be made.

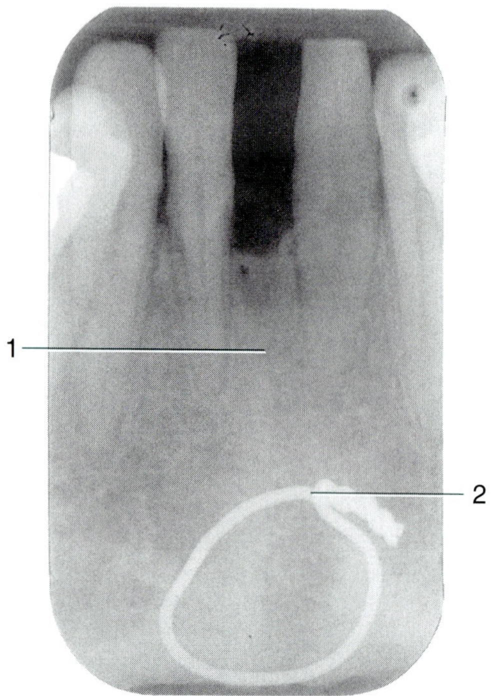

FIGURE 26–24. **Radiograph of mandibular incisor region.** This radiograph shows (**1**) an old fracture line (radiolucent), and (**2**) wire used to reduce the fracture.

Methods of Localization

When examining a radiograph it is generally not possible to determine whether a dental structure or a foreign object embedded within the maxilla or mandible is toward the front (facial or buccal) or behind (lingual) the teeth.

Several localization methods are currently in use. Each requires the exposure of an additional film; either the direction in which the **tube** points is **shifted** or the film is positioned at **right angle** to the position of the first film.

Tube Shift Method

The **oldest** of the localization methods, called the **tube shift method,** was first described by A. C. Clark (**Clark's rule**). Two periapical radiographs are positioned, one after the other, in the area of interest. Both exposures are made with the identical vertical angulation but the horizontal angulation is changed when the second exposure is made.

If the structure or object in question as seen on the second radiograph appears to have moved in the same direction as the horizontal shift of the tube, the structure or object is toward the lingual. Conversely, if the move is in the opposite direction as the shift of the tube, the structure or object must be toward the buccal or facial (see Figure 26–28).

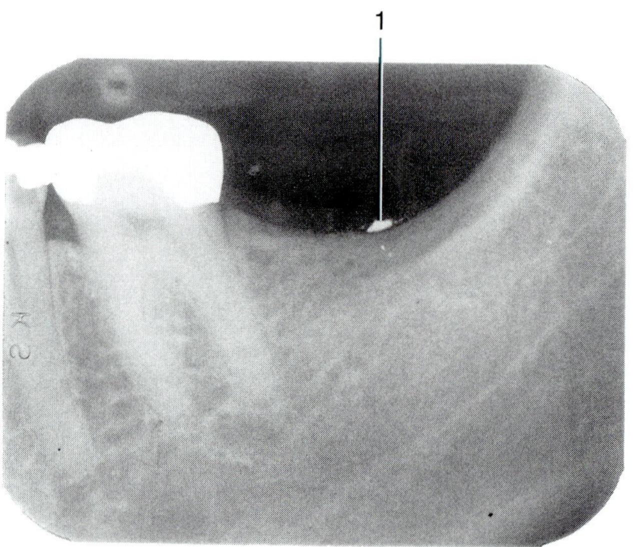

FIGURE 26–25. **Radiograph of mandibular molar region.** Fragments of amalgam (**1**), seen under the soft tissue, probably left after an extraction. Clinically, the gingiva appears bluish-purple and is called amalgam tattoo.

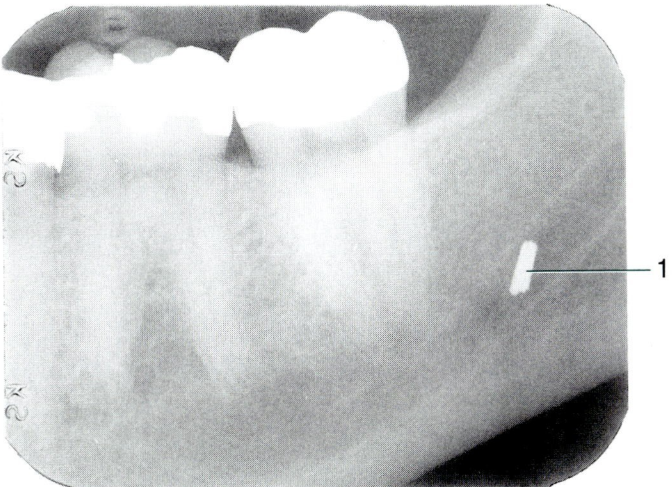

FIGURE 26-26. **Radiograph of mandibular molar region.** This radiograph shows (**1**) a broken burr, which probably occurred when the third molar was removed.

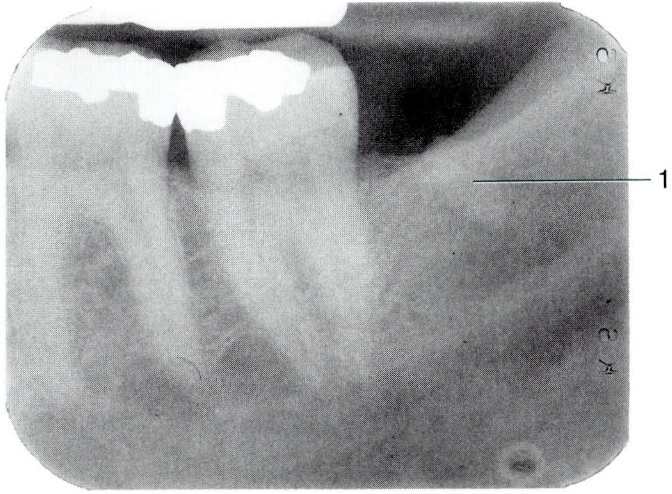

FIGURE 26-27. **Radiograph of mandibular molar region.** Retained root (**1**) is seen.

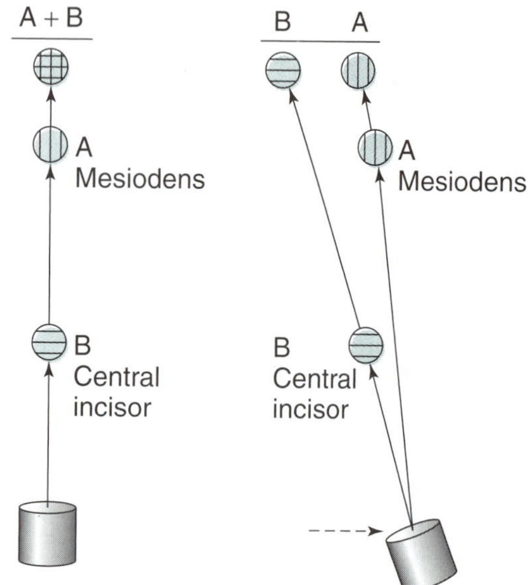

FIGURE 26–28. **In the tube shift localization technique (Clark's rule),** the most lingual object (mesiodens in this case) will move in the same direction as shift of tube. (Courtesy of Eastman Kodak Company and Department of Dental Diagnostic Science, School of Dentistry, University of Texas at San Antonio. Reproduced with permission from Langland OE, Langlais RP, Morris CR: Radiographic localization techniques. *Dent. Radiogr. Photogr. 52*(4): 69–77, 1979.)

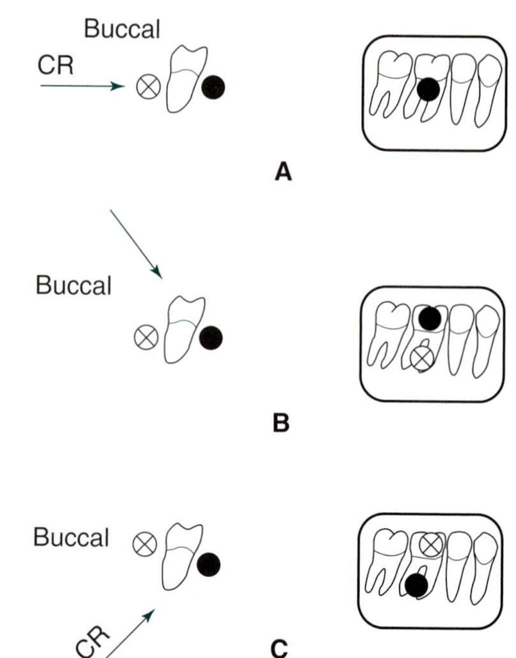

FIGURE 26–29. **Buccal and lingual foreign bodies with a vertical shift of the x-ray beam of 20 degrees.** (**A**) In the original radiograph, buccal and lingual objects are superimposed. (**B**) When the beam is directed inferiorly (positive vertical angulation is explained in Figure 13–13), the buccal object appears to move down while the lingual object appears to move up. (**C**) When the beam is directed superiorly (negative vertical angulation is explained in Figure 13–13), the buccal object appears to move up while the lingual object appears to have moved down. (Courtesy of Eastman Kodak Company and Department of Dental Diagnostic Science, School of Dentistry, University of Texas at San Antonio. Reproduced with permission from Langland OE, Langlais RP, Morris CR. Radiographic localization techniques. *Dent. Radiogr. Photogr.* 52(4): 69–77, 1979)

Two Radiographs at Right Angles to Each Other

The second **method of localization**, first suggested by Bosworth and later refined by Miller, shifts the position of the second film. Two periapical films are used; the first is a conventional radiograph of the area that shows the superior-inferior relation of the object in question to the teeth and the alveolar crest; the second radiograph positioned occlusally at a right (or 90-degree) angle to the first film, shows the buccal- (or facial-) to-lingual relationship. The occlusal technique is described in Chapter 16.

Buccal-Object Rule

A third method was suggested by A. G. Richards to determine the location of the mandibular canal. This technique has been expanded by R. P. Langlais and O. E. Langland and is now known as the **buccal-object rule** (see Figures 26–29 and 26–30).

According to this rule, any buccal object will move when the angulation of the position indicating device (PID), is changed: up or down, right or left. As in the other methods described, two films are used. A 20-degree change of angulation in the desired direction is made when the second film is exposed.

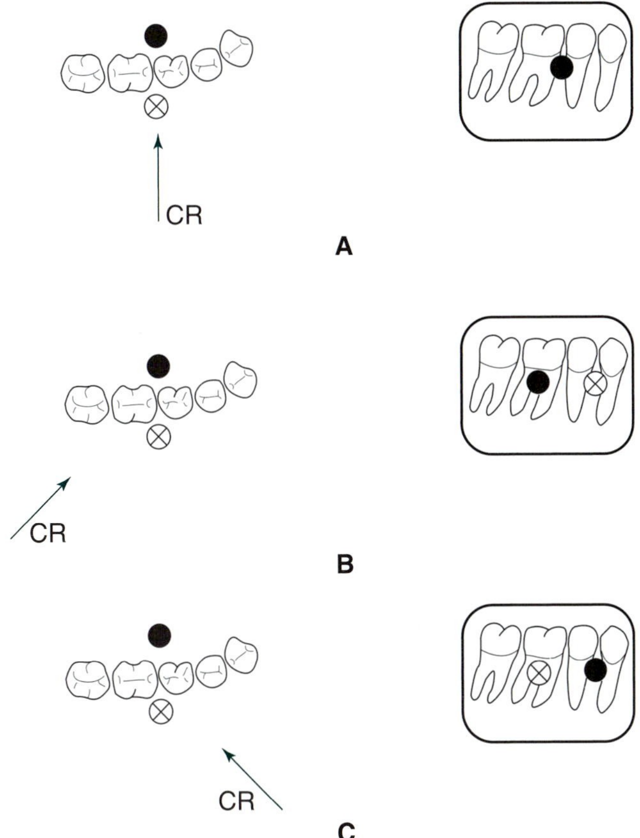

FIGURE 26-30. **Buccal and lingual foreign bodies with a horizontal shift of the x-ray beam of 20 degrees.** (**A**) In the original radiograph, buccal and lingual objects are superimposed. (**B**) When the beam is directed mesially, the buccal object appears to move mesially while the lingual object appears to move distally. (**C**) When the beam is directed distally, the buccal object appears to move distally while the lingual object appears to move mesially. (Courtesy of Eastman Kodak Company and Department of Dental Diagnostic Science, School of Dentistry, University of Texas at San Antonio. Reproduced with permission from Langland OE, Langlais RP, Morris CR: Radiographic localization techniques. *Dent. Radiogr. Photogr.* 52(4): 69–77, 1979)

CHAPTER SUMMARY

The ability to read the radiograph is called interpretation. Some dental radiographers, by virtue of their training, are able to save the dentist time by preparing an interpretation. The final diagnosis, however, is based not only on the radiographs but also on a visual and digital inspection of the teeth, evaluation of clinical tests, and the patient's medicodental history. This task is reserved for dentists and is their sole responsibility.

A skilled dental assistant or hygienist should have little difficulty in differentiating between normal tooth structure, dental caries, and calculus deposits. Other pathological conditions may be more difficult to identify. The dental radiographer should also be able to recognize the radiographic appearance of gold, silver, gutta-percha, dental cement, silicate, acrylic resin, and porcelain. Some restorative materials are easy to identify; others can only be tentatively identified on a radiograph. For example, all metals have a similar radiopaque appearance, whereas silicates and acrylic resins have similar radiolucent appearance. Often a visual inspection is required to distinguish one from the other.

When viewing radiographs it is generally not possible to see whether a dental structure or foreign object is to the facial or to the lingual of the teeth. Two general methods of localization are in use, the tube shift technique and exposure of a second film positioned at a right angle to the first film. With the tube-shift technique, the object in question is to the lingual if it moves in the same direction as the horizontal shift of the tube. With the techniques in which two radiographs are at right angles to each other, one readily observes the location of the object in question.

REVIEW QUESTIONS

1. The competent dental radiographer must be familiar with the more common abnormal or disease conditions in order to make an interpretation of the radiograph.
2. The responsibility to make the final diagnosis remains with the dentist.
3. Which of these materials appears most radiolucent?
   (a) Amalgam
   (b) Dental porcelain
   (c) Silicate
   (d) Acrylic resin
4. Which of these appears radiopaque?
   (a) Lamina dura
   (b) Oral mucosa
   (c) Pulp chamber
   (d) Residual cyst
5. Which of these appears radiolucent?
   (a) Impacted tooth
   (b) Chronic abscess
   (c) Calculus
   (d) Odontoma
6. Radiographically, it is not possible to accurately differentiate between a periapical abscess, a granuloma, or a cyst.
   (a) True
   (b) False
7. All resorptive processes appear:
   (a) In the mandible.
   (b) In the crown of the tooth.
   (c) Radiolucent.
   (d) Radiopaque.

8. Malignant tumors have:
   (a) Well-defined margins and do not metastasize.
   (b) Well-defined margins and metastasize.
   (c) Irregular margins that blend into adjacent bone and do not metastasize.
   (d) Irregular margins that blend into adjacent bone and metastasize.

9. According to Clark's rule for localization:
   (a) The object closest to the film appears to move in the same direction as the shift of the tube.
   (b) The object closest to the film appears to move in the opposite direction as the shift of the tube.
   (c) The object closest to the film does not appear to move in any direction.

10. Hypercementosis causes a:
    (a) Bulbous tooth crown.
    (b) Union between the lamina dura and the tooth root.
    (c) Bulbous tooth root apex.
    (d) Sharp bend in the root.

11. Dens in dente means:
    (a) A tiny tooth.
    (b) A large tooth.
    (c) Twin teeth.
    (d) A tooth within a tooth.

12. A tooth with a sharp bend in the root is called:
    (a) Taurodontia.
    (b) Hypercementosis.
    (c) Dilaceration.
    (d) Concresence.

13. Which of the following appears radiopaque on the radiograph?
    (a) Pulp chamber
    (b) Periapical granuloma
    (c) Periapical abcess
    (d) Gutta-percha point

14. Which of the following appears radiolucent on the radiograph?
    (a) Periapical cyst
    (b) Mesiodens
    (c) Sialolith
    (d) Pulp stone

BIBLIOGRAPHY

Farman A. G., Nortje C. J., & Wood R.E. *Oral and Maxillofacial Diagnostic Imaging*. St. Louis: Mosby, 1993.

Farman A. G., Ruprecht A., Gibbs S. J., & Scarfe W. C. (Eds.). *IADMFR/CMI'97 Advances in Maxillofacial Imaging*. Amsterdam: Elsevier, 1997.

Langlais R. P. & Kasle M. J. *Exercises in Oral Radiographic Interpretation*. 3rd ed. Philadelphia: Saunders, 1992.

Langlais R. P., Langland O. E., & Nortje C. J. *Diagnostic Imaging of the Jaw*. Philadelphia: Williams & Wilkins, 1995.

White S. C. & Pharoah M. J. *Oral Radiology Principles and Interpretation*. 4th ed. St. Louis: Mosby, 2000.

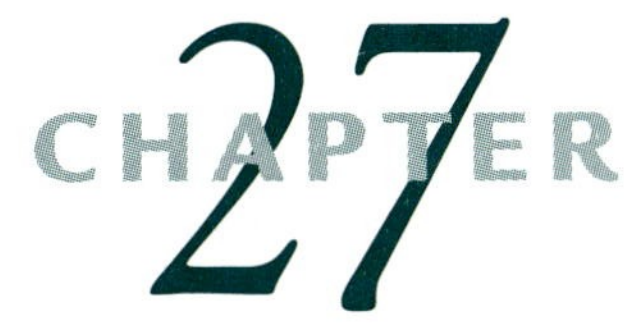

CHAPTER 27

Periodontal Disease

OBJECTIVES

By the end of this chapter the student should be able to:

- Define the key words.
- Describe the radiographic appearance of the healthy periodontium.
- Describe the radiographic appearance of periodontal disease.
- List the four ADA Case Types and describe their radiographic appearance.
- Discuss the clinical examination for periodontal disease.
- Discuss the radiographic examination for periodontal disease.
- Describe the type of radiographs used to interpret periodontal disease and the preferred technique.
- List and describe the limitations of the radiograph in the detection of periodontal disease.

KEY WORDS

Calculus
Furcation
Generalized bone loss
Gingivitis
Horizontal bone loss
Lamina dura
Localized bone loss
Periodontal
Periodontal disease
Periodontal ligament space
Periodontitis
Periodontium
Triangulation
Vertical bone loss
Vertical bitewing radiograph

Introduction

Both clinical and radiographic examinations are needed to diagnosis periodontal disease. While the dental radiographs are an adjunct to the clinical examination they are not a substitute for a good thorough clinical examination. The radiographs allow the dentist to detect changes in bone, identify factors in the dentition which may predispose the patient for periodontal disease, determine the approximate amount and location of bone loss and help the dentist determine a prognosis for treatment of the dentition (see Table 27–1).

The purpose of this chapter is to introduce the dental radiographer to periodontal disease and to its radiographic appearance. Also, radiographic examinations and techniques are presented, along with ADA case types and predisposing factors.

Radiographic Appearance of the Healthy Periodontium

The word **periodontal** (*peri* means "around"; *dontal* means "tooth") literally means "around a tooth." The word periodontium refers to the soft (gingiva) and hard (alveolar bone) tissues that invest and support the teeth. The radiographic appearance of healthy periodontium is described as follows:

Lamina dura: Healthy lamina dura appears as a dense radiopaque line around the roots of the teeth.

Alveolar crest: Normally, the alveolar crest is located 1.0 to 1.5 mm apical to the cementoenamel junctions (CEJ) of the teeth (see Figure 27–1). In the anterior regions of the mouth, the alveolar crest appears pointed and sharp and is very radiopaque (see Figure

TABLE 27-1. Value of Radiographs in Periodontal Assessment

- Amount of bone present.
- Condition of alveolar bone.
- Bone loss in furcation areas.
- Width of the periodontal ligament space.
- Local factors that cause periodontal disease, such as calculus, overhangs, and poorly contoured restorations.

27–2). In the posterior regions of the mouth the alveolar crest is more flat, smooth, and parallel to a line between adjacent cementoenamel junctions (see Figure 27–3). The alveolar crest is usually less radiopaque in the posterior regions than that in the anterior regions of the mouth.

Peridontal ligament space: The healthy peridontal ligament space appears as a thin radiolucent line between the lamina dura and the root of the tooth.

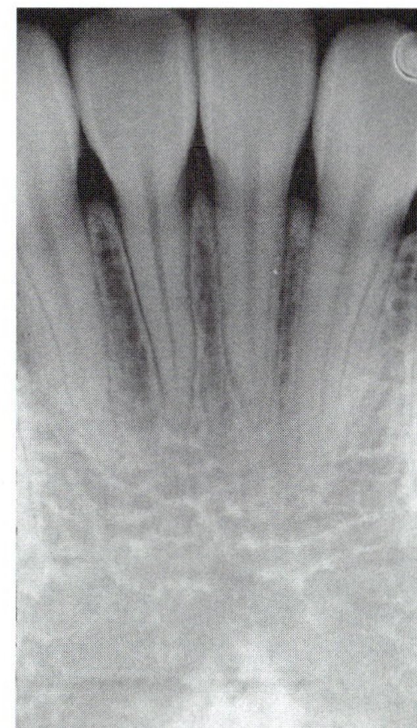

FIGURE 27-2. **Radiograph showing healthy anterior alveolar crest.** Note the normal lamina dura and periodontal ligament space.

Radiographic Appearance of Periodontal Disease

Periodontal disease refers to disease that affects both soft tissues (gingiva) and bone around the teeth. The severity of periodontal disease may range from a simple inflammation of the gingiva to the destruction of supporting bone and the periodontal ligament. The most common periodontal diseases are **gingivitis** and **periodontitis. Gingivitis** is inflammation of the gingiva and limited to the soft tissue (gingiva). **Periodontitis** is also the result of infection, but includes loss of alveolar bone.

The proper diagnosis and evaluation of periodontal disease must be made with a combination of **radiographic** and **clinical examinations.**

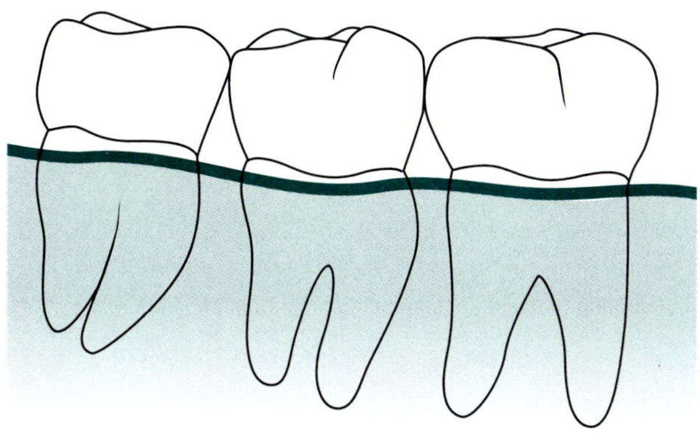

FIGURE 27-1. **Drawing showing normal bone level.** The alveolar crest located 1.5 to 2.0 mm apical to the cementoenamel junctions (CEJ) of the teeth.

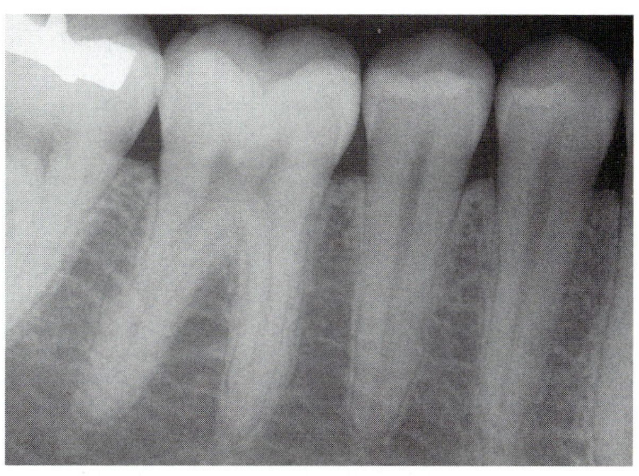

FIGURE 27-3. **Radiograph showing healthy posterior alveolar crest.**

ADA Classification of Periodontal Disease

The American Dental Association (ADA) classifies periodontal disease as follows:

ADA Case Type I (gingivitis): Gingivitis with no bone loss. Therefore, no radiographic change in bone.

ADA Case Type II (early periodontitis): Mild bone loss up to 30%. Radiographs show mild crestal bone loss (see Figure 27–4).

ADA Case Type III (moderate periodontitis): Moderate bone loss (30–50%) may be horizontal or vertical, localized or generalized, and furcation involvement (bone loss between the roots of multirooted teeth). Radiographs show moderate bone loss that may involve the area between the roots of multirooted teeth (see Figure 27–5).

ADA Case Type IV (advanced periodontitis): Advanced bone loss (50% or more). Radiographs show severe bone loss (see Figure 27–6).

Clinical Examination

The **clinical examination** is performed by the dentist and dental hygienist. The soft tissues should be evaluated for signs of inflammation. Normal gingiva appears pink in color, stippled, and firm. Inflamed gingiva appears red, swollen, bleeding and possible pus. A thorough clinical evaluation includes periodontal probing. Whenever periodontal disease is present, radiographs must be made to complete the examination.

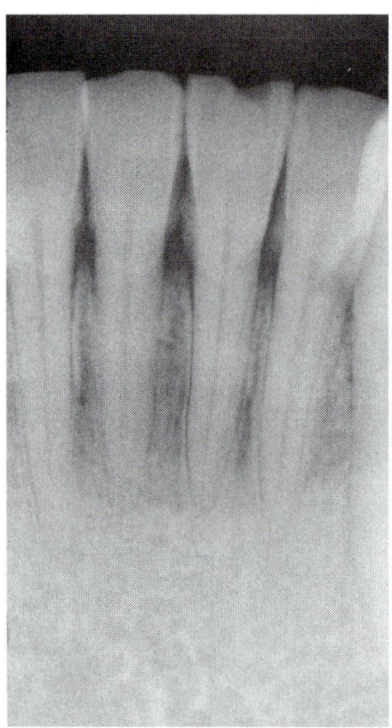

FIGURE 27–4. **Radiograph showing early (mild) bone loss and calculus around the necks of the teeth.**

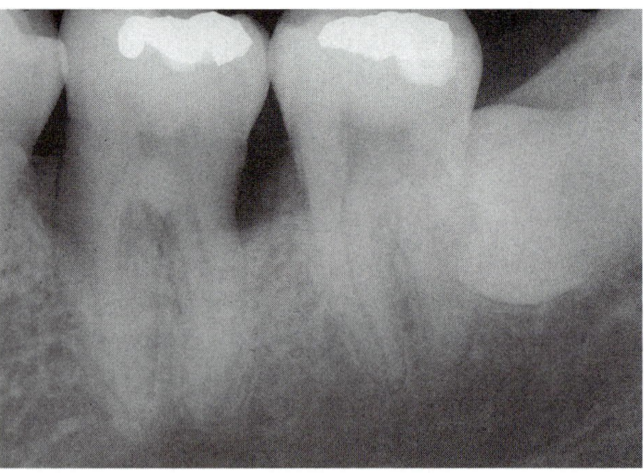

FIGURE 27–5. **Radiograph showing moderate bone loss.**

Radiographic Examination

Radiographs, along with a thorough clinical examination, allow the dental professional to evaluate and document periodontal disease. Bitewing and periapical radiographs, using the paralleling technique, are the films of choice for evaluating periodontal disease. The bisecting technique should not be used because of the vertical angulation used, which may appear to show more or less bone loss than is actually present.

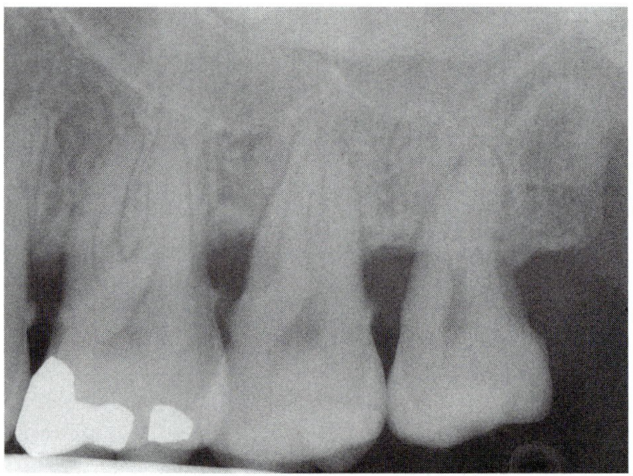

FIGURE 27–6. **Radiograph showing advanced (severe) bone loss.**

Radiographs play an important role in the assessment of periodontal disease. Radiographs help serve to:

1. Detect early to moderate bony changes.
2. Approximate the amount of bone loss.
3. Identify predisposing factors such as overhanging restorations or calculus.
4. Evaluate the prognosis and restorative needs.
5. Serve as a baseline for evaluating the results of treatment.
6. Provide a permanent record of the condition of the bone throughout the course of the disease.

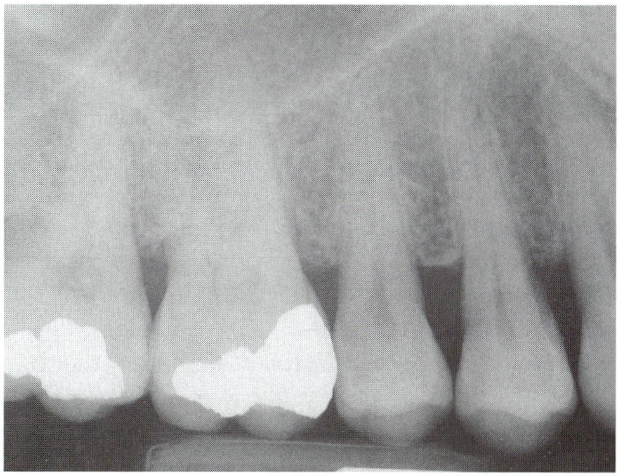

FIGURE 27–8. **Periapical radiograph showing moderate bone loss.**

Radiographic Techniques

Both **bitewing and periapical radiographs** are useful for examining the periodontium (see Figures 27–7 and 27–8). The **paralleling technique** is the best method for evaluating periodontal disease. The film is placed parallel to the long axis of the teeth to ensure that the images of the bone and teeth on the radiograph are not distorted. A high kilovoltage technique is also preferred because it gives long-scale contrast, which allows for better interpretation of the bony structures.

Recently, as we discussed in Chapter 15, some periodontists have recommended the use of **vertical bitewing radiographs** for patients with periodontal disease (see Figure 27–9). This technique uses seven #2 films as vertical bitewing radiographs in the molar, premolar (bicuspid), canine (cuspid), and midline regions. The radiographs are exposed in a standardized and reproducible manor to facilitate comparison of radiographs exposed at different times.

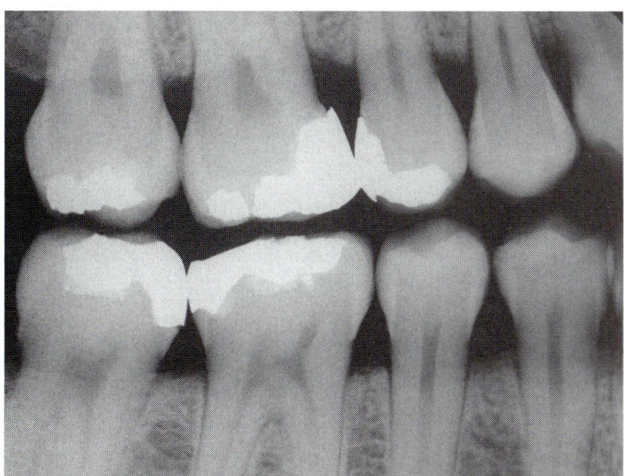

FIGURE 27–7. **Bitewing radiograph showing early bone loss.**

Radiographic Interpretation of Periodontal Disease

The dental radiographer should be familiar with the radiographic appearance of periodontal disease. Radiographs should be viewed and examined for bone loss and any predisposing factors that may contribute to periodontal disease.

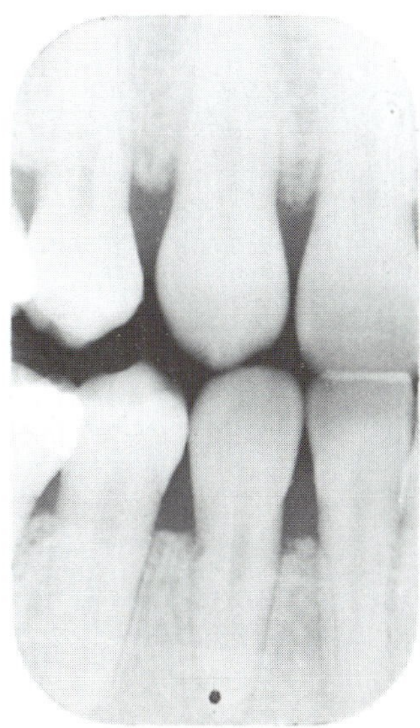

FIGURE 27–9. **Vertical bitewing radiograph showing early bone loss.**

Radiographs are useful diagnostic aids in evaluating **bone loss** in periodontal disease.

Bone Loss

In assessing periodontal disease, the amount of **bone loss** is recorded rather than the amount of bone that remains. However, the radiograph documents the amount bone remaining rather than the amount lost. The amount of bone loss is estimated as the difference between the physiologic bone level and the height of the remaining bone.

Bone loss may be described as either horizontal or vertical. Horizontal bone loss occurs in a plane parallel to the cementoenamel junctions (CEJ) of adjacent teeth. Vertical bone loss, sometimes called angular bone loss, occurs in a vertical plane.

Bone loss may also be described as localized or generalized. **Localized bone loss** occurs in local areas and involves only one or several teeth (see Figures 27–10 and 27–11). **Generalized bone loss** occurs throughout the entire dental arches (see Figure 27–12).

Bone loss as viewed on a dental radiograph can be classified as **early or mild, moderate**, and **advanced (severe)**.

Early or Mild Stage, ADA Case Type II

The **early stage** (ADA Case Type II) of periodontal change is characterized radiographically by changes in the crest of the interproximal bone and by triangulation of the periodontal membrane (see Figures 27–13 and 27–14).

Triangulation is the term given to at widening of the periodontal space at the crest of the interproximal bone. The sides of the triangle are formed by the lamina dura and the root surface while the base is toward the tooth crown.

The normal **crest of interproximal bone** appears radiopaque (white) and runs parallel to a line drawn between the cementoenamel junctions (CEJ) on adjoining teeth at a level 1.0 to 1.5 mm below the CEJ. Normal alveolar crestal bone appears as a radiopaque (white) line and continues around the root of a tooth as the lamina dura. In the early stages of periodontal disease, the radiopaque crest of the septa loses density and appears fuzzy.

Moderate Bone Loss (30–50%), ADA Case Type III

Moderate bone loss (ADA Case Type III) occurs in patients with periodontal disease that has progressed beyond the early stage (see Figures 27–15, 27–16, and 27–17). Moderate bone loss may appear in both the horizontal and vertical planes. Radiolucencies appear in the furcations (branching) of multirooted teeth indicating bone loss (see Figure 27–18).

Horizontal bone loss occurs in a plane parallel to the CEJ of adjoining teeth (see Figures 27–19 and 27–20). Horizontal bone loss describes height loss around adjacent teeth in a region. It may be localized to a quadrant or generalized around the whole mouth. In horizontal

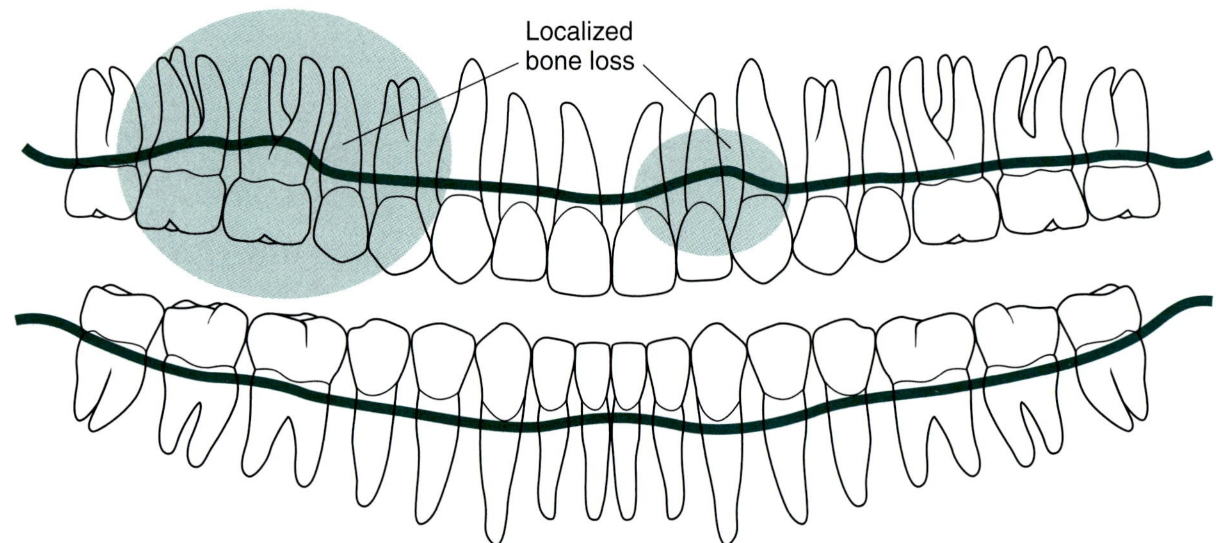

FIGURE 27–10. **Drawing showing localized bone loss.**

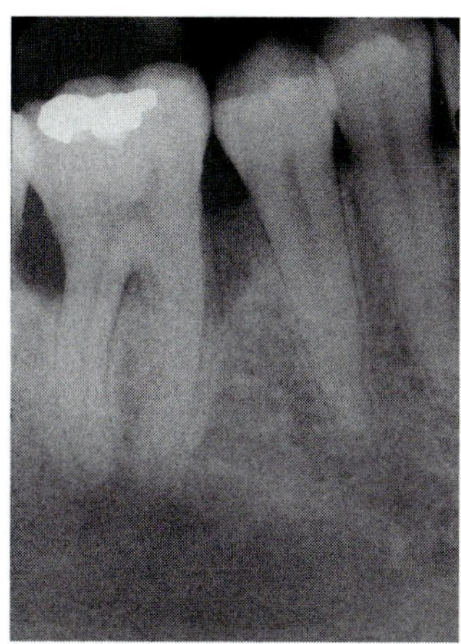

FIGURE 27–11. **Radiograph showing localized bone loss.**

bone loss, both buccal and lingual plates have been resorbed as well as the intervening interdental bone.

Vertical bone loss (angular bone loss or infra-bony pocket) occurs in a vertical direction where the resorption of one tooth root sharing the septum is greater than the other tooth (see Figures 27–21, 27–22, and 27–23).

Advanced (Severe) Bone Loss (50% or more), ADA Case Type IV

The **advanced stage** of periodontal disease (ADA Case Type IV) is characterized radiographically by severe vertical and horizontal bone loss, with furcation involvement, thickened periodontal membranes, and changes in tooth position (see Figures 27–24, 27–25, 27–26, 27–27, 27–28, and 27–29).

Predisposing Local Irritants

Predisposing local irritants such a calculus and defective restorations contribute to periodontal disease and may be detected by radiographs.

Calculus is a stone-like material that forms on the teeth due to calcification of bacterial plaque. Calculus appears as pointed or irregular radiopaque (white) projections on the proximal root surfaces or it may appear as a ring-like radiopacity around the cervical neck of a tooth (see Figure 27–23).

Defective restorations act as food traps and lead to the build-up of bacterial deposits. Radiographs reveal restorations with poor contours, open contacts, overhanging margins, and caries, all of which are local irritants and contribute to periodontal disease (see Figure 27–30).

Limitations of the Radiograph

There are limitations to the use of radiographs in the diagnosis of periodontal disease. Because the radiograph gives a two-dimensional image of three-dimensional structures, the radiograph lacks the third dimension of depth, which results in bone and tooth structures being superimposed over each other. The important limitations

(*text continues on p. 412*)

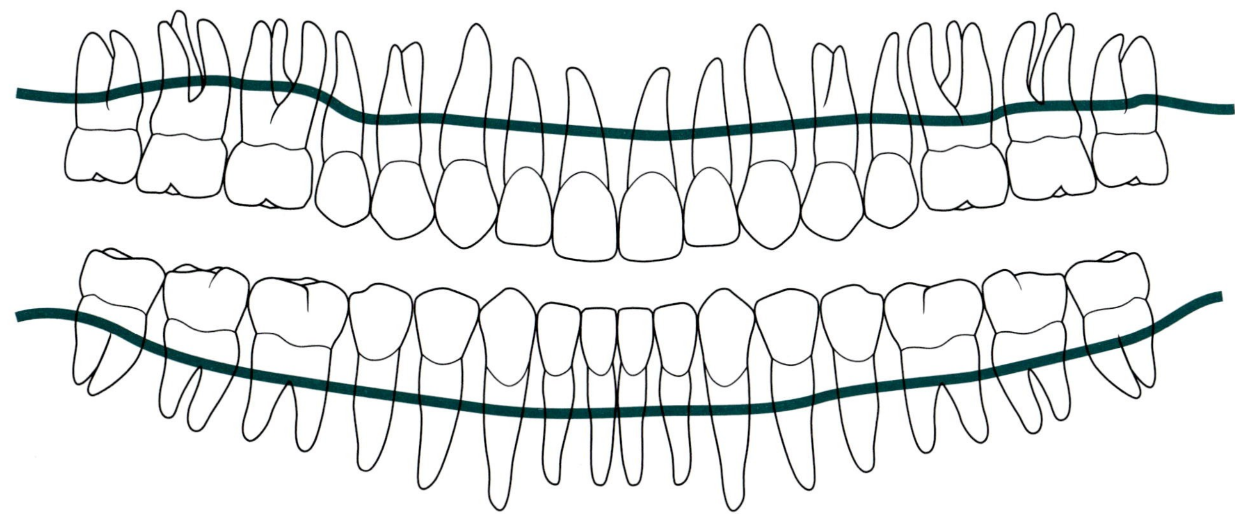

FIGURE 27–12. **Drawing showing generalized bone loss.**

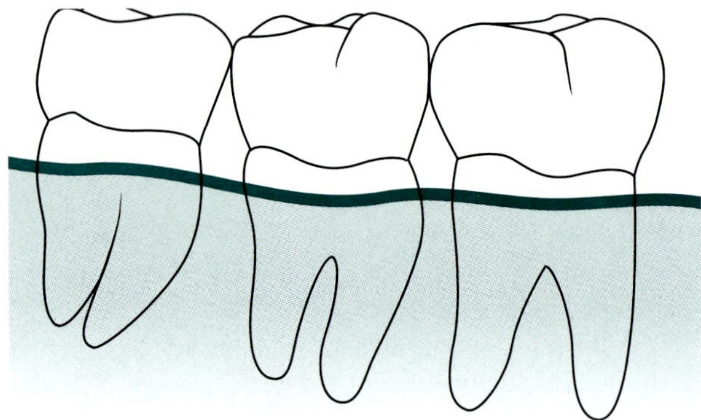

FIGURE 27-13. **Drawing showing early stage or mild bone loss.**

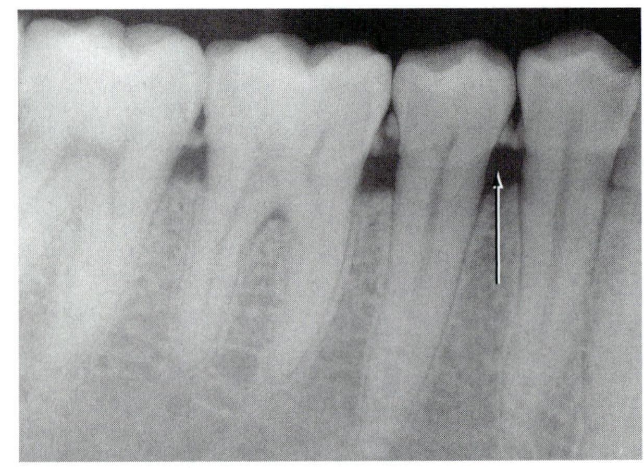

FIGURE 27-14. **Radiograph showing early stage or mild bone loss.** Note the early triangulation on the mesial root of the 2nd premolar (bicuspid).

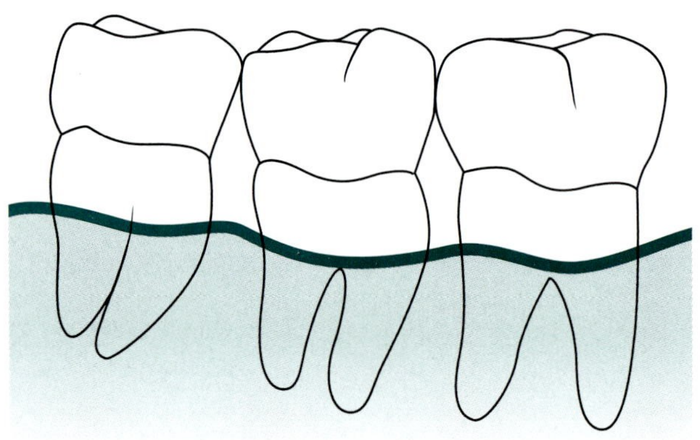

FIGURE 27-15. **Drawing showing moderate bone loss.**

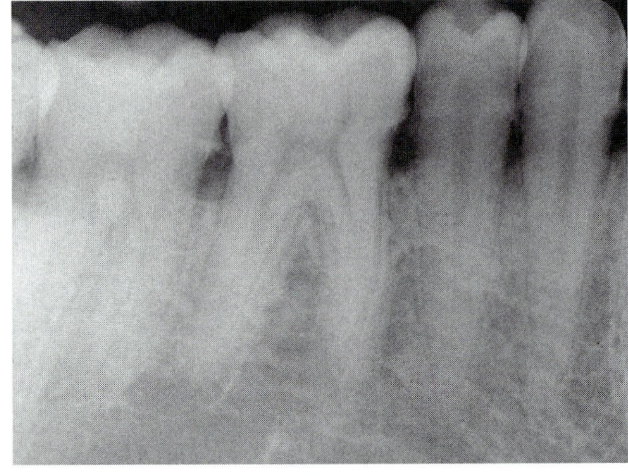

FIGURE 27-16. **Radiograph showing moderate bone loss and heavy calculus.**

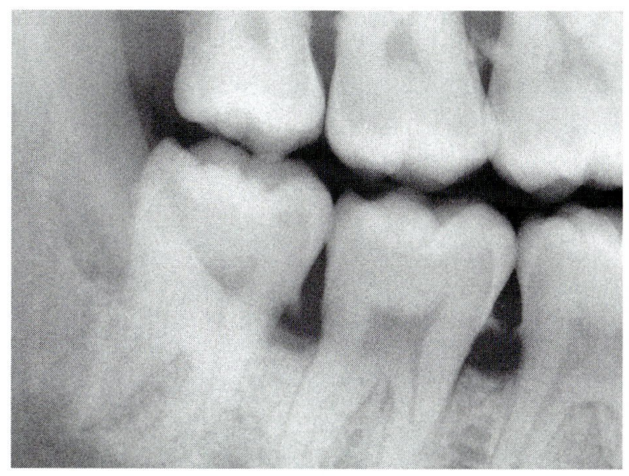

FIGURE 27–17. **Bitewing radiograph showing moderate bone loss and calculus.**

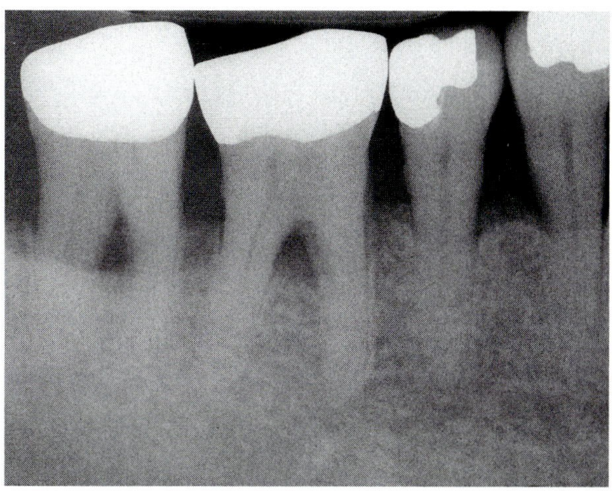

FIGURE 27–18. **Radiograph showing moderate bone loss and furcation involvement of the 1st and 2nd molars.**

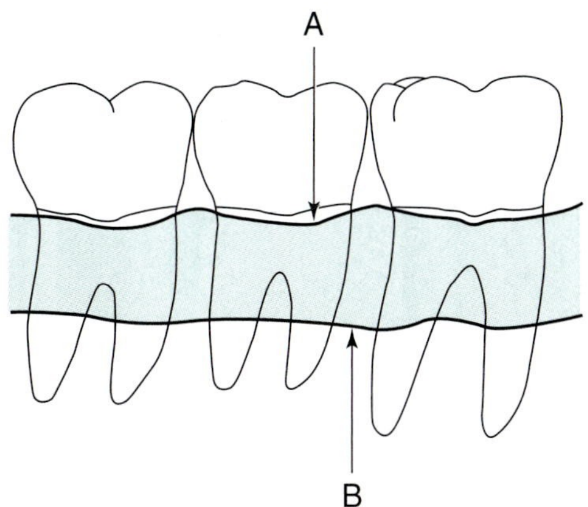

FIGURE 27–19. **Drawing showing horizontal bone loss.** (**A**) Normal (physiologic) level of bone (alveolar bone parallel to the cementoenamel junction) and (**B**) Bone level of patient with periodontal disease. **Horizontal bone loss** is the difference between (**A**) and (**B**) (shaded area).

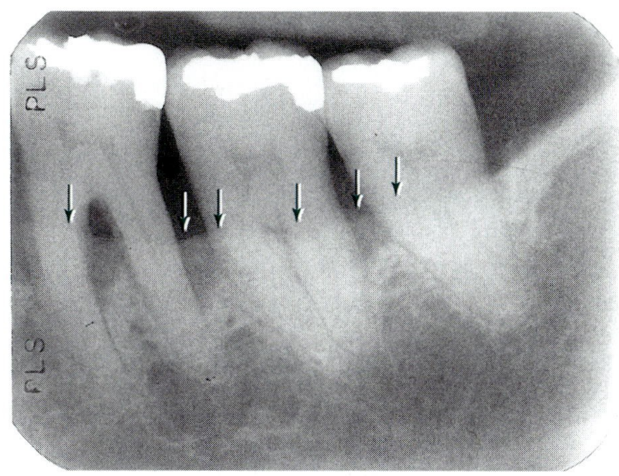

FIGURE 27–20. **Horizontal bone loss.** Arrows show bone level of patient with periodontal disease.

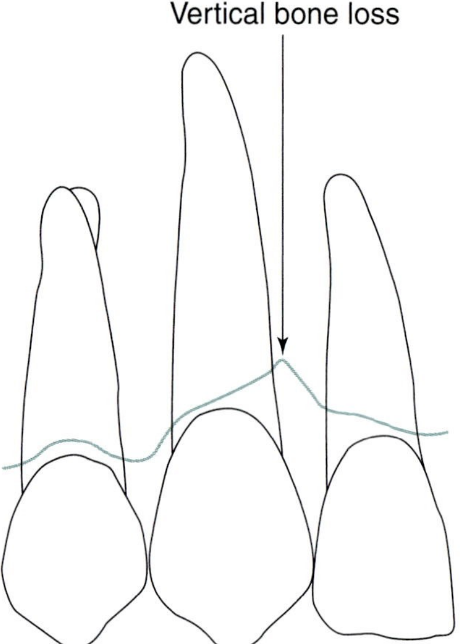

FIGURE 27-21. **Drawing showing vertical bone loss**. Vertical bone loss occurs in a plane that is perpendicular to the cementoenamel junctions of adjacent teeth (up and down).

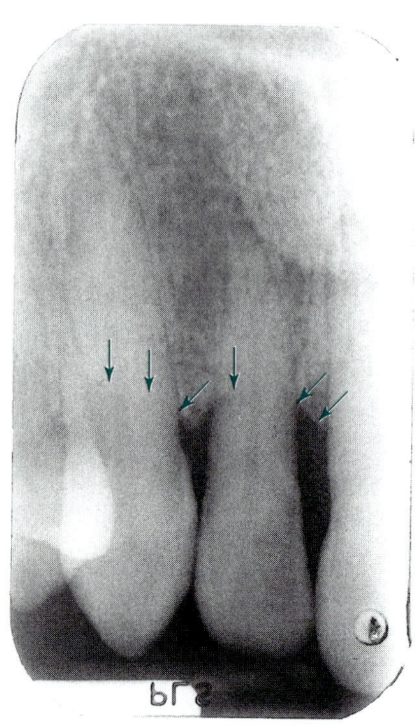

FIGURE 27-22. **Vertical bone loss.** Arrows show bone level of patient with periodontal disease.

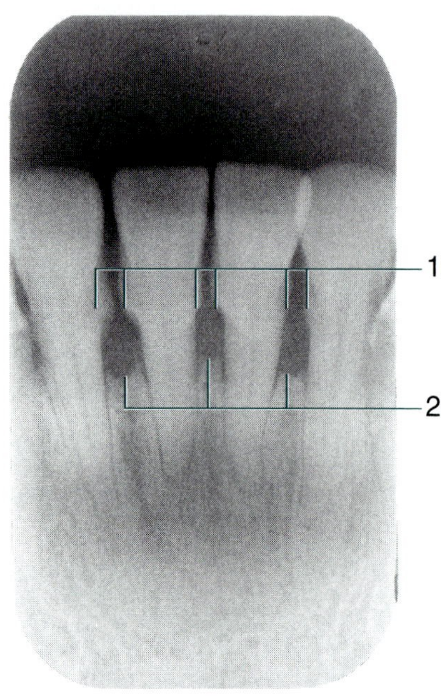

FIGURE 27-23. **Radiograph of mandibular incisor region**. This radiograph shows (**1**) large deposits of calculus around the necks of the teeth and (**2**) radiolucent areas indicating vertical and horizontal bone loss that is typical of periodontal disease.

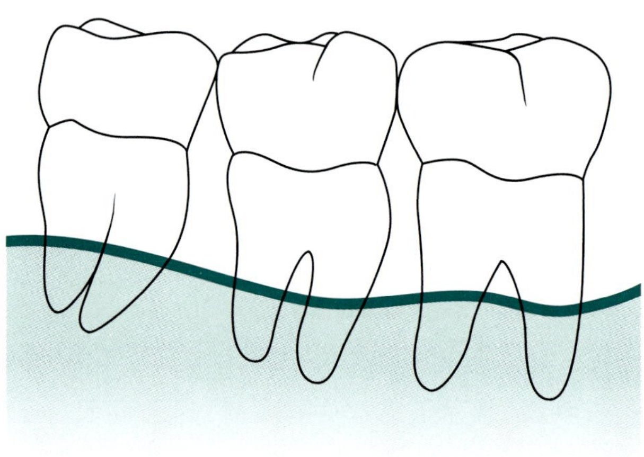

FIGURE 27-24. **Drawing showing advanced stage or severe bone loss.**

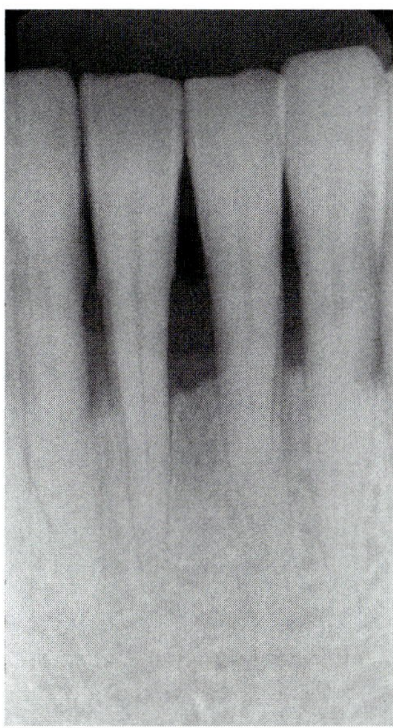

FIGURE 27-25. **Radiograph showing severe bone loss in mandibular anterior region.**

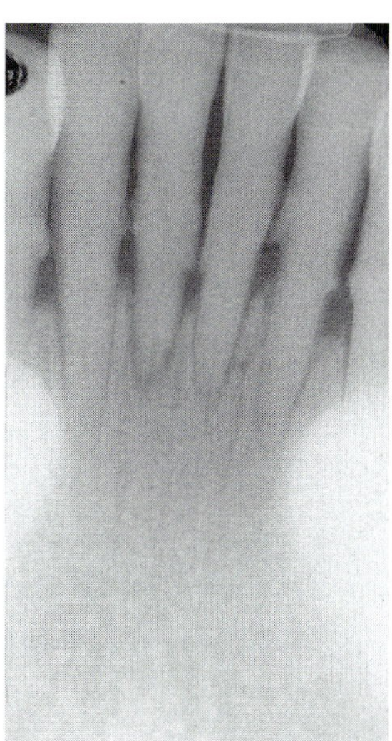

FIGURE 27-26. **Radiograph showing severe bone loss and heavy calculus in mandibular anterior region.**

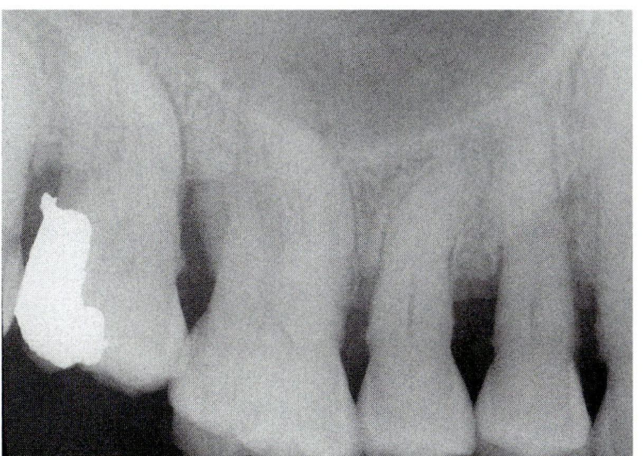

FIGURE 27-27. **Radiograph showing severe bone loss and furcation in maxillary posterior region.**

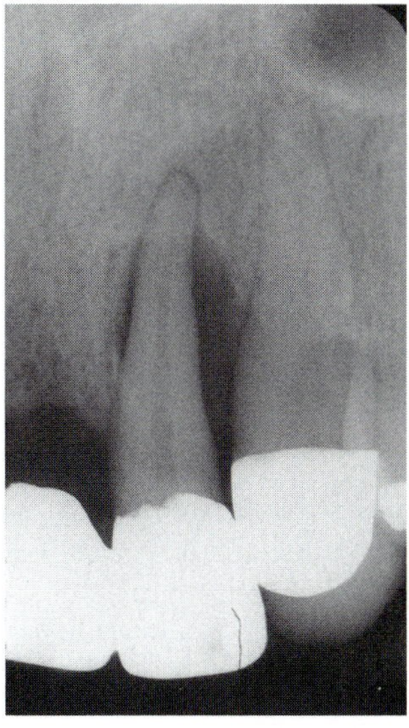

FIGURE 27-28. **Radiograph showing severe vertical bone loss.**

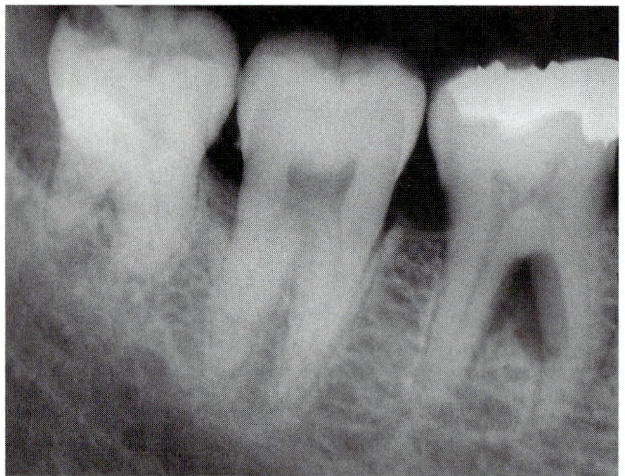

FIGURE 27-29. **Radiograph showing bone loss and furcation involvement of the first molar.**

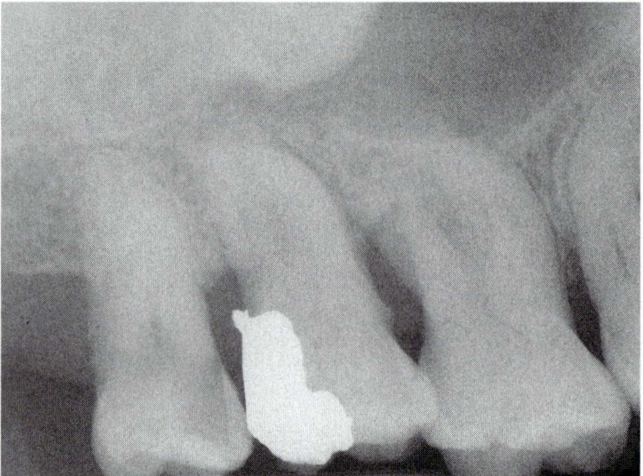

FIGURE 27-30. **Radiograph showing overhang on restoration of maxillary second molar causing periodontal disease.**

are detecting the presence or absence of periodontal pockets, early bone loss, early furcation involvement, calculus, and tooth mobility.

Presence or Absence of Periodontal Pockets

The periodontal pocket is a pathologically deepened gingival sulcus. Because the periodontal pocket consists of soft tissue, it is not visible on the radiograph. Therefore, the only reliable method of locating the pocket and determining its extent is by careful periodontal probing.

Radiopaque material, such as gutta-percha points may be inserted into the pocket so the base of the periodontal pocket can be seen on the radiograph.

Early Bone Loss

Radiographs usually show less bone loss than is actually present. The sensitivity of radiographs in detecting early bone loss is only fair. Usually, bone defects smaller than 3.0 mm cannot be seen on radiographs. Therefore, the earliest signs of periodontal disease must be detected clinically.

Early Furcation Involvement

The furcation area of a tooth should be carefully examined clinically with a probe. The facial and lingual aspects of alveolar bone will often be superimposed over the furcation. Also, improper alignment of the x-ray beam may obliterate the presence or extent of furcation involvement.

Calculus

The detection of dental calculus by the radiograph will depend on the amount of mineralization and on the angulation of the x-ray beam. Therefore, the radiograph cannot be relied on for the thorough detection of calculus.

Tooth Mobility

Obviously, radiographs do not record the mobility of teeth. However, the radiograph may show a widening of the periodontal ligament space, which indicates an increase in tooth mobility.

CHAPTER SUMMARY

Periodontal disease refers to disease that affects both soft tissues (gingiva) and bone around the teeth. The severity of periodontal disease may range from a simple inflammation of the gingiva to the destruction of supporting bone and the periodontal ligament. These according to the ADA can be classified as gingivitis, early periodontitis, moderate periodontitis, or advanced periodontitis. Radiographs, along with a thorough clinical examination, allow the dental professional to evaluate and document periodontal disease.

The dental professional must be able to interpret periodontal disease as seen on a dental radiograph. The interpretation should include the crestal and interseptal bone of the alveolus. Bony changes should be described with regard to location and severity. Also included in the description should be any local irritating factors which may predispose an area of the dentition or the entire dentition to periodontal disease. Local irritating factors may include the presence of calculus and faulty restorations.

There are limitations to the use of radiographs in the diagnosis of periodontal disease. The important limitations are detecting the presence or absence of periodontal pockets, early bone loss, early furcation involvement, calculus, and tooth mobility.

REVIEW QUESTIONS

1. Which of the following terms describes bone loss that occurs in a plane parallel to the cementoenamel junction of adjacent teeth.
   (a) Irregular
   (b) Vertical
   (c) Horizontal
   (d) Periapical
2. The American Dental Association classification for mild bone loss up to 30% is:
   (a) ADA Case Type I (Gingivitis).
   (b) ADA Case Type II (Early Periodontitis).
   (c) ADA Case Type III (Moderate Periodontitis).
   (d) ADA Case Type IV (Advanced Periodontitis).
3. The following term refers to the area between the roots of multirooted teeth:
   (a) Periapical.
   (b) Calculus.
   (c) Cervical.
   (d) Furcation.
4. Local irritating factors may include:
   (a) Enamel.
   (b) Dentin.
   (c) Calculus.
   (d) Lamina dura.
5. Defective restorations may include:
   (a) Open margins.
   (b) Poorly contoured restorations.
   (c) Overhanging margins.
   (d) All of the above.
6. Healthy lamina dura:
   (a) Does not appear on the radiograph.
   (b) Appears only in the furcal areas in posterior teeth.
   (c) Appears as a dense radiopaque line around the roots of the teeth.
   (d) Appears as a dense radiolucent line around the roots of the teeth.

7. To diagnose periodontal disease:
   (a) A clinical exam is unimportant.
   (b) Only use radiographs.
   (c) A clinical exam, periodontal probing, and radiographs are all necessary.
   (d) None of the above.

8. When examining the periodontium, it is best to use:
   (a) Bitewing and periapical films.
   (b) Panoramic films.
   (c) Occlusal films.
   (d) None of the above, radiographs are not useful when examining the periodontium.

9. The best radiographic technique for evaluating periodontal disease is:
   (a) Paralleling.
   (b) Bisecting angle.

10. Radiographs are useful diagnostic aids in evaluating:
    (a) Soft tissue.
    (b) Recession.
    (c) Bone loss.
    (d) Plaque.

11. The term given to a widening of the periodontal space at the crest of the interproximal bone is:
    (a) Triangulation.
    (b) Irritant.
    (c) Open margin.
    (d) Resorption.

12. Limitations of the radiograph include:
    (a) Detecting presence or absence of periodontal pockets.
    (b) Detecting early bone loss.
    (c) Detecting tooth mobility.
    (d) All of the above.

13. Calculus:
    (a) Will always be seen on a radiograph.
    (b) Will never be seen on a radiograph.
    (c) May be seen on a radiograph depending on the amount of mineralization.
    d) May be seen on a radiograph depending on the amount of stain present.

14. Widening of the periodontal ligament space may indicate:
    (a) Tooth mobility.
    (b) Calculus.
    (c) Stain.
    (d) Gingivitis.

BIBLIOGRAPHY

Langlais, R. P. & Kasle, M. J. *Exercises in Oral Radiographic Interpretation*, 3rd ed. Philadelphia: Saunders; 1992.

Langlais, R. P., Langland, O. E., & Nortje C. J. *Diagnostic Imaging of the Jaws*. Philadelphia: Williams & Wilkins; 1995.

White, S. C. & Pharoah M. J. *Oral Radiology Principles and Interpretation*, 4th ed. St. Louis: Mosby; 2000.

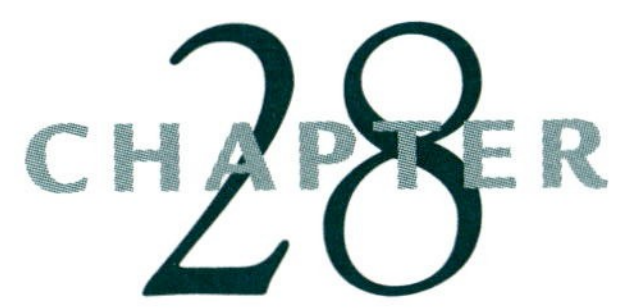

Dental Caries

OBJECTIVES

By the end of this chapter the student should be able to:

- Define the key words.
- Explain the caries process.
- Explain why caries appears radiolucent on the radiograph.
- Discuss both the clinical examination and the radiographic examination for the detection of dental caries.
- Explain the caries depth grading system.
- List the five locations of dental caries and discuss their radiographic appearance.
- Identify the radiographic appearance of dental caries.
- List three conditions that resemble dental caries.

KEY WORDS

Arrested caries
Buccal caries
Caries
Cemental caries
Cervical burnout
Incipient caries
Interproximal caries
Lingual caries
Mach band effect
Nonmetalic restoration
Occlusal caries
Rampant caries
Recurrent caries
Root surface caries

Introduction

Dental caries, also known as tooth decay, is the process by which acids produced by bacteria cause the localized destruction of dental hard tissues. The detection of caries is probably the most common reason for taking dental radiographs. The dental health team should be able to differentiate between normal tooth structures and dental caries on a radiograph.

The purpose of this chapter is to describe dental caries and to introduce the student to the radiographic appearance of dental caries. Also, a caries depth grading system and tips that influence caries interpretation are presented.

Dental Caries

Dental **caries,** or tooth decay, is probably the most frequent reason for taking radiographs. The word caries come from the Latin *cariosus*, which means "rottenness." The term *cavity* is often used to refer to a carious lesion. Dental caries may develop in the enamel and dentin of any tooth surface and occasionally on the cementum, usually near the cementoenamel junction (CEJ).

Description

Dental caries, or tooth decay, is a pathological process consisting of localized destruction of dental hard tissues by organic acids produced by microorganisms. The caries process is one of demineralization of tooth structure (enamel, dentin, cementum) and subsequent destruction. **Caries appears radiolucent** on the radiograph because the decrease in tooth density allows more x-rays to pass through the tooth and darken the film (see Figure 28–1).

Detection

Both a clinical examination and radiographic examination are necessary in the detection of dental caries. Intraoral radiographs can reveal carious lesions that otherwise might go undetected during a thorough clinical examination.

Clinical Examinatiom

Some carious lesions can be detected during a clinical examination using a mirror and explorer. The mirror is used to reflect light, to allow indirect vision, and to re-

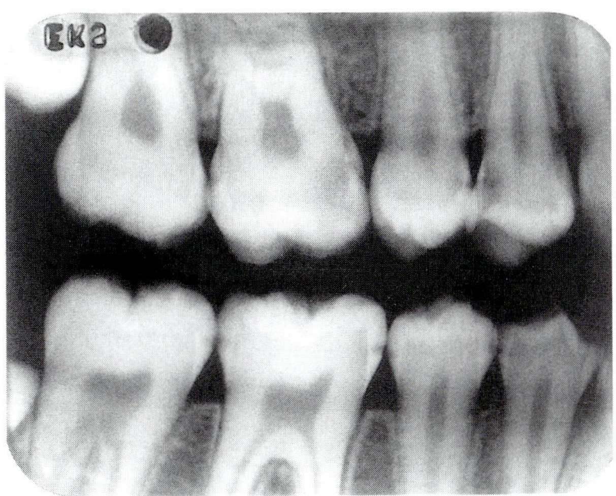

FIGURE 28–1. **Carious lesions.** Radiograph showing multiple carious lesions. Note interproximal caries are found just **gingival to the contact area.**

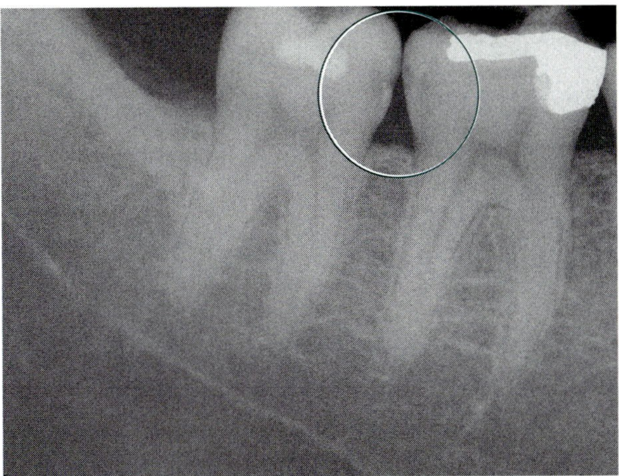

FIGURE 28–2. **Periapical radiograph showing interproximal caries.**

tract the tongue. The explorer is used as a tactile device to detect softness or catches in the grooves, pits, and fissures of the teeth.

The examiner should look for color changes when clinically examining the teeth. Caries may appear as a dark stain in the pits and fissures on the occlusal surfaces of teeth. Smooth surfaces may appear chalky white or opaque. The examiner must remember that the clinical examination alone is not adequate and must be accompanied by a radiographic examination.

Radiographic Examination

Radiographs reveal carious lesions that cannot be seen clinically. To be a useful diagnostic aid the radiographs must be properly angulated, exposed, and processed. Improper horizontal angulation causes overlapping of the contact areas and it is impossible to interpret dental caries.

The bitewing radiograph, described in chapter 15, is the radiograph of choice for the evaluation of caries due to its parallelism to the tooth (see Figure 28–1). However, a properly made periapical radiograph using the paralleling technique may also be used (see Figure 28–2).

Interpreting Dental Caries

Dental caries is a process of decalcification and requires 40 to 50% loss of calcium and phosphorus before the decreased density can be seen on a radiograph. For this reason, the depth of penetration of a carious lesion is deeper than it appears on the radiograph. Also, because the interproximal surfaces of posterior teeth are broad, the loss of small amounts of mineral from incipient lesions may be difficult to see on the radiograph (see Figure 28–3).

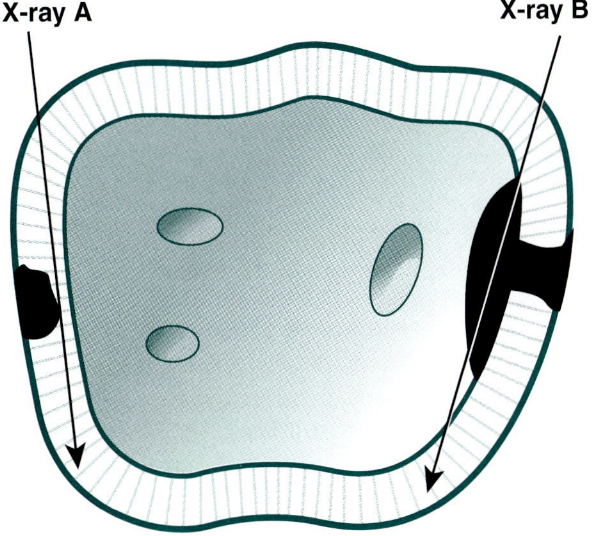

FIGURE 28–3. **Drawing showing ratio of caries to enamel.** This drawing shows (**1**) **x-ray A** passing through a small ratio of caries to enamel, resulting in the caries being difficult to view and (**2**) **x-ray B** passing through a large ratio of caries to enamel, resulting in the caries being easier to view.

The film mounting and viewing techniques described in Chapter 12 are essential when interpreting dental radiographs. This is especially important when interpreting dental caries.

After proper mounting, radiographs should be viewed in a room with subdued lighting. Always use a viewbox and a magnifying glass. Radiographs must be of diagnostic quality to properly evaluate for dental caries. Poor technique may result in nondiagnostic radiographs. Overlapped contact areas caused by improper horizontal angulation make it impossible to detect interproximal caries. Also incorrect exposure factors may result in radiographs that are too light or too dark and are useless for detecting caries.

In recent years, the use of digital imaging technology in place of dental radiographs has increased. Studies show that the digital systems are comparable to the film for interpreting dental caries.

Caries Depth Grading System

Several **systems** are used to **grade** the depth of penetration of caries. This text will use a **grading system** as suggested by Haugejorden and Slack, 1977 (see Figure 28–4). The advantage of this system is that it allows one to accurately grade the penetration of caries (establish a baseline) and to track the progression of the carious lesions at future appointments.

C-1: Enamel caries, penetration less than halfway through the enamel of the tooth. Also called **incipient caries** (incipient means the first stage of existence).

C-2: This **enamel caries** has penetrated over halfway through the enamel.

C-3: Caries of enamel and dentin definitely at or **through the dentinoenamel junction (DEJ)** but less than halfway through the dentin toward the pulp.

C-4: Caries of enamel and dentin that has penetrated **over halfway through the dentin** toward the pulp.

The extent of interproximal caries may be called **incipient, moderate, advanced,** or **severe.**

Incipient Interproximal Caries

Incipient interproximal caries (grade C-1) extends less than halfway through the thickness of enamel (see Figure 28–4, number 1). Incipient lesions are only seen in the enamel.

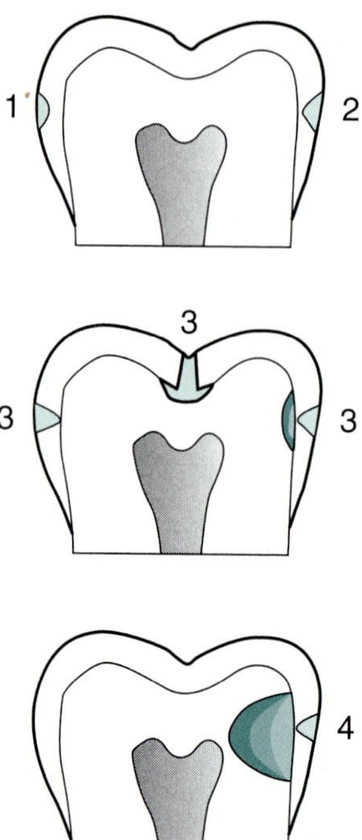

FIGURE 28–4. **Diagram of classification of dental caries as recommended by Haugejorden and Slack. (1) is C-1 caries.** Enamel caries less than halfway through the enamel (incipient caries). **(2) is C-2 caries.** Enamel caries penetrated over halfway through the enamel. **(3) is C-3 caries.** Caries definitely at or through the dentino-enamel junction (DEJ) but less than halfway through the dentin toward the pulp. **(4) is C-4 caries.** Caries that has penetrated over halfway through the dentin toward the pulp.

Moderate Interproximal Caries

Moderate interproximal caries (grade C-2) extends over halfway through the thickness of enamel but does not reach the DEJ (see Figure 28–4, number 2). Moderate lesions are only seen in the enamel.

Advanced Interproximal Caries

Advanced interproximal caries (grade C-3) are those that have reached the DEJ but are less than halfway through the dentin (see Figure 28–4, number 3). Advanced lesions are seen in both the enamel and dentin.

Severe Interproximal Caries

Severe interproximal caries (grade C-4) extends over halfway through the dentin and approaches the pulp chamber (see Figure 28–4, number 4). Severe lesions are seen in both the enamel and the dentin.

Classification of the Radiographic Appearance of Caries

The radiographic appearance of dental caries may be classified according to their location on the tooth.

There are five **locations of caries:**

1. Interproximal
2. Occlusal
3. Buccal
4. Lingual
5. Cemental (root surface)

Also, caries may be recurrent, rampant, or arrested.

Interproximal Caries

Interproximal means between two adjacent surfaces. On dental radiographs, **interproximal caries** are located between the contact point of the tooth and the gingival margin (see Figure 28–1). This is an area in which it is almost impossible to examine clinically and therefore the radiograph is the best tool for the job.

The **shape** of interproximal caries is **triangular** (like a **pyramid**) with the apex toward the DEJ and its base toward the outer surface of the tooth (see Figure 28–4, number 2). At the DEJ the caries spreads, undermining normal enamel, and again takes on a triangular shape as it penetrates toward the pulp. The base of the triangle is along the DEJ and the apex towards the pulp (see Figure 28–4, number 3).

Technical errors such as improper vertical and horizontal angulation will affect interproximal caries detection. Too high or too low vertical angulation obliterates viewing the carious lesion on a radiograph (see Figure 28–5). Improper horizontal angulation causes overlapping of the contact areas of the crowns and makes it impossible to interpret the interproximal surfaces of the teeth for carious lesions (see Figure 28–6).

Occlusal Caries

Occlusal caries are carious lesions located on the chewing surface of the posterior teeth. Because of the superimposition of the buccal and lingual cusps, occlusal caries in its early stages may not be seen on a radiograph (see Figure 28–7). The mirror and explorer clinical examination is the best way to detect occlusal caries in its early stages.

After occlusal caries has reached the DEJ, they may be seen on the radiograph (see Figures 28–8 and 28–9). At the DEJ the caries will appear as a flat radiolucent line. Occlusal caries follows the enamel rods, as does interproximal caries. The shape of occlusal caries is again pyramidal but, with its base toward the pulp and the apex toward the occlusal surface (see Figure 28–4, middle number 3).

Buccal and Lingual Caries

Buccal caries involves the buccal surface of a tooth and **lingual caries** involves the lingual surface (see Figure

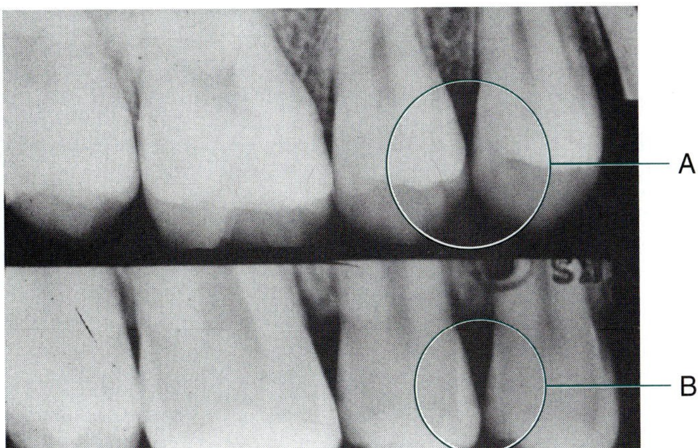

FIGURE 28–5. **Vertical angulation.** (**A**) Improper vertical angulation (too high) obliterates viewing interproximal carious lesion. (**B**) Proper vertical angulation shows interproximal caries.

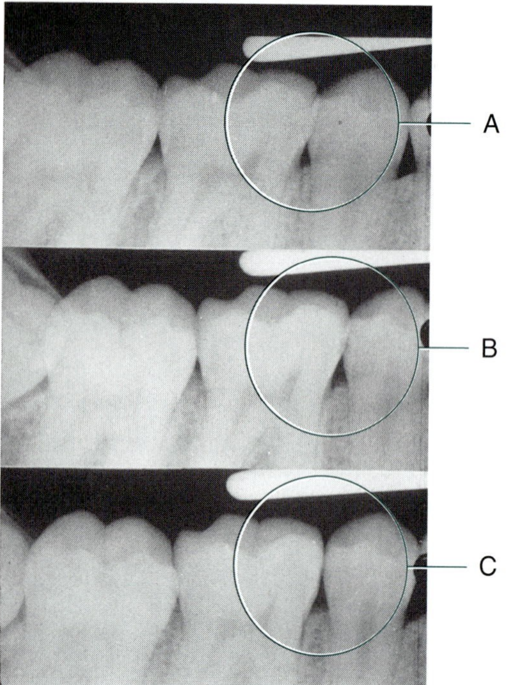

FIGURE 28–6. **Horizontal angulation.** (**A**) Improper horizontal angulation prevents viewing interproximal caries. (**B**) Improved horizontal angulation, but caries difficult to view. (**C**) Proper **horizontal angulation shows interproximal caries.**

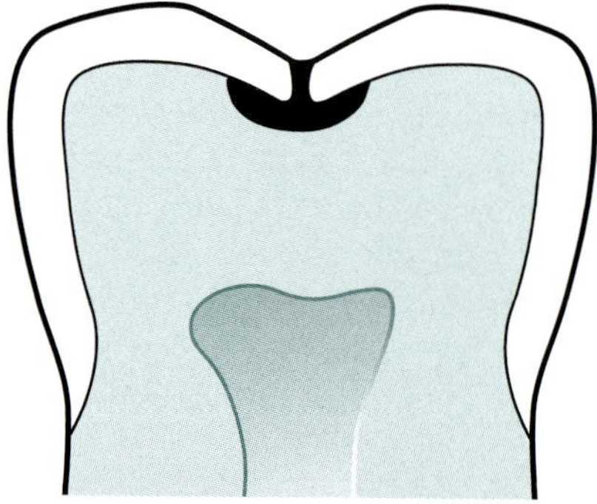

FIGURE 28–7. **Drawing of occlusal caries early stage.** Early occlusal caries extends along the dentinoenamel (DE) junction and may not be seen on the radiograph Early occlusal caries must be detected clinically by mirror and explorer.

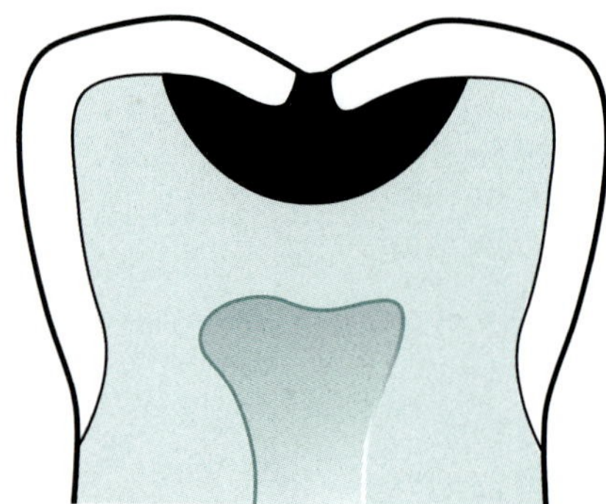

FIGURE 28–8. **Drawing of severe occlusal caries.** Severe or advanced occlusal caries extends well into the dentin.

28–10). Buccal and lingual caries are best detected clinically with a mirror and explorer. Early **buccal and lingual carious lesions** are almost impossible to detect radiographically. This is due to the superimposition of the normal tooth structures over the caries. Later the lesion will appear as a radiolucency characterized by its well-defined borders. This has been characterized as looking into a hole on the radiograph (see Figure 28–11).

Because the radiograph is a two-dimensional image of three-dimensional structures, it is impossible to tell the depth of buccal or lingual caries or its relationship to the pulpal tissue.

Cemental (Root Surface) Caries

Cemental caries (also known as root caries, radicular caries, and senile caries) develops between the enamel border and the free margin of the gingiva on the cemental surface (see Figure 28–12). Bone loss and recession of the gingival tissue are necessary for the caries process to start on the root surfaces. Cemental caries may appear on the buccal, lingual, mesial or distal surface of the tooth.

Radiographically, cemental caries appears as an ill-defined, radiolucent, saucer-shaped area just below the cementoenamel junction (CEJ) (see Figure 28–13). Cemental caries may at times be misinterpreted as cervical burnout. Clinically, cemental caries are easily detected with a mirror and explorer.

Cemental caries occurs in the elderly for the following reasons:

1. The elderly have more **loose contacts** between teeth due to attrition, worn restorations, and periodontal disease. Poor contacts cause food packing.
2. Older persons often have **dry mouth** (**xerostomia**).

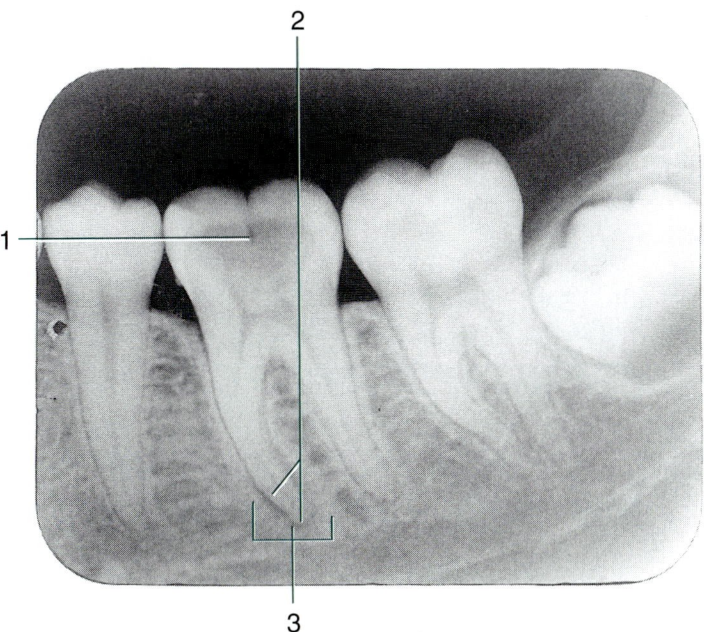

FIGURE 28–9. **Radiograph of occlusal caries.** This radiograph shows (**1**) severe occlusal caries which appears as a large radiolucent lesion in the first molar, (**2**) loss of lamina dura and periapical bone around the mesial root of the first molar, and (**3**) condensing osteitis. Condensing osteitis is a term used when sclerotic (hardened) bone is formed as a result of infection.

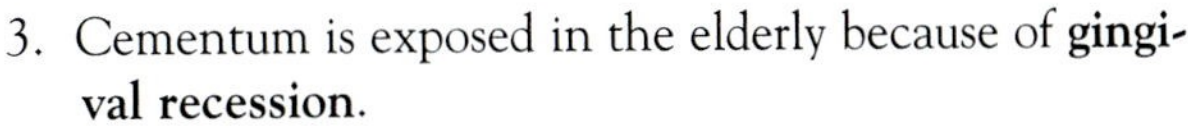

3. Cementum is exposed in the elderly because of **gingival recession.**

Cemental caries is becoming more prevalent as our population ages.

Recurrent (Secondary) Caries

Recurrent or secondary caries is decay that occurs under a restoration or around its margins. Recurrent caries occurs because of poor cavity preparation, defective margins, or incomplete removal of the caries prior to the placement of the restoration.

Recurrent caries appears on a radiograph as a radiolucent area beneath a restoration or apical to the interproximal margin of a restoration (see Figure 28–14).

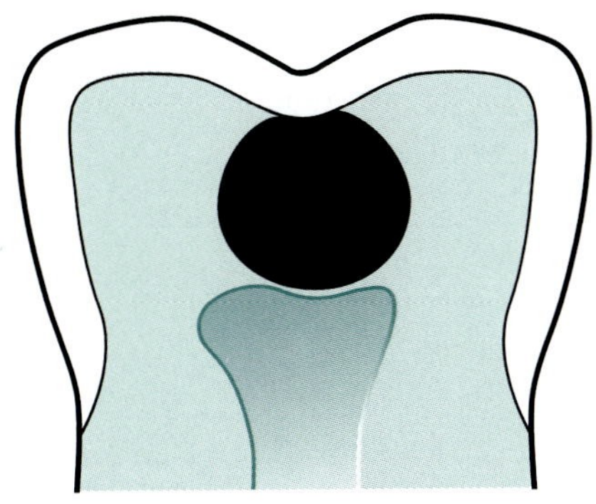

FIGURE 28–10. **Drawing of buccal and lingual caries.** Advanced buccal or lingual caries has well defined borders.

Rampant Caries

The term rampant means growing rapidly or spreading unchecked. **Rampant caries** are severe, unchecked caries that affect multiple teeth. Typically, rampant caries occurs in children with poor dietary and oral hygiene habits. This condition is becoming increasing rare be-

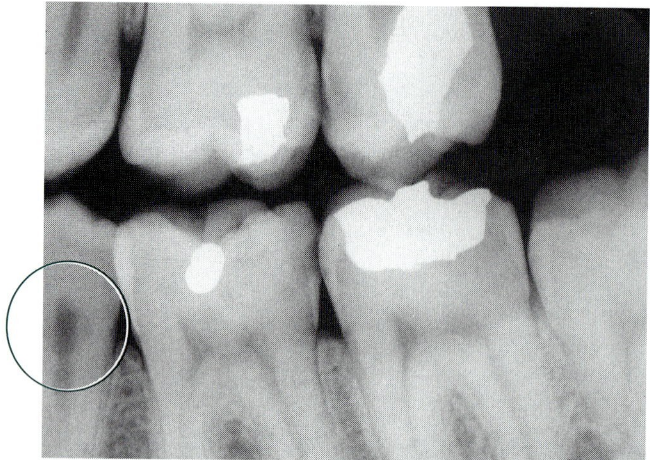

FIGURE 28–11. **Radiograph of buccal caries.** Buccal caries on the mandibular second premolar (bicuspid) appears as a round radiolucency (superimposed over the pulp chamber).

cause of fluoridation of water supplies and the practice of good oral hygiene. Treatment requires extensive dental care and education of the child's parents.

Arrested Caries

The term arrested means stopped or inactive. **Arrested caries** are caries that are no longer active. Carious lesions may become arrested if there is a significant shift in the oral environment from factors that cause caries to those that slow down the caries process. Incipient enamel caries (grade C-1) can remain dormant for long periods of time. Some carious lesions may even be reversed by remineralization.

Conditions Resembling Caries

Three **conditions** that **resemble caries** are nonmetallic restorations, cervical burnout, and mach band effect.

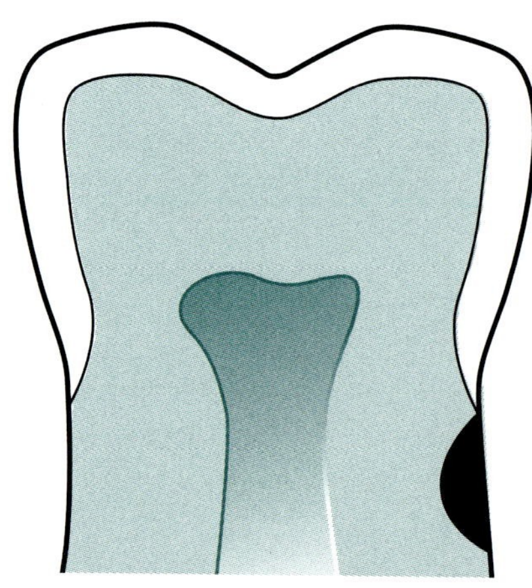

FIGURE 28–12. **Drawing of cemental (root surface) caries.** Cemental caries involves only the roots of teeth. Gingival recession and bone loss precede the caries process to expose the root surfaces.

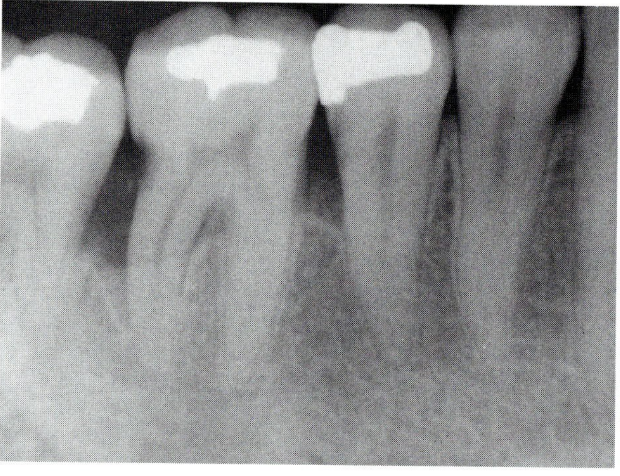

FIGURE 28–13. **Radiograph of cemental (root surface) caries.** Cemental caries appears as a large radiolucency on the distal surface of the distal root of the first mandibular molar. Note the bone loss exposing the root surface.

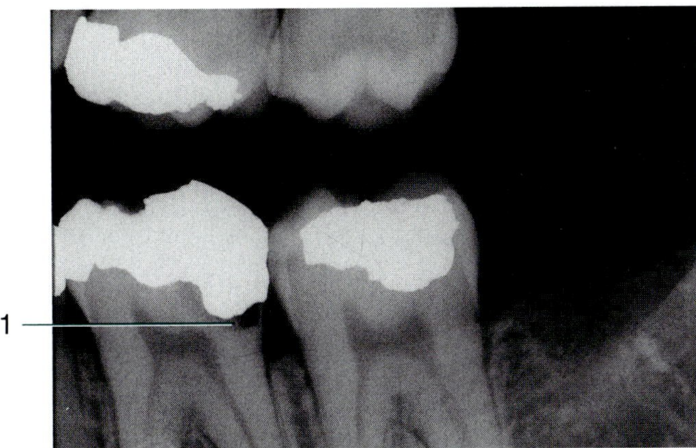

FIGURE 28-14. **Radiograph of recurrent caries.** This radiograph shows (**1**) radiolucent caries under the metallic restoration.

Nonmetallic Restorations

Frequently observed radiolucencies that occasionally are mistaken for caries are nonmetallic esthetic restorations in anterior teeth (see Figures 28–15 and 26–2, number 2). **Nonmetallic restorations** attenuate the x-ray beam so little that the area in question appears radiolucent. Only a clinical examination can make a final determination.

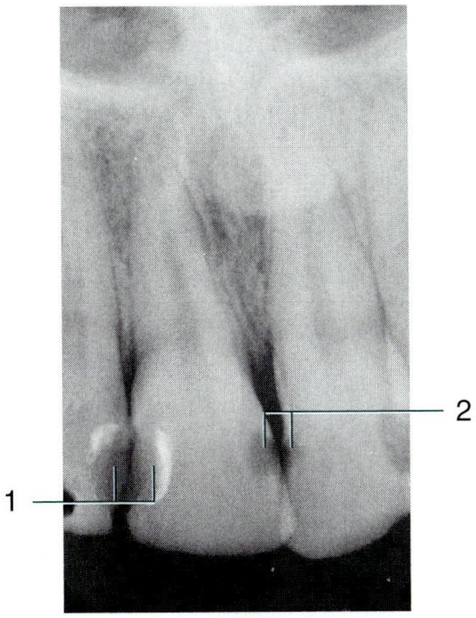

FIGURE 28-15. **Radiograph of nonmetalic restorations and carious lesions in anterior teeth.** This radiograph shows (**1**) radiolucent nonmetalic restorations on the mesial surface of #7 and distal surface of #8. Note both restorations have bases with radiopaque material. (**2**) The radiolucencies on the mesial surfaces of #8 and #9 are carious lesions.

Cervical Burnout

On radiographs on which **cervical burnout** is noted, an irregularly shaped radiolucent area with a fuzzy outline can be seen on both the mesial and distal surfaces along the cervical line. The cause of cervical burnout is the concavity of the root surfaces, which results in greater penetration by the x-rays (see Figure 28–16). Cervical burnout between metalic restorations and the alveolar

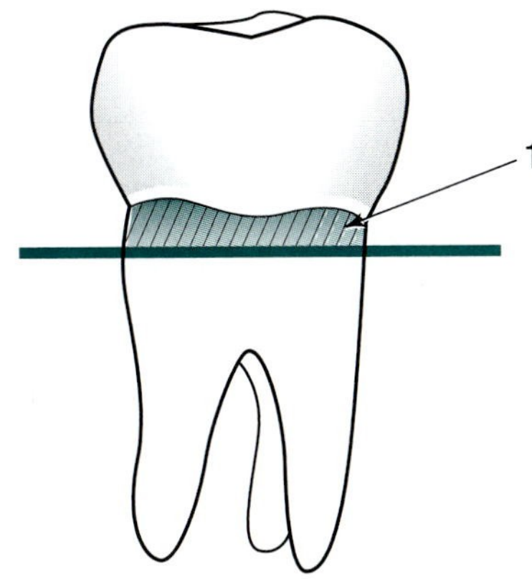

FIGURE 28-16. **Drawing of cervical burnout.** This drawing shows (**1**) cervical root surface between crown and alveolar crest of bone. The thin root surface allows more x-rays to pass than the dense enamel crown and alveolar bone; and therefore is radiolucent.

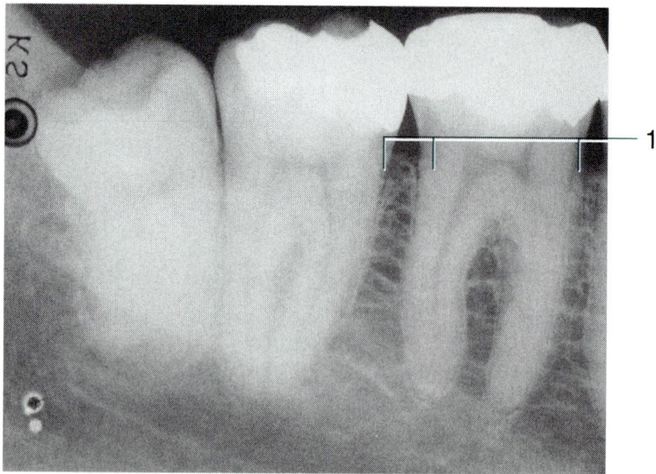

FIGURE 28–17. **Radiograph of cervical burnout.** This radiograph shows (**1**) radiolucent cervical burnout on mesial of the second molar between the restoration and the alveolar crest of bone; and on the mesial and distal of the first molar between the crown and alveolar bone.

crest of bone in posterior teeth is often mistaken for caries (see Figure 28–17).

Mach Band Effect

A radiolucency that frequently occurs, and may be mistaken for caries, is an **optical illusion** caused by overlapping teeth. When two interproximal surfaces overlap (caused by natural overlap of misaligned teeth or by improper horizontal angulation of the x-ray beam) there is a dense radiopaque area surrounded by radiolucent lines. These lines are an optical illusion called the **mach band effect** caused by the high contrast between the normal enamel and the dense overlapped enamel (see Figure 28–18).

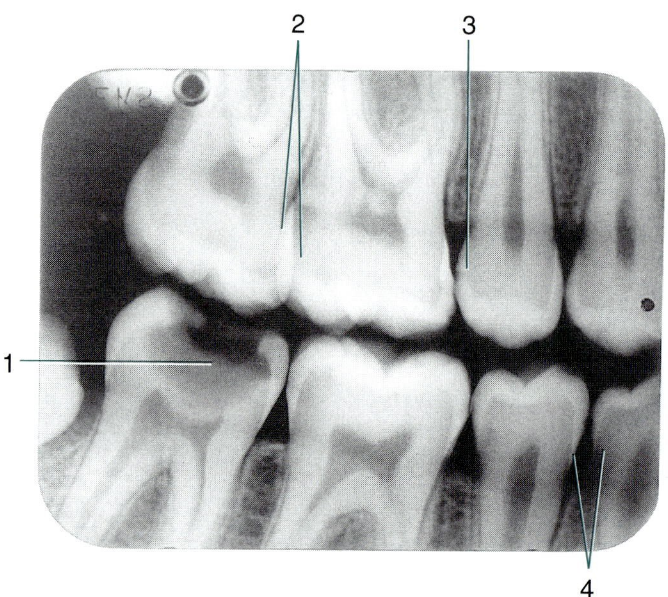

FIGURE 28–18. **Bitewing radiograph.** This radiograph shows (**1**) large occlusal caries, (**2**) radiolucent lines or **mach band effect** (an optical illusion caused by overlapped enamel), (**3**) interproximal caries, and (**4**) cervical burnout.

CHAPTER SUMMARY

Dental caries, also known as tooth decay, is the process by which acids produced by bacteria cause the localized destruction of dental hard tissues. The detection of caries is probably the most common reason for taking dental radiographs. The dental health team should be able to differentiate between normal tooth structures and dental caries on a radiograph.

The caries process is one of demineralization of tooth structure (enamel, dentin, cementum) and subsequent destruction. Caries appears radiolucent on the radiograph because the decrease in tooth density allows more x-rays to pass through the tooth and darken the film. Both a clinical examination and radiographic examination are necessary in the detection of dental caries.

The radiographic appearance of dental caries may be classified according to their location on the tooth. The five locations of caries are interproximal, occlusal, buccal, lingual, and cemental (root surface). Three conditions that resemble caries are nonmetallic restorations, cervical burnout, and mach band effect.

Although never called upon to make a final diagnosis, a skilled dental assistant or hygienist should have little difficulty in differentiating between normal tooth structure and dental caries in its many forms.

REVIEW QUESTIONS

1. Caries in the first stage of existence is called:
   - (a) Senile caries.
   - (b) Cemental caries.
   - (c) Incipient caries.
   - (d) None of the above.
2. The shape of interproximal caries is:
   - (a) Triangular with the apex toward the dentinoenamel junction and its base toward the outer surface of the tooth.
   - (b) Triangular with the apex toward the outer surface of the tooth and its base toward the dentinoenamel junction.
   - (c) Saucer-shaped with the base of the saucer toward the dentinoenamel junction.
   - (d) Round with irregular borders.
3. Caries that occurs under a restoration or around its margins is called:
   - (a) Recurrent caries.
   - (b) Cemental caries.
   - (c) Root caries.
   - (d) Buccal caries.
4. Cemental (root) caries is usually seen on radiographs as a(n):
   - (a) Radiolucent area under a restoration.
   - (b) Ill-defined, radiolucent, saucer-shaped area just below the cementoenamel junction.
   - (c) Black circle on the buccal or lingual surface.
   - (d) Triangular radiolucent area in the enamel just below the contact point.

5. The carious lesion is radiolucent because of:
   (a) Less radiation passing through the lesion than the surrounding tissue.
   (b) More radiation passing through the lesion than the surrounding tissue.
   (c) The mach band effect.
   (d) The carious lesion is radiopaque.

6. If the occlusal carious lesion is seen on a radiographic it will appear:
   (a) As a radiopaque flat line at the DEJ.
   (b) As a radiolucent flat line at the DEJ.
   (c) Only on the buccal cusps.
   (d) Only in the enamel.

7. Cemental caries occurs in the elderly for which of the following reasons?
   (a) Loose contacts.
   (b) Xerostomia.
   (c) Gingival recession.
   (d) All of the above.

8. A condition which may resemble caries radiographically is:
   (a) Xerostomia.
   (b) Amalgam.
   (c) Nonmetallic restoration.
   (d) Incipiency.

9. To be useful aids for caries diagnosis radiographs must be:
   (a) Properly angulated.
   (b) Properly exposed.
   (c) Properly processed.
   (d) All of the above.

10. Which is the radiograph of choice for the evaluation of caries?
    (a) Panoramic
    (b) Bitewing
    (c) Occlusal
    (d) Periapical

11. Two frequently observed radiolucencies that occasionally are mistaken for caries are:
    (a) Esthetic restorations in anterior teeth and cervical burnout.
    (b) Mental foramen and dentigerous cysts.
    (c) Incisive foramen and nutrient canals.
    (d) Cementomas and nutrient canals.

12. The bitewing radiograph clearly identifies:
    (a) Pulp exposures.
    (b) Interproximal carious lesions.
    (c) Periodontal pocket formation.
    (d) Periapical pathology.

BIBLIOGRAPHY

Berry, H. Cervical burnout and mach band: two shadows of doubt in radiologic interpretation of carious lesions. *J. Am. Dent. Assoc.* *106:* 622, 1983.

Langlais, R. P., & Kasle, M. J. *Exercises in Oral Radiographic Interpretation*, 3rd ed. Philadelphia: Saunders; 1992.

Langlais, R. P. Langland, O. E., & Nortje, C. J. *Diagnostic Imaging of the Jaws*. Philadelphia: Williams & Wilkins; 1995.

Langland, O. E. & Langlais, R. P. *Principles of Dental Imaging*. Philadelphia: Williams & Wilkins, 1997.

White, S. C. & Pharoah M. J. *Oral Radiology Principles and Interpretation*, 4th ed. St. Louis: Mosby, 2000.

White, S. C. & Yoon, D. C. Comparative performance of digital and conventional images for detecting proximal surface caries. *Dentomaxillofac. Radiol.* *26*:32, 1997.

Answers to Review Questions

Chapter 1: 1-c, 2-a, 3-e, 4-b, 5-d, 6-c, 7-November 8, 1895, 8-b, 9-a, 10-c, 11-b, 12-c, 13-b, 14-b.

Chapter 2: 1-b, 2-see Figure 2-1, 3-a, 4-d, 5-a, 6-d, 7-a, 8-d, 9-a, 10-c, 11-c, 12-d, 13-c, 14-see glossary, 15-b.

Chapter 3: 1-see Figure 3-4, 2-c, 3-c, 4-(1) a source of free electrons; (2) high voltage to impart speed to the electrons; and (3) a target that is capable of stopping the electrons, 5-c, 6-d, 7-thermionic emission, 8-d, 9-a, 10-b, 11-square, 12-b, 13-a, 14-a, 15-b, 16-d, 17-b, 18-c, 19-(a) 0.5 (b) 0.7 (c) 15 (d) 18, 20-d.

Chapter 4: 1-d, 2-d, 3-c, 4-b, 5-c, 6-a, 7-b, 8-b, 9-a, 10-a, 11-d, 12-d, 13-b and d, 14-central ray, 15-contrast, 16-0.6 seconds, 17-d, 18-10 mR/minute.

Chapter 5: 1-a, 2-a, 3-c, 4-a, 5-c, 6-b, 7-d, 8-d, 9-c, 10-d, 11-d, 12-a, 13-a, 14-b, 15-d, 16-c, 17-d, 18-a, 19-direct hit or target, indirect or poison water, 20-as low as reasonably achievable.

Chapter 6: 1-d, 2-c, 3-b, 4-b, 5-c, 6-d, 7-a, 8-b, 9-c, 10-c, 11-a, 12-inherent, added, aluminum, 13-size, shape, 14-aluminum, 15-longer, 16-d, 17-b, 18-5 mSv (0.5 rem) per year.

Chapter 7: 1-c, 2-b, 3-a, 4-c, 5-b, 6-d, 7-c, 8-d, 9-b, 10-a, 11-d, 12-c, 13-c, 14-b, 15-periapical, bitewing, occlusal, 16-b, 17-a.

Chapter 8: 1-b, 2-b, 3-d, 4-c, 5-c, 6-b, 7-a, 8-d, 9-c, 10-a, 11-c, 12-a, 13-b, 14-d, 15-b, 16-c, 17-b, 18-d, 19-e, 20-c, 21-d, 22-x-ray processing chemicals, intraoral film packets, and discarded radiographs.

Chapter 9: 1-d, 2-c, 3-a, 4-d, 5-c, 6-a, 7-c, 8-c, 9-a, 10-c, 11-c, 12-a, 13-see text, 14-see text.

Chapter 10: 1-a, 2-a, 3-b, 4-b, 5-a, 6-b, 7-a, 8-a, 9-density, 10-b, 11-b, 12-d, 13-b.

Chapter 11: 1-d, 2-c, 3-a, 4-b, 5-c, 6-d, 7-d, 8-a, 9-c, 10-b, 11-i, 12-g, 13-c, 14-e, 15-a, 16-d, 17-f, 18-b, 19-h.

Chapter 12: 1-b, 2-d, 3-b, 4-a, 5-a, 6-b, 7-a, 8-b, 9-d, 10-d, 11-see text, 12-see text.

Chapter 13: 1-c, 2-d, 3-c, 4-d, 5-a, 6-d, 7-b, 8-c, 9-d, 10-c, 11-film, 12-paralleling.

Chapter 14: 1-b, 2-c, 3-b, 4-d, 5-b, 6-a, 7-b, 8-a, 9-see text, 10-see text, 11-c, 12-c, 13-a, 14-b.

Chapter 15: 1-b, 2-c, 3-a, 4-c, 5-d, 6-c, 7-c.

Chapter 16: 1-see text, 2-d, 3-b, 4-c, 5-d, 6-b.

Chapter 17: 1-a, 2-c, 3-b, 4-d, 5-c, 6-b, 7-a.

Chapter 18: 1-d, 2-b, 3-d, 4-b, 5-b.

Chapter 19: 1-a, 2-b, 3-b, 4-a, 5-c, 6-d, 7-d, 8-b, 9-b, 10-e, 11-b, 12-b, 13-e, 14-a, 15-d, 16-c, 17-f.

Chapter 20: 1-b, 2-c, 3-a, 4-d, 5-a, 6-b.

Chapter 21: 1-d, 2-b, 3-a, 4-c, 5-c, 6-b, 7-a, 8-b, 9-b, 10-b, 11-a, 12-c, 13-a, 14-d, 15-d, 16-a, 17-b.

Chapter 22: 1-to prevent the transmission of infectious diseases, 2-see glossary, 3-see text, 4-b, 5-d, 6-c, 7-a, 8-a, 9-c, 10-see text, 11-see text, 12-see text, 13-see text.

Chapter 23: 1-a, 2-a, 3-a, 4-c, 5-d, 6-a, 7-b, 8-c.

Chapter 24: 1-b, 2-a, 3-b, 4-a, 5-a, 6-b, 7-d, 8-c.

Chapter 25: 1-a, 2-a, 3-b, 4-c, 5-c, 6-a, 7-b, 8-dentist.

Chapter 26: 1-interpretation, 2-dentist, 3-c, 4-a, 5-b, 6-a, 7-c, 8-d, 9-a, 10-c, 11-d, 12-c, 13-d, 14-a.

Chapter 27: 1-c, 2-b, 3-d, 4-c, 5-d, 6-c, 7-c, 8-a, 9-a, 10-c, 11-a, 12-d, 13-c, 14-a.

Chapter 28: 1-c, 2-a, 3-a, 4-b, 5-b, 6-b, 7-d, 8-c, 9-d, 10-b, 11-a, 12-b.

GLOSSARY

Abscess: A localized pus formation often accompanied by swelling and pain. In dentistry, an abscess is usually located near the apex of the roots of the infected tooth and may be chronic or acute. Appears radiolucent when large enough to be visible on radiograph.

Absorbed dose: The amount of energy deposited in any form of matter, such as wood, bracket table, air, teeth, muscles, and so forth, by any type of radiation (alpha or beta particles, x- or gamma rays, etc.). The units for measuring the absorbed dose are the gray (Gy) and the rad (radiation absorbed dose).

Absorption: The process through which radiation imparts some or all of its energy to any material through which it passes.

Accelerator (also called an alkalizer): A basic ingredient in the developer solution, usually sodium carbonate, that provides the necessary alkaline medium and softens and swells the gelatin emulsion.

Acetic acid: A chemical in the fixer solution that provides the acid medium to stop further development by neutralizing the alkali of the developer.

Acidifier: A chemical (acetic acid) in the fixer solution that neutralizes the alkali in the developer solution and stops further action of the developer.

Acoustic meatus: The opening at the center of the ear. It is located directly over the temporal bone and shows up on extraoral radiographs as a small radiolucent circle.

Activator: A chemical (usual sodium carbonate) in the developer solution that causes the emulsion on the radiographic film to swell and initiates the reducing action of the developing agents. Sodium carbonate makes the developer alkaline.

Acute: Having a rapid onset, short, severe course, and pronounced symptoms; opposite of chronic.

Acute radiation syndrome: Symptoms of the short-term radiation effects after a massive dose of ionizing radiation.

Added filtration: Added to the inherent filtration built into the x-ray machine. This added filtration is in the form of thin disks of pure aluminum, which can be inserted between the x-ray tube and the lead collimator when the inherent filtration is not sufficient to meet modern radiation safety requirements.

Administrative radiograph. A radiograph taken for other than diagnostic purposes.

Adumbration: The giving forth of a vague shadow.

Aiming device (ring): One of the components of the Rinn XCP and BAI film holders used to determine correct horizontal and vertical alignment (formerly called *locator ring*).

Ala: The wing of the nose. In dental radiography, the depression at which the nostril connects with the cheek.

ALARA: "As low as reasonably achievable," economic and social factors being taken into account.

Ala-Tragus line (Tragus-Ala line): An imaginary plane or line from the ala of the nose (a winglike projection at the side of the nose) to the tragus of the ear (the cartilaginous projection in front of the acoustic meatus of the ear). This plane is important in determining the correct position of the patient's head.

Alkalizer: See **Activator.**

Alpha particle: A common form of particulate (corpuscular) radiation. Alpha particles contain two protons and two neutrons and are positively charged. Symbol α.

Alternating current: A flow of electrons in one direction, followed by a flow in the opposite direction.

Aluminum equivalence: The thickness of aluminum affording the same degree of attenuation, under specified conditions, as the material in question.

Alveolar bone: That portion of the maxillary or mandibular bone that immediately surrounds and supports the roots of the dentition.

Alveolar crest (also called crestal bone): The most coronal portion of the alveolar bone. Appears radiopaque when visible on radiograph.

Alveolar process: That portion of the maxillae or mandible that immediately surrounds and supports the roots of the teeth. Appears radiopaque when visible on radiograph.

Alveolus: In dentistry, that part of the alveolar bone that forms the bony socket in which the roots of the tooth are held in position by fibers of the periodontal ligament.

Amalgam tattoo: The bluish-purple color to the gingival tissue caused by fragments of amalgam under the tissue.

Ameloblastoma: An odontogenic tumor of enamel origin that does not undergo differentiation to the point of enamel formation.

Amelogenesis imperfecta: A hereditary enamel deficiency of the teeth. Believed to be caused by a generalized disturbance of the ameloblasts (enamel-producing cells). Also called *enamel hypoplasia*. The remaining tooth structures are not affected. On radiographs, such teeth lack the radiopaque image of enamel.

Ammeter (milliammeter): A gauge to measure the amount of current flowing through the wires of an electrical circuit.

Amperage: The strength of an electric current measured in amperes.

Ampere: The unit of intensity of an electric current produced by 1 volt (V) acting through a resistance of 1 ohm (Ω).

Analog: Relating to the mechanism in which data is represented by continuously variable physical quantities.

Anatomic order: The order in which the teeth are arranged in the dental arches.

Angle of mandible: The area at the posterior and inferior corners of the mandible, where the body of the mandible meets and joins the ascending ramus of the mandible.

Angstom unit: A unit of measurement that describes the wavelengths of certain high-frequency radiation. One angstrom unit (AU or Å) measures 1/100,000,000 of a centimeter. Most wavelengths used in dentistry vary from about 0.1 AU to a maximum of 1.0 AU.

Angulation: The direction in which the central ray and the PID of the x-ray machine are directed toward the teeth and the film. See **Horizontal angulation, Negative angulation, Positive angulation, Vertical angulation,** and **Zero angulation.**

Ankylosis: A stiffening of a joint caused by a fibrous or bony union. In dentistry the term applies to a union of the tooth to the alveolus caused by mineralization and hardening of the fibers of the periodontal ligament, which normally surrounds the root and separates it from the alveolus.

Anode: The positive electrode (terminal) in the x-ray tube. This is a tungsten block, normally set at a 20-degree angle facing the cathode, imbedded in the copper portion of the terminal. The x-rays emanate from the point of impact of the electronic stream (cathode rays) from the cathode.

Anodontia: A congenital absence of teeth. Any tooth in the dental arch may fail to develop. The teeth most frequently absent are the third molars, the premolars, and the maxillary lateral incisors.

Anomaly: Any deviation from the normal.

Anterior nasal spine (ANS): The most anterior point on the floor of the nasal cavity. This is located at the midsagittal plane.

Antiseptic: Refers to agents used on living tissues to destroy or stop the growth of bacteria.

Aphthous ulcer: Small ulcer in the mouth, characterized by whitish spots around a central core. Commonly known as *canker sore*.

Apical foramen: The opening to the pulp canal at the apex (terminal end) of the root of the tooth. A three-rooted tooth would have three apical foramina.

Apprehensive: Means to be anxious or fearful about the future.

Area monitoring: The routine monitoring of the level of radiation in an area such as a room, building, space around radiation-emitting equipment, or outdoor space.

Arrested caries: Caries that are no longer active.

Asepsis: The absence of septic matter, or freedom from infection.

Atom: The smallest particle of an element that has the properties of that element. Atoms are extremely minute and are composed of a number of subatomic particles. See **Proton, Electron,** and **Neutron.**

Atomic number (also called Z number): The total number of protons in the nucleus of an atom.

Atomic weight (also called A number or mass number): The total number of protons and neutrons in the nucleus of an atom.

Attenuation: In radiography, the process by which a beam of radiation is reduced in energy when passing through matter.

Attitude: The position assumed by the body in connection with a feeling or mood.

Autotransformer: A special single-coil transformer that corrects fluctuations in the current flowing through the x-ray machine.

Background radiation: Ionizing radiation that is always present. It consists of cosmic rays from outer space, naturally occurring radiation from the earth, and radiation from radioactive materials.

Backscatter: Radiation that is deflected by scattering processes at angles greater than 90 degrees to the original direction of the beam of radiation.

Barrier: Any material that is used to prevent the transmission of infective microorganisms to the patient.

Beam indicating device (BID): A device attached to the tube head at the aperture to direct the useful beam of radiation.

Benign: Not recurrent; favorable for recovery.

Beta particle: A form of particulate radiation. High-speed negative electrons. Symbol β.

Binding energy: The internal energy within the atom that holds its components together.

Bisecting technique (bisecting-angle or short-cone technique): An exposure technique in which the central beam of radiation is directed perpendicularlv toward an imaginary line that bisects the angle formed by the recording plane of the film and the long axis of the tooth.

Bisector: The imaginary line that bisects the angle formed by the film and tooth. See **Bisecting technique.**

Biteblock: A small device, usually made of plastic, Styrofoam, or wood, which can be inserted between the teeth and held in place by biting pressure. It functions to hold the x-ray film in position while it is being exposed.

Bitewing radiograph: A radiograph that shows the crowns of both the upper and lower teeth on the same film.

Bitewing tab (bitetab): A piece of heavy paper or linen and paper that is attached at the center of the film packet and on which the patient bites to stabilize the film during a bitewing exposure.

Bloodborne pathogens: Pathogens present in blood that causes disease in humans.

Bremsstrahlung: German word for "braking radiation." The stopping or slowing of the electrons of the cathode stream as they collide with the nuclei of the target atoms.

Buccal caries: Caries that involves the buccal surface of a tooth.

Buccal-object rule: See **Clark's rule.**

Calcifications: The deposition of calcium salts from the saliva into the tissues surrounding the teeth.

Calculus: In dentistry, a deposition of mineral salts to form a concretion or ring around the root of a tooth or to cover parts of the crown. Also known as *scale* or *tartar*.

Canal: A tube-like passageway through bone that contains nerves and blood vessels. Appears radiolucent in radiographs.

Cancellous bone: See **Trabecular bone.**

Canthus: The angle at either end of the slit that separates the eyelids. In radiography, the inner canthus is the part of the slit nearest to the nose; the outer canthus is the part farthest from the nose.

Cardboard cassette: Two pieces of cardboard that are hinged on one end and have a metal clasp on the other end to tightly lock the holder after an extraoral film is inserted into a paper envelope within the holder. Used to make extraoral exposures. (Formerly called *exposure holder*.)

Caries: A disease of the calcified tissues of the teeth. The inorganic portion is demineralized and the organic tissues are destroyed.

Cassette: A rigid film holder consisting of a case with a hinged lid. Cassettes may be designated extraoral or intraoral. Most cassettes contain a pair of intensifying screens and are intended for extraoral use. Intraoral cassettes have a very limited use.

Cassette holder: The part of a panoramic-type x-ray machine that holds the cassette.

Cathode: The negative electrode (terminal) in the x-ray tube. The cathode consists of a tungsten filament wire that is set in a molybdenum focusing cup that directs the cathode stream toward the target on the anode.

Cathode stream (beam or ray): The stream of electrons traveling from the heated filament of the cathode toward the target on the anode inside the x-ray tube. This beam of electrons travels at approximately half the speed of light. The speed depends on the electromotive force (kilovoltage) that is applied.

Cemental caries (root surface caries): Caries that develops on the roots of teeth between the enamel border and the free margin of the gingiva.

Cementoma: A tumor derived from the periodontal ligament of a fully developed and erupted tooth, usually a mandibular incisor. Early cementomas are radiolucent and appear identical to radicular cysts. In the later stages of development, calcification occurs and cementomas appear as radiopaque masses surrounded by a radiolucent line. The teeth associated with cementomas are vital and need no treatment.

Cementum: One of the four basic tooth structures. The thin layer of bony tissue that covers the root of a tooth. It differs in structure from bone in that it contains a large number of Sharpey's fibers. Because the cementum layer is so thin that it blends into the dentin of the tooth, it is generally radiographically indistinguishable from dentin. When the mass of cementum is large, as in hypercementosis, it appears radiopaque.

Central beam (ray): The central portion of the primary beam of radiation.

Cephalometer: A headholder or precision instrument used to stabilize the patient's head during exposure. This usually has cephalostats or craniostats, devices used to standardize the procedure so that identical results may be obtained each time. This holds the head parallel to the film and at right angles to the radiation beam.

Cephalometric radiographs (headplates): Lateral and posteroanterior extraoral head films. Frequently used in orthodontic treatment, they are used less often in prosthodontic treatment.

Cephalometric tracings: Tracings from a cephalometric headplate made on acetate. These tracings indicate the location of various planes and points of interest to the orthodontist. The data are used to measure existing conditions and compare them with future or desirable conditions.

Cephalostat: A device used to stabilize the patient's head in a plane that is parallel to the film and at right angles to the central rays of the x-ray beam. Ear rods that can be pushed into the openings of the acoustic meatus of the ear help to accomplish this. Also called **craniostats.**

Cervical burnout: A radiolucency often observed on the mesial and distal root surfaces near the cementoenamel junction. The radiolucent appearance is caused by the concave shape of the root at the cervical line and is frequently mistaken for caries when radiographs are being diagnosed.

Chairside manner: Refers to the conduct of the dental radiographer while working at the patient's chairside.

Characteristic radiation: A form of radiation originating from an atom following removal of an electron or excitation of the atom. The wavelength of the emitted radiation is specific for the element concerned and the particular energy levels that are involved.

Charge-couple device (CCD): A CCD is a solid-state detector used in many electronic devices such as the video camera, surgical microscope, and fax machine. A CCD used in digital radiography is an image receptor found in the intraoral sensor, which converts x-rays to electrons.

Chromosomes: Structures found in the cell nuclei, which carry the hereditary materials. These are constant in number for each species.

Clark's rule (buccal-object rule): A rule for the orientation of structures portrayed in two or more radiographs exposed at a different angle.

Collimation: The restriction of the useful beam to an appropriate size; generally, to a diameter of 2 3/4 in. (7 cm) at the skin surface.

Collimator: A diaphragm, usually lead, designed to restrict the dimensions of the useful beam.

Compton effect (Compton scattering): An attenuation process for x- and gamma radiation in which a photon interacts with an orbital electron or an atom to form a displaced electron and a scattered photon (x-ray) of reduced energy.

Concrescence: A condition where the cementum of adjacent teeth is united.

Condensing osteitis: A term used to describe the formation of compact sclerotic bone within the jaws. Such areas of hardened bone are frequently seen on dental radiographs and appear more radiopaque than the surrounding bone areas. Such areas are generally irregular in shape or location. See **Osteitis.**

Condyle: A rounded knob or projection on a bone, usually where that bone articulates (joins) with another bone. In dental radiography, the condyle of the mandible articulates with the glenoid fossa (depression) of the temporal bone.

Cone (PID): A cone or cylindrical position-indicating device (PID) to indicate the direction of the central beam of radiation. The length of the cone helps to establish the desired target-surface distance. The term cone originated because formerly all PIDs were cone-shaped. The closed, pointed cone caused interference with the passage of the x-ray beam and produced a large amount of scatter radiation. All modern PIDs are open-ended. Although no longer appropriate, some still refer to the PID as a cone.

Cone cut: A term used to describe a technique error in which the central beam is not directed toward the center of the film. This produces a blank area in that part of the radiograph that was not reached by the radiation.

Contact area: The area of a tooth surface that touches another tooth. This generally refers to the mesial surface of one tooth making contact with the distal surface of the tooth behind it in the dental arch. The spot where the teeth actually touch is the contact point and the area between the contact point and the gingiva (gum) is called the embrasure.

Contamination: The soiling by contact or mixing.

Contrast: The visual differences between shades ranging from black to white in adjacent areas of the radiographic film. A radiograph that shows few shades is said to have short-scale contrast, while one that shows many variations in shade is said to possess long-scale contrast. The use of increased kilovoltage results in the production of a radiograph with long-scale contrast.

Control factors: The three factors on a x-ray machine control panel are milliamperage, exposure time, and kilovoltage.

Control panel: That portion of the x-ray machine that houses the major controls. Includes the timer, milliamperage and kilovoltage selectors.

Controlled area: A defined area in which the occupational exposure of personnel to radiation is under the supervision of the radiation protection supervisor. The dental office is designated as a controlled area.

Corpuscular radiation (particulate radiation): Minute subatomic particles such as protons, electrons, and neutrons; also alpha and beta particles. These particles occupy space; have mass and weight; and, with the exception of neutrons, have an electrical charge.

Cortical bone: The solid, outer portion of the bone. Also known as dense or compact bone. Such bone appears very radiopaque (white) on radiographs.

Coulomb (C): A unit of electrical charge; the quantity of electrical charge transferred by 1 ampere in 1 second (equal to 6.25×10^{18} electrons).

Coulombs per kilogram (C/kg): A coulomb is a unit of electrical charge (equal to 6.25×10^{18} electrons). The unit C/kg measures electrical charges (ion pairs) in a kilogram of air.

Crest: In radiation, the peak of an electromagnetic wave. The distance from crest to crest determines the wavelength—hence its penetration ability.

Cross-contamination: To contaminate from one place or person to another place or person.

Cross-sectional technique: A technique used in occlusal radiography, in which the central ray is directed toward the area of interest and parallel to the long axes of the teeth and adjacent areas.

Current: In radiation, a flow of electricity from a point of higher potential to a point of lower potential. The electric current used in most homes and dental offices is spoken of as "line current."

Cutting reducer: A chemical used to lighten a radiograph that has been accidentally overexposed or overdeveloped. The chemical removes layer after layer of the metallic silver on the radiograph until the desired density is produced.

Cyst: An epithelium-lined sac containing fluid or other fibrous or solid material. If filled with fluid or fibrous materials, cysts appear radiolucent. Common cysts in dental radiography are dentigerous, follicular, radicular (apical or periapical), and residual.

Darkroom: A room with controlled lighting where x-ray film is handled and processed.

Daylight loader: A light-shielded compartment attached to an automatic processor so films can be unwrapped in a room with white light.

"Dead-man" switch: A switch so constructed that a circuit-closing contact can only be maintained by continuous pressure by the operator.

Decay process: In radiography, the radioactive disintegration of the nucleus of an unstable atom by the emission of particles, photons of energy, or both.

Deciduous teeth: The primary dentition. Teeth that fall out or are exfoliated naturally. The deciduous dentition consists of 20 teeth—8 incisors, 4 canines, and 8 molars.

Definition: In radiography the sharpness and clarity of the outline of the structures on the image shown on the film. Poor definition is generally caused by movement of the patient, film, or the tube head during exposure.

Dens in dente: A developmental anomaly in which the enamel invaginates within the body of the tooth.

Densitometer: An instrument for measuring the amount of darkening of x-ray film, based on a photocell measuring the light transmitted through a given area of the film.

Density: In radiography, film blackening (the amount of light transmitted through a film). The simplest way to increase or decrease the density of a radiograph is to increase or decrease the milliamperage and exposure time (milliampere/second).

Dentigerous cyst: A cyst derived from the enamel organ and always associated with the crown of a tooth.

Dentin: One of the four basic tooth structures. The chief substance or tissue of the tooth that surrounds the tooth pulp. It is covered by enamel on the crown of the tooth and by cementum on the root. Appears radiopaque, but not as dense as enamel.

Dentinoenamel junction (DEJ): The junction between the dentin and enamel of a tooth.

Dentinogenesis imperfecta: A hereditary condition characterized by imperfectly formed dentin that has an opalescent or amber color.

Dentulous: With teeth; areas of the jaws having teeth.

Depth dose: The total amount of radiation absorbed at any given point inside the patient or object.

Detail: The point-by-point delineation of the minute structures visible in the shadow images on the radiograph.

Developer: The chemical solution used in film processing that makes the latent image visible.

Developer agent: Elon and hydroquinone, substances that reduce the halides in the film emulsion to metallic silver. Elon brings out the details and hydroquinone brings out the contrast in the film.

Diagnosis: The art of differentiating and determining the nature of a problem or disease. Dental radiographs are an important factor in evaluating the condition of the dentition and help in finalizing the diagnosis.

Diaphragm: A plate, usually lead, with a central aperture so placed as to restrict the useful beam. See **Collimator.**

Digital imaging: A method of making a radiographic image using a computer. A filmless imaging system. The difference between digital images and radiographs is that digital images have no physical form. Digital images exist only as bits of information in a computer file which tells the computer how to construct an image to place upon a monitor or other viewing device.

Digital radiography: A method of producing a filmless radiographic image using a sensor (instead of film) and transmitting the electronic information directly into a computer, which serves to acquire, process, store, retrieve, and display the radiographic image.

Digital subtraction: A reversing of the gray-scale as an image is viewed. Radiolucent images appear radiopaque and radiopaque images appear radiolucent.

Digitize: To convert an image into a digital form that can be processed by a computer.

Dilaceration: A tooth with a sharp bend in the root.

Direct digital imaging: A method of directly obtaining a digital image by exposing an intraoral sensor to x-rays to produce an image that can be viewed on a computer monitor.

Direct current: Electric current that flows continuously in one direction. Unidirectional current is produced in batteries but cannot be used in x-ray machines unless they are modified.

Direct theory: A theory that states cell damage results when ionizing radiation directly hits critical areas within the cell.

Disability: A physical or mental impairment that substantially limits one or more of an individual's major life activities.

Disclosure: The process of informing the patient about the risks and benefits of a treatment procedure.

Disinfect: A term used to describe those efforts made to reduce the disease-producing microorganisms to an acceptable level.

Disinfection: The act of disinfecting.

Dispenser: In radiography, a lead-lined chute or container from which unexposed film packets can be removed one at a time.

Distortion: The variation in the true size and shape of the object being radiographed.

Dosage: The radiation absorbed in a specified area of the body measured in grays or rads.

Dose: The amount of absorbed radiation in grays or rads at any given point. Measurements inside the body are difficult to make. Doses are often spoken of as absorbed, depth, entrance, erythema, exposure, skin, or surface doses.

Dose equivalent: A term used for radiation protection purposes to compare the biological effects of the various types of radiation. Dose equivalent is defined as the product of the absorbed dose times a biological effect modifying factor. Since the modifying factor for x-rays is one, the absorbed dose and the dose equivalent are equal. The units for measuring the dose equivalent are the sievert (Sv) and the rem.

Dose rate: The radiation dose received per unit of time.

Dose-response curve: A curve that shows the dose given to tissues and the response of the tissues to that dose.

Dosimeter: A small device, usually the size of a fountain pen, used to measure radiation. This device contains a small ionizing chamber and an electrometer that can be read by the person wearing the dosimeter.

Drum: A part of some panoramic-type x-ray machines to which a flexible cassette can be attached. The drum and attached film rotate when the machine is in operation.

Duplicating film: A photographic film that appears similar to x-ray film and is used to duplicate x-ray films in a contact-printer-type x-ray duplicating unit.

Duty cycle: The length of time that the x-ray tube can be energized. A consecutive series of long exposures can overheat and damage the tube.

DXTTR (dental x-ray teaching and training replica): A skull with complete dentition that is covered with simulated plastic skin to resemble the head. Contains a hinge mechanism to open and close the mouth. Used by students to practice making radiographic exposures. Also known as a *mannequin* or *phantom*. Sometimes written *Dexter*.

Dysphagia: Difficulty in swallowing.

Edentulous: Without teeth; areas of the jaws with no teeth.

Edentulous survey: A radiographic examination of the mouth of a patient without teeth. The mouth may be totally or partially edentulous.

Electric circuit: A path of electrical current.

Electric current: The flow of electrons through a conductor.

Electrical potential: See **Potential.**

Electricity: Electrons in motion.

Electrode: Either of two terminals of an electric source; in the x-ray tube, either the anode or the cathode.

Electromagnetic radiation: Forms of energy propelled by wave motion as photon. This is a combination of electric and magnetic energy. This radiation has no charge, mass, or weight and travels at the speed of light. These forms of energy differ tremendously in wavelength, frequency, and properties. For convenience they are arranged in diagrammatic form as the electromagnetic spectrum.

Electromagnetic spectrum: Types of electromagnetic energies arranged in diagrammatic form on a chart. These include radio and television waves, infrared waves, visible light, ultraviolet waves, x-rays, gamma rays, and cosmic radiations. The longer wavelengths are measured in meters and the shorter ones in centimeters or angstroms.

Electromotive force: The difference in potential between the cathode and the anode in the x-ray tube (generally expressed in kilovolts).

Electron: A small, negatively charged particle of the atom containing much energy and little mass.

Electron cloud: A mass of free electrons that hovers around the filament wire of the cathode when it is heated to incandescence. The number of free electrons increases as the milliamperage is increased.

Electron shells: See **Energy levels.**

Electrostatic: Electric charges at rest (static electricity).

Element: In chemistry, a simple substance that cannot be decomposed by chemical means.

Elongation: A term used in radiography to refer to a distortion of the image in which the tooth structures appear longer than the anatomical size. This is most often caused by insufficient vertical angulation of the central beam.

Embrasure: The space between the sloping proximal surfaces of the teeth. The space may diverge facially, lingually, occlusally, or apically. The interdental papillae normally fill most of the apical embrasures.

Empathy: The ability to share in another's emotions or feelings.

Emulsion: The coating on radiographic film, a gelatinous solution containing silver halides.

Emulsion speed: The sensitivity of the film to the radiation exposure.

Enamel: One of the four basic tooth structures. The white, compact, and very hard substance that covers the dentin of the crown of the teeth. Appears very radiopaque on the radiographs.

Endodontia: The branch of dentistry concerned with the prevention, diagnosis, and treatment of diseases and injuries of the dental pulp and periapical tissues.

Energy: In physics, the ability to do work and overcome resistance.

Energy levels (electron shells or orbits): A term used in chemistry and physics to denote spherical levels containing the electrons of the atom.

Enhancement: Intensification of detail, making a radiograph easier to interpret.

Enhancer: A device that brings out details on a radiograph. Contains focusing devices and magnifying lenses.

Entrance dose (skin dose): Radiation dosage at the point where it enters the patient.

Erythema dose: Radiation overdose that produces temporary redness of the skin.

Exit dose: The absorbed dose delivered by a beam of radiation to the surface through which the beam emerges from an object.

Exostosis: A bony growth projecting outward from the surface of a bone or tooth. Occasionally encountered on the palate or the lingual surface of the mandible

Exposure: A measure of ionization produced in air by x- or gamma radiation. It is the sum of the electrical charges of all of the ions of one sign produced in air when all electrons liberated by photons in a volume element of air are completely stopped in air, divided by the mass of air in the volume present. The units of exposure are coulombs per kilogram (C/kg) and the roentgen (R).

Exposure chart: A chart listing the exposure factors (milliamperage, exposure time, and kilovoltage) for each radiographic procedure.

Exposure factors: The exposure factors are milliamperage (mA), exposure time, and kilovoltage (kVp).

Exposure incident: An incident that involves contact with blood or other potentially infectious materials and that results from procedures performed by dental personnel.

Exposure rate: The exposure per unit of time.

Exposure time: The time interval, expressed in seconds or impulses, that x-rays are produced.

Extension arm: Flexible arm from which the tube head of the x-ray machine is suspended.

Extension cone (extension tube): A long cone- or tube-shaped position indicating device.

External auditory meatus: An opening in the temporal bone located superior and anterior to the mastoid process.

Extraoral: Outside the mouth.

Extraoral radiograph: A radiograph exposed outside the mouth.

Farmer's solution: A chemical reducer used to lighten a dark overexposed or overdeveloped film.

Fast film (high speed): Fast film requires less radiation for exposure.

Filament: The spiral tungsten coil in the focusing cup of the cathode of the x-ray tube.

Film badge: A monitoring device containing a special type of film, which when properly developed and interpreted, gives a measurement of the exposure received during the time the badge was worn. The film badge has been replaced by the thermoluminescent dosimeter (TLD).

Film hanger: A stainless steel hanger equipped with clips used to hold films during processing.

Film holder: A mechanical device used to hold and stabilize dental x-ray film in the mouth.

Film loop: A thin, stiff paper constructed in such a manner that a film packet can be slid into the loop portion to hold the film in position while the patient bites on the tab portion. Used in bitewing radiography. Also known as a *bitewing loop*.

Film mount: A celluloid, plastic, or cardboard holder with frames or windows so arranged that any desired size and number of radiographs can be fastened to the mount for display and viewing of the films.

Film mounting: The placement of dental radiographs in a film mount.

Film packet: The intraoral film that is wrapped and enclosed for dental use by the manufacturer. It contains one or two films, a dark protective paper on either side, a thin sheet of lead foil on the back side of the film, and a semi-moistureproof outer wrap.

Film placement: The act of positioning the film packet in the patient's mouth. In horizontal placement, the widest dimension of the film is positioned horizontally, whereas in vertical film placement, the widest film dimension is positioned vertically.

Film safe: A lead-lined receptacle for storing exposed dental film packets.

Film sensitivity: See **Emulsion speed.**

Filter: Absorbing material, usually aluminum, placed in the path of the beam of radiation to remove a high percentage of the low energy (longer wavelength) x-rays.

Filtration: The use of absorbers for selectively absorbing or screening out the low-energy x-rays from the primary beam. See **Added filtration, Inherent filtration,** and **Total filtration.**

Fistula: A narrow canal or tubular channel leading from an abscess or a diseased lesion within the alveolar bone or soft tissues to the outside of the oral membrane. Fluid in the form of pus or some other serous exudate may be contained within the fistula. Often the fistula leads to a parulis, also known as a *gumboil.*

Fixer: In radiography or photography, a solution of chemicals that stops the action of the developer and makes the image permanently visible.

Fixing agent: Sodium thiosulfate, also known as "hypo" or hyposulfite of sodium. It is one of several chemical ingredients of the fixer solution and functions to remove all unexposed and any remaining undeveloped silver bromide grains from the emulsion.

Flexible cassette: A cassette made of plastic or other flexible material so that it can be wrapped around the drum of certain types of panoramic x-ray machines.

Fluorescence: The emission of a glowing light by certain mineral salts when they are struck by particular wavelengths. In radiography, the calcium tungstate that is in the emulsion of the intensifying screen of cassettes glows and gives off a bluish light when the crystals are struck by the x-ray photons.

Focal spot: A small area on the target on the anode toward which the electrons from the focusing cup of the cathode are directed. X-rays originate at the focal spot.

Focal trough: A term describing that area of the dental anatomy that is reproduced distinctly on a panoramic radiograph. The size and shape of the focal trough vary with each panoramic x-ray machine.

Focusing cup: A curved device around the cathode wire filament that is designed to focus the free electrons toward the tungsten target of the anode.

Fog: A darkening of the finished radiograph caused by any of several factors such as old or contaminated processing solutions, exposure to chemical fumes, faulty safelight, or scatter radiation.

Follicular cyst (dentigerous cyst): A cyst associated with the enamel follicle.

Foramen: A naturally formed hole or passage through a bone or tooth. Often the opening for a canal through which blood vessels and nerves pass. Appears radiolucent on radiograph.

Foreign body: Any object or material not normally found in the area.

Foreshortening: A term used in radiology to refer to a distortion of the image in which the tooth structures appear shorter than their actual anatomical size. This is most often caused by excessive vertical angulation of the central beam.

Fossa: A depression or hollow area on a tooth or bone. If large enough, it will appear as a radiolucent area on a radiograph.

Fracture: The breaking of a part, usually appears as a radiolucency.

Fracture line: A break in a bone that appears radiolucent on the radiograph.

Frankfort plane: The horizontal plane between the porion and orbitale.

Frequency: The number of crests of a wavelength passing a given point per second.

Full-mouth survey: The complete radiographic examination of the mouth in which a film is positioned periapically in each major tooth area. This normally entails a minimum of 14 films, and may be over 20 films. Generally such a survey also includes bitewing films.

Furcation: The area between the roots of multirooted teeth.

Fusion: A condition where the dentin and one other dental tissue of adjacent teeth are united.

Gag reflex: A protective mechanism that serves to clear the airway of obstruction.

Gagging: Making an involuntary effort to vomit.

Gamma rays: A form of electromagnetic radiation with properties identical to x-rays. Usually produced spontaneously in the form of emission from radioactive substances.

Gelatin: A component of the film emulsion coating the film base in which the halide crystals are suspended.

Geiger counter: A radiation monitoring device that counts the ionizing particles that pass through it. A needlelike electrode inside a gas-filled chamber sets up a current in an electrical field whenever the gas is ionized by radiation.

Gemination: A single tooth bud divides and forms two teeth.

Generalized bone loss: Bone loss that occurs evenly throughout the dental arches.

Genes: The fundamental units of inheritance, arranged on the chromosomes and carrying the individual traits of the organisms.

Genetic cells: The cells contained within the testes and ovaries, containing the genes.

Genetic effects: Radiation effects upon the genes and hence upon future generations. It is known that massive exposure of the genes to radiation may produce mutations.

Genial tubercles: An anatomical landmark situated near the midline on the lingual surface of the mandible about halfway between the alveolar crest and the inferior border of the mandible. There are four of them, and on a radiograph they appear like a very small doughnut-shaped, radiopaque ring. The lingual foramen is located in the center of this ring.

Geometric unsharpness: Poor image definition due to the penumbra.

Gingivitis: Inflammation of the gingiva.

Glenoid fossa: A depression on the temporal bone. The condyle of the mandible fits into this fossa to form the temporomandibular joint. This landmark is seen only on extraoral radiographs.

Globulomaxillary cyst: A cyst arising between the maxillary lateral incisor and the canine (cuspid).

Granuloma: A tumor or neoplasm made up of granulation tissue. Often follows an abscess. Is usuallv round or oval and surrounded by a fibrous capsule. Appears radiolucent on a radiograph.

Gray (Gy): A unit for measuring absorbed dose. One gray equals 1 joule (unit of energy) per kilogram of tissue. One gray equals 100 rads.

Gray scale: Refers to the total number of shades of gray visible in an image.

Grenz rays: The longest wavelength of the x-rays, known as soft radiation because they have little penetrating power.

Grid: A device used in extraoral radiography to prevent scatter radiation from affecting the film.

Half-life: The period required for the disintegration of half of the atoms in a sample of some specific radioactive substance.

Half-value layer (HVL): The thickness of a specified material that, when introduced into the path of a given beam of radiation, reduces the exposure rate by half.

Halide: A compound of a halogen (astatine, bromine, chlorine, fluorine, or iodine) with another element or radical. In radiography a halide, usually bromide of silver, is suspended in the gelatin that coats the film base.

Hamular process (hamulus): A very small hooklike process of bone that extends downward and slightly backward from the sphenoid bone. It appears radiopaque and can occasionally be seen posterior to the maxillary tuberosity.

Hardening agent (hardener): Potassium alum, one of the chemicals of the fixing solution. It functions to shrink and harden the wet emulsion.

Hard radiation: Rays of high energy and extremely short wavelengths. Essential for dental radiography.

Head positioner: A device used on panoramic and cephalometric x-ray machines to stabilize the head into the most favorable position.

Hemostat: A surgical instrument used as an intraoral film holder.

Herpes labialis: An inflammatory skin disease characterized by the formation of small vesicles in clusters on the lips. Often called *fever sores* or *blisters*.

Herringbone pattern (also called tire-track pattern): An image on a radiograph when the film has been placed in the mouth backwards and exposed.

High-voltage transformer (step-up transformer): A device consisting of two metal cores and coils so positioned within the circuitry of the tube head that it is capable of increasing the potential of the line current to the high kilovoltage that is required to produce x-radiation.

Horizontal angulation: The direction of the central beam in a horizontal plane. Faulty horizontal angulation is the main cause of overlapping the proximal structures during exposure.

Horizontal bone loss: Bone loss that occurs in a plane parallel to the cementoenamel junctions of adjacent teeth.

Horizontal placement: See **Film placement.**

Hypercementosis: An excessive development of the cementum of the tooth. It is usually, but not necessarily, confined to the apical portion of the root. Only occurs on vital teeth and is most frequently encountered on premolars. Area involved appears radiopaque.

Identification dot: A small circular embossed mark on the corner of each x-ray film. The raised side of this convexity is always placed toward the side facing the x-ray beam. The identification dot makes it possible to determine whether the exposure was made on the patient's right or left side.

Image: In radiography, the duplicate in outline form of the structures exposed to radiation. A latent (invisible) image forms on the film when it is exposed. This latent image becomes visible after development and final processing.

Image magnification: An enlargement of the structures shown on the radiograph over their actual size. Such enlargement is greatest when the target of a x-ray machine is closer to the structures being x-rayed, and is decreased when distance is greater.

Image receptor: The component of an imaging system that the x-rays strike. In radiography, the image receptor is the film.

Impacted tooth (impaction): A tooth that is embedded in the alveolar bone in such a manner that its eruption is prevented. An impaction may be partial or total.

Impulse: In dental radiography, a measure of exposure time. Many x-ray machines are calibrated to make the exposure in impulses instead of fractions of a second. There are 60 impulses per second.

Incandescence: In radiography, the stage in which the tungsten filament in the cathode becomes red-hot with heat and glows, thus liberating free electrons that swarm around the glowing wire to form the electron cloud.

Incipient: Beginning to appear or exist.

Incipient caries: Caries beginning to appear or exist.

Incisive foramen: An important maxillary landmark. It is situated at the midline of the palate immediately behind the central incisors. The nasopalatine nerve and vessels emerge from it. The shape varies but is usually seen as a round pea-shaped radiolucent area. When faulty horizontal angulation is used, the image of the foramen may be superimposed over the apex of the root of the central incisor. It may then be mistaken for an abscess or a cyst.

Indicator light: A light on the control panel of an x-ray machine that illuminates when the machine is turned on.

Indicator rod (arm): One of the components of the Rinn XCP and BAI film holders. When properly assembled and positioned in the mouth, this metal rod serves as a guide in determining the correct angulation of the position indicating device (PID).

Indirect digital imaging: A method of obtaining a digital image in which an existing radiograph is scanned or photographed and then converted into a digital image.

Indirect theory: A theory that states cell damage results indirectly when x-rays cause the formation of toxins in the cell; the toxins in turn cause the cell damage.

Infection control: The prevention and reduction of disease-causing (pathogenic) microorganisms.

Infectious waste: Waste (such as blood, blood products, and contaminated sharps) that may contain pathogens.

Inferior border of the mandible: The dense layer of cortical bone that forms the lower portion of the body of the mandible. It appears very radiopaque on the radiograph.

Informed consent: Permission given by a patient after being informed of the details of a treatment procedure.

Inherent filtration: The filtration built into the machine by the manufacturer. This includes the glass x-ray tube envelope, the insulating materials of the tube head, and the materials that seal the port.

Intensifying screen: A card or plastic sheet coated with calcium tungstate or similar fluorescent salt crystals and positioned in the cassette so that it contacts the film. When exposed to radiation, the fluorescent salts glow, giving off a blue or green light that along with the radiation causes the latent image to form faster than is possible when radiation alone is used.

Intensity: Intensity is the total energy of the x-ray beam. Intensity of the x-ray beam is the product of the number of x-rays (quantity) and energy of each x-ray (quality) per unit of area per time of exposure.

Interpret: To explain or to disclose meaning.

Interpretation: In dental radiography, the ability to read what is revealed by the radiograph. The final interpretation is the responsibility of the dentist. Dental auxiliaries should be capable of making a preliminary interpretation.

Interproximal: Between two adjacent surfaces.

Interproximal caries: Caries found between two adjacent teeth.

Interproximal radiograph (bitewing radiograph): A radiograph that shows the crowns of both the upper and lower teeth on the same film.

Intraoral: Inside the mouth.

Intraoral cassette: A very small cassette holding an occlusal film. Its purpose is to reduce exposure time through the action of the intensifying screens.

Intraoral radiograph: A radiograph produced when the film is placed within the mouth and exposed.

Intrex™: Trade name of an x-ray machine that has the tube in a recessed position within the tube head.

Inverse square law: A rule stating that the intensity of radiation is inversely proportional to the square of the distance from the source of the radiation to the point of measurement.

Ion: An electrically charged particle, either negative or positive.

Ion pair: A pair of ions, one positive and one negative.

Ionization: The formation of ion pairs.

Ionization chamber: An instrument for measured ionizing radiation.

Ionizing radiation: Radiation that is capable of producing ions.

Irradiation: The exposure of an object or a person to radiation. This term can be applied to radiations of various wavelengths, such as infrared rays, ultraviolet rays, x-rays, and gamma rays.

Isotope: An alternate form of an element, having the same number of protons but a different number of neutrons inside the nucleus. Many isotopes are radioactive.

Kilovolt (kV): A unit of electromotive force, equal to 1,000 volts. High kilovoltage is essential for the production of dental x-rays.

Kilovolt peak (kVp): The crest value in kilovolts of the potential difference of a pulsating generator.

Kinetic energy: The energy possessed by a mass because of its motion.

Lamina dura: A thin, hard layer of cortical bone that lines the dental alveolus. Appears as a thin radiopaque line around the roots of the teeth on dental radiograph.

Laminography: A type of body-section radiography (tomography). *Lamina* means "thin layer" and *graphy* means "to record."

Landmarks: In dental radiography this term refers to a number of structures located on the bones of the head or face and certain points on the soft tissues of the face or the oral cavity.

Latent image: The invisible image produced when the film is exposed to the x-ray photons. This image remains invisible until the film is processed.

Latent period: The time between exposure to radiation and the first clinically observable symptoms. The word latent means "hidden."

Lateral headplate: Large extraoral film placed against either side of the head and parallel to it.

Lateral jaw survey: An extraoral exposure of either side of the patient's face that produces an image of both the maxilla and mandible on the same film.

Lateral skull survey: A large radiograph of either side of the skull. See **Lateral headplate.**

Law of B and T (Bergonie and Tribondeau): States "the radiosensitivity of cells and tissues is directly proportional to their reproductive capacity and inversely proportional to their degree of differentiation."

LD 50-30 (median lethal) dose: The dose of radiation that will be lethal for 50% of a large population during a specified length of time, usually 30 days.

Lead equivalence: The thickness of a material that affords the same degree of attenuation to radiation as a specified thickness of lead.

Lead protective apron: Apron made of lead or lead-equivalent materials. This covers patients' gonadal areas to protect them from radiation.

Leakage radiation: The x-rays that escape out of the tube head at places other than the port.

Lethal dose: The amount of radiation that is sufficient to cause the death of an organism.

Liable: To be legally obligated to make good any loss or damage that may occur.

Light fog: Clouding or darkening of radiographic film through accidental exposure to light or prolonged exposure to a safelight.

Line current: The electric current normally passing through the electric lines in most homes and offices. In the United States, this is generally a 110-volt alternating current.

Line focus principle: The method by which the size of the focal spot is reduced to the desired size by the manufacturer. By facing the target at an angle toward the cathode filament, the electron beam is focused into a narrow rectangle on the anode. When viewed from below, as from the position of the film packet, the rectangular area looks like a small square.

Line switch: The toggle switch that is used to turn the x-ray machine on or off.

Lingual caries: Caries that involves the lingual surface of a tooth.

Lingual foramen: A very small opening through which a branch of the incisive artery emerges. It is located in the center of the genial tubercles on the lingual side of the mandible. See also **Genial tubercles.**

Localized bone loss: Bone loss that occurs in isolated areas.

Long-scale contrast: The variations in contrast, with many shades of gray, shown on radiographs exposed with high kilovoltage.

Low-voltage transformer (step-down transformer): A device consisting of two metal cores and coils so positioned within the circuitry of the tube head that it is capable of decreasing the line voltage to between 3 and 12 volts. Such voltage is required in the cathode to warm up the filament wire.

Mach band effect: An optical illusion first described by Ernst Mach in 1865. This effect occurs along boundaries of sharp contrast. There appears to be a darker band along the edge of radiolucent areas and, similarly, a lighter band along the edge of radiopaque areas. The mach band effect is an edge enhancement, created in the eye, which does not result from an actual density change in the film emulsion

Macrodontia: Very large teeth.

Magnification (enlargement): Refers to a radiographic image that appears larger than the actual size of the object it represents.

Malignant: Tendency to progress in virulence; tendency to spread and go from bad to worse.

Malpractice: Improper practice. Malpractice results when one is negligent.

Malposed tooth: A tooth not in normal location.

Mandibular canal: A long canal extending from the mandibular foramen on the medial aspect of the ramus of the mandible to the mental foramen on the lateral aspect of the body of the mandible. The canal carries nerves and blood vessels that supply most of the teeth in the mandible. The canal appears radiolucent. A thin radiopaque line above and below it on the radiograph outline the cortical bone that lines the canal.

Mandibular plane: A term used in cephalometric radiography. The line of the inferior border of the mandible from the gonion to the menton.

Maxillary sinus: The radiolucent cavity seen within the maxilla apical to the maxillary posterior teeth.

Maxillary tuberosity: A radiopaque prominence of bone on the distal portion of the maxillary alveolar ridge.

Maximum permissible dose (MPD): The maximum accumulated dose that persons who are occupationally exposed may have at any given time of their life.

Maximum permissible dose equivalent: For radiation purposes, the maximum dose equivalent that a person or body part is allowed to receive in a stated period of time. It is the dose of ionizing radiation that, in the light of present knowledge, is not expected to cause detectable body damage to average persons at any time during their lifetime. For whole-body radiation, this is currently established at 0.05 Sv/y (5 rems/y) for radiation workers. Sometimes called radiation protection guide (RPG).

Mean tangent: The average point where several curved surfaces touch if a ruler is held against them. The labial or buccal surfaces of all teeth have their most prominent point toward the lips or the cheeks and curve toward the mesial or distal. A mean tangent could be established by using a small ruler or any straight edge and attempting to align as many of the teeth as possible. Occasionally four or even five of the posterior teeth will touch the ruler at some point. An imaginary line can be substituted for the ruler, and that is the mean tangent. To establish correct horizontal angulation, the central rays are directed at right angles to the mean tangent

Meatus: An opening in the bone. The acoustic meatus (the outer opening of the canal of the ear) is often observed on extraoral dental radiographs as a small radiolucent circle.

Median palatine suture: An irregular line formed by the junction of the palatine processes of the right and left maxillae. On radiographs it appears as a thin radiolucent line running vertically between the roots of the maxillary incisors.

Mental foramen: An opening through which the mental nerve and related blood vessels emerge on the lateral aspect of the body of the mandible. The location of this foramen varies and is often not shown on radiographs. When visible, it appears as a small round radiolucent area near the roots of the mandibular premolars.

Microdontia: Very small teeth.

Midsagittal plane (midsagittal line): An imaginary vertical line or plane passing through the center of the body that divides it into a right and left half.

Milliammeter: A device on the control panel of many x-ray machines for determining and controlling the number of milliamperes of electric current.

Milliampere (mA): The milliampere is one thousandth of an ampere. In radiography, the milliamperage determines the number of electrons available at the filament. See **Ampere.**

Milliampere second (mAs): The relationship between the milliamperage used and the exposure time in seconds. When one is increased, the other must be correspondingly decreased if the density of the exposed radiograph is to remain the same.

Milliroentgen (mR): One-thousandth of a roentgen. See **Roentgen.**

Modifying factor (quality factor): A factor used for radiation protection purposes and in radiation biology to account for the difference in the biological effectiveness of the various types of radiation (x-, gamma, alpha, beta, etc). Some radiations (such as alpha particles) cause more biological damage than others (such as x-rays). The modifying (quality) factor is used to convert absorbed dose to dose equivalent. The modifying factor for x-rays is 1, for alpha particles it is 10.

Molecule: A chemical combination of two or more atoms that forms the smallest particle of a substance that retains the properties of that substance.

Monitoring: In radiation, the use of any of several devices to determine whether an area is within safe radiation limits or whether a person's exposure is within permissible limits. See **Area monitoring** and **Personnel monitoring.**

Monitoring badge: A device worn by a radiation worker to measure the amount of radiation received in a given period of time. This is most often accomplished by wearing a **thermoluminescent dosimeter (TLD).**

Mount: To place radiographs in the film mount for display purposes.

Movement: Movement or motion of the film, patient, or tube head during radiographic exposure that results in a less sharp image.

Mutation: A change in the hereditary pattern of an organism. The change itself, if the organism survives, becomes hereditary. It is currently believed that any radiation exposure to the reproductive cells is capable of causing some form of mutation.

Mylohyoid ridge: A ridge of bone running diagonally downward and forward on the medial aspect of the ramus of the mandible to near the apices of the molar roots. This bony ridge serves for muscle attachments and parallels the oblique ridge, but on the lingual surface and about 1/4 in (6 mm) lower. This ridge is not always seen on radiographs; when visible, the ridge is radiopaque.

Negative: A photographic or radiographic film wherein light and dark areas of the subject are shown in reverse.

Negative angulation (negative vertical angulation or **minus angulation):** Angulation achieved by pointing the tip or end of the PID upward from a horizontal plane.

Negative ion: An ion that has a negative electric charge. See **Ion.**

Negligence: Failure to use a reasonable amount of care when failure results in injury or damage to another.

Neutron: One form of corpuscular radiation (particulate), or subatomic particle. A neutron has no electric charge and has about the same mass as a proton.

Nonmetalic restoration: A restoration that does not contain metal and appears radiolucent on the radiograph.

Nonodontogenic cyst: A cyst that arises from epithelium other than that associated with tooth formation.

Nonscreen film (no-screen film): A form of extraoral film that has an extra-thick coating of emulsion and is sensitive to radiation. See **Screen film.**

Nutrient canal: A small tube-like passageway through bone that contains blood vessels and nerves. It appears radiolucent in radiographs.

Object: In dental radiography, whatever is being radiographed, usually a tooth or teeth.

Object-film distance: The distance between the object being radiographed and the film.

Oblique ridge: A diagonal ridge of bone on the lateral aspect of the mandible. The ridge runs downward and forward from the anterior border of the ramus to the level of the cervical portion of the molar and premolar roots. This landmark appears very radiopaque.

Occipital protuberance: A bulge or prominence at the center of the outer surface of the squamous portion of the occipital bone. The location of this protuberance can be determined by palpating the back of the patient's head.

Occlusal caries: Caries found on the occlusal (chewing) surface of posterior teeth.

Occlusal plane: The plane between the maxillary and the mandibular teeth.

Occlusal radiographs: Radiographs produced by placing the film along the incisal or occlusal plane and having the patient stabilize it by biting down on it. In addition to the teeth, occlusal radiographs may show surrounding maxillary or mandibular bone structures. Depending on the film placement and angle of exposure, cross-sectional or topographic radiographs are produced. See **Cross-sectional technique** and **Topographical technique.**

Occupational exposure (infection control definition): A worker (dental personnel) coming in contact with blood, saliva, or other infectious material that involves the skin, eye, or mucus membrane.

Odontogenic cyst: A cyst that arises from epithelial cells associated with the development of a tooth.

Odontoma: A tumor of odontogenic origin in which enamel and dentin are formed. The odontoma may contain soft tissues that appear radiolucent and also contain a hard calcified mass, sometimes resembling a tooth, which appears radiopaque on the radiograph. *Compound odontoma* refers to odontogenic tissues in normal relationship that resemble teeth. *Complex odontoma* denotes odontogenic tissues arranged in a haphazard manner with no resemblance to normal tooth formation. *Compound-complex odontoma* is a mixture of the two types.

Operator (radiographer): The person operating any x-ray equipment to make exposures.

Oral radiographic survey: An examination of the teeth based on one or more radiographs of the dental area of interest.

Oral radiography: All the procedures needed to produce radiographs of the teeth or head. These include adjustments of the x-ray machine, preparation of the patient, generation of x-radiation, and film processing interpretation.

Orbitale (Or): The lowest point on the contour of the boney orbit.

Orthopantomograph™: A trade name for a panoramic-type x-ray machine produced by Siemens Corporation.

Ossifications: The pathological or abnormal conversion of soft tissues into bone.

Osteitis: A bone inflammation. In radiography, the term refers to changes in bone density resulting from disease, trauma, or infection. In **rarefying osteitis,** the bone appears more radiolucent, whereas in **condensing osteitis,** the bone structures appear more radiopaque.

Osteoma: Benign tumors composed of bone. They vary greatly in size and appear radiopaque.

Osteomyelitis: An acute or chronic inflammation of the bone or bone marrow, which may sometimes be visible on radiographs.

Output: The amount of radiation that an x-ray machine produces, calculated in coulombs per kilogram per second (roentgens per second), measured at the open end of the PID.

Overlapping: A term used in radiography to refer to a distortion of the tooth image in which the structures of one tooth are superimposed over the structures of the adjacent tooth. This is most often caused by faulty horizontal angulation of the central beam.

Oxidation: In dental radiography, the process during which the chemicals of the developing and fixing solutions combine with oxygen and lose their strength.

Oxidizing agent: Any substance that produces oxidation in another substance.

Panelipse™: A trade name for a panoramic-type x-ray machine produced by the Gendex Corporation.

Panoramic radiography: Radiographic procedures with a special-purpose x-ray machine that uses a fixed position of the x-ray source, object, and film to produce a radiograph of the entire dentition and surrounding structures on a single film.

Panorex™: A trade name for a panoramic x-ray machine produced by Keystone X-ray, Inc. The radiographs taken by this machine can be easily recognized by a .5-in. (12-mm) white area in the middle of the film.

Pantomography: The art of making graphic recordings of tissue contours on radiographic film.

Paralleling technique (long-cone technique or right-angle technique): In radiography, an intraoral technique that requires a biteblock or some type of film holder to hold the film packet parallel to the teeth while the central beam of radiation is directed perpendicularly (at right angles) toward the teeth and the film.

Parenteral exposure: Exposure to blood that results from puncturing the skin barrier.

Particulate radiation: See **Corpuscular radiation.**

Parulis: A raised swollen area indicating an abscess of the gum. Often called a *gumboil.* A fistula often connects the parulis with the core of the abscess at the apex of the root.

Pathogen: A disease-causing microorganism.

Patient education: This term refers to the duty and responsibility of every member of the dental health team—informing the public, specifically dental patients, about benefits of oral health, preventive dentistry, and good dental care. As used in this text, patient education refers to providing the patient with necessary information on the value of dental radiography and the safety measures employed in the dental office to limit the effects of radiation exposure.

Pediatric film: The smaller sizes of film packets commonly used for radiographs of children's teeth.

Penumbra: In radiography, a partial shadow or fuzzy outline around the image.

Periapical: Around the apex of a tooth.

Periapical abscess: A collection of pus located around the apex of a nonvital tooth (appears radiolucent).

Periapical cyst: An epithelial-lined sac located around the apex of a nonvital tooth (appears radiolucent).

Periapical granuloma: A localized mass of granulation tissue located around the apex of a nonvital tooth (appears radiolucent).

Periapical radiograph: A radiograph that shows the entire tooth or teeth and surrounding tissues. *Peri* means "around" and *apical* is the root end of the tooth.

Periodontal: Around a tooth.

Periodontal disease: Disease that affects the tissues around the teeth.

Periodontal ligament: A thin but very dense and strong fibrous tissue that binds the cementum of the tooth to the lamina dura that lines the alveolus. It not only attaches the tooth to the alveolar bone but also acts as a cushion. Radiographically, the periodontal ligament appears as a thin radiolucent line between the lamina dura and the root.

Periodontal ligament space: The space between the root of a tooth and the lamina dura.

Periodontitis: Inflammation of the periodontium.

Periodontium: Tissues that invest and support the teeth (gingiva and alveolar bone).

Personnel monitoring: The occasional or routine measuring of the amount of radiation to which a person working around radiation has been exposed during a given period of time. This is most often accomplished by wearing a monitoring badge, such as a thermoluminescent dosimeter (TLD).

Phantom: In dental radiography, a device the size and shape of the head and usually containing parts of the skull and all of the teeth. This is covered with plastic and other materials that resemble the lips, cheeks, tongue, and other facial structures. These materials scatter x-radiation in the same ways as the tissues of the body do. The jaws are opened and closed by means of mechanical devices to enable the student to position and expose films in lieu of patients. See **DXTTR.**

Phleboliths: Calcified masses that are observed as round or oval bodies in the soft tissues of the cheeks.

Phosphors: Fluorescent crystals, usually calcium tungstate, used in the emulsion that coats the intensifying screens. These give off light when subjected to radiation.

Photoelectric effect: An attenuation process for x- and gamma radiation in which a photon interacts with an orbital electron of an atom. All of the energy of the photon is absorbed by the displaced electron in the form of kinetic energy.

Photon (x-ray photon): A quantum of energy. Both x-rays and gamma rays are photons.

PID: See **Position-indicating device.**

Pixel (*pix*, plural of *pic*ture; *el*, *el*ement): Any of the small discrete elements that together constitute an image. Discrete units of information (also termed *picture element*). Any of the detecting elements of a charge-coupled device used as an optical sensor.

Plane: In dental radiography, a level surface or a straight line connecting two anatomic landmarks.

Pocket dosimeter: A small personal monitoring device that resembles a fountain pen in size and can be clipped to the garment to measure radiation received. See **Dosimeter.**

Point of entry: The spot on the surface of the face toward which the central beam of radiation is directed when making intraoral exposures.

Polychromatic: A term derived from the Greek meaning, "having many colors." This term is used in dental radiography to describe the x-ray beam that is composed of many different wavelengths.

Porion (P): The midpoint on the upper edge of the external auditory meatus.

Port: An opening in the tube head that is covered with a permanent seal of glass, beryllium, or aluminum through which the x-rays leave the tube head. The port is opposite the window in the x-ray tube and is the place where the PID attaches to the tube head.

Position indicating device (PID): Any device attached to the tube head at the aperture to direct the useful beam of radiation. It can be long or short, pointed, cylindrical or rectangular, and open or closed.

Positive angulation (positive vertical angulation or plus angulation): Angulation achieved by pointing the end of the PID downward from a horizontal plane.

Positive ion: An ion that has a positive electric charge. See **Ion.**

Posteroanterior radiograph: A radiograph of the head in which the x-ray film is in front of the face and the x-ray machine is behind the patient; the x-ray beam is directed at the occipital bone and passes through the skull from the back to the front.

Potential: In radiography and electricity, the difference in relative voltage or amount of electric pressure between the negative and positive electrodes.

Preservative: In radiography and photography, one of the chemicals (sodium sulfite) used in both the developer and fixer solutions to slow down the rapid rate of oxidation and prevent spoilage of the solution.

Pressure mark: A black (radiolucent) line that appears on a processed film at a point where the film packet has been bent or subjected to excessive pressure.

Preventive radiation: X-rays, through their ability to penetrate tissues, enable the dentist to look within the jaws and the teeth to discover conditions that can be remedied when recognized in time, thus preventing greater future problems to the dental patient. Preventive radiation is also practiced by the medical profession for diagnosis and therapy.

Primary beam (primary radiation or useful beam): The original undeflected useful beam of radiation that emanates at the focal spot of the x-ray tube and emerges through the aperture of the tube head.

Primary protective barrier: A barrier sufficient to attenuate the useful beam to the required degree.

Primary radiation: See **Primary beam.**

Process: In dental anatomy, any prominent outgrowth of bone. May be rounded or pointed. Processes of dental importance include alveolar, coronoid, hamular, (hamlets), mastoid, and styloid. These appear radiopaque.

Processing: The act of bringing out the latent image and making it permanently visible. Includes the following darkroom procedures: developing, rinsing, fixing, washing, and drying. See **Developer** and **Selective reduction.**

Processing tank: A metal or hard rubber receptacle divided into compartments for developer solution, water rinse, and fixer solution and used to process radiographs.

Profile radiographs (lateral head plates): Radiographs that record the shadow images of the soft tissues forming the facial curves and the features of the profile and those forming the tongue and palate of the oral cavity. They are used to indicate the facial contours and to indicate the relationship of the soft to the bony tissues.

Protection survey: An evaluation of the radiation hazards incidental to the production, use, or existence of sources of radiation under a specific set of conditions.

Protective apron: An apron made of radiation-absorbing material (lead equivalent), used to protect the patient from unnecessary radiation exposure. See **Lead protective apron.**

Protective barrier: A barrier of radiation-absorbing material used to reduce radiation exposure. See **Primary protective barrier** and **Secondary protective barrier.**

Protective tube housing (diagnostic tube housing): An x-ray tube housing so constructed that the leakage radiation measured at a distance of 1 m from the target does not exceed 1 millisievert (100 millirems) in 1 hour when the tube is operated at its maximum, continuous-rated current for the maximum-rated tube potential.

Proton: A subatomic particle of the atom. The proton is contained in the nucleus and has a positive electrical charge. The proton has mass and weight. The number of protons determines the chemical element.

Pulp polyp: A vascular outgrowth of the pulp into the oral cavity when the crown of the tooth is largely destroyed by dental caries. Polyps are frequently observed on children between the ages of six and ten. As a rule such polyps are easily seen on visual examination but have no specific outline on the radiograph because they blend into the radiolucency as an occlusal extension of the pulp chamber.

Pulp stone: Calcifications that appear in the pulp chamber of the teeth, caused by an abnormal disposition of calcium salts. Often described as nodules or denticles. Seen on radiographs as one or more small radiopaque irregularly shaped rounded masses within the pulp chamber.

Qualified expert: In dental radiation-monitoring terminology, a person having the knowledge and training to measure ionizing radiation, to evaluate safety techniques, and to advise regarding radiation protection needs of dental x-ray installations.

Quality control: A term used to describe a series of tests to assure that the radiographic system is functioning properly and that the radiographs produced are of an acceptable level of quality.

Quality factor (Q): A factor used for radiation protection purposes that accounts for differences in biological effectiveness among the different kinds of radiation, For x-rays, $Q = 1$.

Quantum: In quantum theory, an elemental unit of energy. The theory holds that energy is not absorbed or radiated continuously but discontinuously in definite units called *quanta*.

Rad (roentgen-absorbed dose): A special unit of absorbed dose equal to 0.01 joule (unit of energy) per kilogram of tissue (which is equal to the old terminology of 100 erg/g of tissue). For x-rays, the rad is approximately numerically equivalent to the roentgen. Doses smaller than a rad are expressed in millirads, with 1,000 millirads equaling 1 rad. The rad has been replaced by a new unit for measuring absorbed dose, the gray (Gy). One rad equals 0.01 Gy.

Radiation: The emission and propagation of energy through space or through a material medium in the form of electromagnetic waves, corpuscular emissions such as alpha and beta particles, or rays of mixed and unknown types such as cosmic rays. Most radiations used in dentistry are capable of producing ions directly or indirectly by interaction with matter.

Radiation field: The region in which energy is being propagated.

Radiation hazard: The risk of exposure to radiation in an area where x-ray equipment is operating or where radioactive material is stored. Any uncontrolled source of radiation presents a potential danger.

Radiation hygiene: Methods protecting persons from accidental injury from exposure to radiation. Also includes techniques used to reduce and control the amounts of radiation used in medical and dental installations.

Radiation monitoring: See **Monitoring, Area monitoring,** and **Personnel monitoring.**

Radiation protection supervisor: The person directly responsible for radiation protection and safety measures. In dental offices, it is usually the dentist.

Radiation protection survey: In dentistry, an evaluation of the radiation safety in and around a dental office.

Radiator: A large mass of copper just outside the x-ray tube and connected to the anode terminal. The radiator functions to carry off the excess heat produced in the energy exchange that takes place when the electrons of the cathode stream are converted into about 1% x-rays and 99% heat. The radiator conducts the heat away from the target and cools the tube.

Radicular cyst: A cyst around the apex of a tooth. Generally seen as a small radiolucent circular area that extends away from the apical portions of the root. The sac of the cyst has a distinct wall or capsule that surrounds it and can be distinguished as a faint radiopaque thin line.

Radioactivity: The process whereby certain unstable elements undergo spontaneous disintegration (decay). The process is accompanied by emissions of one or more types of radiation and generally results in the formation of a new isotope.

Radiograph: An image produced on photosensitive film by exposing the film to x-rays and then developing the film so that a negative is produced. Also called an **x-ray film,** *radiogram*, *roentgenogram*, or *roentgenograph*.

Radiographer: Person who operates a x-ray machine. See **Operator.**

Radiographic fog: A darkening or clouding of the radiographic film image caused by exposure of the film to stray radiation during storage or by failure to protect the film from radiation while other exposures are made.

Radiography (roentgenography): The making of radiographs by exposing and processing x-ray film.

Radiology: That branch of medical science that deals with the use of radiant energy in the diagnosis and treatment of disease.

Radiolucent: That portion of the processed radiograph that is dark because the exposed structures lack density; also refers to a substance that permits the passage of x-rays with little or no resistance.

Radio-osteosclerosis: An increase in density to the bone that appears radiopaque due to excessive ionizing radiation.

Radiopaque: That portion of the radiographic film that appears light; also refers to a substance that resists the passage of radiation.

Radioresistant: Refers to a substance or tissue that is not easily injured by ionizing radiation.

Radiosensitive: Refers to a substance or tissue that is relatively susceptible to injury by ionizing radiation.

Rampant caries: Severe, unchecked caries that affect multiple teeth.

Ramus: The ascending portion of each end of the mandible.

Rarefaction: The state of being or becoming less dense, usually as a result of some disease process, indicated by radiolucent areas in the bone structures shown on radiographs.

Rarefying osteitis: A term used to describe a demineralization of the trabecullae within the alveolar bone. The causes are often difficult to determine and vary considerably. Appears on a radiograph as an irregularly shaped radioluncent area.

Rectification: In radiography, the unidirectional current inside the x-ray tube from the cathode to the anode.

Rectifier: A device within the vacuum tube for converting the alternating to direct current.

Recurrent caries: Caries that occurs under a restoration or around its margins.

Reducer: A chemical capable of bringing a salt into its metallic state by removing the nonmetallic elements.

Reduction: In dental radiography, a process in which an overexposed or overdeveloped radiograph is placed in a reducing solution. This lightens the radiographic image by removing one layer of metallic silver at a time from the film surface.

Rem (roentgen equivalent man): A unit used to measure the dose equivalent. It is used to compare the biological effects of the various types of radiation. One rem equals 1 rad times a biological effect modifying factor. Since the modifying factor for x- and gamma radiation equals 1, the number of rems is identical to the absorbed dose in rads for these radiations. The rem has been replaced by a new unit for measuring the dose equivalent, the sievert (Sv). One rem equals 0.01 Sv.

Replenisher: A superconcentrated solution of developer or fixer that is added daily, or as indicated, to the developer or fixer in the processing tank to compensate for loss of volume and loss of strength from oxidation. The act of adding replenisher to the processing solutions is known as replenishment.

Residual cyst: This is a cyst that remains in the jaw after the tooth that caused the cyst to form is no longer attached to it. During surgical removal of the root or during exfoliation, cysts may become detached from the root and remain within the bone for many years, often undiscovered. Such cysts may become encapsulated with an epithelial lining or may undergo considerable growth. Radiographically the cyst appears radiolucent and the lining of the cyst appears as a thin radiopaque line.

Resolution: The discernable separation of closely adjacent image details.

Resorption: Removal by absorption. In radiography, resorption generally refers to a loss of bone or tooth structure. Resorption may originate from natural causes such as the gradual reduction of size of the roots of deciduous teeth, or it may be idiopathic (the result of unknown causes), as may occasionally be observed by internal or external changes in the size of the pulp chamber or the length of the roots of permanent teeth.

Restrainer: In radiography, the potassium bromide in the developer solution. It slows down the action of the Elon and hydroquinone in the developer and inhibits the tendency of the solution to chemically fog the films.

Retained root: A root remaining after the tooth has been extracted.

Reticulation: Cracking of the film emulsion caused by a large temperature difference between the developer and the rinse water.

Reverse-Towne projection: An extraoral projection used to view the condylar neck of the mandible.

Rhinoliths: Calcifications within the maxillary sinuses.

Ridge (alveolar): A ridge is an extended elevation or crest of bone. In dental radiography, the term ridge generally refers to the alveolar crests of the mandible or the maxillae. The alveolar ridge may be partially or fully edentulous. On dental radiographs the ridges appear radiopaque.

Right-angle technique: See **Paralleling technique.**

Risk: The chance or likelihood of adverse effects or death resulting from exposure to a hazard.

Risk management: The policies and procedures to be followed by the radiographer to reduce the chances that a patient will file legal action against the dentist and staff.

Roentgen (R): The special unit of exposure to radiation measured in air. This is the exposure required to produce in air 2.58^{10} coulombs per kilogram of air. A simpler definition of the roentgen is that it is the amount of x-radiation or gamma radiation required to ionize 1 cc of air at standard conditions of pressure and temperature (2.083 billion ion pairs).

Roentgen ray: See **X-ray.**

Root surface caries: See **Cemental caries.**

Rotational center: In tomographic radiology, the axis on which the tube head and the drum rotate.

Rotational panoramic radiography: A specific radiographic projection technique that utilizes a narrow beam of x-rays to image a curved layer.

Rule of isometry: A geometric theorem stating that two triangles with two equal angles and a common side are equal triangles. The application of this theorem to the bisecting technique was suggested by Cieszynski in 1907 (Cieszynski's law).

Safelight: A special type of filtered light that can be left burning in the darkroom while films are processed. The safelight rays do not affect the film emulsion unless the filter is defective, they are too close to the film being exposed, or they are allowed to shine on the unprocessed film for too long.

Safelight filter: A filter covering the safelight that removes the short wavelengths in the blue-green region of the visible light spectrum that expose x-ray film. The longer wavelength red-orange light is allowed to pass through the filter illuminating the darkroom.

Sagittal plane: An imaginary vertical line or plane that bisects the body into a right and left portion. If the plane is exactly at the middle, it is referred to as the midsagittal plane. This is a very important orientation line in determining the ideal position of the patient's head during radiographic exposure.

Sanitation: A term used when microorganisms are reduced to a level of concentration considered to be safe.

Scatterguard: A steel cylinder inserted by the manufacture into the center of the PID where the PID attaches to the aperture of the tube head. Its purpose is to absorb scattered radiation.

Scatter radiation: Radiation that has been deflected from its path by impact during its passage through matter. This form of secondary radiation is scattered in all directions by the tissues of the patient's head during exposure to x-radiation.

Scintillation counter: An area-monitoring device containing a photoelectric cell that helps to measure the flashes of visible light emitted when the radiation that bombards certain salt crystals causes them to fluoresce.

Sclerosis: A hardening of the body tissues as a result of inflammation or an excessive growth of fibrous tissue and deposition of mineral salts. In dental radiography, sclerosis generally refers to a stiffening of the temporomandibular articulation or a mineralization of the alveolar bone. See **Condensing osteitis.**

Screen film: A type of extraoral film for use in cassettes with intensifying screens. This film has an emulsion that is more sensitive to the green, blue, and violet lights, emitted when the radiation strikes the phosphors in the intensifying screens than to the x-radiation.

Secondary protective barrier: A barrier sufficient to attenuate stray radiation to the required degree.

Secondary radiation: The radiation given off by any matter irradiated with x-rays. This form of radiation is created at the instant the primary beam interacts with matter and gives off some of its energy, forming new and less powerful wavelengths. This is often referred to as scatter radiation.

Selective reduction: A chemical change that takes place within the film emulsion during development. During this change, the nonmetallic elements are separated from the silver halide of the exposed grains, leaving a coating of metallic silver on the film emulsion while the bromide is removed. The process is called selective because the unexposed grains are not reduced.

Self-determination: The legal right of an individual to make choices concerning health care treatment.

Self-induction: An electrical term referring to the ability of a single coil in an autotransformer to vary the current and potential in a nearby circuit.

Self-rectification: In radiography, the ability of the x-ray machine to produce x-rays only during the portion of the alternating current cycle when the cathode has a negative charge and the anode has a positive charge.

Sensitivity: See **Emulsion speed.**

Sensitometer: An instrument used to measure the sensitivity of films to x-rays.

Sensor: An electronic or specially coated plate that is sensitive to x-rays. A small detector that is placed intraorally to capture a radiographic image when exposed to x-rays.

Sepsis: Infection, or the presence of septic matter.

Septum: In dental radiography, a thin wall of bone that acts as a partition to separate the nasal cavity or the maxillary sinuses. Appears radiopaque.

Sharp: Any object that can penetrate the skin, such as needles or scalpels.

Sharpness (see Definition): The distinct outlines of the structures on the image shown on a radiograph.

Shells: See **Energy levels.**

Shield (shielding): A protective barrier of structural materials.

Short-scale contrast: Variations in contrast, with few shades of gray as when the differences between blacks and whites on the radiograph are great. Fewer shades are produced when low kilovoltage is used.

Sialolith: A salivary calculus or hardened, stonelike mass that forms within the passage of the salivary ducts. If sufficiently large, such masses appear slightly radiopaque on the radiograph.

Sievert (Sv): A new unit for measuring the dose equivalent that has replaced the rem. The sievert is used to compare the biological effects of the various types of radiation. One sievert equals one gray times a biological effect modifying factor. Because the modifying factor for x- and gamma radiation equals 1, the number of sieverts is identical to the absorbed dose in grays for these radiations. One sievert equals 100 rems.

Sinus (maxillary): A cavity within the body of the maxilla that communicates with the middle meatus of the nose. It is also called the *antrum of Highmore*. All sinuses are lined with a mucous membrane and are filled with air or fluid. The apices of some of the maxillary teeth may occasionally protrude into the maxillary sinus. Sinuses may also be located on the ethmoid, frontal, and sphenoid bones. The sinuses reduce the weight of the skull without greatly weakening it.

Sinus survey: An extraoral radiograph exposed in such a manner that the maxillary sinus can be examined. This projection is similar to the posteroanterior survey.

Skin dose: See **Entrance dose.**

Slit: In rotational panoramic radiography, a vertical opening on the tube head through which the narrow x-ray beam exits or the narrow vertical opening on the cassette where the x-ray beam enters to record the image.

Soft radiation: Rays of low energy and long wavelengths that have little penetrating power. These have no value in producing dental radiographs and are removed from the polychromatic beam by filtration.

Somatic cells: All body cells except the reproductive cells.

Somatic effect: In radiography, the effect of radiation on all body cells except the reproductive cells, especially the effect on the blood, the soft muscular tissues, and the bone.

Source: In radiography, the place where the x-ray photons originate. This is the focal spot on the target of the anode inside the x-ray tube.

Source-film distance: See **Target-film distance.**

Source-surface distance (source-skin distance, target-skin distance, or target-surface distance): The distance measured along the path of the central ray from the center of the focal spot (front surface of the target) to the surface of the skin or irradiated object.

Statute of limitations: The time period during which a person may bring a malpractice action against another person.

Step wedge (penetrometer): A device consisting of increments of absorber through which a radiographic exposure is made on film to permit determination of the amounts of radiation reaching the film by measurements of film density. From such data, conclusions may be drawn as to the initial intensity and penetrative power of the radiation.

Sterilization: The total destruction of spores and disease-producing microorganisms.

Stray radiation: The sum of the leakage and scattered radiation; radiation that emanates from parts of the tube other than the focal spot.

Structural shielding: The protection afforded by building materials, such as the thickness of a stucco wall.

Subject contrast: The area-to-area difference in density in a radiograph caused by the differing thicknesses of the tissues or the object radiographed.

Submandibular fossa: A depression near the angle on the lingual of the mandible, irregular in size, usually below the area of the roots of the molars and extending forward as far as the premolar region. The basal bone of the mandible is so thin and offers so little resistance to the passage of the x-rays that it appears radiolucent.

Submentovertex projection: An extraoral projection showing the base of the skull, the position of the mandibular condyles, and the zygomatic arches.

Supernumerary teeth: These are extra teeth not normally a part of the dentition. Such teeth may be deciduous but are usually permanent. Many supernumerary teeth resemble normal teeth but the majority have conical crowns and are smaller than the tooth they resemble. Some bear no resemblance to normal tooth. These are often unerupted and malpositioned. Radiographically the tooth structures appear the same as any other tooth.

Surface dose: The dose of radiation at the skin surface measured in grays or rads.

Survey: A term used in dental radiography to indicate an examination of a complete area with radiography. For example, a complete radiographic inspection of all the teeth is called a full-mouth survey, whereas a single film of one specific area could be a lateral jaw survey, a mandibular molar survey, and so forth.

Suture: A line of union of adjacent cranial or facial bones that appears radiolucent on radiographs.

Symphysis: In dental radiography, the prominent bone area where the right and left sides of the mandible fuse at midline.

Syndrome: A group of symptoms that together characterize a disease or lesion.

Target: The small block of tungsten imbedded in the face of the anode, bombarded by the electrons streaming toward it from the cathode. The fiscal spot is located on the target.

Target-film distance (source-film distance or focus-film distance): The distance between the focal spot on the target and the recording plane of the film.

Target-object distance (source-object distance or focus-object distance): The distance between the target on the anode in the x-ray tube and the object being radiographed.

Target-surface distance (source-surface distance): The distance between the target and the surface of the object being radiographed.

Taurodontia: Teeth characterized by very large pulp chambers and very short roots.

Temporomandibular joint (TMJ) radiograph: An extraoral film use to show in profile the articulation of the head of the mandibular condyle with the glenoid fossa of the temporal bone and the surrounding structures.

Thermionic emission: The release of electrons when a material such as tungsten is heated to incandescence; specifically, the boiling off of electrons from the cathode filament in the x-ray tube when electric current is passed through it.

Thermoluminescent dosimeter (TLD): A monitoring device containing certain crystalline compounds (usually lithium fluoride) that store energy when struck by x-rays and then, when heated, give off light in proportion to the amount of radiation exposure.

Threshold dose: The minimum exposure that will produce a detectable degree of any given effect.

Time delay: The short interval between the moment the activator button on the x-ray machine is depressed and the instant that the high-voltage current begins to flow across the x-ray tube.

Timer: A mechanical, electrical, or electronic device that can be set to predetermine the duration of the interval that the current flows through the x-ray machine to produce x-rays.

Tomograph: A radiograph made using the tomography technique.

Tomography: A special radiographic technique used to show detailed, images of structures located within a predetermined plane of tissue while eliminating or blurring those structures in the planes not selected.

Tooth-bearing areas: Areas of the jaws in which teeth are normally located.

Topographical technique: A method used in occlusal radiography, in which the rules of bisecting are followed and the radiation beam is directed through the apices of the teeth perpendicularly toward the bisector.

Torus: An outgrowth of bone.

Total filtration: The combination of the inherent and added filtration in a x-ray machine. Many states require a total filtration of 2.5 mm of aluminum equivalent for x-ray machines operating at or above 70 kVp.

Trabecular bone (cancellous bone): The softer spongy bone that makes up the bulk of the inside portion of most bones. The cells of trabecular bone vary in size and density.

Tragus: The small cartilaginous prominence of tissues located neat the center and in front of the acoustic meatus (outer ear opening).

Trait: A distinguishing quality or characteristic.

Transcranial projection: An extraoral projection used to view the temporomandibular joint (TMJ) in both an open and closed position.

Transformer: One of several types of electrical devices capable of increasing or decreasing the voltage of an alternating current by mutual induction between primary and secondary coils or windings on cores of metal. See **High-voltage transformer** and **Low-voltage transformer.**

Triangulation: Widening of the periodontal space at the crest of the interproximal bone.

Trough: The low spot in the wave form; the opposite of the crest of the wave.

Tube head (tube housing): The protective metal covering that contains the x-ray tube, the high-voltage and low-voltage transformers, and insulating oil. It is attached to the flexible extension arm by a yoke. The PID attaches to the tube head at the port.

Tube side: A term used to describe the side of the film packet or the cassette that must be positioned facing the source of x-rays coming from the tube.

Tubercle: A rounded eminence on a bone.

Tuberosity: A broad eminence situated on a bone.

Tumor: A swelling; a growth of tissue.

Tungsten (Wolfram): An element with an atomic number of 74. Owing to its high melting point, this metal is extremely suitable to use as the cathode filament and as the anode target in the production of x-rays.

Universal precautions: A method of infection control in which blood and certain body fluids are treated as if known to be infectious for HIV, HBV, and other blood-borne pathogens.

Useful beam (useful radiation): That part of the primary beam that is permitted to emerge from the housing of the tube and is limited by the port, and the collimator, or other collimating device such as a lead-lined PID.

Vertical angulation: The direction of the central beam in an up or down direction achieved by directing the tip of the PID upward or downward. See **Negative angulation** and **Positive angulation.**

Vertical bone loss: Bone loss that occurs in a vertical direction (also called angular bone loss).

Vertical bitewing radiograph: A bitewing radiograph made with the long axis of the film placed in a vertical direction.

Vertical placement: See **Film placement.**

Viewbox: A light source used to view dental radiographs.

Viewer (viewbox or illuminator): A device for concentrating or reflecting light; generally, a lamp behind an opaque glass used for viewing radiographs.

Viewing: Examining dental radiographs using a view box for a light source.

Volt: A unit of electromotive force or potential that is sufficient to cause a current of 1 ampere (A) to flow through a resistance of 1 ohm (Ω).

Voltage: Electrical pressure or force that drives the electric current through the circuit of the x-ray machine. See **Kilovolt** and **Kilovolt peak.**

Voltmeter: A device for measuring the electromotive force (the difference in potential or voltage) across the x-ray tube.

Wavelength: In radiography, the length in angström units or centimeters of the electromagnetic radiations produced in the x-ray machine.

Wetting agent: A chemical preparation similar to a detergent that reduces the surface tension of film. A small amount may be added to the developer or the final rinse water to facilitate development and drying of the radiograph.

Wharton's duct: The excretory duct of the submaxillary gland. The opening of this duct is located under the tongue near the lingual frenulum—the small fold that limits the movement of the tongue. On rare occasions the opening of this duct may be blocked by the formation of a stone or mass of calculus called a sialolith.

Window: In radiography, the thin wall of glass in an x-ray tube opposite the focal spot. The primary x-ray beam leaves the tube through this thin area of the tube envelope.

Work load: In radiography, the total time that the x-ray machine is used, expressed in milliampere seconds per week.

Xeroradiography: A technique combining exposure to x-rays by a conventional x-ray machine with a special dry-processing system resulting in a photolike image rather than a transparent radiograph.

Xerostomia: Dryness of the mouth from lack of normal secretion.

X-ray (roentgen ray): The radiant energy of short wavelength discovered by Wilhelm Conrad Roentgen in Germany in 1895 and designated as x-ray by him. This form of radiant energy has the power to penetrate substances that are ordinarily opaque and to record shadow images on photographic film. The term roentgen ray is more technical than the more commonly used term x-ray.

X-ray film: See **Radiograph** or **Film packet.**

X-ray film hanger: Mechanical device for holding x-ray film during the processing procedures.

X-ray timer: A clocklike device that can be set for the time intervals required in film processing. It is activated by a lever and rings when the interval has elapsed.

X-ray tube: An electronic tube, located in the tube head, which generates x-rays.

Yoke: The curved portion of the x-ray machine that can revolve 360 degrees horizontally where it is connected to the extension arm. The tube head is suspended within the yoke and can be rotated vertically within it.

Zero angulation (zero vertical angulation): Angulation achieved by directing the tip of the PID so that the entire PID is parallel with the plane of the floor. When directed in this manner, the central beam travels parallel with the plane of the floor. See **Negative angulation** and **Positive angulation.**

Zygomatic arch: The arch formed by the temporal process of the malar (zygomatic) bone and the zygomatic process of the temporal bone. This forms the outer margin of the cheek prominence.

INDEX

A

B

K

L

M

N

S

Z